U0188406

汉英对照黄帝内经常用语辞典

Chinese-English Dictionary of Common Terms
in Huang Di Nei Jing
（Yellow Emperor's Internal Classic）

主编译　王尔亮　杨　渝

上海科学技术出版社

内 容 提 要

中医古籍，灿若星辰。《黄帝内经》作为中医药学的奠基之作，是中医药学术传承的知识载体，也体现出中华民族特有的精神价值和思维方式。

本辞典以 2017 年版《实用内经词句辞典》为底本，精选《黄帝内经》常用术语，在多年中医典籍英译研究成果的基础上，参考中外《黄帝内经》经典译本和相关术语英译的国际标准，进行专业解读与翻译。本辞典考源有据、文医兼备、汉英对照，有较强的学术性和实用性。英文翻译既坚持中医经典的原汁原味，又适当考虑现代中外读者的阅读和接受习惯，便于检阅与学习。

本书可供从事中医药工作人员、英语翻译及中医药国际传播专业人员，以及海外中医药学习者使用。

图书在版编目（ＣＩＰ）数据

汉英对照黄帝内经常用语辞典 / 王尔亮，杨渝主编译. -- 上海 ：上海科学技术出版社，2022.10
　ISBN 978-7-5478-5834-9

　Ⅰ. ①汉… Ⅱ. ①王… ②杨… Ⅲ. ①《内经》—词典—汉、英 Ⅳ. ①R221-61

中国版本图书馆CIP数据核字（2022）第159196号

本书为上海中医药大学《黄帝内经》国际研究院立项项目

汉英对照黄帝内经常用语辞典
主编译　王尔亮　杨　渝

上海世纪出版（集团）有限公司
上海科学技术出版社　　出版、发行
（上海市闵行区号景路 159 弄 A 座 9F - 10F）
邮政编码 201101　　www.sstp.cn
山东韵杰文化科技有限公司印刷
开本 889×1194　1/32　印张 22.75
字数 700 千字
2022 年 10 月第 1 版　2022 年 10 月第 1 次印刷
ISBN 978 - 7 - 5478 - 5834 - 9/R·2582
定价：168.00 元

本书如有缺页、错装或坏损等严重质量问题，请向印刷厂联系调换

编译委员会

顾 问
王庆其

主 审
陈 晓

主编译
王尔亮 杨 渝

英文审校
Natasha Lee（李美莲，Canada）

编译者
（按姓氏汉语拼音顺序排列）

陈 晓 金 珏 Natasha Lee

潘 霖 王尔亮 杨 渝 张淑娜

作 者 简 介

王尔亮

编辑,医学博士。主要从事医学英文期刊的编辑出版工作及中医药典籍翻译研究。现工作于上海交通大学医学院附属瑞金医院。主持科研课题 4 项,参与国家级、省部级科研项目 10 余项,发表学术论文 30 余篇。参与点校和整理《伤寒活人指掌图》《医门法律》,译著《黄帝内经素问新译:汉英对照》,参编《精编常用中医英语字典:汉英对照》《中医临床经典语录荟萃:汉英对照》《上海地区馆藏未刊中医钞本提要》《内经实用词句辞典》等专著 10 余部。曾获"第七届上海市高等学校学报优秀编辑""第五届上海市高校科技期刊优秀编辑"等荣誉称号。

杨 渝

博士,上海中医药大学外语教学中心副教授,硕士生导师,近年来在 CSSCI、CSCD 等核心期刊上发表论文近 30 篇,主编、副主编、参编"十二五""十三五""十四五"国家规划等英文教材 4 部,词典 2 部;主译"十二五""十三五"国家规划图书、海外汉学家著作等相关中医英文教材及著作 6 部。近年来主持研究省部级等各级别项目 30 余项,参与国家重大社科、国家社科冷门绝学及省部级课题 10 余项。曾多次在上海市和校级教学竞赛中获得一、二、三等奖。为上海中医药大学"骨干教师""金牌教师",*Chinese Medicine and Culture* 英文刊审稿人及青年编委。现担任世界中医药学会联合会内经分会理事,中华中医药学会翻译分会委员,上海市中医学会中医基础分会委员,世界中医药学会联合会中医文献及流派分会理事,中医药翻译与国际传播专业委员会常务理事。

前　言

　　成书于两千多年前的《黄帝内经》，上承生命启智之文明，下启医学发展之风格，为中医学四大经典之首。正如"西方医学之父"希波克拉底的学说为现代西方医学拉开序幕，《黄帝内经》亦为中医学奠定了坚实的基础，超越时空，历久弥新。

　　回顾自然科学的发展史，科学的发展呈现这样的特征：初期的研究是就对象的各个侧面进行个案的研究，随着各个研究领域的深入，在某一历史阶段，对研究对象有了综合性的认识，这种综合对科学研究的发展往往具有决定性的作用。《黄帝内经》成书的意义就不局限于一本经典著作的问世，更在于它实现了对各个医学观点、学派和研究成果的综合和统一，促进多学科的渗透和融合，建立了中医理论体系。

　　《黄帝内经》孕育于春秋秦汉中国优秀传统文化的母体，在先人的灵感、哲思、智慧的滋养和抚育下，将累积数千年的、散在而又极为丰富的临床经验上升为规律、法则和思想体系。从全球视野看，它是人类对生命奥秘和健康疾病不同于西方的另一种认识和解读，今天看来仍然不乏真知灼见，值得我们研读和深思。

　　在西方，早在 1925 年，美国学者 Percy Millard Dawson 就用英文向读者介绍了《素问》这部著作；1949 年美国学者 Emerita ILza Veith 的 *The Yellow Emperor's Classic of Internal Medicine* 成为第一部《黄帝内经》的英译本。进入 21 世纪，著名的德国医史学家文树德（Paul Ulrich Unschuld）及国内学者李照国的《黄帝内经》全译本，为《黄帝内经》的国际传播发挥了重要作用。

　　然而，《黄帝内经》毕竟是一部两千多年前的著作，由于思维方式、遣词用句的古今差异，对于母语是汉语的读者都颇为困难，更不用说非母语的读者了。因此,推出一部汉英对照的《黄帝内经》工具书就显得十分必要。

本辞典的中文条目,主要参照王庆其、陈晓主编的《实用内经词句辞典》,英译部分由王尔亮、杨渝主译。王尔亮博士毕业于上海中医药大学,是医学英文期刊的资深编辑,主要从事医学英文期刊的出版和中医药典籍的译介研究;杨渝博士系上海中医药大学外语中心英语副教授,主要致力于中医翻译和中医药国际传播研究。得益于两位英语专业科班出身,又先后成为中医学(《黄帝内经》研究方向)博士的青年才俊,本辞典才得以面世。

书稿编译中,参考了诸多《黄帝内经》译本和词典,在本书后列出,在此向这些译本和词典的作者致谢。初稿完成后,陈晓教授对全书做了审阅,外籍专家 Natasha Lee(李美莲)负责对英译部分审阅并提出修改意见,金珏博士对全书汉语、英文进行了仔细的校对。本项目属于跨文化、跨时空的艰巨工作,编委会虽竭尽全力,仍觉得有许多力不从心的地方,疏漏难免,恳请海内外同道指正。

编译委员会
2021 年 12 月

Preface

Huang Di Nei Jing (*Yellow Emperor's Internal Classic*), written over 2000 years ago, heads the four classics of traditional Chinese medicine (TCM). It encompasses the enlightened quest to understand the human body in ancient times and expedites later developments in medical science. As Hippocrates is proclaimed to have heralded modern western medicine, *Huang Di Nei Jing* (*Yellow Emperor's Internal Classic*) has been credited to have laid the solid foundation for TCM. Furthermore, this classic is recently becoming recognized as a timeless work full of greatness and vitality.

The development of science always follows a pattern in which the earlier research cases become the case studies of each of the target's aspects, and eventually evolves into a comprehensive understanding at a certain phase, thus playing a fundamental role in the development of research. This classic, as such, epitomizes an integrated and unified presentation of each medical view, school of thought and research outcome, facilitating the infiltration and fusion of different disciplines and establishing the theoretical system of TCM.

Inspired by the philosophy and wisdom of the pre-Qin and the Han dynasty forebears, *Huang Di Nei Jing* (*Yellow Emperor's Internal Classic*) highlights the rich and rather non-methodical clinical experience accumulated over a thousand years into rules and systems, offering an interpretation of life's mysteries and concepts of disease different from its western counterparts, all the while radiating truth and foresight worthy of continued research up to present.

As early as 1925, the American scholar Percy M. Dawson introduced *Plain Questions* translated in English to Western readers. Following this, the American author Ilza Veith produced the first English translation of *Huang Di Nei Jing* (*Yellow Emperor's Internal Classic*) in 1949. Moreover, in the 21st century the translation by Paul U. Unschuld, a famous German medical historian, and the Chinese scholar Li Zhaoguo, fueled international diffusion of this outstanding Chinese classic.

Considering that this classic dates back to more than 2000 years ago, the original diction, sentence patterns and thinking modes are remarkably different from those in modern times. This creates much difficulty not only for foreign readers but also for native audiences, thus rendering this publication of a Chinese-English bilingual dictionary instrumental to the understanding of it.

The Chinese entries in the dictionary drew reference mainly from *A Practical Dictionary of Expressions in Huang Di Nei Jing* edited by Wang Qinqi and Chen Xiao, and the English entries were mainly done by Wang Erliang and Yang Yu. Dr. Wang graduated from Shanghai University of Traditional Chinese Medicine. She is a senior editor of English medical journals, and is highly experienced in the research of English translations of TCM classics and their overseas publicity. Dr. Yang is an associate professor of English at the Foreign Languages Education Centre of SHUTCM, teaching and doing in-depth and extended research in the translation of TCM works and the TCM international communication. The above-named scholars made their vision of this dictionary become a reality not only due to their academic credentials as English majors, but also having attained additional TCM doctorates specifically focused on the research of *Huang Di Nei Jing* (*Yellow Emperor's Internal Classic*).

Acknowledged within are the various translated versions of *Huang Di Nei Jing* (*Yellow Emperor's Internal Classic*) and previous dictionaries, referred to during the endeavour of this present dictionary. A thousand thanks go to Professor Chen Xiao, who reviewed the whole dictionary; Dr. Natasha Lee from Canada, who gave precious counsel regarding the English sections; Dr. Jin Jue, who proofread the two languages meticulously. This is a formidable project spanning cultures and times, with inevitable compromises and omissions despite the arduous efforts of the editorial committee, for which we humbly request the tolerance and rectification of fellow scholars at home and abroad.

Editorial Board

December, 2021

总 目

凡　　例

一、音译不同表示的形式

在采用音译时,对于已经广泛使用、约定俗成的术语,采用英语普通名词形式表示。如"气""阴阳",表示为"qi""yin and yang"。对于使用较少、尚未形成共识的单词,则用小写斜体,每字独立音译,如"宫""商""角""徵""羽"译为"*gong*""*shang*""*jue*""*zhi*""*yu*";"少徵"译为"*shao zhi*";若上述单词与其他词组成中文复合词时,则用合体音译表示,如"少徵之人"译为"*shaozhi*-type people"。十二经络名核心名词统一译为合体音译,如"阳明"译为"*yangming*"。

二、不同符号的意义

《黄帝内经》术语存在一词多义与不同注家不同释义的现象,对此凡在《黄帝内经》中有多种含义的词条,均以①②③……圈号表示;若历代注家有不同注解的词,择要列出,并用(1)(2)(3)……表示。若不同含义又分不同释义的区别,用〈〉表示。

三、检索编排

汉语词条检索提供部首笔画和汉语拼音两种排列方式。为避免《素问》《灵枢》冗长的英文篇名反复出现问题,正文释义不英译具体篇名,只标记篇名序号,在书末专列序号与英文篇名索引,以备查考。

General Notices

1. Principles of transliteration

There are two fundamental principles of transliteration in this book. First, for the terms which are commonly accepted and widely used in the West, such as "qi" and "yin and yang", the regular form of an English word is used. Second, for the terms yet to be adopted by the West, lowercase italics are chosen. For example, "宫""商""角""徵" and "羽" have been translated as "*gong*""*shang*""*jue*""*zhi*" and "*yu*"; "少徵" has been translated as "*shao zhi*". However, when dissyllables such as "*shao zhi*" are formed into a Chinese compound word with other words, a combined transliteration form is used, for example, "少徵之人" is translated as "*shaozhi*-type people". The core of the names of twelve meridians are translated into combined transliteration form, for example, "阳明" is translated as "*yangming*".

2. Function of symbols

For polysemants, ①②③... is used to list the various meanings; for words illustrated in different ways by annotators of different times, the most important illustrations are chosen and listed as (1)(2)(3)...; if each meaning of a polysemant has been illustrated by different annotators into different ways, 〈〉is used to specify each meaning.

3. Methods of retrieval

Radical-stroke order and pinyin order of the Chinese characters has been provided. Furthermore，only the sequence number of each chapter in the body of the dictionary has been kept in order to avoid the repetition of the chapter names of *Huang Di Nei Jing*. The Chinese-English chapter titles in detail can be found with their corresponding numbers in the index part.

拼音检字表

qǔ
曲…………266
蛐…………627

qù
去…………221

quán
权…………258
颧…………639

quē
缺…………500

què
雀…………529
阙…………594

R

rán
然…………568
髯…………612

rè
热…………488

rén
人…………21

rèn
任…………282

rì
日…………148

róng
荣…………439

róu
柔…………483

ròu
肉…………276

rú
濡…………631

rǔ
乳…………401

ruǎn
软…………382

ruí
蕤…………612

ruì
锐…………556

rún
腘…………553

ruò
弱…………519
烳…………537

S

sāi
塞…………597

sān
三…………

sàn
散…………545

sǎng
颡…………621

sè
涩…………516

shàn
疝…………415
善…………570

shāng
伤…………283
商…………537

shàng
上…………63

shǎo
少…………136

shào
少…………136

shé
舌…………278
折…………336

shēn
伸…………352
身…………353

shén
神…………479

shèn
肾…………383
甚…………438
胂…………463

shēng
升…………178
生…………238

shéng
绳…………542

shèng
圣…………254
胜…………463
盛…………525

shī
尸…………77
失…………240
师…………265
湿…………571

笔画检字表

(所注页码为目录之页码)

目　录

七画

十画

十二画

一　画

一阳　①肝。肝为阴中之阳脏，故称一阳。出《素问·逆调论》。②少阳经脉。出《素问·经脉别论》《素问·阴阳类论》等。③三阳经脉协调如一。出《素问·阴阳离合论》。

一阳（yī yáng）　① Liver. The liver is the yang organ within the yin, hence the name the first yang. See *Su Wen* chapter 34. ② *Shaoyang* meridian. See *Su Wen* chapter 21 and *Su Wen* chapter 79. ③ Unity of three yang meridians. The integration of three yang meridians as a unity, thus called the first yang. See *Su Wen* chapter 6.

一阳为纪　一阳，即少阳。纪，会。言少阳出入于太阳阳明之间，为阳之交会，故称之为纪。出《素问·阴阳类论》。

一阳为纪（yī yáng wéi jì）　**the first yang as the convergence** *Yī yáng* or the first yang, meaning *shaoyang*. *Jì* means convergence. It is said that *shaoyang* enters and exits both the *taiyang* and *yangming* meridians as the convergence of the three yang meridians, therefore called convergence. See *Su Wen* chapter 79.

一阳为游部　一阳，即少阳。游，游行。部，身形部分。因少阳经行人身之侧，出入于太阳、阳明之间，故称为游部。出《素问·阴阳类论》。

一阳为游部（yī yáng wéi yóu bù）　**the first yang as the wandering part** *Yī yáng* or the first yang, meaning *shaoyang*. *Yóu* meaning wandering. *Bù* or parts, meaning body parts. The *shaoyang* meridian travels along the side of the human body, passing through *taiyang* and *yangming*, thus called wandering part. See *Su Wen* chapter 79.

一阴　①指太阴、少阴、厥阴三阴合一。出《素问·阴阳离合论》。②指厥阴。出《素问·经脉别论》。③单指或统指手足厥阴心包、肝及其经脉。出《素问·阴阳别论》。④指微阴。出《素问·阴阳别论》。

一阴（yì yīn）　① The unity of

taiyin, *shaoyin* and *jueyin*. See *Su Wen* chapter 6. ② *Jueyin*. See *Su Wen* chapter 21. ③ The pericardium meridian of hand *jueyin* and liver meridian of foot *jueyin* solely or unified. See *Su Wen* chapter 7. ④ Slight yin. See *Su Wen* chapter 7.

一阴为独使　一阴即厥阴,因其阴尽阳生,交通终始,故谓独使。出《素问·阴阳类论》。

一阴为独使(yì yīn wéi dú shǐ) **the first yin as the sole facilitator** The first yin, here, refers to *jueyin*. *Jueyin* is at the junction of the end of yin and at the beginning of yang, hence is named the sole facilitator. See *Su Wen* chapter 79.

一纪　指三十年的节气。一年二十四节气,三十年共七百二十个节气,为一纪。出《素问·阴阳类论》。

一纪(yí jì)　**one solar era** Representing 30 years in solar terms. There are twenty-four solar terms in a year. In 30 years, there are 720 solar terms, referred to as one solar era. See *Su Wen* chapter 79.

一备　天之六气循环一周之谓,为六年。出《素问·天元纪大论》。

一备(yí bèi)　**one completeness** The circulation of heaven's six kinds of qi, indicating six years. See *Su Wen* chapter 66.

一宫　九宫之一。北方坎宫,属水位。出《素问·六元正纪大论》。

一宫(yì gōng)　**one mansion** One of the nine mansions. The northern Kan mansion, belonging to the water position. See *Su Wen* chapter 71.

二　画

二十八会　两侧手足十二经脉，合二跷、督、任脉交相会。会，会合。出《灵枢·玉版》。

二十八会（èr shí bā huì）**twenty-eight convergences** The twelve bilateral meridians of the hands and feet，integrated with the *yinqiao*，*yangqiao*，governor and conception vessels. *Huì* means convergence. See *Ling Shu* chapter 60.

二十八星　即二十八宿。出《灵枢·卫气行》。

二十八星（èr shí bā xīng）**twenty-eight stars** Twenty-eight constellations. See *Ling Shu* chapter 76.

二十八脉　指人体二十八条经脉。即手足十二经脉，左右共计二十四条，合阴跷、阳跷、任、督四条经脉，凡二十八脉。出《灵枢·五十营》。

二十八脉（èr shí bā mài）**twenty-eight meridians** Twenty-eight meridians in the human body，including the twelve hand and foot meridians，totaling twenty-four meridians bilaterally. That combined with the four meridians of *yinqiao*，*yangqiao*，conception and governor vessels，altogether twenty-eight meridians. See *Ling Shu* chapter 15.

二十八宿　宿（xiù 秀），星宿。古代天文学家把黄道的恒星划分为二十八个星座的名称，又称二十八星。东、西、南、北各有七宿。东方苍龙七宿：角、亢、氐、房、心、尾、箕；西方白虎七宿：奎、娄、胃、昴、毕、觜、参；南方朱雀七宿：井、鬼、柳、星、张、翼、轸；北方玄武七宿：斗、牛、女、虚、危、室、壁。出《灵枢·五十营》。

二十八宿（èr shí bā xiù）**twenty-eight constellations** Ancient astronomers divided the fixed stars of the zodiac into twenty-eight constellations，also called the twenty-eight stars. There are seven constellations in the east，west，south and north respectively. The seven Black Dragon constellations of the east sky are *jiao*，*kang*，*di*， *fang*，*xin*，*wei*，*ji*；the seven White Tiger constellations of the west sky are *kui*，*lou*，*wei*，*mao*，*bi*，*zi*，*shen*；the seven Vermilion Bird constellations of the south sky are *jing*，*gui*，*liu*，*xing*，*zhang*，*yi*，*zhen*；and the seven Black Tortoise constellations of the north sky are *dou*，*niu*，*nv*，*xu*，*wei*，*shi*，*bi*. See *Ling Shu* chapter 15.

二十五人 即阴阳二十五人。详见该条。出《灵枢·阴阳二十五人》。

二十五人（èr shí wǔ rén） **twenty-five types of people** Refers to the physical appearance of twenty-five types of people. See *Ling Shu* chapter 64.

二十五阳 阳，即指胃气。指五脏与五时相应，各有五种胃气之脉。出《素问·阴阳别论》。

二十五阳（èr shí wǔ yáng） **twenty-five yang** Here yang refers to stomach-qi, and indicates the five viscera corresponding with the five seasons, each having five kinds of stomach-qi pulse，in total twenty-five yang. See *Su Wen* chapter 7.

二十五变 ① 人的体质按五行分类，每一行又分五型，计二十五种体质类型。出《灵枢·阴阳二十五人》。② 五脏病按五行生克规律各有五种传变方式，合为二十五变。出《素问·玉机真藏论》。③ 五脏按形态及位置，各有大小、高下、坚脆、端正、偏倾等五种变化，合为二十五变。出《灵枢·本藏》。

二十五变（èr shí wǔ biàn）① The constitution of the human body can be classified into five types according to the five elements，and every type is further divided into five types，in total manifested as twenty-five types. See *Ling Shu* chapter 64. ② The five visceral diseases each have five kinds of transformations according to the law of generation and inhibition of the five elements，altogether twenty-five changes. See *Su Wen* chapter 19. ③ According to the shape and position of the five viscera，each is classified as either small or big，is located above or below，hard or brittle to the touch，and stands upright or inclined，in total twenty-five changes. See *Ling Shu* chapter 47.

二十五腧 五脏各有井、荥、输、经、合五腧穴，计二十五腧穴。

出《灵枢·九针十二原》。

二十五腧(èr shí wǔ shū) **twenty-five acupoints** Each of the five viscera have five *shu*-acupoints, *jing*, *xing*, *shu*, *jing*, *he*, adding up to twenty-five *shu*-acupoints in total. See *Ling Shu* chapter 1.

二火 ① 指少阴君火和少阳相火。出《素问·六微旨大论》。② 指代阳性脏腑。出《素问·示从容论》。③ 指心、肝。出《素问·逆调论》。

二火(èr huǒ) ① The sovereign fire of the *shaoyin* meridian and the ministerial fire of the *shaoyang* meridian，the so-called two fires. See *Su Wen* chapter 68. ② The yang viscera. See *Su Wen* chapter 76. ③ The heart and the liver. See *Su Wen* chapter 34.

二阳 ① 心。出《素问·逆调论》。心为阳中之阳脏，故称二阳。② 单指或统指手、足阳明经脉。出《素问·阴阳类论》。

二阳(èr yáng) ① The heart. See *Su Wen* chapter 34. The heart is the yang viscera in yang，the so-called the second yang. ② The hand or foot *yangming* meridians independantly or in unity. See *Su Wen*

chapter 79.

二阳为卫 二阳，即阳明。卫，捍卫。阳明为阖，其脉维络于前，能却御诸邪，卫扶生气。出《素问·阴阳类论》。

二阳为卫(èr yáng wéi wèi) **the second yang as the guard** *Èr yáng* refers to *yangming*. *Wèi* means to guard. *Yangming* is the door and its meridians connect together in front of the door. It can defend against the evils and protect the healthy qi. See *Su Wen* chapter 79.

二阳为维 二阳，即阳明。维，维络。出《素问·阴阳类论》。

二阳为维(èr yáng wéi wéi) **the second yang as the connector** *Èr yáng* refers to *yangming*. *Wéi* means to connect. See *Su Wen* chapter 79.

二阳结谓之消 二阳，即阳明，包括手阳明大肠与足阳明胃。结，谓阳热搏结。消，消渴善饥，即后世所谓"消证"。阳明热结，故善消水谷。见《素问·阴阳别论》。

二阳结谓之消(èr yáng jié wèi zhī xiāo) **The second yang accumulating is called consumption.** *Èr yáng* refers to *yangming*，including the large intestine meridian of hand *yangming* and the stomach meridian of foot *yangming*. *Jié* refers to the accumulation of yang heat. *Xiāo* refers to consumptive thirst with rapid hungering, also named *xiāo zhèng*（consumption syndrome）in later generations. Therefore，heat accumulation in *yangming* leads to the rapid digestion of food and water. See *Su Wen* chapter 7.

二阴　① 单指或统指手足少阴心肾及其经脉。出《素问·阴阳类论》《素问·经脉别论》《素问·阴阳别论》。② 指前、后阴。出《素问·金匮真言论》。

二阴（èr yīn）　① Refers to the heart，kidney and their hand and foot *shaoyin* meridians individually or unified. See *Su Wen* chapter 79，*Su Wen* chapter 21，and *Su Wen* chapter 7. ② Refers to the anterior yin（external genitalia）and the posterior yin（anus）. See *Su Wen* chapter 4.

二阴为里　二阴，即少阴。少阴属肾主水，其气沉，故为里。出《素问·阴阳类论》。

二阴为里（èr yīn wéi lǐ）　the second yin as the interior *Èr yīn* refers to *shaoyin*. *Shaoyin* belongs to the kidney and corre-

sponds to water，its qi is sinking in property，thus it is characterized as interior. See *Su Wen* chapter 79.

二阴为雌　二阴，即少阴。少阴属肾主水，其位在下而主里，水能生物，故称之为雌。出《素问·阴阳类论》。

二阴为雌（èr yīn wéi cí）　the second yin as feminine *Èr yīn* refers to *shaoyin*. *Shaoyin* belongs to the kidney and corresponds to water. Its position is low and it governs the interior，and because water can generate all things，hence the name feminine. See *Su Wen* chapter 79.

二间　经穴名。属手阳明大肠经，在食指桡侧当掌指关节前下方凹陷处。出《灵枢·本输》。

二间（èr jiān）　Er Jian（LI 2）Acupoint name. Belonging to the large intestine meridian of hand *yangming*，and located on the radial side of the index finger in the depression at the anterior-inferior part of the metacarpophalangeal joint. See *Ling Shu* chapter 2.

二皇　指伏羲、神农。出《素问·著至教论》。

二皇（èr huáng）　Two Rulers

Two rulers refer to Fu Xi and Shen Nong. See *Su Wen* chapter 75.

十一焦　即第十一胸椎。焦，《太素·输穴》作"椎"。出《灵枢·背腧》。

十一焦（shí yī jiāo）　**eleventh jiao** The eleventh *jiao* refers to the eleventh thoracic vertebra. "焦"（*jiāo*）is recorded as "椎"（*zhuī*, vertebra）in the *Tai Su（Grand Plain）* "Acupoints". See *Ling Shu* chapter 51.

十一藏　即五脏六腑。指心、肺、肝、肾、脾、胃、大肠、小肠、三焦、膀胱、胆十一个脏器。出《素问·六节藏象论》。

十一藏（shí yī zàng）　**eleven viscera** Refers to the five viscera and six bowels, including the heart, lung, liver, kidney, spleen, stomach, large intestine, small intestine, triple *jiao*, bladder and gallbladder, eleven visceral organs in total. See *Su Wen* chapter 9.

十二支　即子、丑、寅、卯、辰、巳、午、未、申、酉、戌、亥十二地支。十二支的原意是古代物候的符号。说明一年中生物发展过程形象的变化。自夏代始用十二地支计月。支，即分的意思。以十二地支分建于十二

个月份。运气学说中以十二地支配十天干纪年，以推算每年运气变化的情况。出《素问·本病论》。

十二支（shí èr zhī）　**twelve branches** Including the twelve earthly branches：*zi*，*chou*，*yin*，*mao*，*chen*，*si*，*wu*，*wei*，*shen*，*you*，*xu* and *hai*. The original meaning of the twelve branches is the symbol of ancient phenology, which used to explain the changes in the course of development of living things in one year. Since the Xia dynasty however，the twelve branches have been used to count the months. *Zhī* means division，so the twelve branches are used to identify the 12 months of the year. In the theory of circuits and qi，the twelve Earthly Branches match the ten Heavenly Stems used to mark the year and calculate the changes in movement and qi in every year. See *Su Wen* chapter 73.

十二从　出《素问·阴阳别论》
（1）十二辰。见《素问》王冰注。
（2）十二经脉。见《素问注证发微》。

十二从（shí èr cóng）　**See *Su Wen**

chapter 7.（1）**twelve two-hour periods** See *Su Wen* annotated by Wang Bing.（2）**twelve meridians** See *Su Wen Zhu Zheng Fa Wei*（*Annotation and Elaboration on Su Wen*）.

十二分　见《素问·五藏生成》。（1）四肢各有三节,合为十二节。见《类经·经络二十一》。（2）十二经脉之分部。见《素问》王冰注。

十二分（shí èr fēn）　**twelve divisions** See *Su Wen* chapter 10.（1）The four limbs each have three joints，thus twelve joints overall. See *Lei Jing*（*Classified Classic*）"Meridians and Collaterals Chapter 21". (2) Subdivisions in the twelve meridians. See *Su Wen* annotated by Wang Bing.

十二节　① 指双侧肩、肘、腕、髋、膝、踝十二大关节。出《灵枢·邪客》。② 十二节气。出《灵枢·经别》。③ 指偶刺、报刺、恢刺、齐刺、扬刺、直针刺、输刺、短刺、浮刺、阴刺、傍针刺、赞刺十二种针刺方法。出《灵枢·官针》。

十二节（shí èr jié）　① Indicating the twelve larger joints of the shoulder，elbow，wrist，hip，knee and ankle bilaterally. See

Ling Shu chapter 71. ② Twelve seasonal sections See *Ling Shu* chapter 11. ③ Refers to twelve kinds of needling methods，including paired needling，trigger needling，relaxing needling，triple needling，dissemination needling，perpendicular needling，transport point needling，short thrust needling，superficial needling，yin needling，proximate needling and repeated shallow needling. See *Ling Shu* chapter 7.

十二邪　十二种病邪。欠、哕、唏、振寒、噫、嚏、亸、泣出、太息、涎下、耳鸣、啮舌等病症皆是十二邪乘正气之虚入于空窍而致。出《灵枢·口问》。

十二邪（shí èr xié）　**twelve evils** Twelve kinds of pathological evils. Yawning，retching，sobbing，quivering from cold，belching，sneezing，drooping，tearing，sighing，drooling，tinnitus and tongue biting are the diseases and symptoms all caused by the twelve evils passing into the hollow orifices when healthy qi is deficient. See *Ling Shu* chapter 28.

十二辰　古时一日分为十二时辰,即子时、丑时、寅时、卯时、辰时、巳时、午时、未时、申时、酉时、戌时、亥时。出《灵枢·卫气行》。

十二辰（shí èr chén） **twelve double-hour periods** In ancient times，one day was divided into twelve double-hour periods：*zi*，*chou*，*yin*，*mao*，*chen*，*si*，*wu*，*wei*，*shen*，*you*，*xu* and *hai*. See *Ling Shu* chapter 76.

十二时 古代一日的计时单位，即十二时辰：夜半为子时，鸡鸣为丑时，平旦为寅时，日出为卯时，食时为辰时，隅中为巳时，日中为午时，日昳为未时，晡时为申时，日入为酉时，黄昏为戌时，人定为亥时。出《灵枢·经别》。

十二时（shí èr shí） **twelve double-hour units** The daily unit of time in ancient times，that is，the twelve double-hours：*zi* (from 11 p.m. to 1 a.m.)；*chou* (from 1 a.m. to 3 a.m.)；*yin* (from 3 a.m. to 5 a.m.)；*mao* (from 5 a.m. to 7 a.m.)；*chen* (from 7 a.m. to 9 a.m.)；*si* (from 9 a.m. to 11 a.m.)；*wu* (from 11 a.m. to 1 p.m.)；*wei* (from 1 p.m. to 3 p.m.)；*shen* (from 3 p.m. to 5 p.m.)；*you* (from 5 p.m. to 7 p.m.)；*xu* (from 7 p.m. to 9 p.m.)；*hai* (from 9 p.m. to 11 p.m.).

See *Ling Shu* chapter 11.

十二疟 即足太阳、足少阳、足阳明、足太阴、足少阴、足厥阴之疟，及肺、心、肝、脾、肾、胃疟之总称。出《素问·刺疟》。

十二疟（shí èr nüè） **twelve Nüe Syndromes** The general term for the Nüe Syndromes of the foot *taiyang*，foot *shaoyang*，foot *yangming*，foot *taiyin*，foot *shaoyin*，and foot *jueyin* meridians，as well as the Nüe Syndromes of the lung，heart，liver，spleen，kidney and stomach. See *Su Wen* chapter 36.

十二官 即十二藏。见该条。出《素问·灵兰秘典论》。

十二官（shí èr guān） **twelve officials** Namely the twelve viscera. See "十二藏". See *Su Wen* chapter 8.

十二经之海 即血海，指冲脉。出《灵枢·海论》。参"四海"条。

十二经之海（shí èr jīng zhī hǎi） **sea of the twelve meridians** That is the sea of blood. It refers to the thoroughfare vessel. See *Ling Shu* chapter 33. See "四海".

十二经水 指清、渭、海、湖、汝、渑、淮、漯、江、河、济、漳十二条河川湖海。出《灵枢·经水》。

十二经水（shí èr jīng shuǐ）

twelve rivers The twelve rivers include Qing River, Wei River, Hai River, Hu River, Ru River, Sheng River, Huai River, Luo River, Jiang River, He River, Ji River and Zhang River. See *Ling Shu* chapter 12.

十二经脉 又称十二正经,包括手足三阴三阳经脉,共十二条,是经络系统中的主体部分。即手太阴肺经,手厥阴心包经,手少阴心经,手阳明大肠经,手少阳三焦经,手太阳小肠经,足太阴脾经,足厥阴肝经,足少阴肾经,足阳明胃经,足少阳胆经,足太阳膀胱经。它们内属于十二脏腑,分布于全身,是气血运行的主要通道,有一定的流注次序,循环传注,周流不息。各条经脉都有一定的循行路线,与体内一定的脏腑相络属。出《灵枢·海论》。

十二经脉(shí èr jīng mài) **twelve meridians** Also named the twelve regular meridians, including three yang meridians and three yin meridians of both feet and hands, in total twelve meridians which make up the main part of the meridian system. That is, lung meridian of hand *taiyin*, pericardium meridian of hand *jueyin*, heart meridian of hand *shaoyin*, large intestine meridian of hand *yangming*, triple *jiao* meridian of hand *shaoyang*, small intestine meridian of hand *taiyang*, spleen meridian of foot *taiyin*, liver meridian of foot *jueyin*, kidney meridian of foot *shaoyin*, stomach meridian of foot *yangming*, gallbladder meridian of foot *shaoyang*, bladder meridian of foot *taiyang*. They belong to the twelve viscera and bowels and are distributed all over the body. They are the main channels for the movement of qi and blood and reflect a certain order of flowing, circulating and continuous flowing. Each meridian has a certain route and is connected to a corresponding internal organ. See *Ling Shu* chapter 33.

十二俞 十二脏腑在背部的俞穴,如心俞、肺俞、肝俞、脾俞、肾俞等,均为足太阳膀胱经的经穴。出《素问·五藏生成》《素问·大奇论》。

十二俞(shí èr shū) **twelve acupoints** The twelve viscera and bowels correspond to acupoints located on the back, that is the heart acupoint (BL 15), the lung acupoint （BL 13）, the liver acupoint （BL 18）, the spleen acupoint （BL 20）, the kidney acupoint （BL 23）etc. All the acupoints belong to the bladder meridian of foot *taiyang*. See *Su Wen* chapter 10. See *Su Wen* chapter 48.

十二络脉 十二经脉分别从络穴分出一络,其中阴经的络脉走向与它相为表里的阳经,阳经的络脉走向与它相为表里的阴经,以沟通表里两经的联系。出《素问·气穴论》。

十二络脉（shí èr luò mài） **twelve network vessels** The twelve meridians have their collaterals as ramifications from the collateral acupoints respectively. The yin meridians move towards the yang meridians that internally-externally related, and vice versa, hence to promote the communication of internal and external meridians. See *Su Wen* chapter 58.

十二原 十二经脉在腕、踝关节附近各有一个原穴,是脏腑原气经过和留止的部位。其名称是太渊（肺）、神门（心）、大陵（心包）、太白（脾）、太冲（肝）、太溪（肾）、合谷（大肠）、腕骨（小肠）、阳池（三焦）、冲阳（胃）、丘墟（胆）、京骨（膀胱）。脏腑有病变,可取十二原穴。出《灵枢·九针十二原》。

十二原（shí èr yuán） **twelve original acupoints** Each of the twelve meridians has a source acupoint near the wrist and ankle joints, the places where the original visceral qi passes through and remains. Their names are Tai Yuan （LU 9）, Shen Men （HT 7）, Da Ling （PC 7）, Tai Bai （SP 3）, Tai Chong （LV 3）, Tai Xi （KI 3）, He Gu （LI 4）, Wan Gu （SI 4）, Yang Chi （SJ 4）, Chong Yang （ST 42）, Qiu Xu （GB 40）, Jing Gu （BL 64）. When there are pathological changes in the viscera and bowels, the twelve source acupoints can be selected. See *Ling Shu* chapter 1.

十二部 指十二经脉在皮肤上的分属部位。出《素问·皮部论》。

十二部（shí èr bù） **twelve sections** Refers to the classified sections of the twelve meridians on the skin. See *Su Wen* chapter 56.

十二盛 盛,有余之意。即阴气盛、阳气盛、阴阳俱盛、上盛、下盛、甚饥、甚饱、肝气盛、肺气盛、心气盛、脾气盛、肾气盛，共计十二。出《灵枢·淫邪发梦》。

十二盛（shí èr shèng） **twelve abundances** *Shèng* means abundance, or excessive. There are twelve excessive conditions: excessive yin qi, excessive yang qi, excess of both yin and yang, upper excess, lower excess, excessively hungry, excessively full, excessive liver qi, excessive lung qi, excessive heart qi, excessive spleen qi, and excessive kidney qi. See *Ling Shu* chapter 43.

十二禁 指新行房事、已醉、新怒、新劳、已饱、已饥、已渴、大惊恐、乘车来、步行来等十二种情况属禁刺之例。出《灵枢·终始》。

十二禁（shí èr jìng） **twelve prohibitions** Refers to sexual intercourse, inebriation, rage, overexertion, gorged, starving, thirsty, fright, commuting by vehicle, commuting on foot, etc. See *Ling Shu* chapter 9.

十二藏 又称十二官，指心、肺、脾、肝、肾、膻中、胆、胃、小肠、大肠、三焦、膀胱十二个内脏的总称。《灵枢·经脉》将膻中作心包络。后世一般统称五脏、六腑及心包络为十二藏。出《素问·灵兰秘典论》。

十二藏（shí èr zàng） **twelve viscera** Also known as the twelve governors, namely the heart, lung, spleen, liver, kidney, Danzhong (pericardium), gallbladder, stomach, small intestine, large intestine, triple *jiao* and bladder. This denoted the general term for the twelve internal organs including Danzhong which indicated the pericardium as recorded in *Ling Shu* chapter 10. In later generations, it was generally referred to as the five viscera, six bowels, and pericardium. See *Su Wen* chapter 8.

十干 即甲、乙、丙、丁、戊、己、庚、辛、壬、癸十天干。十干原本是古代物候的符号。自殷代始用来计算天、日次第的符号。运气学说中以十干配十二地支纪年，以推算每年运气变化的情况。出《素问·本病论》。

十干（shí gān） **ten stems** Refers to the ten Heavenly Stems: *jia*, *yi*, *bing*, *ding*, *wu*, *ji*, *geng*, *xin*, *ren* and *gui*. The origin of the ten stems is the symbol of ancient phenology, and the calculation of the days and sequences began in the Yin dynasty. In the movement and qi theory, the ten Heavenly Stems paired with the twelve Earthly Branches marked the year and was used to calculate the changes of the movement and qi in every year. See *Su Wen* chapter 73.

十五络 即十五络脉，又称十五别络。是十四络脉和脾之大络的合称。别络，是从经脉中分出来的支脉，大多分布于体表。在四肢部，从十二经脉各分出一络，其中阴经的络脉走向与它相为表里的阳经，阳经的络脉走向与它相为表里的阴经。以加强表里两经的联系。在躯干部，有任脉络（身前）、督脉络（身后）及脾之大络（身侧）。各络脉均有一络穴及所主病症（见表1）。出《灵枢·经脉》。

表1　十五络脉表

十五络	穴名	分　布	实　症	虚　症
手太阴络	列缺	走手阳明	手锐掌热	呵欠、小便遗数
手少阴络	通里	走手太阳	支膈	不能言
手厥阴络	内关	走手少阳	心痛	心烦
手太阳络	支正	走手少阴	节弛、肘废	生疣
手阳明络	偏历	走手太阴	龋齿、耳聋	齿寒、痹隔
手少阳络	外关	走手厥阴	肘挛	不收
足太阳络	飞阳	走足少阴	鼻窒、头背痛	衄、蚓
足少阳络	光明	走足厥阴	厥	痿躄、坐不能起
足阳明络	丰隆	走足太阴	喉痹体猝哑狂癫	足不收，胫枯
足太阴络	公孙	走足阳明	霍乱、腹中切痛	鼓胀
足少阴络	大钟	走足太阳	烦闷、闭癃	腰痛
足厥阴络	蠡沟	走足少阳	睾肿、猝疝、挺长	暴痒
任脉络	鸠尾	散于腹	腹内痛	痒瘙
督脉络	长强	挟脊上项散头上	脊强	头重
脾之大络	大包	布胸腹	身尽痛	百节皆纵

十五络(shí wǔ luò)　**fifteen collaterals** Also known as the fifteen divergent collaterals, and is the collective name of the fourteen collaterals plus the large collateral of the spleen. Divergent collaterals refer to the branch vessels separated from the meridians, which are mostly distributed on the surface of the body. In the four extremities, the twelve meridians divide into twelve collaterals separately, in which the collaterals of the yin meridians correspond to the yang meridians both internally and externally, and the reverse is true for the collaterals of the yang meridians. The result is the overall strengthening of the connection between the exterior and interior meridians. In the body, there is a conception vessel (anterior), a governor vessel (posterior) and a large spleen collateral. Each collateral corresponds to one collateral acupoint and governs several disease patterns (See Table 1). See *Ling Shu* chapter 10.

Table 1　Fifteen Collaterals

Fifteen Collaterals	Name of acupoint	Distribution	Excess symptoms	Deficiency symptoms
Hand *taiyin* collateral	Lie Que (LU 7)	Hand *yangming* meridian	feverish sensation over the ulna head and the palm	yawning, incontinence of urine or frequent urination
Hand *shaoyin* collateral	Tong Li (HT 5)	Hand *taiyang* meridian	epigastric flatulence	difficulty to speak
Hand *jueyin* collateral	Nei Guan (PC 6)	Hand *shaoyang* meridian	heartache	dysphoria
Hand *taiyang* collateral	Zhi Zheng (SI 7)	Hand *shaoyin* meridian	difficulty of the elbow to move, weakness of the joints	wart
Hand *yangming* collateral	Pian Li (LI 6)	Hand *taiyin* meridian	dental caries, deafness	coldness of teeth, obstruction of diaphragm

续　表

Fifteen Collaterals	Name of acupoint	Distribution	Excess symptoms	Deficiency symptoms
Hand *shaoyang* collateral	Wai Guan (SJ 5)	Hand *jueyin* meridian	spasm of the elbow	flaccidity
Foot *taiyang* collateral	Fei Yang (BL 58)	Foot *shaoyin* meridian	nasal obstruction, headache and backache	nosebleed
Foot *shaoyang* collateral	Guang Ming (GB 37)	Foot *jueyin* meridian	coldness of limbs	flaccidity of foot, inability to stand up
Foot *yangming* collateral	Feng Long (ST 40)	Foot *taiyin* meridian	obstruction of the throat, sudden loss of voice, mania	flaccidity of foot, atrophy of muscles around the tibia
Foot *taiyin* collateral	Gong Sun (SP 4)	Foot *yangming* meridian	cholera, sharp pain in the abdomen	drum-like flatulence of the abdomen
Foot *shaoyin* collateral	Da Zhong (KI 4)	Foot *taiyang* meridian	dysphoria and depression, difficulty to urinate and defecate	lumbago
Foot *jueyin* collateral	Li Gou (LR 5)	Foot *shaoyang* meridian	persistent erection of penis	sudden pruritus vulvae
Conception vessel	Jiu Wei (CV 15)	In the abdomen	abdominal pain	itching
Governor vessel	Chang Qiang (DU 1)	Beside the spine upward to the neck and spreads to the head	stiffness of spine	heaviness of head
Large collateral of the spleen	Da Bao (SP 21)	In the chest and abdomen	general pain of the body	looseness of all the joints

十六部　指形体十六部。出《素问·调经论》。(1) 两肘、两臂、两䯏、两股、身之前后左右、头之前后左右也。见《素问直解》。(2) 九窍、五脏及手、足。见《太素·气穴》。(3) 任、督、阴跷、阳跷及手足三阴三阳经脉。见《素问集注》。

十六部（shí liù bù）　**sixteen sections** Refers to the sixteen sections of the human body. See *Su Wen* chapter 62.（1）Two elbows，two arms，two popliteal spaces，two thighs，the front back left and right aspects of the body and head. See *Su Wen Zhi Jie*（*Direct Interpretation on Su Wen*）.（2）Nine orifices，five viscera，hands and feet. See *Tai Su*（*Grand Plain*）"Qi Point".（3）Conception vessel，governor vessel，*yinqiao* meridian，*yangqiao* meridian as well as the three yang meridians and the three yin meridians of the hands and feet. See *Su Wen Ji Zhu*（*Collected Annotation of Su Wen*）.

十四络脉　又称十四别络。是从本经脉的络穴分出的支脉，大多分布于体表。有加强十二经脉中相为表里的两条经脉之间联系的功能。十二经脉各有一条，加督脉、任脉的络脉，合称十四络脉。出《素问·气穴论》。参"络脉"条。

十四络脉（shí sì luò mài）　**fourteen collaterals** Also known as the fourteen divergent collaterals，it refers to the branch vessel being separated from the col-lateral acupoints of its meridians and mostly distributed on the surface of the body. It can strengthen the communication function between the two meridians which are internally and externally related to each other. The fourteen collaterals comprise one collateral for each of the twelve meridians，as well as the collaterals of the conception vessel and governor vessel. See *Su Wen* chapter 58. See "络脉".

十脉　五脏之脉，左右各五，合之为十。出《素问·气穴论》。

十脉（shí mài）　**ten meridians** The meridians of the five viscera on both left and right sides，ten meridians altogether. See *Su Wen* chapter 58.

十度　即脉度、藏度、肉度、筋度、俞度，合左右为十度。出《素问·方盛衰论》。

十度（shí dù）　**ten measurements** The measurements for the meridians，viscera，muscles，sinews and acupoints bilaterally，in total ten measurements. See *Su Wen* chapter 80.

七节　出《素问·刺禁论》。（1）指第七椎骨。见《素问注证发微》。（2）椎骨自下而上的第七节。

见《类经·针刺六十四》。

七节（qī jié）　**seventh joint** See *Su Wen* chapter 52. (1) Refers to the seventh vertebra. See *Su Wen Zhu Zheng Fa Wei*（*Annotation and Elaboration on Su Wen*）. (2) The seventh vertebra measured from bottom to top. See *Lei Jing*（*Classified Classic*）"Needling Chapter 64".

七诊　指三部九候脉中,一候之脉见有独小、独大、独疾、独迟、独热、独寒、独陷下等七种异常的脉象。出《素问·三部九候论》。

七诊（qī zhěn）　**seven pulses** Refers to the seven abnormal pulses of the three sections and nine indicators, such as one division's pulse can be small, large, rapid, delayed, hot, cold or sunken. See *Su Wen* chapter 20.

七疝　指七种疝。出《素问·骨空论》(1) 指五脏疝及狐疝、㿉疝。见《素问注证发微》。(2) 指心风疝、肝风疝、脾风疝、肺风疝、肾风疝、狐风疝、癀疝。见《类经·疾病七十》。(3) 指寒疝、水疝、筋疝、血疝、气疝、狐疝、癞疝。见《素问》吴崑注。

七疝（qī shàn）　**seven hernias** Refers to seven kinds of hernias. See *Su Wen* chapter 60. (1) Refers to hernias of the five viscera, inguinal hernias and scrotum hernias. See *Su Wen Zhu Zheng Fa Wei*（*Annotation and Elaboration on Su Wen*）. (2) Refers to heart-wind hernias, liver-wind hernias, spleen-wind hernias, lung-wind hernias, kidney-wind hernias, inguinal-wind hernias and scrotum hernias. See *Lei Jing*（*Classified Classic*）"On Diseases Chapter 70". (3) Refers to cold hernias, water hernias, sinew hernias, blood hernias, qi hernias, inguinal hernias and scrotum hernias. See *Su Wen* annotated by Wu Kun.

七星　又名七曜。即太阳、月亮、木星、火星、土星、金星和水星等七大行星。出《素问·针解》。

七星（qī xīng）　**seven stars** Also named the seven luminaries referring to the the seven large planets, that is the Sun, the Moon, Jupiter, Mars, Saturn, Venus and Mercury. See *Su Wen* chapter 54.

七宫　指西方属金之位。出《素问·六元正纪大论》。

七宫（qī gōng）　**seventh mansion** Refers to the position of metal in the Western direction. See

Su Wen chapter 71.

七损八益　出《素问·阴阳应象大论》。(1)指古代的房中术。据湖南长沙马王堆出土竹简《养生方·天下至道谈》载,八种房中术有益于养生保精,七种房中术有损精气,不利于养生。(2)指阴阳消长的变化规律。见《类经·阴阳二》。

七损八益(qī sǔn bā yì)　**seven injuries and eight benefits** See *Su Wen* chapter 5. (1) Refers to ancient sexology. According to bamboo slips unearthed at Mawangdui, Changsha in Hunan Province, *Formula for Health-preservation*(*Yang Sheng Fang*), eight kinds of sexology are beneficial for health-preservation and essence-protection, while seven kinds of sexology are harmful to essential qi and are adverse for health-preservation. (2) Refers to the waning and waxing of yin and yang as outlined by the law of change. See *Lei Jing*(*Classified Classic*) "Yin and Yang Chapter 2".

七窍　两目、两耳、鼻、口、舌。其分别与五脏相通,能反映五脏的生理、病理。出《灵枢·脉度》。

七窍(qī qiào)　**seven orifices** Two eyes, two ears, a nose, a mouth and a tongue. These correspond with the five viscera, and can reflect the physiology and pathology of the viscera. See *Ling Shu* chapter 17.

七焦　指第七胸椎。焦,《太素·输穴》作"椎"。出《灵枢·背腧》。

七焦(qī jiāo)　**the seventh *jiao*** Refers to the seventh thoracic vertebra. *Jiao* refers to "vertebra" in *Tai Su*(*Grand Plain*) "Acupoint". See *Ling Shu* chapter 51.

七曜　七曜,即日、月、金、木、水、火、土七星。出《素问·天元纪大论》。

七曜(qī yào)　**seven luminaries** Notably the Sun, the Moon, Venus, Jupiter, Mercury, Mars and Saturn. See *Su Wen* chapter 66.

八风　为古代气象术语,指从八个方面刮来的风。即《灵枢·九宫八风》所说南方来的大弱风,西南方来的谋风,西方来的刚风,西北方来的折风,北方来的大刚风,东北方来的凶风,东方来的婴儿风,东南方来的弱风。出《灵枢·九宫八风》。

八风(bā fēng)　**eight winds** Ancient meteorological term. It refers to winds originating from eight different orientations as mentioned in *Ling Shu* chapter 77. They include the *da ruo* wind from the south, the *mou* wind from the south-west, the *gang* wind from the west, the *zhe* wind from the northwest, the *da gang* wind from the north, the *xiong* wind from the northeast, the *ying er* wind from the east, and the *ruo* wind from the southeast. See Ling Shu chapter 77.

八正 ① 指春分、秋分、夏至、冬至、立春、立夏、立秋、立冬八个节气的正常气候。出《素问·八正神明论》。② 指东、南、西、北、东南、西南、东北、西北八方正位。出《灵枢·九针论》。

八正(bā zhèng) ① Refers to normal weather conditions in the eight solar terms, namely the Spring Equinox, the Autumn Equinox, the Summer Solstice, the Winter Solstice, the Beginning of Spring, the Beginning of Summer, the Beginning of Autumn, and the Beginning of Winter. See *Su Wen* chapter 26. ② Refers to the correct location of the eight directions: east, south, west, north, southeast, southwest, northeast and northwest. See *Ling Shu* chapter 78.

八正神明论 《素问》篇名。八正,又称八纪,指立春、立夏、立秋、立冬、春分、夏至、秋分、冬至八个节气。神明,万物变化莫测谓之神,显露于外谓之明。此篇主要阐述四时八正之气,针法神明之用,故名。其内容有四时八正、日月星辰的变化与人体气血盛衰以及针刺补泻用"方"用"圆"的关系;四诊与四时阴阳变化结合的诊断方法等。

八正神明论(bā zhèng shén míng lùn) **The Theory of Spirit Brilliance in the Eight Directions** Chapter title in *Su Wen*. The eight directions, also known as the eight disciplines, referring to the Beginning of Spring, the Beginning of Summer, the Beginning of Autumn, the Beginning of Winter, the Spring Equinox, the Summer Solstice, the Autumn Equinox, and the Winter Solstice. As to spirit brilliance, all things unpredictable, refers to the spirit, and all things exposed outwardly refers to the brilliance. This chapter elaborates on healthy qi coming from the eight directions during the four seasons, and the technique of spirit brilliance acupuncture, hence the name. The content includes the four seasons and eight directions, the relationship between the changes of the sun, moon and stars with the rise and fall of qi and blood in the human body, the relationship between techniques and effects during needling that reducing techniques should be used with Fang, and reinforcing techniques should be used with Yuan, the diagnostic method combining the four methods of diagnosis and the four seasons with the changes in yin and yang.

八节　指四肢两侧的肘、腕、膝、踝八个关节。出《灵枢·九针论》。

八节（bā jié）　**eight joints** Refers to the eight joints of the four extremities bilaterally, namely the elbows, wrists, knees and ankles. See *Ling Shu* chapter 78.

八动　指春分、秋分、夏至、冬至、立春、立夏、立秋、立冬八个节气之风的变化。出《素问·宝命全形论》。

八动（bā dòng）　**eight movements** Refers to the wind changes in the eight solar terms: the

Spring Equinox, the Autumn Equinox, the Summer Solstice, the Winter Solstice, the Beginning of Spring, the Beginning of Summer, the Beginning of Autumn, and the Beginning of Winter. See *Su Wen* chapter 25.

八达　远及八方之外。达，通达。出《素问·上古天真论》。

八达（bā dá）　**eight reaches** Remote areas beyond the eight orientations. *Dá* means reaches. See *Su Wen* chapter 1.

八纪　即立春、立夏、立秋、立冬、春分、夏至、秋分、冬至八个节气。出《素问·阴阳应象大论》。

八纪（bā jì）　**eight seasonal turning points** Refers to the Beginning of Spring, the Beginning of Summer, the Beginning of Autumn, the Beginning of Winter, the Spring Equinox, the Summer Solstice, the Autumn Equinox and the Winter Solstice, the eight solar terms. See *Su Wen* chapter 5.

八极　极，极限。八极，八方的远际。出《素问·阴阳类论》。

八极（bā jí）　**eight limits** *Jí* means limit or extreme boundary. The eight limits refer to the remotest regions in the eight directions. See *Su Wen*

chapter 79.

八虚　指两肘、两腋、两髀、两腘，皆筋骨之隙，气血所流注者，故名。出《灵枢·邪客》。

八虚（bā xū）　**eight *xu*** Refers to the space where the qi and blood flow between the sinews and bones in the eight joints, including the elbows, axillae, hips and popliteal fossae bilaterally. See *Ling Shu* chapter 71.

八溪　指两肘、两腋、两骱、两腘。出《素问·五藏生成》。

八溪（bā xī）　**eight *xi*** Refers to the elbows, the axillae, the hips and the popliteal fossae bilaterally. See *Su Wen* chapter 10.

八髎　髎（liáo 辽）穴总称，即上髎、次髎、中髎、下髎，左右各有一穴。属足太阳膀胱经之穴。在腰以下骶后孔中。出《素问·骨空论》。

八髎（bā liáo）　**eight Liao acupoints** The general name for the Liao acupoints belonging to the bladder meridian of foot *taiyang*, including the upper Liao acupoint, the secondary Liao acupoint, the middle Liao acupoint and the lower Liao acupoint bilaterally and located on the posterior sacral foramen below the waist. See *Su Wen*

chapter 60.

人与天地相应　天地，指自然界。人与自然是一个统一的整体，人是自然万物之一，赖大自然而生存，自然界的变化可直接或间接地影响人体而产生相应的变化。人犹一小天地，与自然界遵循着同一变化规律。这是中医学的基本学术思想，它贯穿于生理、病理、诊断、治疗、养生诸方面。出《灵枢·邪客》。

人与天地相应（rén yǔ tiān dì xiāng yìng）　**the relevance of man with Heaven and Earth** Heaven and Earth refer to nature. Man and nature are a unified whole. Man is one part of nature and the existence of human beings depend on nature. Changes in nature can affect the human body directly or indirectly, thus the corresponding changes can be found in the human body. Human beings in themselves are their own small Heaven and Earth and therefore follow the same laws as nature does regarding changes. This is the fundamental academic thought of chinese medicine linking the aspects of physiology, pathology, diagnosis, treatment and health preservation. See *Ling Shu*

chapter 71.

人之常数　指人体血气的正常数量。人体经脉血气因阴阳的变化而有多寡之分。在《内经》诸篇中有关六经血气多少的记载稍有出入。出《素问·血气形志》《灵枢·五音五味》《灵枢·九针论》。所谓血气的多少，仅是古人对人体生理功能的一种经验的推测，有待进一步研究。

人之常数（rén zhī cháng shù）
regular count in the human body Refers to the normal count of blood and qi in the human body. The amount of blood and qi in the vessels of the human body varies due to changes in yin and yang. There are some discrepancies recorded in the different chapters of *Nei Jing*（*Internal Classic*）as to the amount of blood and qi in the six meridians. See *Su Wen* chapter 24，*Ling Shu* chapter 65，and *Ling Shu* chapter 78. Here the amount of blood and qi is merely speculation on the part of the ancients derived from their experience regarding the physiological function of the human body，which needs further study.

人中　部位名。鼻下方与唇上方中央凹陷部分，又称人中沟、水沟。足阳明经、督脉行经此处。出《灵枢·经脉》。后世指人中沟上 1/3 交点处为水沟穴，别名人中，属督脉，是手、足阳明经脉与督脉的会穴。

人中（rén zhōng）　**Ren Zhong** Body part name. The sunken middle region between the nose and lips，located on the foot *yangming* meridian and governor vessel，also named Ren Zhong Gou（GV 26），or Shui Gou（GV 26）. See *Ling Shu* chapter 10. In later generations it was referred to as Renzhong and located at the intersection of Shui Gou（GV 26）and the upper 1/3 section of Ren Zhong Gou（GV 26）. It belongs to the governor vessel and is the meeting point of the hand and foot *yangming* meridians and the governor vessel.

人气　①指人与天地相应之生气。出《素问·诊要经终论》。②指卫气，见《灵枢·卫气行》。③指阳气，出《素问·生气通天论》。④指经气。见《灵枢·五十营》。⑤指正气。出《灵枢·顺气一日分为四时》。

人气（rén qì）　① Refers to the qi produced by the human body through its correspondence with Heaven and Earth. See *Su Wen* chapter 16. ② Refers to defensive qi. See *Ling Shu* chapter 76. ③ Refers to yang qi, See *Su Wen* chapter 3. ④ Refers to qi of the meridians. See *Ling Shu* chapter 15. ⑤ Refers to healthy qi, vital qi. See *Ling Shu* chapter 44.

人伤于寒而传为热　寒邪外束，阳气内郁，故传而为热。出《素问·热论》《素问·水热穴论》。

人伤于寒而传为热（rén shāng yú hán ér chuán wéi rè）**pathogenic cold attacking the body and transforming into heat** Pathogenic cold binds the exterior as yang qi becomes stagnant internally, therefore transforming into heat. See *Su Wen* chapter 31 and chapter 61.

人迎　① 经穴名。属足阳明胃经，在结喉两旁一寸五分处的动脉。出《素问·气府论》。② 指人迎脉，即颈部结喉旁的动脉。是古人代诊脉的重要部位。通过人迎脉和寸口脉的对比来确定脏腑气血的盛衰。出《灵枢·四时气》《灵枢·禁服》。

人迎（rén yíng）　① Ren Ying (ST 9) Acupoint located on the stomach meridian of foot

yangming，1.5 *cun* bilateral to the prominentia laryngea. See *Su Wen* chapter 59. ② Refers to the *ren ying* pulse，that is the artery on both sides of the neck and throat. In ancient times，it was an important anatomical part for pulse diagnosis. The exuberance or insufficiency of qi and blood in the viscera and bowels is determined by comparing the *ren ying* and *cun kou* vessels. See *Ling Shu* chapter 19 and *Ling Shu* chapter 48.

人饮食劳倦即伤脾　饮食不节，脾失健运。劳力过度，脾气受损，阻碍水谷精微的生化与输布。出《素问·本病论》。

人饮食劳倦即伤脾（rén yǐn shí láo juàn jì shāng pǐ）**If a person's diet is improper, and he suffers from exhaustion, the spleen is harmed.** Improper diet triggers transportation dysfunction of the spleen. Excessive fatigue and impaired spleen-qi obstructs the generation, transformation and transportation of grain and water essence. See *Su Wen* chapter 73.

人忧愁思虑即伤心　忧愁思虑，泛指七情所伤。心藏神，忧愁思虑过度,心神受伤。出《素问·本病论》。

人忧愁思虑即伤心(rén yōu chóu sī lù jí shāng xīn) **the heart impaired by excessive anxiety, grief, overthinking and preoccupation** Anxiety, grief, overthinking and preoccupation generally refers to impairment by the seven emotions. As the heart stores the spirit, excessive anxiety, grief, overthinking and preoccupation damages heart-spirit. See *Su Wen* chapter 73.

人卧血归于肝　指肝藏血和调节血运的功能。见《素问·五藏生成》。

人卧血归于肝(rén wò xuě guī yú gān) **Blood flows to the liver when people lie on the bed.** Refers to the function of the liver to store blood and regulate blood circulation. See *Su Wen* chapter 10.

人定　即夜卧入睡安定之时。出《素问·标本病传论》。

人定(rén dìng) Refers to the time when people are at rest and fall asleep. See *Su Wen* chapter 65.

九九制会　九九,在地指九州九野,在人指九窍九脏。制,正也;会,会通。九九制会,指人之九窍九脏,地之九州九野,与天度气数相应。出《素问·六节藏象论》。

九九制会(jiǔ jiǔ zhì huì) **nine-nine system** Nine-nine refers to nine administrative regions and nine states on the earth, and in the human body it refers to nine orifices and nine viscera. *Zhì* refers to set up, and *huì* refers to correspondence. Nine-nine system refers to nine orifices and nine viscera in human body, and nine administrative regions and nine states on the earth, with this information one can establish a correspondence with the degrees of heaven and the numbers of qi. See *Su Wen* chapter 9.

九气　由怒、喜、悲、恐、思、惊、寒、热、劳等因素引起气的九种病理变化。出《素问·举痛论》。

九气(jiǔ qì)　**nine kinds of qi** Refers to the qi undergoing nine kinds of pathological changes due to anger, joy, sorrow, fear, overthinking, fright, cold, hot, and overstrain. See *Su Wen* chapter 39.

九节　指第九胸椎。出《灵枢·杂病》。

九节(jiǔ jié)　**nine joints** Refers

to the ninth thoracic vertebra. See *Ling Shu* chapter 26.

九州 古代行政区划。出《素问·生气通天论》。

九州(jiǔ zhōu) **nine regions** Refers to the administrative regions in ancient China. See *Su Wen* chapter 3.

九针 ①古代针具分类名。即镵针、员针、锓针、锋针、铍针、员利针、毫针、长针、大针。出《灵枢·官针》。②古医籍名。已佚。出《素问·离合真邪论》。③九针中的第九种针,即大针。出《素问·针解》。

九针(jiǔ zhēn) ① Classification names of needles in ancient China, such as arrow-head needle, round needle, lift needle, sharp-edged needle, sword-shaped needle, round-sharp needle, filiform needle, long needle and big needle. See *Ling Shu* chapter 7. ② Title of an ancient book, already gone missing. See *Su Wen* chapter 27. ③ The ninth needle among the nine needles, the big needle. See *Su Wen* chapter 54.

九针十二原 《灵枢》篇名。九针,指镵针、员针、锓针、锋针、铍针、员利针、毫针、长针、大针等九种针具;十二原,十二经脉的原穴,为经气输注之地,分布于肘、膝、胸、脐等处。此篇主要论述了九针的概念、作用及操作方法,十二原穴的部位与主治,故名。

九针十二原(jiǔ zhēn shí èr yuán) **Nine Needles and Twelve Origins [Openings]** Chapter title in *Ling Shu*. Nine needles refer to nine kinds of needles: arrow-head needle, round needle, lift needle, sharp-edged needle, sword-shaped needle, round-sharp needle, filiform needle, long needle and big needle. Twelve origins refer to the original acupoints of the twelve meridians, the places where the meridians and qi are infused and distributed in the elbows, knees, chest, and navel. This chapter mainly discusses the concept, function and manipulation techniques of the nine needles, and the locations and indications of the twelve original acupoints, hence the name.

九针论 《灵枢》篇名。九针,指镵针、员针、锓针、锋针、铍针、员利针、毫针、长针、大针九种针具。此篇主要论述九针的形状、大小、长短及治疗的适应证、注意事项等,故名。

九针论(jiǔ zhēn lùn) **Discussion on Nine Needles** Chapter title in *Ling Shu*. Nine needles refer to arrow-head needle, round needle, lift needle, sharp-edged needle, sword-shaped needle, round-sharp needle, filiform needle, long needle and big needle, nine kinds of needles. This chapter mainly discusses the shape, size, length, therapeutic indications and precautions of nine needles, thus its name.

九宜 对九针的理论有明确的认识,并能恰当加以运用,谓之九宜。出《灵枢·五禁》。

九宜(jiǔ yí) **nine adequacies** The nine adequacies entails a definite understanding of the nine needles theory in order to apply it appropriately. See *Ling Shu* chapter 61.

九星 指天蓬、天芮(守)、天冲、天辅、天禽、天心、天任、天柱、天英九星。出《素问·天元纪大论》。

九星(jiǔ xīng) **nine stars** Refers to the *tian peng*, *tian rui* (*shou*), *tian chong*, *tian fu*, *tian qin*, *tian xin*, *tian ren*, *tian zhu*, and *tian ying* stars. See *Sun Wen* chapter 66.

九宫 ① 离、艮、兑、乾、巽、震、坤、坎八卦之宫,加上中央,合为九宫,用以表示四方四隅中央九个方位。出《灵枢·九宫八风》。② 指南方离宫。见《素问·六元正纪大论》。

九宫(jiǔ gōng) ① The eight divinatory trigrams of *li* (fire), *gen* (mountain), *dui* (lake), *qian* (heaven), *xun* (wind), *zhen* (thunder), *kun* (earth) and *kan* (water), in addition to the central part, make up the nine palaces, which are used to express the nine directions, including the four corners, the four regions and the central part. See *Ling Shu* chapter 77. ② Refers to the southern *li* (fire) palace. See *Su Wen* chapter 71.

九宫八风 《灵枢》篇名。九宫,指离、艮、兑、乾、巽、震、坤、坎八卦之宫,加上中央,合为九宫,用以表示四方四隅中央的方位,以及二分、二至、四立的八个节气。八风,指四方四隅八方所来的风,即大弱风、谋风、刚风、折风、大刚风、凶风、婴儿风、弱风。该篇主要论述九宫的运转与八风虚实的关系,以及对人体的影响,故名。

九宫八风(jiǔ gōng bā fēng)

Nine Palaces and Eight Winds
Chapter title in *Ling Shu*. Nine palaces refers to the eight divinatory trigrams of *li* (fire), *gen* (mountain), *dui* (lake), *qian* (heaven), *xun* (wind), *zhen* (thunder), *kun* (earth) and *kan* (water), in addition to the central part, which make up the nine palaces, and used to express the central part of the four corners, four regions, and eight solar stems, including the two Equinoxes (spring, autumn), two Solstices (summer, winter) and four Beginnings (spring, summer, autumn, and winter). Eight winds refers to winds coming from eight directions, including the *da ruo* wind, the *mou* wind, the *gang* wind, the *zhe* wind, the *da gang* wind, the *xiong* wind, the *ying er* wind, and the *ruo* wind. This chapter mainly discusses the relationship between the movement of the nine palaces and the deficiency and excess of the eight winds, and its influence on the human body, thus named Nine Palaces and Eight Winds.

九候 候，脉候。全身有上、中、下

三部，每部之中又有天、地、人三个候脉部位，三而三之，称为九候。分别是：上部天为两额之动脉，"候头角之气"；上部地为两颊之动脉，"候口齿之气"；上部人为耳前之动脉，"候耳目之气"。中部天为手太阴寸口，"以候肺"；中部地为手阳明合谷，"以候胸中之气"；中部人为手少阴神门，"以候心"。下部天为足厥阴五里，"以候肝"；下部地为足少阴太溪，"以候肾"；下部人为足太阴箕门，"以候脾胃之气"。出《素问·三部九候论》。

九候（jiǔ hóu） **nine indicators**
Hóu Refers to the condition of the pulse. The whole body has three parts: upper, middle, and lower, and each part contains heaven, earth and man, the three pulse indicator sections. Three on three is also known as the nine indicators. They are differentiated as: the upper sky is the artery on both sides of the forehead, "the qi of the corner of the head indicator"; the upper earth is the artery at both sides of the cheeks, "the qi of the mouth and teeth indicator"; the upper man is the artery at the anterior of both ears, "the qi

of the ears and eyes indicator". The middle sky is hand *taiyin cun kou*, "as lung indicator"; the middle earth is hand *yangming he gu*, "as the qi in the central chest indicator"; the middle man is the hand *shaoyin shen men*, "as the heart indicator". The lower sky is foot *jueying wu li*, "as the liver indicator"; the lower earth is foot *shaoyin tai xi*, "as the kidney indicator"; the lower man is foot *taiyin ji men*, "as the qi of the spleen and stomach indicator". See *Su Wen* chapter 20.

九窍 两耳、两鼻孔、两目、口及前后阴的总称。出《灵枢·邪客》。

九窍(jiǔ qiào)　**nine orifices** The general name for both ears, both nostrils, both eyes, the mouth, the external genitals and the anus. See *Ling Shu* chapter 71.

九野 ① 即九州之分野。出《素问·六节藏象论》。② 九宫。出《灵枢·九针论》。

九野(jiǔ yě)　① Namely nine administrative regions. See *Su Wen* chapter 9. ② Nine palaces. See *Ling Shu* chapter 78.

九窒 窒,即抑塞。言天之五星天蓬、天柱、天冲、天英、天芮,地之五星地苍、地阜、地晶、地玄、地彤的抑塞情况,此云九窒,乃合九星之数。出《素问·本病论》。

九窒(jiǔ zhì)　**nine obstructions** *Zhì* means obstruction and refers to the obstruction of *tian peng*, *tian zhu*, *tian chong*, *tian ying*, *tian rui*, the five stars of heaven, and *di cang*, *di fu*, *di jing*, *di xuan*, *di tong*, the five stars of earth, this is to say that the nine obstructions are thus in conjunction with the numbers of the nine stars. See *Su Wen* chapter 73.

九焦 即第九胸椎。焦,《太素》作"椎"。出《灵枢·背腧》。

九焦(jiǔ jiāo)　**nine jiao** That is the ninth thoracic vertebra. *Jiāo* is written as "椎" in *Tai Su（Grand Plain）*. See *Ling Shu* chapter 51.

九藏 指肝、心、脾、肺、肾与胃、小肠、大肠、膀胱九个脏器。见《素问·三部九候论》。

九藏(jiǔ zàng)　**nine viscera** Refers to the liver, the heart, the spleen, the lung, the kidney, the stomach, the small intestine, the large intestine and the bladder, altogether nine viscera. See *Su Wen* chapter 20.

三　画

三十六输　六腑经脉各有井、荥、输、经、合及原穴，共计三十六输穴，故名，亦称三十六腧。出《灵枢·顺气一日分为四时》。

三十六输（sān shí liù shū）**thirty-six acupoints** Each meridians of the six bowels have its own well points，brook points，stream points，river points，sea points and source points，in total thirty-six acupoints，hence its name；also known as the thirty-six *shu* acupoints. See *Ling Shu* chapter 44.

三水　指肝、脾、肾三阴脏。出《素问·示从容论》。

三水（sān shuǐ）**three waters** Refers to the liver，the spleen and the kidney，as the three yin viscera. See *Su Wen* chapter 76.

三气　运气术语。指平气、不及、太过三者。出《素问·五常政大论》。

三气（sān qì）**three qi** Term for the circuits and qi and refers to the three states which are normality，deficiency and excess. See *Su Wen* chapter 70.

三毛　又称丛毛。大趾爪甲后二节间背上有毛的部位。出《灵枢·经脉》。

三毛（sān máo）**three hairs** Also known as cluster of hair. It is the hairy part on the dorsal aspect of the big toe between the posterior two internodes. See *Ling Shu* chapter 10.

三百六十五节　出《素问·六节藏象论》。（1）指人体三百六十五个骨节。见《素问识》。（2）指三百六十五气穴。见《素问绍识》。

三百六十五节（sān bǎi liù shí wǔ jié）**three hundred and sixty-five joints** See *Su Wen* chapter 9. （1）Refers to three hundred and sixty-five joints in the human body. See *Su Wen Zhi* (*Understanding Su Wen*). （2）Refers to three hundred and sixty-five qi acupoints. See *Su Wen Shao Zhi* (*Continuation of Understanding Su Wen*).

三百六十五穴　全身经穴之约数。考《内经》所载穴位数与此不符。出《素问·气穴论》。

三百六十五穴（sān bǎi liù shí wǔ

xuè) **three hundred and sixty-five acupoints** The approximate number of all the acupoints in the human body. According to textual research，the number of acupoints recorded in *Nei Jing*（*Internal Classic*）does not accord with this. See *Su Wen* chapter 58.

三百六十五会　即三百六十五穴。会,会合,穴位是经气会合之处,故名。出《灵枢·小针解》。见"三百六十五穴"条。

三百六十五会(sān bǎi liù shí wǔ huì)　**three hundred and sixty-five meeting points** Another name for the three hundred and sixty-five acupoints. *Huì* means meeting, and the location where the qi and meridians meet are at the acupoints, thus called three hundred and sixty-five meeting points. See *Ling Shu* chapter 3. See "三百六十五穴".

三百六十五脉　即三百六十五穴会。出《素问·气穴论》。

三百六十五脉(sān bǎi liù shí wǔ mài)　**three hundred and sixty-five meridians** Another name for the three hundred and sixty-five acupoints. See *Su Wen* chapter 58.

三百六十五络　全身细小络脉的约数。出《灵枢·邪气藏府病形》。

三百六十五络(sān bǎi liù shí wǔ luò)　**three hundred and sixty-five collaterals** The approximate number of all the minute collaterals in the human body. See *Ling Shu* chapter 4.

三百六十节　即三百六十五节之约数。出《灵枢·邪客》。

三百六十节(sān bǎi liù shí jié)　**three hundred and sixty joints** That is the approximate number for the three hundred and sixty-five joints. See *Ling Shu* chapter 71.

三合　① 运气术语。也称太乙天符。出《素问·天元纪大论》。② 指胀病邪正相合,有合于血脉,合于五脏,合于六腑之不同。出《灵枢·胀论》。③ 指表里经脉相互络属的第三种配合。出《灵枢·经别》。

三合(sān hé)　① Terminology of the circuits and qi. Also called *tai yi tian fu*（heavenly complement）. See *Su Wen* chapter 66. ② Refers to the combination of pathogenic and positive factors in distension diseases, differently combined with blood vessels，the five viscera and the six bowels. See *Ling Shu* chapter 35. ③ Refers to three kinds of mutual cooperation between the internal and external meridians with the corresponding collaterals. See *Ling Shu* chapter 11.

三阳 ① 运气学说六气中一阳、二阳、三阳(少阳、阳明、太阳)之总称。出《素问·天元纪大论》。② 统指太阳、少阳、阳明之经脉脏器。出《素问·阴阳离合论》。③ 指太阳。出《素问·阴阳类论》。④ 单指或合指手、足太阳小肠、膀胱及其经脉。见《素问·阴阳别论》《素问·阴阳类论》。

三阳(sān yáng) ① The general name for the first, second and third *yang* (*shaoyang*, *yangming*, *taiyang*) among the six qi in the circuits and qi theory. See *Su Wen* chapter 66. ② Generally refers to the meridians and viscera of *taiyang*, *shaoyang* and *yangming*. See *Su Wen* chapter 6. ③ Refers to *taiyang*. See *Su Wen* chapter 79. ④ Refers solely or in combination to the meridians of the small intestine meridian of hand *taiyang* and the bladder meridian of foot *taiyang*. See

Su Wen chapter 7 and *Su Wen* chapter 79.

三阳为父 三阳,即太阳。总督诸经,有高尊之意,故称之为父。出《素问·阴阳类论》。

三阳为父(sān yáng wéi fù) **the third *yang* as the father** The third *yang*, another name for *taiyang*, governs all the meridians with a sense of nobleness and respect, thus called the father. See *Su Wen* chapter 79.

三阳为表 出《素问·阴阳类论》。(1) 三阳,即太阳,又称巨阳,主一身之表,为诸阳主气。见《素问集注》。(2) 当作"三阴为表"。见《类经·疾病七》。

三阳为表(sān yáng wéi biǎo) **the third *yang* as the exterior** See *Su Wen* chapter 79. (1) The third yang, or *taiyang*, also named giant yang, governs the entire body's exterior and acts as the master of yang qi. See *Su Wen Ji Zhu* (*Collected Annotation of Su Wen*). (2) Should be regarded as "the third yin as the exterior". See *Lei Jing* (*Classified Classic*) "On Diseases Chapter 7".

三阳为经 三阳,足太阳。太阳为开,循身之背,犹大经之经于外。出《素问·阴阳类论》。

三画

三阳为经（sān yáng wéi jīng）
the third *yang* as the meridian
The third *yang* refers to the foot *taiyang* meridian. *Taiyang* as the opening is distributed along the back of the body, and is the giant meridian of the exterior meridians. See *Su Wen* chapter 79.

三阳结谓之隔　三阳即太阳。包括手太阳小肠经与足太阳膀胱经。结，热结不解之谓。隔，隔塞不通，包括胸腹痞塞不畅，上不能食，下不得便等病证，小肠属火，膀胱属水，小肠热结则火不化，膀胱热结则津液涸，故为隔塞不通之病。出《素问·阴阳别论》。

三阳结谓之隔（sān yáng jié wèi zhī gé）　**stagnation of the third yang meaning obstruction** The third yang, another name for *taiyang*, includes the small intestine meridian of hand *taiyang* and the bladder meridian of foot *taiyang*. *Jié* refers to the stagnated heat failing to resolve. *Gé* refers stagnation and inability to move, and includes obstruction of the chest and abdomen, inability to eat in the upper digestive tract, and inability to defecate in the lower aspect of the digestive tract. The small intestine belongs to fire, and the bladder belongs to water, thus when there is heat stagnation in the small intestine, the fire cannot be transformed, as well as when the heat stagnates in the bladder, body fluids will dry up. Therefore it is called stagnation-disease. See *Su Wen* chapter 7.

三阴　① 运气学说六气中一阴、二阴、三阴（厥阴、少阴、太阴）之总称。出《素问·天元纪大论》。② 统指厥阴、少阴、太阴之经脉脏器。出《素问·阴阳离合论》。③ 指太阴。出《素问·阴阳类论》。④ 单指或合指手、足太阴之经脉脏器。出《素问·太阴阳明论》《素问·阴阳类论》。

三阴（sān yīn）　① The general name for the first *yin*, second *yin* and third *yin*（*jueyin*, *shaoyin* and *taiyin*）among the six qi in the circuits and qi theory. See *Su Wen* chapter 66. ② Generally refers to the meridians and viscera of *jueyin*, *shaoyin* and *taiyin*. See *Su Wen* chapter 6. ③ Refers to *taiyin*. See *Su Wen* chapter 79. ④ Refers solely or in combination to the meridians and viscera of hand or foot *taiyin*. See *Su Wen* chapter 29 and *Su Wen* chapter 79.

三阴为母 三阴，即太阴，能滋养诸经，故称之为母。出《素问·阴阳类论》。

三阴为母(sān yīn wéi mǔ) **The third *yin* as the mother.** The third yin，another name for *taiyin*，can nourish all the meridians，thus called the mother. See *Su Wen* chapter 79.

三阴结谓之水 三阴，即太阴，包括手太阴肺与足太阴脾。结，寒结不解。水，水湿不化之病。寒结三阴，阳气不运，肺不化水，脾不制水，故为水病。出《素问·阴阳别论》。

三阴结谓之水(sān yīn jié wèi zhī shuǐ) **stagnation of the third *yin* meaning water** The third yin，another name for *taiyin*，includes the lung meridian of hand *taiyin* and the spleen meridian of foot *taiyin*. *Jié* refers to the cold failing to resolve，and *shuǐ* refers to water and dampness failing to transform and causing disease. When cold stagnates in three yin，yang qi fails to move，the lung fails to transform water，and the

spleen fails to restrain water，therefore it is called water-disease. See *Su Wen* chapter 7.

三里 ① 经穴名。即足三里，为足阳明胃经的合穴，在膝下三寸胫骨前髃外一横指处。出《素问·针解》。② 面之上、中、下三部，俗称三停。出《灵枢·天年》。

三里(sān lǐ) ① Name of acupoint. Also named Zu San Li (ST 36)，which is the *he*-sea acupoint on the stomach meridian of foot *yangming*. It is located three *cun* below the knee at a transverse finger from the anterior border of the tibia. See *Su Wen* chapter 54. ② The upper，middle and lower parts of the face，commonly called "*san ting*". See *Ling Shu* chapter 54.

三员 指人体上、下、中外三部。出《灵枢·百病始生》。

三员(sān yuán) **three sections** Refers to three external sections of the human body，that is upper，lower，center. See *Ling Shu* chapter 66.

三间 经穴名。属手阳明大肠经输穴。位于第二掌骨小头桡侧后凹陷中。出《灵枢·本输》。

三间(sān jiān) **San Jian (LI 3)**

Name of acupoint belonging to the large intestine meridian of hand *yangming*. Located in the posterior radial depression of the second metacarpal capitulum. See *Ling Shu* chapter 2.

三刺 ① 即齐刺,在病变部位正中一刺,并在两边各一刺,故名三刺。出《灵枢·官针》。② 指针刺皮肤、肌肉、分肉三种深浅部位的方法。出《灵枢·官针》。

三刺(sān cì) ① Namely simultaneous piercing where one needle is inserted straight into the location of the disease as well as two needles inserted at both sides respectively, therefore it is called triple piercing. See *Ling Shu* chapter 7. ② Refers to the method of piercing at different depths at three locations: the skin, the muscles and the partings of the flesh. See *Ling Shu* chapter 7.

三变 指三种不同的刺法。即刺营、刺卫、刺寒痹。刺营是刺静脉出血,刺卫是疏泄卫气,刺寒痹是针后药熨。出《灵枢·寿夭刚柔》。

三变(sān biàn) **three changes** Refers to three different needling methods, namely piercing the nutrient qi, piercing the defensive qi and piercing the area where there is cold-blockage illness. Piercing the nutrient qi means venous bleeding. Piercing the defensive qi means dredging the defensive qi. Piercing the area where there is cold *bi* (impediment) illness refers to applying medicated compresses after needling. See *Ling Shu* chapter 6.

三实 指岁气旺盛、月亮盈满、时令调和的气候。人体在上述气象条件下,虽有贼风邪气,不会致病。出《灵枢·岁露论》。

三实(sān shí) **three excesses** Refers to the condition where in a whole year the qi is plentiful, the moon is full and harmony exists among seasonal changes. Under the abovementioned meteorological conditions, the human body will not fall ill regardless there is pathogenic wind or evil qi. See *Ling Shu* chapter 79.

三品 即上、中、下三品。是最早的药物分类法。详载《神农本草经》。该书以药性为依据,把没有毒性、可久服者列为上品;没有毒性或毒性较小而可治病补虚者列为中品;有毒或性较峻烈而不能久服者列为下品。出《素问·至真要大论》。

三品（sān pǐn） **three ranks** Known as the top, medium and low grade medicines, which was the earliest method for medicine classification recorded in detail in *Shen Nong Ben Cao Jing*（*Shennong's Herbal Classic*）. Based on their medicinal properties, top grade drugs are those non-toxic drugs which can be taken for a long period of time; medium grade drugs are those non-toxic or less toxic drugs which can treat diseases as well as tonify deficiency; low grade drugs are those toxic or relatively powerful drugs which cannot be taken for a long period of time. See *Su Wen* chapter 74.

三脉 指手足三阳经脉。出《灵枢·九针十二原》。

三脉（sān mài） **three meridians** Refers to the three hand and foot yang meridians. See *Ling Shu* chapter 1.

三结交 经穴名。即任脉经关元穴，在脐下三寸，腹中线上，出《灵枢·寒热病》。

三结交（sān jié jiāo） **San Jie Jiao（BL 26）** Name of acupoint, that is the acupoint Guan Yuan（BL 26）on the conception vessel, which is three *cun* below the navel and located on the ventral median line. See *Ling Shu* chapter 21.

三候 诊脉的三个部位。谓候脉部位分天、地、人三个部分。出《素问·三部九候论》。参见"九候"条。

三候（sān hóu） **three indicators** The three locations for pulse-taking. It is said that each location for pulse diagnosis can be divided into three regions: heaven, earth and man. See *Su Wen* chapter 20. Refers to "九候".

三部 ① 诊脉的三个部位。上部指额、颊、耳前动脉搏动处；中部指寸口，合谷、神门处；下部指五里，太溪、箕门处。是古代遍身诊法的三个切脉部位。出《素问·三部九候论》。② 额、鼻、颌三停。见《灵枢·天年》。③ 起病的上、中、下三个部位。见《灵枢·百病始生》。

三部（sān bù） ① The three locations for pulse-taking. The upper section refers to the location of the frontal, buccal, and anterior auricular arteries; the medium section refers to the location of *cun kou*, He

三画

Gu (LI 4), and Shen Men (HT 7); the lower section refers to the location of Wu Li (LR 10), Tai Xi (KI 3), and Ji Men (SP 11). They are the three ancient pulse-taking locations for the whole body. See *Su Wen* chapter 20. ② The three regions: forehead, nose and jaw. See *Ling Shu* chapter 54. ③ The upper, middle and lower parts where disease originates. See *Ling Shu* chapter 66.

三部九候 诊脉方法。其特点是遍诊全身上、中、下三部有关动脉。上为头部，中为手部，下为足部。上中下各部又分为天、地、人三候，三三合而为九（见表2）。出《素问·三部九候论》。

表 2　三部九候的部位

三部	九候	相应经脉和穴位	所属动脉	诊断意义
上部 （头）	天	足少阳经（两额动脉）太阳穴	颞浅动脉	候头角之气
	地	足阳明经（两颊动脉）巨髎穴	面动脉（颌内动脉）	候口齿之气
	人	手少阳经（耳前动脉）耳门穴	颞浅动脉	候耳目之气
中部 （手）	天	手太阴寸口部的太渊穴、经渠穴	桡动脉	候肺
	地	手阳明合谷穴	拇主动脉	候胸中之气
	人	手少阴神门穴	尺动脉	候心
下部 （足）	天	足厥阴五里或太冲穴	蹠背动脉	候肝
	地	足少阴太溪穴	胫后动脉跟支	候肾
	人	足太阴箕门穴或冲阳穴	股动脉或足背动脉	候脾胃之气

三部九候(sān bù jiǔ hóu) **three sections and nine indicators** The pulse diagnosis method which is characterized by the general inspection of the related upper, medium and lower arteries of the whole body. The upper section is the head, the medium the hand, and the lower the foot. The upper, medium, and lower sections are divided into three indicators respectively, namely heaven, earth, and man. Therefore the combination of three times three is also the nine indicators (Table 2). See *Su Wen* chapter 20.

Table 2   Locations of the three sections and nine indicators

Three Sections	Nine Indicators	Relative Meridians and Acupoints	Artery it pertains to	Diagnostic Significance
Upper Section (Head)	Heaven	Temple (EX-HN 5) of the foot *shaoyang* meridian (Bilateral Frontal Arteries)	Superficial Temporal Artery	Reflecting the qi of the frontal eminences
	Earth	Ju Liao (ST 3) of the foot *yangming* meridian (Bimalar Arteries)	Facial Artery (Internal Maxillary Artery)	Reflecting the qi of the mouth and teeth
	Human	Er Men (SJ 21) of the hand *shaoyang* meridian (Preauricular Artery)	Superficial Temporal Artery	Reflecting the qi of the ears and eyes
Medium Section (Hand)	Heaven	Tai Yuan (LU 9), Jing Qu (LU 8) of the *cun kou* of the hand *taiyin* meridian	Radial Artery	Reflecting the lung
	Earth	He Gu (LI 4) of the hand *yangming* meridian	Principal Artery pf Thumb	Reflecting the qi in the chest
	Human	Shen Men (HT 7) of the hand *shaoyin* meridian	Ulnar Artery	Reflecting the heart
Lower Section (Foot)	Heaven	Wu Li (LR 10) or Tai Chong (LR 3) of the foot *jueyin* meridian	Dorsal Metatarsal Artery	Reflecting the liver
	Earth	Tai Xi (KI 3) of the foot *shaoyin* meridian	Calcaneal Branches of Posterior Tibial Artery	Reflecting the kidney
	Human	Ji Men (SP 11) or Chong Yang (SP 12) of the foot *taiyin* meridian	Femoral Artery or Dorsal Pedal Artery	Reflecting the spleen and stomach

三部九候论 《素问》篇名。三部九候，为古人的全身诊脉方法。此篇专论三部九候脉的诊法，故名。

三部九候论（sān bù jiǔ hóu lùn）**Discussion on the Three Sections and Nine Indicators** Chapter title in *Su Wen*. Three sections and nine indicators refers to the ancient pulse-taking method for the whole body. This chapter specializes in the diagnostic methods for the vessels of the three sections and nine indicators. Hence its name.

三部九候皆相失者死 三部，指人体头面部、手腕部、足踝部三个诊脉部位。九候，指上述三个诊脉部位中又各分为天、地、人三个诊候之处,三而三之,则为九候。相失,言三部九候的脉象相互不协调,参差不一致。死,谓预后极凶险。出《素问·三部九候论》。

三部九候皆相失者死(sān bù jiǔ hóu jiē xiāng shī zhě sǐ) **three sections and nine indicators in disharmony indicate impending death** The three sections refer to the three pulse-taking regions of the human body,namely the head and face,the wrists,and the ankles. The nine indicators refer to the above-mentioned three pulse-taking regions further divided into three indicators,namely heaven,earth,and man,thus three times three making nine indicators. *Xiāng shī* means that the pulses of the three sections and nine indicators are uncoordinated and inconsistent. *Sǐ* indicates a very dangerous prognosis. See *Su Wen* chapter 20.

三虚 指年虚、月虚、时虚。年虚,指当年岁气不及;月虚,指月缺无光;时虚,指失时之和,即四时气候反常。三虚时,人易受外邪侵袭。出《灵枢·岁露论》。

三虚(sān xū) **three deficiencies** Refers to deficient yearly, monthly and seasonal conditions. A deficient yearly condition refers to a year with a weakness in qi. A deficient monthly condition refers to an imperfect and dim moon. A deficient seasonal condition refers to an abnormal climate of the four seasons. When the above three deficiencies occur, people will easily be invaded by exogenous evils. See *Ling Shu* chapter 79.

三焦 ① 六腑之一。主要功能为疏通水道。分为上焦、中焦、下焦三部分。其经脉为手少阳三焦经,与手厥阴心包经相表里。出《素问·灵兰秘典论》。② 焦,通椎。三焦即背部第三椎。出《灵枢·背腧》。

三焦(sān jiāo) ① Triple *jiao*. One of the six bowels whose major function is to dredge water passages. It is divided into three parts, the upper *jiao*, the middle *jiao* and the lower *jiao*. It pertains to the triple *jiao* meridian of hand *shaoyang*, which is internally and externally related to the pericardium meridian of hand *jueyin*. See *Su*

Wen chapter 8. ② "焦" is the same as "椎" in ancient Chinese. The triple *jiao* was the name given to the third vertebra of the back. See *Ling Shu* chapter 51.

三焦下腧 即足太阳之别络，自踝上五寸间别入腨阳，以出于委阳穴，乃并太阳之正脉。出《灵枢·本输》。

三焦下腧（sān jiāo xià shū）**lower acupoint of triple *jiao*** Namely the connecting collateral of foot *taiyang* meridian, which enters into the calf at five *cun* above the ankle，exits at Wei Yang（BL 39）acupoint and then merges into the regular *taiyang* meridian. See *Ling Shu* chapter 2.

三焦手少阳之脉 即手少阳三焦经，为十二经脉之一。其循行路线从环指指尖开始，向上沿小指和环指的中间，沿手背至腕部，上行于前臂外侧两骨中间，向上穿过肘，沿上臂外侧上肩，交出足少阳经之后，经过缺盆向下，分布于两乳之间的膻中，散络于心包，穿过横膈，依次属上、中、下三焦。一支从膻中，向上出缺盆，至肩部项后，沿耳后，直上耳上角，然后屈曲下行，绕颊至眼眶下。另一支

从耳后，入耳中，再出耳前，过上关穴前，和原来在颊前一支脉相交，至目外眦（眼外角），这一支脉接足少阳经。出《灵枢·经脉》。

三焦手少阳之脉（sān jiāo shǒu shào yáng zhī mài） **triple *jiao* meridian of hand *shaoyang*** Belonging to one of the twelve meridians，the triple *jiao* meridian's route starts from the tip of the ring finger, reaches the wrist upward along the middle of the little finger and ring finger as well as the back of the hand. Then it ascends to the middle of the two lateral bones of the forearms, passes upward through the elbow and reaches the shoulder along the lateral aspect of the upper arm. After merging into the foot *shaoyang* meridian, it goes downward through the supraclavicular fossa, spreads over Dan Zhong（CV 17）between the two breasts, scatters its collaterals around the pericardium, passes through the diaphragm and pertains to the upper *jiao*, middle *jiao* and lower *jiao* respectively. One branch parts from Dan Zhong

（CV 17） and goes upward through the supraclavicular fossa. After reaching the nape of the shoulder，it goes straight to the upper and posterior aspect of the ear along the postauricular region. Then it descends circuitously and comes to the area beneath the eye socket around the cheeks. Another branch originates from the posterior border of the ear，enters into the center of the ear to the preauricular region. Before passing through Shang Guan (GB 3)，it intersects with the malar branch and reaches the lateral angle of the eyes. This branch connects with foot *shaoyang* meridian. See *Ling Shu* chapter 10.

三焦胀 病症名。六腑胀之一。症见皮肤中气胀，按之轻虚而空软。出《灵枢·胀论》。

三焦胀(sān jiāo zhàng) **triple** *jiao* **distension** Disease pattern name and one of the six-fu organ distensions. Symptoms include fullness of qi in the skin, and appears mildly deficient and empty and soft with palpation. See *Ling Shu* chapter 35.

三焦咳 六腑咳之一。由五脏六腑咳久不愈，传变而成。出《素问·咳论》。

三焦咳(sān jiāo ké) **triple** *jiao* **cough** One of the six-fu organ coughs caused by disease transmission of a long-term unrecovered cough of the five viscera and six bowels. See *Su Wen* chapter 38.

三焦理 腠理。出《灵枢·论勇》。

三焦理(sān jiāo lǐ) **skin structure of the triple** *jiao* The interstices. See *Ling Shu* chapter 50.

三隧 指糟粕、津液、宗气三种物质的通道。出《灵枢·邪客》。

三隧(sān suì) **three channels** Refers to the thoroughfare for waster matters，body fluids and pectoral qi. See *Ling Shu* chapter 71.

三膲 膲通焦，即三焦。出《灵枢·经脉》。

三膲(sān jiāo) **triple** *jiao* "膲" is the same as "焦"，namely the triple *jiao*. See *Ling Shu* chapter 10.

三藏 指肝、脾、肾三脏。出《素问·示从容论》。

三藏(sān zàng) **three viscera** Refers to the three organs of the liver，spleen and kidney. See *Su Wen* chapter 76.

干姜 药名。性味辛热，有温中

散寒通阳的作用。出《灵枢·
寿夭刚柔》。

干姜（gān jiāng）　**dried ginger**
（*Rhizoma Zingiberis*）Medicinal
name. It is pungent in flavor
and hot in property，with the
function of warming the
middle，dispersing the cold and
unblocking the yang. See *Ling
Shu* chapter 6.

工巧神圣　指高超的医疗技术。
出《素问·至真要大论》。

工巧神圣（gōng qiǎo shén shèng）
master practitioner Refers to
superb medical skills. See *Su
Wen* chapter 74.

土　五行之一。由自然界的"土"
抽象而来。其特性是稼穑。因
有播种和收获农作物的作用，
因而引申为具有生化、承载、受
纳等作用或性质的事物，故有
"土载四行""土为万物之母"之
说。根据五行归类的方法，归
属于土的，在五脏为脾，在气候
为湿，在季节为长夏，在方位为
中央，在五味为甘，在五色为黄。
出《素问·阴阳应象大论》。

土（tǔ）　**earth** One of the five el-
ements，which came about by
the notion of earth in nature.
It is characterized by sowing
and reaping，and thus extends
its meaning to all the substances

with the function or nature of
generation， transformation，
support and reception. It is said
that earth carries all the other
four elements and that it refers
to the mother of all things on
Earth. According to the classification of the five elements，
things pertaining to the element
of earth are the spleen among
the five viscera，dampness regarding climate， the late
summer among the seasons，
the center direction among the
directions，sweetness among
the five flavors and yellow
among the five colors. See *Sun
Wen* chapter 5.

土曰卑监　土运不及曰卑监。
卑，卑下，衰微之意。监，监制，
土气不达，则作用低下，化物作
用亦受到抑制。故称。出《素
问·五常政大论》。

土曰卑监（tǔ yuē bēi jiàn）
Earth is known as degradation.
It is said that if there is inadequate qi during an earth year，
there will be inferior supervision.
Bēi means inferiority and dec-
lination while *jiàn* means supervision. Thus if earth qi is
obstructed，it will cause ineffi-
ciency and its function of

transformation will also be inhibited. See *Su Wen* chapter 70.

土曰备化　土运平和曰备化，以土含万物，无所不备，土生万物，无所不化之故。出《素问·五常政大论》。

土曰备化（tǔ yuē bèi huà）**Earth is known as preparation and transformation** It is said that if the qi is balanced during an earth year, there will be perfect transformation as earth contains and generates all things on earth, and there is nothing that cannot be embraced and transformed by earth. See *Su Wen* chapter 70.

土曰敦阜　敦，厚也；阜，高也。土运太过曰敦阜，是土气有余高厚尤盛。出《素问·五常政大论》。

土曰敦阜（tǔ yuē dūn fù）　**Earth is known as thickness and highness.** It is said that if there is excessive qi during an earth year, there will be a prominent mound. *Dūn* means thickness and *fù* means mound. What is known as a prominent mound refers to an excessive earth qi, one being especially thick and abundant. See *Su Wen* chapter 70.

土气　① 运气概念中的六气之一，主气六步中的四之气，主大暑后六十日，湿土主令。出《素问·六微旨大论》。② 五行中之土气，与脾相应，主长夏。出《素问·六节藏象论》。

土气（tǔ qì）　① Earth qi, one of the six qi in the movement of qi concept. It governs the fourth qi in the theory of six qi, controls the sixty days after Great Heat (12th solar term) and corresponds to damp earth among the four seasons. See *Su Wen* chapter 68. ② It refers to earth qi among the five elements. It is associated with the spleen governing the late summer. See *Su Wen* chapter 9.

土形之人　体质名。又称上宫。阴阳二十五人之一。土形之人在五音属宫，宫音之中有正、偏、太、少的区别，分为上宫，左宫，大宫，加宫，少宫，以此类比土形人中的五种体质类型，上宫得土气之全者，左宫、大宫、加宫、少宫得土气之偏者，故上宫之人为标准土形人，其体形特征：面圆，头大，肤黄，肩背丰厚，腹大，大腿至足胫部壮实，手足不大，肌肉丰满，全身上下匀称，步履稳重，举足轻。其禀性是：内心安定，助人为乐，不喜依附权势，爱结交人。该体质大多能耐于秋冬,不耐于春夏,故春夏易发病。出《灵枢·阴阳二十五人》。

土形之人（tǔ xíng zhī rén) **people pertaining to earth element** Name of constitution. It is also known as upper *gong*. It also refers to one of the twenty-five types of people divided according to yin and yang. People pertaining to earth element belong to the *gong* tone in the five sounds. Within the *gong* tone, the sound is further differentiated into regular, partial, excess and less, and then divided into upper *gong* tone, left *gong* tone, large *gong* tone, added *gong* tone and lesser *gong* tone, thereby comparing the five kinds of constitutions pertaining to the people belonging to earth element. People of upper *gong* tone obtain complete earth qi and people of left *gong* tone, large *gone* tone, added *gong* tone and lesser *gong* tone obtain partial earth qi, therefore people of upper *gong* tone are referred to as standard people pertaining to earth element. Their body features include round face, big head, yellow skin, shapely shoulders and back, big belly, sturdy thighs and legs, small hands and feet, well-developed muscles, symmetry between the upper and lower parts of the body as well as taking stable and light steps when walking. Their character includes mental calmness, preference for helping others, disliking to rely on power and loving to make friends. These people can tolerate the weather in autumn and winter, but are intolerant to the weather in spring and summer, therefore they are vulnerable to fall ill in spring and summer. See *Ling Shu* chapter 64.

土运 五运之一。根据天干化五运之理,凡逢甲、逢己之年时,由土运主事。其时,气候偏潮湿,偏热,湿气流行;物候表现为万物充分成熟;疾病多见伤脾的症候等。出《素问·天元纪大论》。

土运（tǔ yùn) **earth movement** One of the five circuits. According to the theory of the ten Heavenly Stems transforming the five circuits, during the *jia* and *ji* years, the earth movement will take charge. At that time, the climate will be slightly damp and hot with prevalence of damp qi. All things on Earth will be fully ripe. As for disease, symptoms pertaining to spleen damage will be more common. See *Su Wen* chapter 66.

土位　即太阴湿土旺盛所主之时令。出《素问·六微旨大论》。

土位（tǔ wèi）　**earth position** Namely the season dominated by *taiyin* and with an exuberance of damp earth. See *Su Wen* chapter 68.

土郁　土运之气被郁遏。运气学说中，按五行相克规律，由于一方太盛或所克一方太弱而使受克一方被抑制，不能正常发挥作用的现象，称为郁。五行中木能克土，若木太过或土不及时则会发生木偏旺而使土气被郁。出《素问·六元正纪大论》。

土郁（tǔ yù）　**earth depression** The qi of earth circuit has been restrained causing depression. In the circuits and qi theory, according to the principles of mutual restriction of the five elements, depression refers to the phenomenon that when one element is too excessive or the restricted element is too weak,

the restricted one will be inhibited and unable to function normally. In the five elements, wood can restrict earth. If wood is too excessive or earth is insufficient, wood will become exuberant, causing depression of earth qi. See *Su Wen* chapter 71.

土郁夺之　土郁，即土气被郁。从自然气候变化言，长夏应湿而不湿，应化而不化；从人体言，脾为湿困，壅滞不通，皆称为土郁。夺，劫夺。凡土气抑郁之病应该用吐、下等劫夺的方法治疗。出《素问·六元正纪大论》。

土郁夺之（tǔ yù duó zhī）　**When the earth qi is depressed, just take it away.** Earth depression, that is the earth qi has become depressed. According to natural climate changes, the late summer should be a damp period when actually it is not, also transformation should take place while it doesn't. In relation to the human body, the spleen has become obstructed and is stagnant due to dampness. *Duó* means pillage. For diseases of depressed earth qi, methods for vomiting and purgation should be taken in order to recover. See *Su Wen* chapter 71.

土疫　湿温之类的传染病。出《素问·本病论》。

土疫（tǔ yì）　**earth pestilence** Infectious diseases of the damp warm type. See *Su Wen* chapter 73.

下　① 泻下。出《素问·至真要大论》。② 陷下。出《素问·举痛论》。③ 消退。出《素问·诊要经终论》。④ 进针。出《素问·诊要经终论》。⑤ 在泉之气。出《素问·五运行大论》。⑥ 客主加临中客气的五行属性为主气之子时，谓之下。出《素问·五运行大论》。⑦ 与上相对而言。出《素问·脉要精微论》。

下（xià）　① Purgation. See *Su Wen* chapter 74. ② Sinking. See *Su Wen* chapter 39. ③ Retrogression. See *Su Wen* chapter 16. ④ Inserting Needles. See *Su Wen* chapter 16. ⑤ The qi located in the spring. See *Su Wen* chapter 67. ⑥ In the comprehensive analysis of dominant qi and guest qi，and while considering the five element properties of the guest qi，if the guest qi is the son of the dominant qi，it is called *xià*. See *Su Wen* chapter 67. ⑦ Lower position or in opposition to the upper position. See *Su Wen* chapter 17.

下工　指诊疗技术较低的医生。这种医生不注重对疾病的预防以及早期诊断、治疗。而且在诊察病情时，缺乏全面的观点，故治愈率较低。出《素问·八正神明论》。

下工（xià gōng）　**inferior practitioner** It refers to doctors with inferior diagnostic skills，who don't pay attention to the prevention as well as the early stage diagnosis and treatment of diseases. When examining the patient's condition，they usually lack comprehensive opinions；therefore，their recovery rate is low. See *Su Wen* chapter 26.

下气上争不能复　言寒厥的病机。出《素问·厥论》。（1）下焦阴寒之气上争，阳气不和，阴阳不能恢复协调。见《太素·寒热》。（2）阴阳交争，身半以下之气引而上争，不能复归其经脉之中。见《素问》吴崑注。（3）在下之肾气虚损而与上焦之气相争，不能恢复正常。见《素问注证发微》。

下气上争不能复（xià qì shàng

zhēng bù néng fù) **Struggle between qi in the lower upwards cannot recover.** Refers to the pathogenesis of cold-impediment syndrome. See *Su Wen* chapter 45. (1) *Yin* cold qi in the lower *jiao* fights upwards while yang qi is disharmonized，and yin and yang cannot restore coordination. See *Tai Su*（*Grand Plain*）"Cold and Heat". (2) In the struggle between yin and yang，the qi in the lower part of the body moves upwards to fight and cannot return to its original meridian. See *Su Wen* annotated by Wu Kun. (3) The lower part of kidney qi is deficient and fights with qi of the upper *jiao*，thus unable to return to its normal state. See *Su Wen Zhu Zheng Fa Wei*（*Annotation and Elaboration on Su Wen*）.

下毛　阴毛。出《灵枢·四时刺逆从论》。

下毛（xià máo）　**lower hair** *Yin* hair，refers to hair in the lower section of the body. See *Ling Shu* chapter 64.

下白　大便色白。出《素问·至真要大论》。

下白（xià bái）　**lower white** White

stools. See *Su Wen* chapter 74.

下加　运气术语，下，指在泉之气。下加，把中运加于在泉之气。出《素问·六元正纪大论》。

下加（xià jiā）　*xia jia* Circuits and qi terminology. *Xià* refers to the qi in spring. *Xià jiā* means incorporating the middle circuit qi into the qi in spring. See *Su Wen* chapter 71.

下血　便血。出《素问·大奇论》。

下血（xià xuě）　**lower blood** Hematochezia. See *Su Wen* chapter 48.

下关　经穴名。属足阳明胃经穴名。在上关下，耳前动脉凹陷处，合口有空，张口即闭。出《素问·气穴论》。

下关（xià guān）　**Xia Guan (ST 7)** Name of acupoint. It pertains to the acupoint on the stomach meridian of foot *yangming*. It is below Shang Guan（GB 3）acupoint and located in the concavity of the anterior auricular artery. With a closed mouth，there is a hole，however with an open mouth the hole closes. See *Su Wen* chapter 58.

下纪　指关元穴，一名次门，为小肠的募穴，在脐下三寸。出《素问·气穴论》。

下纪（xià jì）　**lower regulator** Refers to Guan Yuan（BL 26）acupoint，and also called Ci Men. It is the front-mu acupoint of the small intestine and is located three *cun* below the navel. See *Su Wen* chapter 58.

下极　两目之间的部位。面部色诊用以测候心的功能状况，出《灵枢·五色》。

下极（xià jí）　**lower region** The extremely low region between the eyes. During facial colour inspection，it is used to detect the condition of the heart's function. See *Ling Shu* chapter 49.

下利　泄泻。出《素问·六元正纪大论》。

下利（xià lì）　**lower diarrhea** Diarrhea. See *Su Wen* chapter 71.

下者不以偶　指下法要用药味少、药力专的奇方，避免用偶方攻下太过而致药毒伤正。出《素问·至真要大论》。

下者不以偶（xià zhě bù yǐ ǒu）　**Purgation is not for the even-drug formula.** Refers to the method of purging，and not using an even prescription. It means that in purgation，formulas should contain an odd and fewer number of drugs，with a single efficacy，in order to avoid medicinal toxicity，which in turn damages healthy qi caused by the strong purgative effect of even-drugged prescriptions. See *Su Wen* chapter 74.

下者举之　治法。病变出现正气下陷的，应以升提补虚之法治疗。出《素问·至真要大论》。

下者举之（xià zhě jǔ zhī）　**raising method for the sinking** Therapeutic method. When pathological changes manifest in the sinking of healthy qi，methods should be taken to treat with raising and supplementing the deficiency. See *Su Wen* chapter 74.

下实上虚　言下部邪气盛实，正气为邪气所阻，不能上达，故上部正气虚弱。可出现头晕目眩，振摇不定，视物不清，耳聋等症。出《素问·五藏生成》。

下实上虚（xià shí shàng xū）　**lower excess and upper deficiency** It is said that when evil qi in the lower part of the body is excessive，it blocks the healthy qi and it cannot go upwards，therefore weakness in the healthy qi of the upper part results in symptoms of dizziness，vertigo，trembling，blurred vision，and deafness. See *Su Wen* chapter 10.

三画

三画

下经　古医籍名,已佚。推测它可能是一本关于病理学的专著。见《素问·病能论》。

下经(xià jīng)　*The Lower Classic* Name of an ancient medical book（Already missing）. Presumably it was a treatise on pathology. See *Su Wen* chapter 46.

下临　运气术语。降临之意。出《素问·五常政大论》。

下临(xià lín)　*xia lin* circuits and qi terminology meaning to arrive. See *Su Wen* chapter 70.

下俞　指足经下部之俞穴。其名称是:太阳(束骨),少阴(太溪),少阳(临泣),厥阴(太冲),阳明(陷谷),太阴(太白)。出《素问·经脉别论》。

下俞(xià shū)　lower transporter Refers to the transport points in the lower part of the foot meridian. Their names are: *taiyang*（Shu Gu, BL 65）, *shaoyin*（Tai Xi, KI 3）, *shaoyang*（Lin Qi, GB 41）, *jueyin*（Tai Chong, LR 3）, *yangming*（Xian Gu, ST 43）and *taiyin*（Tai Bai, SP 3）. See *Su Wen* chapter 21.

下窍　统指前后阴便、溺两窍。出《素问·阴阳应象大论》。

下窍(xià qiào)　lower orifice Refers to the anterior and posterior orifices for passing urine and stools respectively. See *Su Wen* chapter 5.

下陵　经穴名,又名足三里,属足阳明胃经。在膝下三寸胫骨外缘。出《灵枢·本输》。

下陵(xià líng)　Xia Ling（ST 36）Name of acupoint. Xia Ling（ST 36）, also called Zu San Li（ST 36）, belongs to the stomach meridian of foot *yangming*. It is located 3 *cun* below the knee on the external aspect of the tibia. See *Ling Shu* chapter 2.

下陵三里　简称下陵,即足三里。出《灵枢·九针十二原》。见"三里"条。

下陵三里(xià líng sān lǐ)　Xia Ling San Li（ST 36）Short form Xia Ling, that is Zu San Li（ST 36）. See *Ling Shu* chapter 1. Please refer to the phrase of "三里".

下盛则气胀　下,指三部九候诊法中的下部之脉,即下肢五里穴,太溪穴,箕门穴等脉动应手之处。下部脉气盛是邪滞于下,气不得升,故为气胀。出《素问·脉要精微论》。

下盛则气胀(xià shèng zé qì zhàng)　lower excess leads to distension of qi *Xià* refers to the pulse in the lower part within the diagnostic method of three sections and nine indicators，namely the pulsating regions of Wu Li（LR 10），Tai Xi（KI 3）and Ji Men（SP 11）acupoints of the lower extremities. Exuberant pulse qi in the lower part results from stagnation of evil in the lower and qi failing to go upwards，leading to the distension of qi. See *Su Wen* chapter 17.

下虚上实 ① 下虚，指肾气虚；上实，指涕泣俱出。出《素问·阴阳应象大论》。或可出现头痛等巅顶部疾患。出《素问·五藏生成》。② 指阳气下虚上实，可见癫狂等疾患。出《素问·脉解》。

下虚上实（xià xū shàng shí）① *Xià xū* refers to the deficiency of kidney qi，while *shàng shí* means running nose and tears. See *Su Wen* chapter 5. Lower deficiency and upper excess may also lead to headaches or other disorders at the apex of the head. See *Su Wen* chapter 10. ② It refers to the lower deficiency and upper excess of yang qi，where madness disorders can arise. See *Su Wen*

chapter 49.

下晡 晡（bǔ 补），申时，下午三时至五时。出《素问·藏气法时论》。

下晡（xià bǔ） **late afternoon** Shen subdivision from 3 p.m. to 5 p.m. used in ancient times. See *Su Wen* chapter 22.

下脘 胃脘下口幽门部。今有下脘穴，在脐上二寸处。出《灵枢·四时气》。

下脘（xià wǎn） **lower duct** The pylorus area of the lower opening of the gastric cavity. Currently，Xia Wan（CV 10）acupoint is located two *cun* above the navel. See *Ling Shu* chapter 19.

下厥上冒 下厥，指气血逆上而四肢厥冷。上冒，指因浊气不降而胸腹冒闷膜胀。与脾胃升降失调有关。出《素问·五藏生成》。

下厥上冒（xià jué shàng mào） **lower reversal and upper veiling** *Xià jué* refers to reversal cold in the four extremities due to the counterflow of qi and blood. *Shàng mào* refers to oppression and distension in the chest and abdomen due to turbid qi not descending. This is related to the disharmony among the ascending and descending of the spleen and stomach. See *Su Wen* chapter 10.

下焦　三焦之一,位于下部,是肾、膀胱、大肠所居之处。与水液糟粕排泄有密切关系。出《灵枢·营卫生会》。参"下焦如渎"及"三焦"条。

下焦(xià jiāo)　**lower *jiao*** One of the three *jiao* located in the lower part of the body, in the area of the kidney, bladder and large intestine. It is closely related to the discharge of water fluids and waster matters. See *Ling Shu* chapter 18. Please refer to the phrases "下焦如渎" and "三焦".

下焦如渎　言下焦的功能。渎,指沟渠,形容下焦肾、大肠、膀胱注泄水液糟粕,如同沟渠。出《灵枢·营卫生会》。

下焦如渎(xià jiāo rú dú)　**The lower *jiao* is like a ditch.** Refers to the functions of the lower *jiao*. *Dú* refers to ditch and describes the lower *jiao*'s kidney, large intestine and bladder which have ditch-like appearances as they drain water fluids and waster matters. See *Ling Shu* chapter 18.

下焦溢为水　下焦,指肾与膀胱。溢,满溢。水,水肿病。肾为气化之主,膀胱为气化之所,病者功能失常,则气不化水,溢于肌肤而为水肿之病。出《素问·宣明五气》。

下焦溢为水(xià jiāo yì wéi shuǐ)　**Overflow of the lower *jiao* leads to edema.** *Xià jiāo* refers to the kidney and bladder. *Yì* means overflow. *Shuǐ* refers to edema. The kidney acts as the governor of qi transformation and the bladder acts as the place where qi transformation occurs. For dysfunctional patients, the qi fails to transform water causing it to overflow into the skin and resulting in edema. See *Su Wen* chapter 23.

下廉　穴位名,即下巨虚,在上廉穴下三寸。出《素问·针解》。

下廉(xià lián)　**Xia Lian (ST 39)** Acupoint name and known as Xia Ju Xu (ST 39), located three *cun* below Shang Lian (ST 37) acupoint. See *Su Wen* chapter 54.

下管　下脘,胃脘下部。出《灵枢·六微旨大论》。

下管(xià guǎn)　**lower duct** Namely lower gastric cavity. See *Ling Shu* chapter 68.

下膈　病证名,指食后一定时间,

仍反吐而出的病证,相当于反胃。出《灵枢·六微旨大论》。

下膈(xià gé) **lower barrier** Disease name. Refers to a certain period of time after eating, patients continue regurgitating, which is equivalent to vomiting. See *Ling Shu* chapter 68.

寸口 又名气口、脉口,是切脉的主要部位,在两手桡骨头内侧桡动脉搏动处,属太阴肺经。该处太渊穴去鱼际仅一寸,故名。出《素问·平人气象论》。

寸口(cùn kǒu) **cun kou** Also called qi opening or pulse opening and refers to the major region for pulse-taking. It is located at the medial radial heads of both hands in the radial artery pulse pertaining to the *taiyin* lung meridian. It indicates Tai Yuan (LU 9) acupoint being one *cun* apart from Yu Ji (LU 10), thus its name. See *Su Wen* chapter 18.

寸脉 即寸口脉。又称"气口""脉口"。两手桡骨头内侧桡动脉的诊脉部位,属于太阴肺经,该处太渊穴去鱼际一寸,故名。寸口脉是切脉的主要部位。出《素问·通评虚实论》。

寸脉(cùn mài) **cun pulse** Namely *cun kou* pulse, and also known as "qi opening" or "pulse opening". It belongs to the lung meridian of hand *taiyin*, and is located at the pulse-taking region of the radial artery at the radial aspect. It is so called due to the one *cun* apart distance between Tai Yuan (LU 9) acupoint and Yu Ji (LU 10). *Cun kou* pulse is the primary pulse-taking location. See *Su Wen* chapter 28.

大 ① 指大脉。脉体宽大,其来和缓从容,为气血充盈的正常脉象。若脉大而实数,为实证;大而无力为虚证,皆是病势发展之象。出《素问·脉要精微论》。② 指大方。药量大而药味少的方剂。出《素问·至真要大论》。③ 指大针。古代九针之一。出《灵枢·玉版》。

大(dà) ① It refers to a large pulse. The pulse is powerful but moderate, indicating the normal pulses for engorged qi and blood. If the pulse is large but replete and rapid, it indicates an excess pattern. If the pulse is large but feeble, it indicates a deficiency pattern. Both are indications of the progress of a disease. See *Su Wen* chapter 17. ② Refers to a large formula with just a few drugs all in large quantities. See *Su Wen* chapter 74. ③ Refers to big needle，one kind of needle amongst nine used in ancient times. See *Ling Shu* chapter 60.

大丁　即大疔。泛指痈疡肿毒。出《素问·生气通天论》。

大丁（dà dīng）　**large boil** Namely *dà dīn* and generally refers to an abscess with pyogenic infection. See *Su Wen* chapter 3.

大小为制　大小，指方剂之大与小，即大方、小方。大方，或药味少而分量重，或药味多而药力大，其作用较为强烈。小方，或药味多而药量轻，或药味少而药力薄，其作用较轻微。治病制方，或大或小，须以适合病情为标准，病轻者用小方，重者用大方。出《素问·至真要大论》。

大小为制（dà xiǎo wéi zhì）　**large or small formulas according to the severity of the disease** *Dà xiǎo* refers to large and small formulas. Large formulas indicate either formulas with a few drugs dispensed in large quantities，or formulas with plenty of drugs all of strong efficacy，thus intensifying effectiveness. Small formulas indicate either formulas with a variety of drugs dispensed in small quantities，or formulas with just a few drugs of weak efficacy，where effectiveness is lighter. When writing prescriptions to treat disease，the patients' conditions should be taken into consideration when choosing large or small formulas. Small formulas should be used for patients with mild illnesses while large formulas should be used for those with severe ones. See *Su Wen* chapter 74.

大气　① 大邪气。出《素问·热论》。② 宗气。出《灵枢·五味》。③ 太虚之气。见《素问·五运行大论》。④ 经气。出《素问·离合真邪论》。

大气（dà qì）　① Great evil qi. See *Su Wen* chapter 31. ② Ancestral qi. See *Ling Shu* chapter 56. ③ Qi of greater deficiency. See *Su Wen* chapter 67. ④ Meridian qi. See *Su Wen* chapter 27.

大分　分，分界，引申为肌肉会合处的分理间隙。大分，即大肌肉间的分理间隙。出《素问·长刺节论》。

大分（dà fēn）　**large parting** *Fēn* means boundary，extending to the interstice at the junction of muscles. *Dà fēn* refers to the interstice between large muscles. See *Su Wen* chapter 55.

大仓 穴名，即中脘穴，又称太仓。出《灵枢·根结》。

大仓（dà cāng） **Da Cang（CV 12）** Acupoint name，also called Zhong Wan（CV 12）acupoint，or Tai Cang（CV 12）. See *Ling Shu* chapter 5.

大风 ① 凌厉的风邪。能导致中风等各种风疾。出《灵枢·刺节真邪》。② 疬风病，即后世所称的麻风病。出《素问·长刺节论》。参"疬风"条。

大风（dà fēng） ① Swift and fierce evil wind which can lead to a variety of wind diseases such as strokes. See *Ling Shu* chapter 75. ② Pestilent wind，namely leprosy in later generations. See *Su Wen* chapter 55. See "疬风".

大包 足太阴脾经之大络穴，在腋中线上，当第六肋间隙中。脾经别出的最大络脉即起于此。出《灵枢·经脉》。

大包（dà bāo） **Da Bao（SP 21）** A large collateral acupoint on the spleen meridian of foot *taiyin* located on the mid-axillary line at the sixth intercostal space，from which the largest collateral of the spleen meridian diverges. See *Ling Shu* chapter 10.

大则病进 大，指脉大，脉体宽大之谓。在疾病时出现大脉，提示病情的发展。脉大而实为邪实，大而无力为正虚。出《素问·脉要精微论》。

大则病进（dà zé bìng jìn） **large pulse indicates the progress of disease** *Dà* refers to large pulse，indicating that the pulse is broad with a bigger amplitude than normal. If a disease manifests itself with a large pulse，this indicates the progress of the disease. If the pulse is large and replete，it indicates evil excess. If the pulse is large but weak，it indicates deficiency of healthy qi. See *Su Wen* chapter 17.

大刚风 八风之一，指由北方刮来的风。出《灵枢·九宫八风》。

大刚风（dà gāng fēng） *da gang wind* It belongs to one of the eight winds and refers to the wind coming out of the north. See *Ling Shu* chapter 77.

大肉 泛指大块隆盛的肌肉。多分布于臂、臀、腿处。见《素问·玉机真藏论》。

大肉（dà ròu）　**major flesh** It generally refers to the massive muscles，usually distributed on the arms，hips and legs. See *Su Wen* chapter 19.

大羽　体质名。阴阳二十五人中水形人之一种。出《灵枢·五音五味》。见"大羽之人"。

大羽（dà yǔ）　**major yu** Name of constitution. It refers to water-shaped people，one of the twenty-five types of people divided according to yin and yang. See *Ling Shu* chapter 65. See "大羽之人".

大羽之人　体质名。大，即太；羽，五音之一，五行属水。大羽，羽音之一，此代表阴阳二十五人中水形人之一种，其特征是神情自得。出《灵枢·阴阳二十五人》。参"水形之人"。

大羽之人（dà yǔ zhī rén）　**people pertaining to the major *yu* tone** Name of constitution. *Dà* means grandness. *Yǔ* belongs to one of the five sounds and pertains to water in the five elements. *Dà yǔ*，one of the *yu* tones，refers to water type of people，out of the twenty-five types of people divided according to yin and yang. It represents water-shaped people，who are char-

acterized by self-satisfied expressions. See *Ling Shu* chapter 64. Please refer to the phrase of "水形之人".

大豆黄卷　黄豆芽。出《灵枢·五味》。

大豆黄卷（dà dòu huáng juǎn）　**soybean sprout** Soybean sprout. See *Ling Shu* chapter 56.

大针　九针之一。长四寸，粗大而头尖，形如杖，锋微圆，用于泻关节积液。出《灵枢·九针十二原》《灵枢·官针》。

大针（dà zhēn）　**big needle** One of the nine needles. It is 4 *cun* long，thick and big with a pointed end. Its pointed end resembles a club and its sharp point is slightly rounded，which serves to drain water from the joints. See *Ling Shu* chapter 1 and *Ling Shu* chapter 7.

大谷　出《素问·五藏生成》。（1）手足大关节处。见《类经·经络二十一》。（2）肉之大分。见《素问集注》。（3）大经所会之处。见《素问》王冰注。

大谷（dà gǔ）　**large valley** See *Su Wen* chapter 10. (1) The large joints of the hands and feet. See *Lei Jing*（*Classified Classic*）" Meridians and Collaterals Chapter 21". (2) Large interstice of flesh. See *Su Wen Ji Zhu*（*Collected Annotation of Su Wen*）.（3）The convergence area of large meridians. See *Su Wen* annotated by Wang Bing.

大肠 六腑之一。上与小肠相接,下连魄门。其受小肠移下之食物残渣糟粕,吸收部分水分,变化成粪便,通过魄门排出体外,是传道之腑。其经脉为手阳明大肠经,与手太阴肺经相表里。出《灵枢·本输》《素问·灵兰秘典论》。

大肠（dà cháng） **large intestine** One of the six bowels. The upper part is connected to the small intestine and the lower part of is connected to the anus. The large intestine receives food residue and waster matters transported by the small intestine, partially absorbs water, transforms all this into faeces and excretes it out of the body through the anus, making it the *fu* organ, namely, bowel, responsible for transportation. It pertains to the large intestine meridian of hand *yangming* and is internally and externally related to the lung meridian of hand *taiyin*. See *Ling Shu* chapter 2 and *Su Wen* chapter 8.

大肠手阳明之脉 即手阳明大肠经,为十二经脉之一。其循行路线从大指次指之端开始,向上沿食指桡侧上行,经过合谷穴,沿前臂上方,进入肘外侧,再沿上臂外侧前缘,上肩,出肩峰前缘,与诸阳经相会于柱骨的大椎上,再向下入缺盆,进入胸腔络于肺,向下通过膈肌下行至脐旁天枢穴处,属于大肠。一支从缺盆上行,经颈部至面颊,过大迎穴,入下齿中,又从内外出挟口角两旁,过地仓穴,左脉向右,右脉向左,交叉于人中,上行夹于鼻孔两侧(接足阳明胃经)。出《灵枢·经脉》。

大肠手阳明之脉（dà cháng shǒu yáng míng zhī mài） **large intestine meridian of hand *yangming*** Namely the large intestine meridian of hand *yangming*, belonging to one of the twelve meridians. Its pathway starts from the tip of the forefinger, goes upwards along the radial side of the forefinger, passes He Gu（LI 4）acupoint, reaches the lateral side of the elbow along the interior aspect of the forearm, then comes to the shoulder along the anterior lateral aspect of the upper arm and comes out of the anterior border of the acromion，meeting all the yang meridians at Da Zhui（DU 14）on the spine. Then it descends to the supraclavicular fossa，comes into the thoracic cavity to closely connect to the lung. It then descends to Tian Shu（ST 25）acupoint next to the navel through the diaphragm，pertaining to the large intestine. One branch goes upwards from the supraclavicular fossa，to the cheeks through the neck，passes Da Ying（ST 5）acupoint，enters the gums of the lower teeth，curves around the upper lip，comes out of the corner of the mouth and passes through Di Cang（ST 4）acupoint. The left vessel goes to the right and the right vessel goes to the left，crossing at the philtrum，and ascends along both sides of the nose（connecting to the stomach meridian of foot *yangming*）. See *Ling Shu* chapter 10.

大肠者皮其应　应，应合之意。肺与大肠相表里，肺外合皮毛，故大肠与皮相应。出《灵枢·本藏》。

大肠者皮其应（dà cháng zhě pí qí yìng）　**the large intestine corresponds to the skin** *Yìng* means coordination. The lung is internally and externally related to the large intestine. The lung corresponds to the skin and hair externally，therefore the large intestine corresponds to the skin. See *Ling Shu* chapter 47.

大肠胀　病证名。六腑胀之一。症见肠鸣、腹痛、泄泻。出《灵枢·胀论》。

大肠胀（dà cháng zhàng）　**large intestine distention** Disease name. One of the six bowels distentions. Symptoms include borborigmus，abdominal pain and diarrhea. See *Ling Shu* chapter 35.

大肠咳　六腑咳之一，由肺咳不愈传变而成。证候特点为咳而大便遗出。出《素问·咳论》。

大肠咳（dà cháng ké）　**large intestine cough** One of the six-bowel coughs. It is caused by the transmutation of incessant lung coughing. Its pattern is characterized by encopresis when coughing. See *Su Wen* chapter 38.

大角　体质名。阴阳二十五人中木形人之一种。见《灵枢·五音五味》，见"大角之人"。

大角（dà jiǎo）　**major** *jiao* Name of constitution. Refers to the wood-shaped people，one of the twenty-five types of people divided according to yin and yang. See *Ling Shu* chapter 65. See "大角之人".

大角之人　体质名。角，五音之一，五行属木。大角，角音之一，此代表阴阳二十五人中木形人之一种，其特征是柔顺美长。出《灵枢·阴阳二十五人》，参"木形之人"。

大角之人（dà jiǎo zhī rén）　**major** *jiao***-type people** Name of constitution. *Jiǎo* refers to one of the five sounds，pertaining to wood in the five elements. *Dà jiǎo* is one kind of *jiao* tone，representing wood-shaped people，and is one out of the twenty-five types of people divided according to yin and yang. Their features are calm，amiable and pleasant. See *Ling Shu* chapter 64. Please refer to "木形之人".

大迎　经穴名。又名髓孔，属足阳明胃经。在曲颔前一寸三分，骨陷者中动脉。出《灵枢·寒热病》。

大迎（dà yíng）　**Da Ying (ST 5)** Acupoint name，also called Sui Kong (ST 5) or medullary hole. It pertains to the stomach meridian of foot *yangming*，and is located one *cun* and three *fen* anterior to the angle of the mandible，in the bone concavity of the median artery. See *Ling Shu* chapter 21.

大杼　经穴名。属足太阳膀胱经。在项第一椎下两旁各一寸五分陷者中。出《素问·水热穴论》。

大杼（dà zhù）　**Da Zhu (BL 11)** Acupoint name，pertaining to the bladder meridian of foot *taiyang*. It is located in the concavity that is one *cun* and five *fen* from each side of the first cervical vertebra. See *Su Wen* chapter 61.

大杼脉　当指大杼穴。出《灵枢·癫狂病》。

大杼脉（dà zhù mài）　*Dazhu* **meridian** Actually refers to Da Zhu (BL 11) acupoint. See *Ling Shu* chapter 22.

大奇论　《素问》篇名。此篇着重以脉象的变化论述了疝、瘕、肠澼、偏枯、暴厥病机症状及预后，因其所论都是比较少见的奇病，故名。

大奇论（dà qí lùn）　**Discussion on Unusual Diseases** The title

of a chapter in *Su Wen*. It discusses the pathogenic symptoms and prognosis of hernias, conglomerations, diarrhea, hemiplegia, and sudden fainting by focusing on the changes of pulses. The contents of this chapter all belong to uncommon diseases. Hence the name.

大明　太阳。出《素问·六元正纪大论》。

大明（dà míng）　**great brilliance** *Taiyang*. See *Su Wen* chapter 71.

大泻　针刺的泻实之法。在病人吸气时入针,呼气时出针,出针时则左右摇大其针孔而不按闭,以利邪气外出。出《素问·调经论》。

大泻（dà xiè）　**massive drainage** The needling method for draining excess. When the patient is inhaling, insert the needle and when exhaling, remove the needle. When removing the needle, move the needle around to enlarge the acupoint hole in order to allow the evil qi to disperse out of the body. See *Su Wen* chapter 62.

大泻刺　九刺法之一,用铍针切开引流以治脓性痈疡。出《灵枢·官针》。

大泻刺（dà xiè cì）　**massive drainage needling** One of the nine needling methods which uses sword-shaped needles to cut a lesion and drain the pus out of a purulent abscess and ulcer. See *Ling Shu* chapter 7.

大经　即经脉,相对于络脉而言,故称大经。出《素问·痿论》。

大经（dà jīng）　**large meridian** Namely the meridians, in comparison with the collaterals, hence it is named the large meridian. See *Su Wen* chapter 44.

大要　古医籍名。内容涉及运气、方药、病机、诊法诸方面,已佚。出《素问·六元正纪大论》。

大要（dà yào）　*The Great Essential* Name of ancient medical book, which has already gone missing. Its contents include movement of qi, formulae and medicines, pathogenesis and diagnosis. See *Su Wen* chapter 71.

大骨　泛指人体四肢及腰、脊、肩等长大骨骼。出《素问·玉机真藏论》。

大骨（dà gǔ）　**large bone** It generally refers to the long and large bones of the four extremities, waist, spine and shoulders of the human body. See *Su Wen* chapter 19.

大骨之会　肩贞穴。见《素问·通评虚实论》。

大骨之会（dà gǔ zhī huì）**meeting point of large bones** Jian Zhen（SI 9）acupoint. See *Su Wen* chapter 28.

大钟　经穴名。为足少阴肾经的络穴。位于内踝后下方，跟腱内侧缘与跟骨交角处，太溪穴下0.5寸稍后。出《灵枢·经脉》。

大钟（dà zhōng）**Da Zhong（KI 4）** Acupoint name，pertaining to the collateral acupoint of the kidney meridian of foot *shaoyin*. Located at the posterior-inferior aspect of the medial malleolus, at the intersection between the medial aspect of the achilles tendon and the calcaneus，approximately 0.5 *cun* inferior to Tai Xi（KI 3）acupoint. See *Ling Shu* chapter 10.

大宫　体质名。阴阳二十五人中土形人之一种。出《灵枢·五音五味》。见"大宫之人"。

大宫（dà gōng）**major gong** Name of constitution. Refers to the people pertaining to the earth element，one of the twenty-five types of people divided according to yin and yang. See *Ling Shu* chapter 65.

Please refer to the phrase of "大宫之人".

大宫之人　体质名。大即太；宫，五音之一，五行属土。大宫，宫音之一，此代表阴阳二十五人中土形人之一种，其特征是平和柔顺。出《灵枢·阴阳二十五人》。参"土形之人"。

大宫之人（dà gōng zhī rén）**major gong-type people** Name of constitution. *Dà* means grandness. *Gōng* belongs to one of the five sounds，and pertains to earth in the five elements. *Dà gōng* is one of the *gong* tones representing earth-shaped people，one out of the the twenty-five types of people divided according to yin and yang. Their features are gentle and agreeable. See *Ling Shu* chapter 64. Please refer to "土形之人".

大神灵　对黄帝的赞美之称。出《素问·六节藏象论》。

大神灵（dà shén líng）**the great spirit** Magnificent praise for the Yellow Emperor. See *Su Wen* chapter 9.

大络　①十二经之别络。见《素问·缪刺论》。②经脉。出《灵枢·玉版》。③经气通行的道路。络，通路。出《灵枢·动输》。

三画

大络（dà luò）　① The divergent collateral of the twelve meridians. See *Su Wen* chapter 63. ② The meridians. See *Ling Shu* chapter 60. ③ The passage for meridian circuits and qi. *Luò* means passage. See *Ling Shu* chapter 62.

大都　经穴名。是太阴脾经的荥穴。在足大趾本节后内侧，当第一蹠趾关节前缘赤白肉际处。出《灵枢·本输》。

大都（dà dū）　**Da Du（SP 2）** Acupoint name of the brook acupoint of the *taiyin* spleen meridian. It is located at the medial posterior aspect of the bump of the great toe，actually at the border of the red and white flesh，at the anterior aspect of first metatarsophalangeal joint. See *Ling Shu* chapter 2.

大息　较深的呼吸。出《素问·刺热》。

大息（dà xī）　**deep breath** Rather deep breathing. See *Su Wen* chapter 32.

大海　指胃。又称水谷之海。出《灵枢·决气》。

大海（dà hǎi）　**large sea** Refers to the stomach and is also called the sea of water and grains. See *Ling Shu* chapter 30.

大弱风　八风之一，指由南方刮来的风。出《灵枢·九宫八风》。

大弱风（dà ruò fēng）　*da ruo* **wind** One of the eight winds. Refers to the wind coming out of the south. See *Ling Shu* chapter 77.

大陵　经穴名。手厥阴心包经的原穴，输穴，在掌后横纹中点两筋之间凹陷处。出《灵枢·九针十二原》《灵枢·本输》。

大陵（dà líng）　**Da Ling（PC 7）** Acupoint name. It is source acupoint on the pericardium meridian of hand *jueyin* pertaining to the transport acupoint. It is located in the concavity between the two tendons at the midpoint of the transverse line posterior to the palm. See *Ling Shu* chapter 1 and *Ling Shu* chapter 2.

大晨　早晨天大亮之时。出《素问·标本病传论》。

大晨（dà chén）　**early morning** The time in the morning with burning daylight. See *Su Wen* chapter 65.

大偻　形体伛偻之病。因阳气开合失度，寒邪侵袭，筋脉拘急而致。出《素问·生气通天论》。

大偻（dà lóu）　**severe bending** A disease involving a bent back caused by tendon rigidity due to the abnormal opening and closing of yang qi as well as the invasion of cold evil. See *Su Wen* chapter 3.

大椎 ① 骨骼名。指第七颈椎，因其棘突较为高大，故名。出《素问・气府论》。② 经穴名。属督脉经。在第七颈椎棘突与第一胸椎棘突之间，别名百劳，上杼。出《素问・气穴论》。

大椎（dà zhuī）　① Name of a bone. Refers to the seventh cervical vertebra due to its large acantha. See *Su Wen* chapter 59. ② Name of Da Zhui (SI 6) acupoint pertaining to the governor vessel. It is located between the seventh cervical and first thoracic spinous processes，and is also called Bai Lao（SI 6）acupoint or Shang Zhu（SI 6）acupoint. See *Su Wen* chapter 58.

大惑 指医生对三部九候诊法迷惑不解，而进行错误的施治。出《素问・离合真邪论》。

大惑（dà huò）　**great perplexity** Refers to a doctor who is confused about the diagnostic method of three sections and nine indicators，thus leading to the wrong treatment. See *Su Wen* chapter 27.

大惑论 《灵枢》篇名。大，甚也；惑，迷乱眩晕。此篇主要论述了眼睛的构造及其与五脏的关系。说明了登高而惑的道理，以及善忘、善饥、不得卧、多卧等病的病机。因其篇首即论关于大惑的内容，故名。

大惑论（dà huò lùn）　**Discussion on Great Perplexity** The title of a chapter in *Ling Shu*. *Dà* means extreme and *huò* means confusion. This chapter mainly discusses eye structure as well as their relationship with the five viscera. It explains that the reason for confusion is due to ascension and is the pathogenesis for amnesia, rapid hungering, the inability to sleep and somnolence，etc. The content regarding the Great Perplexity is at the beginning of the chapter, hence its name.

大厥 病证名。指突然昏厥，为厥证之一种。由于血与气并于上，致上实下虚，下虚则阴脱，阴脱则阳越，阴阳不相承接，故昏厥。出《素问・调经论》。

大厥（dà jué）　**massive syncope** Disease name. Refers to sudden fainting and belonging to one of the syncope patterns. It is due to the qi and blood co-existing in the upper part, leading to upper excess and lower deficiency. Lower deficiency brings about yin collapse and yin collapse leads to yang floating. Yin and yang cannot connect with each other and finally fainting comes about. See *Su Wen* chapter 62.

大敦　经穴名。足厥阴肝经井穴,在足大趾外侧去爪甲根部一分处,或取于大趾背侧三毛中。出《灵枢·本输》。

大敦(dà dūn)　**Da Dun (LR 1)** Acupoint name, belonging to the well acupoint of the liver meridian of foot *jueyin*. It is located one *fen* from the toenail root at the lateral side of the great toe or it can be located at the dorsal aspect of the great toe in the three hair region. See *Ling Shu* chapter 2.

大腹　① 部位名。脐周及脐上腹部。出《素问·藏气法时论》。② 腹部膨大。出《灵枢·经脉》。

大腹(dà fù)　① Name of body part on the abdomen at the peri-umbilicus and above the umbilicus. See *Su Wen* chapter 22. ② Enlarged abdomen. See *Ling Shu* chapter 10.

大腧　指大杼穴。属足太阳膀胱经,为《难经·四十五难》八会穴中的骨会穴。在背腧穴之中,其高居于五脏六腑各腧穴之上,所以称为大腧。出《灵枢·背腧》。

大腧(dà shū)　**Da Shu (BL 11)** Refers to Da Shu acupoint pertaining to the bladder meridian of foot *taiyang*. It refers to the bone meeting acupoint of the eight meeting acupoints in *Nan Jing* (*Classic of Difficult Issues*) "The 45th Difficult Issue". Located in the back transport acupoint, it is higher than any of the transport acupoints of the five viscera and six bowels, thus called Da Shu. See *Ling Shu* chapter 51.

大痹　病证名。严重的痹证。由于冬季针刺不当,使脏气虚而邪痹于五脏所致。出《素问·四时刺逆从论》。

大痹(dà bì)　**massive impediment** Disease name for one with a severe impediment pattern. It is caused by visceral qi deficiency and evil obstructing the five viscera due to improper needling in winter. See *Su Wen* chapter 64.

大瘕　出《素问·刺热》。(1)指腹中结块之病证。见《素问经注节解》。(2) 指大瘕泄，即痢疾。见《素问集注》《难经·五十七难》。

大瘕(dà jiǎ)　serious conglomeration See *Su Wen* chapter 32. (1) Refers to a disease with abdominal lumps. See *Su Wen Jing Zhu Jie Jie*(*Excerpts of Annotations of Su Wen*). (2) Refers to the drainage of a large obstruction，namely diarrhea. See *Su Wen Ji Zhu*(*Collected Annotation of Su Wen*) and *Nan Jing*(*Classic of Difficult Issues*) "The 57th Difficult Issue".

大藏　出《素问·长刺节论》。(1) 五脏。见《素问注证发微》。(2) 肺脏。见《太素·杂刺》。

大藏(dà zàng)　large depot See *Su Wen* chapter 55. (1) Five viscera. See *Su Wen Zhu Zheng Fa Wei*(*Annotation and Elaboration on Su Wen*). (2) Lung. See *Tai Su*(*Grand Plain*) "Miscellaneous Needling".

上　① 指运气中的司天。因其位在正南位(在上方)主气的三之气上，故称。见《素问·天元纪大论》。② 指高明的医生，亦称上工。出《灵枢·九针十二原》。③ 指天。出《素问·金匮真言论》。④ 与下相对而言。出《素问·脉要精微论》。⑤ 指

吐法。出《素问·至真要大论》。⑥ 上逆。出《素问·举痛论》。⑦ 指君火。出《素问·五运行大论》。参"不当位"条。

上(shàng)　① Refers to Celestial control within the five circuits and qi. It is so called due to its southern position（located in the upper area）above the third qi in a year. See *Su Wen* chapter 66. ② Refers to outstanding doctors，also called upper *gong*. See *Ling Shu* chapter 1. ③ Refers to heaven. See *Su Wen* chapter 4. ④ The opposite of "下"（xià：bottom，down）. See *Su Wen* chapter 17. ⑤ Refers to emetic therapy. See *Su Wen* chapter 74. ⑥ Upward reversal（of qi）. See *Su Wen* chapter 39. ⑦ Refers to sovereign fire. See *Su Wen* chapter 67. See "不当位".

上七窍　即七窍。参该条。因其均在颜面部故曰"上"。出《灵枢·脉度》。

上七窍(shàng qī qiào)　seven upper orifices Namely seven orifices. Reference entry "七窍". It is so called as all seven orifices are located at the facial region. See *Su Wen* chapter 17.

上工　指高明的医生。这类医生

十分注重对疾病的预防,强调早期诊断,早期治疗。见《素问·八正神明论》。并且具有高超的诊疗技术,能将察色、辨脉、诊尺肤多种方法结合起来,治愈率可达十分之九。见《灵枢·邪气藏府病形》。

上工(shàng gōng)　**master doctor** Refers to outstanding doctors who pay particular attention to disease prevention and diagnosis as well as treatment in early stage. See *Su Wen* chapter 26. With superb diagnosis and treatment skills, they combine examination of countenance, pulse identification and palpation of forearm skin all together so that nine out of ten patients can restore health. See *Ling Shu* chapter 4.

上工治未病　言高明的医生,是在未病之前,先行防治,而不是在发现病症之后,才去治疗。出《灵枢·逆顺》。参"治未病"条。

上工治未病(shàng gōng zhì wèi bìng)　**Master doctors treat the disease before its onset.** Indicates that master doctors will take preventive measures before disease onset rather than perform treatment afterwards. See *Ling Shu* chapter 55. See "治未病".

上天　九宫中之离宫,又称天宫。位在正南方,主夏至、小暑、大暑三个节气。出《灵枢·九宫八风》。

上天(shàng tiān)　*shang tian* Li gong（*li* palace）within the Nine Palaces（nine directions in ancient China）, also called the Heavenly Palace（*tian gong*）. It is located at due south and governs three seasonal terms, namely Summer Solstice（*xia zhi*）, minor summer heat（*xiao shu*）and massive summer heat（*da shu*）, for 46 days in total. See *Ling Shu* chapter 77.

上气　①气喘。出《素问·五藏生成》。②人体上部之气,包括头部清阳之气。出《灵枢·口问》。

上气(shàng qì)　① Asthma. See *Su Wen* chapter 10. ② Qi in the upper part of the body, including lucid *yang* qi of the head. See *Ling Shu* chapter 28.

上丹田　部位名。出《素问·本病论》。(1)眉心间。见《抱朴子·地真》。(2)脑。见《类经·运气四十四》。

上丹田(shàng dān tián)　**upper dan tian** Name of body part.

See *Su Wen* chapter 73 (The original contents were lost in history and the present text was supplemented by scholars in the Song dynasty). (1) Place between the eyebrows. See *Bao Pu Zi* chapter 18 "Di Zhen". (2) Brain. See *Lei Jing* (*Classified Classic*) "Circuits and Qi Chapter 44".

上古 指远古时代,即人类生活的原始时代。出《素问·上古天真论》。

上古(shàng gǔ) **remote antiquity** Refers to ancient times, in other words the primitive age of human activity. See *Su Wen* chapter 1.

上古天真论 《素问》篇名。上古,指远古时代;天真,一指自然纯朴的天性,一指先天真元之气,即篇中所说的肾气。该篇主要讨论了上古之人由于重视保养天真的养生方法,因而得以健康长寿的道理,以及肾气在人体生长发育过程中的重要作用。

上古天真论(shàng gǔ tiān zhēn lùn) **Theory on Ancient Ideas on How to Preserve Natural Healthy Energy** The title of a chapter in *Su Wen*. *Shàng gǔ* refers to an era of remote antiquity,while *tiān zhēn* means plain nature on one hand and primordial qi on the other,or kidney qi mentioned in this chapter. This chapter primarily discusses how ancient people managed to attain health and longevity through thinking highly of preserving *tiān zhēn* and the importance of kidney qi in the growth and development of humans.

上关 经穴名。属足少阳经,别名客主人。在颧弓上缘,距耳廓前缘约一寸处,与下关直对。出《素问·气穴论》。

上关(shàng guān) **Shang Guan (GB 3)** Name of acupoint belonging to the gallbladder meridian of foot *Shaoyang*,and also known as *Ke Zhu Ren*. It is located at the superior border of the zygomatic arch,one *cun* from the front edge of the pinna directly opposite to Xia Guan (ST 7). *Su Wen* chapter 58.

上羽 ① 体质名。羽,五音之一,五行属水。上羽,羽音之一,此代表阴阳二十五人中水形之人。出《灵枢·阴阳二十五人》。见"水形之人"。② 运气名。指水运太过。出《素问·五常政大论》。

三画

三画

上羽（shàng yǔ）　① Name of constitution. *Yu*，one of the five tones，belongs to water according to the five-element theory. *Shang yu*，one of *yu* tones，refers to people whose physical appearance resembles that of "water" among the twenty-five types of people divided according to yin and yang. See *Ling Shu* chapter 64. See "水形之人". ② Name of circuits and qi and refers to the excess movement of water. See *Su Wen* chapter 70.

上纪　指中脘穴，一名太仓，为胃的募穴。在上脘下一寸属任脉。出《素问·气穴论》。

上纪（shàng jì）　**Shang Ji（CV 12）**Refers to Zhong Wan（CV 12）acupoint，also named Tai Cang and is the front-mu acupoint of the stomach（and one of the conception vessel points）. It is located one *cun* below Shang Wan（CV 13）acupoint and belongs to conception vessel. See *Su Wen* chapter 58.

上角　① 体质名。角，五音之一，五行属木。上角，角音之一，此代表阴阳二十五人中木形之人。出《灵枢·阴阳二十五人》。参"木形之人"。② 运气名。指木运太过。出《素问·五常政大论》。

上角（shàng jué）　① Name of constitution. *Jué*，one of the five tones，belongs to wood according to the five-element theory. *Shang jue*，one of the *jue* tones，represents those people with the physical appearance of "wood" among the twenty-five types of people divided according to yin and yang. See *Ling Shu* chapter 64. Please refer to "木形之人". ② Name of the movement of qi and refers to the excess movement of wood. See *Su Wen* chapter 70.

上经　古医籍名，已佚。其内容可能讨论有关人与自然关系的问题，《素问·病能论》有"上经者，言气之通天也"之言，推测似与《素问·生气通天论》较为接近。

上经（shàng jīng）　*The Remote Classic* Name of ancient medical classic（already gone missing）. It most likely discussed the relationship between man and nature. See *Su Wen* chapter 46. It is said that the upper classic discussed the interrelation between life and nature，and it has been speculated that it may have been similar to *Su Wen* chapter 3.

上临 运气术语。上,指司天之气。上临,把值年中运与司天之气相会,根据两者五行属性的关系,确定该年是否属于运气同化之年。临,会合。出《素问·六元正纪大论》。

上临(shàng lín) *shang lin* Terminology of circuits and qi. *Shàng* refers to qi of Celestial control. *Shàng líng*, in the year when the qi of *zhong yun* and Celestial control meet, and according to the relationship between both corresponding elements in the five element theory, it is decided whether or not the year is one of circuits and qi assimilation. See *Su Wen* chapter 71.

上帝 上古时代的帝君。出《素问·移精变气论》。

上帝(shàng dì) **superior emperor** Emperor in ancient times. See *Su Wen* chapter 13.

上宫 ① 体质名。宫,五音之一,五行属土。上宫,宫音之一,此代表阴阳二十五人中土形之人。出《灵枢·阴阳二十五人》。参"土形之人"。② 运气名。指土运太过。出《素问·

五常政大论》。

上宫(shàng gōng) ① Name of constitution. *Gong* refers to one of the five ancient Chinese tones belonging to the earth element according to the five-element theory. Upper *gong*, one of the *gong* tones, refers to those people whose physical appearance resembles "earth" among the twenty-five types of people divided according to yin and yang. See *Su Wen* chapter 64. Please refer to "土形之人". ② Name of the movement of qi and refers to the excess of earth movement. See *Su Wen* chapter 70.

上窍 耳目鼻口等头面部七孔窍之统称。出《素问·阴阳应象大论》。

上窍(shàng qiào) **upper orifices** The general name of the seven facial orifices including the ears, eyes, nostrils and mouth. See *Su Wen* chapter 5.

上盛则气高 上,指三部九候诊法中的上部之脉,即两额、两颊、耳前之动脉。此部之脉盛大,是邪壅于上,故见气盛喘满之证。出《素问·脉要精微论》。

上盛则气高(shàng shèng zé qì gāo) **excessive upper pulse**

leads to upper flow of qi *Shàng* refers to the upper pulses in the diagnostic methods of the three sections and nine indicators, namely the throbbing pulses of the forehead, cheeks and preauricular area. These strong and large pulses indicate pathogens of congestion in the upper part of the body, with symptoms of qi exuberance, panting and fullness. See *Su Wen* chapter 17.

上虚下实　①指脉象。上部脉象虚弱，下部脉象壅实。出《素问·脉要精微论》。②指病机。肺气虚弱而气积胸中。出《素问·五藏生成篇》。

上虚下实（shàng xū xià shí）　① Refers to a pulse where the upper part is deficient and the lower part is excessive. See *Su Wen* chapter 17. ② Refers to the pathogenesis where deficient lung qi leads to an accumulation of qi in the chest. See *Su Wen* chapter 10.

上脘　胃脘上口贲门部。今有上脘穴，在脐上五寸。出《灵枢·四时气》。

上脘（shàng wǎn）　**epigastrium** Cardia area at the upper part of the stomach. At present it refers to Shang Wan（CV 13） acupoint, located five *cun* above the navel. See *Ling Shu* chapter 19.

上商　①体质名。商，五音之一，五行属金。上商，商音之一，此代表阴阳二十五人中金形之人。出《灵枢·阴阳二十五人》。见"金形之人"。② 运气名。指金运太过。出《素问·五常政大论》。

上商（shàng shāng）　① Name of constitution. *Shāng*, one of the five tones, belongs to metal according to the five-element theory. *Shàng shāng*, one of the *shang* tones, here represents people whose physical appearance is that of "metal" among the twenty-five types of people divided according to yin and yang. See *Su Wen* chapter 64. See "金形之人". ② Name of circuits and qi, refers to the excess of metal movement. See *Su Wen* chapter 70.

上焦　三焦之一，位于上部，是心、肺所居之处，与气液的输布有密切关系。出《灵枢·营卫生会》。参"三焦"条。

上焦（shàng jiāo）　**upper *jiao*** One of the triple *jiao* located in the upper part of the body where the heart and lung dwell. It is closely connected to the distribution of qi and fluids. See *Ling Shu* chapter 18. See "三焦".

上焦出气 上焦能将中焦化生的水谷精气敷布至全身。出《灵枢·痈疽》。

上焦出气（shàng jiāo chū qì） **The upper *jiao* transports qi.** The upper *jiao* distributes the essential qi, essence, food and water produced by the middle *jiao*, all over the body. See *Ling Shu* chapter 81.

上焦如雾 言上焦的功能。上焦心肺,布散宣发水谷之精气,若雾露之气遍溉周身。出《灵枢·营卫生会》。

上焦如雾（shàng jiāo rú wù） **The upper *jiao* is like fog.** Speaking about the function of the upper *jiao*. The heart and lung located in the upper *jiao* can diffuse essential qi, essence, food and water like fog and dew, all over the body. See *Ling Shu* chapter 18.

上管 上脘,即胃之上口。出《灵枢·本藏》。

上管（shàng guǎn） **epigastrium** Refers to *shang wan*, the upper opening of the stomach. See *Ling Shu* chapter 47.

上膈 ①《灵枢》篇名。该篇阐述噎膈证中属于下脘虫积成痈的病因、证候及治法。② 病证。指食入即吐的噎膈证。出《灵枢·上膈》。

上膈（shàng gé） ① Chapter title in *Ling Shu*. This chapter elaborates on the causes, symptoms and treatment of worm accumulation in the lower stomach duct causing abscess in dysphagia syndrome. ② Name of syndrome. Refers to dysphagia characterized by vomiting right after ingesting food. See *Ling Shu* chapter 68.

上徵 ① 体质名。徵（zhǐ 指）,五音之一,五行属火。上徵,五音之一,此代表阴阳二十五人中火形之人。出《灵枢·阴阳二十五人》。见"火形之人"。② 运气名。指火运太过。出《素问·五常政大论》。

上徵（shàng zhǐ） ① Name of constitution. *Zhǐ* is one of the five tones in the ancient Chinese five-tone scale and belongs to fire in terms of the five elements. *Shàng zhǐ*, one of the five tones, refers to people with the physical appearance of "fire" among the twenty-

三画

five types of people divided according to yin and yang. See *Ling Shu* chapter 64. See "火形之人". ② Name of circuits and qi. Refers to excessive fire movement. See *Su Wen* chapter 70.

上膲　膲通焦，即上焦。出《灵枢·大惑论》。

上膲（shàng jiāo）　**upper *jiao*** "膲" is the same as "焦", so it is the same as "上焦", the upper *jiao*. See *Ling Shu* chapter 80.

小　① 指六岁以下者。出《灵枢·卫气失常》。② 形体瘦小。出《灵枢·卫气失常》《灵枢·禁服》。③ 少。即病变轻浅者，用针要少。出《灵枢·卫气失常》。④ 小方，指药味少或药味多而分量轻的方剂。出《素问·至真要大论》。⑤ 指小便。出《素问·标本病传论》。⑥ 指小脉。脉来细小如线。出《素问·离合真邪论》。⑦ 指病轻微。出《灵枢·官针》。⑧ 指小针。出《灵枢·玉版》。⑨ 细密。出《灵枢·本藏》《灵枢集注》。

小（xiǎo）　① Refers to children under the age of six. See *Ling Shu* chapter 59. ② Thin and tiny body shape. See *Ling Shu* chapter 59 and chapter 48. ③ Fewer. As the disease gets milder，the patient receives fewer acupuncture treatments. See *Ling Shu* chapter 59. ④ A small formula，namely one with fewer medicinal herbs or more medicinal herbs in smaller quantities. See *Su Wen* chapter 74. ⑤ Urine. See *Su Wen* chapter 65. ⑥ Refers to a thin thread-like pulse. See *Su Wen* chapter 27. ⑦ Refers to a mild disease. See *Ling Shu* chapter 7. ⑧ Refers to small needles. See *Ling Shu* chapter 60. ⑨ Fine and closely woven. See *Ling Shu* chapter 47 and *Ling Shu Ji Zhu* (*Collected Annotation of Ling Shu*).

小子　雷公的自谦之称。出《灵枢·五色》。见"雷公"。

小子（xiǎo zǐ）　*xiao zi* A youngling，what Lei Gong calls himself out of modesty. See *Ling Shu* chapter 49. See "雷公".

小分　分，分界，引申为肌肉会合处的分理间隙。小分，即小肌肉间的分理间隙。出《素问·长刺节论》。

小分（xiǎo fēn）　**small parting** *Fēn* means dividing line，and its extended meaning is subcutaneous interstitial space. Small parting therefore means the subcutaneous interstitial space between small muscles. See *Su Wen* chapter 55.

小心　出《素问·刺禁论》。《太素》作"志心"。(1)心包络。见《素问注证发微》。(2)命门。刘完素、张介宾、吴崑、汪昂等认为是指命门。(3)膈俞穴心气所出之处。见《素问直解》。

小心（xiǎo xīn）　**xiao xin** See *Su Wen* chapter 52. It is written as "志心" in *Tai Su*（*Grand Plain*）. (1) Pericardium collateral. See *Su Wen Zhu Zheng Fa Wei*（*Annotation and Elaboration on Su Wen*）. (2) Life gate. Master physicians including Liu Wansu, Zhang Jiebin, Wu Kun and Wang Ang consider *xiao xin* as the life gate in TCM. (3) Ge Shu（BL 17）acupoint，where the qi of the heart exits. See *Su Wen Zhi Jie*（*Direct Interpretation on Su Wen*）.

小针　针具名。亦称微针，相当现代之毫针。出《灵枢·九针十二原》。

小针（xiǎo zhēn）　**small needles** Name of needling instruments，also called microneedles. They are the counterpart of the modern day filiform needles. See *Ling Shu* chapter 1.

小针解　《灵枢》篇名。小针，指微小的针刺工具。此篇主要是对《九针十二原》中有关针刺内容进行注解和补充说明，故名。

小针解（xiǎo zhēn jiě）　**Explanatory Remarks on the Small Needles** Chapter title in *Ling Shu*. *Xiǎo zhēn* refers to microneedling instrument and this chapter mainly expounds on contents over needling from chapter 1，thus its name.

小肠　六腑之一。上与胃相通，下与大肠相接。主要功能是受盛、化物。其承受胃中初步腐熟之水谷，继续消化，分别清浊，在吸收其精华养料后，将糟粕下送大肠，水液渗入膀胱。其经脉为手太阳小肠经，与手少阴心经相表里。出《素问·灵兰秘典论》。

小肠（xiǎo cháng）　**small intestine** One of the six bowels. At the superior aspect，it is connected to the stomach and at the inferior aspect，it joins with the large intestine. The major functions of the small intestine are reception and transformation：it receives preliminarily decomposed food from the stomach and continues to digest it. After separating the clear and the turbid and absorbing the essentials from the food, the small intestine transfers waste matters to the large intestine and conveys water to the bladder. It pertains to the small intestine meridian of hand *taiyang* and it connects to the heart meridian of hand *shaoyin* both internally and externally. See *Su Wen* chapter 8.

小肠手太阳之脉　即手太阳小肠经,为十二经脉之一。其循行路线从小指外侧端(少泽穴)开始,沿手外侧至腕,过锐骨直上,沿前臂骨下缘,出肘后内侧两筋之间,再沿上臂外侧后缘,出肩后骨缝,绕行肩胛,相交于肩上入缺盆,络于心,沿食道,穿过横膈,至胃部,下行,属于小肠。一支从缺盆沿颈上颊,主眼外角,转入耳内。再一支从面颊走眼眶下部,至鼻,行眼内角,斜行而络于颧部,接足太阳膀胱经。出《灵枢·经脉》。

小肠手太阳之脉(xiǎo cháng shǒu tài yáng zhī mài)　**small intestine meridian of hand** *taiyang* Refers to the small intestine meridian of hand *taiyang* which is one of the twelve meridians. It starts from the lateral end of the little finger (Shao Ze, SI 1), goes along the lateral side of the hand to the wrist and runs past the styloid process of the radius and goes straight upward along the lower edge of the forearm bone. Then it exits from the space between the two sinews inside the outer margin of the elbow, runs along the lower edge of the lateral aspect of the upper arm, exits from the sutura behind the shoulder, passes around the scapula and meets over the shoulder before going into the supraclavicular fossa. Next it connects to the heart and goes through the diaphragm along the esophagus to the stomach and then runs downwards and connects to the small intestine. A branch vessel, along the neck, runs upwards from the supraclavicular fossa to the tempora, passes the paropia and enters into the ear. Another branch vessel goes from the cheek to the bottom of the eye socket and then to the nose, next, it runs past the inner corner of the eye and begins to move diagonally to connect to the cheekbone and join the bladder meridian of foot *taiyang*. See *Ling Shu* chapter 10.

小肠胀　病证名。六腑胀之一。症见少腹胀，引腰而痛。出《灵枢·胀论》。

小肠胀（xiǎo cháng zhàng）　**small intestine distention** Disease Name. It manifests with a distended lower abdomen which pulls and causes pain in the lower back. See *Ling Shu* chapter 35.

小肠咳　六腑咳之一。由心咳不愈传变而成。证候特点为咳而随出屎气。出《素问·咳论》。

小肠咳（xiǎo cháng ké）　**small intestine cough** One of the six bowel coughs. It is caused by the transmutation of incessant heart cough, and characterized by a cough accompanied with foul-smelling qi. See *Su Wen* chapter 38.

小金丹　《内经》十三方之一。由辰砂二两，雄黄一两，雌黄一两，紫金半两组成，用火煅之，取出研细，炼白沙蜜为丸，如梧桐子大，每天用冷水送服一丸，连服十天，古人认为可预防疫疠等传染病。出《素问·刺法论》。

小金丹（xiǎo jīn dān）　**Small Golden Pallet** One of the thirteen formulas in *Nei Jing* (*Internal Classic*). It consists of two *liang* (one *liang* = 50 g) of cinnabar, one *liang* of realgar, one *liang* of orpiment and a half *liang* of purple gold. After being calcined with fire, it is removed and pulverized. Pellets are made with whitish honey, the same size as phoenix tree seeds. The ancients believed that infectious diseases such as epidemic diseases and pestilence could be prevented if people took one pellet orally with cold water every day for ten consecutive days. See *Su Wen* chapter 72.

小络　指孙络。出《素问·调经论》。参"孙络"条。

小络（xiǎo luò）　**small collateral** Name of a tertiary collateral. See *Su Wen* chapter 62. Please refer to "孙络".

小海　经穴名。手太阳小肠经之合穴。在肘内大骨外，去肘端五分陷者中。出《灵枢·本输》。

小海（xiǎo hǎi）　**Xiao Hai (SI 8)** Acupoint name. Refers to the *he*-sea acupoint of the small intestine meridian of hand *taiyang*. Located in the outer part of the major bone in the elbow, it is in the concavity that is five *fen* to the end of the elbow. See *Ling Shu* chapter 2.

小腹 ① 又称少腹,指脐下两侧腹部。或指腹部脐下部分。出《素问·藏气法时论》。② 腹部平束不隆起。出《灵枢·阴阳二十五人》。

小腹（xiǎo fù）　① Refers to the area of the abdomen on both sides below the navel or the area of the abdomen below the navel. See *Su Wen* chapter 22. ② An abdomen that is flat and not bulging. See *Ling Shu* chapter 64.

小溪　出《素问·五藏生成》。(1) 周身骨节。见《类经·经络二十一》。(2) 肉之小分处。见《素问集注》。(3) 小络之会。《素问》王冰注。

小溪（xiǎo xī）　**small ravine** See *Su Wen* chapter 10. (1) Body condyles. See *Lei Jing*（*Classified Classic*）"Meridians and Collaterals Chapter 21". (2) Small parting of the flesh. See *Su Wen Ji Zhu*（*Collected Annotation of Su Wen*）. (3) Meeting point of small collaterals. See *Su Wen* annotated by Wang Bing.

口问　《灵枢》篇名。口问,由口头问答所传授的医学知识。该篇论述了外感六淫,内伤七情及饮食起居失常为致病因素,还对欠、哕、唏、振寒、噫、嚏、嚲、泣涕、太息、涎下、耳鸣、啮舌十二种疾病的病因病机、治则治法作了具体的阐述,最后分别讨论了上中下三气不足的症状表现。由于这些内容系口问得于先师,故名。

口问（kǒu wèn）　**Oral Inquiry** Chapter title in *Ling Shu*. Oral inquiry suggests that medical knowledge is passed on orally. This chapter discusses pathogenic factors such as the external contraction of the six excesses, the internal damage of the seven emotions and irregular lifestyle habits. It also expounds on the etiology, disease mechanisms, and therapeutic principles of the twelve diseases, namely, insufficiency, hiccups, shortness of breath, quivering with cold, belching, slackening of meridians and vessels, tearing and snivelling, deep sighing, drooling, tinnitus and tongue biting. In addition, it discusses qi insufficiency, manifestations in the upper, middle and lower body respectively, at the end of the passage. As the masters of older generations imparted this knowledge to others orally, the chapter was named *kǒu wèn*, or oral inquiry. Hence its name.

口疮　病名。口腔患疮疡。出《素问·气交变大论》。

口疮(kǒu chuāng)　**oral ulcer** Disease name. Ulcer inside oral cavity. See *Su Wen* chapter 69.

口喎　口歪斜。出《灵枢·经脉》。

口喎(kǒu wāi)　**Wry mouth**, refers to a deviated mouth. See *Ling Shu* chapter 10.

口僻　口歪斜。又称口喎。出《灵枢·经筋》。

口僻(kǒu pì)　**wry mouth** Wry mouth, refers to a deviated mouth, or *kǒu wāi*. See *Ling Shu* chapter 13.

口糜　口舌糜烂。出《素问·气厥论》。

口糜(kǒu mí)　**aphthous stomatitis** The erosion of the mucous membrane in the mouth and on the tongue. See *Su Wen* chapter 37.

巾针　古代生活用针，长一寸六分，离针头半寸处突呈尖锐。镵针的形状仿此针。出《灵枢·九针论》。

巾针(jīn zhēn)　**jin needle** A one *cun* and six *fen* long needle used in ancient times in daily life. Half a *cun* from the pin-

head it becomes sharp, and the spade needle is modeled after this needle. See *Ling Shu* chapter 78.

久风为飧泄　因久受风邪，内伤脾土，而变为完谷不化的泄泻。出《素问·脉要精微论》。

久风为飧泄(jiǔ fēng wéi sūn xiè)　**Long-term exposure to wind causes diarrhea.** Long-term exposure to wind evil causes internal damage to the spleen and diarrhea with undigested food results. See *Su Wen* chapter 17.

久立伤骨　骨为干，支撑形体，久立易劳伤骨。出《素问·宣明五气》《灵枢·九针论》。

久立伤骨(jiǔ lì shāng gǔ)　**Standing for a long period of time harms the bones.** The bones support the body, and standing for extended periods of time tends to harm them. See *Su Wen* chapter 23 and *Ling Shu* chapter 78.

久行伤筋　筋的功能是利机关，司运动。久行则劳累过度而伤筋。出《素问·宣明五气》《灵枢·九针论》。

久行伤筋(jiǔ xíng shāng jīn)　**walking for a long period of time harms the sinews** The sinews are responsible for the free movement of the joints and govern activity. Fatigue resulting from walking for long periods of time harms the sinews. See *Su Wen* chapter 23 and *Ling Shu* chapter 78.

久坐伤肉 久坐不动,肌肉软弱乏力,故称伤肉。出《素问·宣明五气》《灵枢·九针论》。

久坐伤肉（jiǔ zuò shāng ròu）**Sitting for a long time harms the flesh.** Sitting for prolonged periods of time would lead to muscle weakness，thus it is said that sitting for a long time harms the flesh. See *Su Wen* chapter 23 and *Ling Shu* chapter 78.

久卧伤气 久卧则阳气不伸,气运不健,故称伤气。临床常见久卧而神疲乏力等。出《素问·宣明五气》《灵枢·九针论》。

久卧伤气（jiǔ wò shāng qì）**Lying down for a long time harms qi.** Lying down for prolonged periods of time will disturb the expansion of yang qi and cause dysfunction of qi movement，thus lying down for extended periods of time harms qi. Mental fatigue and lack of strength due to sleeping for longer periods of time are com-mon clinical manifestations. See *Su Wen* chapter 23 and *Ling Shu* chapter 78.

久视伤血 目之视觉功能赖血以濡养,故久视可伤血。出《素问·宣明五气》《灵枢·九针论》。

久视伤血（jiǔ shì shāng xuě）**Straining the eyes for a long time harms the blood.** Good vision relies on the blood nourishing the eyes，therefore straining the eyes for an extended period of time harms the blood. See *Su Wen* chapter 23 and *Ling Shu* chapter 78.

广肠 直肠,大肠之末段。出《灵枢·肠胃》。

广肠（guǎng cháng）**broad intestine** The rectum, the end of the large intestine. See *Ling Shu* chapter 31.

广明 《素问·阴阳离合论》。（1）即大明,指阳气盛明。见《素问》王冰注。（2）指心。见《素问注证发微》。

广明（guǎng míng）**broad brilliance** See *Su Wen* chapter 6. (1) Refers to the great brightness of yang qi. See *Su Wen* annotated by Wang Bing. (2) Refers to the heart. See *Su Wen Zhu Zheng Fa Wei*（*Annotation and Elaboration on Su*

门　① 指经气在经络的出入之处。出《灵枢·九针十二原》《灵枢·小针解》。② 针刺的针孔。出《素问·离合真邪论》。

门(mén)　① Refers to the place where qi enters and leaves the meridians and collaterals. See *Ling Shu* chapter 1 and chapter 3. ② Refers to the hole the acupuncture leaves behind in the skin. See *Su Wen* chapter 27.

尸厥　病证名。指突然昏倒不省人事,其状若尸的病证。出《素问·缪刺论》。

尸厥(shī jué)　**unconsciousness** Name of the disease in which the patient suddenly falls down with loss of consciousness, like a corpse. See *Su Wen* chapter 63.

巳亥之纪　指纪年地支是巳、亥之年,为厥阴风木司天。纪,纪年。出《素问·六元正纪大论》。参"厥阴之政"条。

巳亥之纪(sì hài zhī jì)　**year of si and hai** In the years si and hai as recorded by the Earthly Branches, *jueyin* wind wood controls the heaven. *Jì* means to record the years. See *Su Wen* chapter 71. See "厥阴之政".

子门　子宫颈口。出《灵枢·水胀》。

子门(zǐ mén)　**cervix** The opening of the uterus. See *Ling Shu* chapter 57.

子午之纪　指纪年地支是子、午之年,为少阴君火司天。纪,纪年。出《素问·六元正纪大论》。参"少阴之政"条。

子午之纪(zǐ wǔ zhī jì)　**year of zi and wu** In the zi and wu years recorded according to the Earthly Branches, *shaoyin* monarch fire controls the heaven. *Ji* means recording the years. See *Su Wen* chapter 71. Refers to the phrase "少阴之政".

子处　指子宫。出《灵枢·五色》。

子处(zǐ chù)　**uterus** Refers to womb. See *Ling Shu* chapter 49.

卫气　① 具有温煦护卫、抗邪作用的气。由水谷精气化生而成,性质慓悍滑利,行于脉外,内而胸腹脏腑,外而皮肤肌肉,遍及全身。出《素问·痹论》。②《灵枢》篇名。主要论述脏腑营卫的生理功能,强调十二经脉之标本虚实及六腑气街,对预防治疗的重要意义。这些内容皆与卫气的功能有关,故名。

卫气(wèi qì)　① Defensive qi. It is the qi having the function of warming, protecting, and resisting pathogens. It is generated by the essential qi of water and food, and it moves quickly and smoothly outside the vessels. It reaches every part of the body including the chest, abdomen, internal organs, skin and muscles. See *Su Wen* chapter 43. ② Chapter title in *Ling Shu*. This chapter mainly explains the physiological functions of nutrient qi, defensive qi, viscera and bowels, and emphasizes the significance of root, branch, deficiency, and excess of the twelve meridians, and the qi routes of the six bowels in preventing and treating diseases. All these are related to the function of defensive qi, thus the chapter named Defensive Qi.

卫气失常　《灵枢》篇名。此篇主要讨论卫气运行失常所引起的各种病变及其针刺治法,故名。篇中还提出了人体的小、少、壮、老的四个发展阶段以及膏、肥、肉三种不同体质类型的特点。

卫气失常（wèi qì shī cháng）**Defensive Qi Abnormality** Chapter title in *Ling Shu*. This chapter mainly discusses various diseases caused by the abnormal movement of defensive qi and their methods of treatment with acupuncture. It also discusses the four stages of growth in people (small, young, strong and old) and the three different types of body constitutions (greasy, fat and muscular).

卫气行　《灵枢》篇名。此篇主要论述了卫气在人体的运行规律,以及掌握这种规律对治疗疾病的重要意义,故名。

卫气行（wèi qì xíng）**Movement of Defensive Qi** Chapter title in *Ling Shu*. This chapter mainly expounds the laws according to which defensive qi moves inside the body and the great significance of mastering these laws for treating diseases, thus its name.

卫气虚则不用　出《素问·逆调论》。见“荣气虚则不仁”条。

卫气虚则不用（wèi qì xū zé bú yòng）**When defensive qi is deficient, it loses its function.** See *Su Wen* chapter 34. See “荣气虚则不仁”.

卫出于下焦　出《灵枢·营卫生会》。（1）卫气为阳气的一部分,其化源根于下焦命门,其运行起始于下焦肾和膀胱两经,故称。见《类经·经络二十三》。（2）“下”为“上”之误,当是

"卫出于上焦"。见《灵枢集注》。

卫出于下焦(wèi chū yú xià jiāo) **Defensive qi originates in the lower** *jiao*. See *Ling Shu* chapter 18. (1) Defensive qi, a part of yang qi, originates from the life gate of the lower *jiao* and its movement starts from the meridians of the kidney and bladder in the lower *jiao*. See *Lei Jing* (*Classified Classic*) " Meridians and Collaterals Chapter 23". (2) "下" should be corrected with "上" and the corrected expression should read "卫出于上焦". See *Ling Shu Ji Zhu* (*Collected Annotation of Ling Shu*).

女子胞 即子宫，属奇恒之腑。出《素问·五藏别论》。见"胞"条。

女子胞(nǚ zǐ bāo) **uterus** Meaning the uterus and belonging to the extraordinary fu-organs. See *Su Wen* chapter 11. See "胞".

飞阳 ① 足太阳膀胱经在小腿部的别络，即飞阳之脉。出《灵枢·经脉》。② 经穴名。足太阳膀胱经的络穴，在足外踝上七寸。出《素问·刺腰痛》。

飞阳 (fēi yáng) **flying yang** (1) The diverging collateral located at the calves of the bladder meridian of foot *taiyang*，namely the flying *yang* vessel. See *Ling Shu* chapter 10. (2) Acupoint name. Refers to Fei Yang（BL 58），located 7 *cun* above the ankle，on the bladder meridian of foot *taiyang*. See *Su Wen* chapter 41.

飞阳之脉 出《素问·刺腰痛》。(1) 由足太阳膀胱经飞阳穴分出，走向足少阴经之络脉，为足太阳之别络。见《类经·针刺四十九》。(2) 指阴维脉。见《素问》王冰注。

飞阳之脉(fēi yáng zhī mài) **flying yang vessel** See *Su Wen* chapter 41.（1）Refers to the collateral divergent from Fei Yang（BL 58）acupoint of the bladder meridian of foot *taiyang*，going towards the foot *shaoyin* meridian. It pertains to the divergent collateral of the foot *taiyang* meridian. See *Lei Jing*（*Classified Classic*）"Needling Chapter 49". (2) Refers to the *yinwei* meridian. See *Su Wen* annotated by Wang Bing.

马刀侠瘿 病证名。结核瘰疬之属，多生于颈项腋下。出《灵枢·经脉》。

马刀侠瘿(mǎ dāo xiá yīng) **scrofula** Disease name pertaining to tuberculosis scrofula, and usually appearing below the neck and armpits. See *Ling Shu* chapter 10.

马矢煴 燃烧而无火焰的干马粪。出《灵枢·寿夭刚柔》。

马矢煴(mǎ shǐ yūn) **dry horse dung** Dry horse dung which burns without flaming. See *Ling Shu* chapter 6.

马膏 即马脂。出《灵枢·经筋》。

马膏(mǎ gāo) **horse fat** Refers to horse fat. See *Ling Shu* chapter 13.

四 画

丰隆 经穴名。属足阳明胃经。在外踝上八寸。出《灵枢·经脉》。

丰隆（fēng lóng） **Feng Long (ST 40)** Acupoint name，belonging to the stomach meridian of foot *yangming*，and located eight *cun* above the external malleolus. See *Ling Shu* chapter 10.

王气 王，通旺。王气，亢盛之气。出《素问·至真要大论》。

王气（wáng qì） **flourishing qi** "王" is the same as "旺". Flourishing qi refers to exuberant qi. See *Su Wen* chapter 74.

王宫 又称下极。居两目之中，是面部色诊测候心的部位。心为君主之宫。故曰王宫。出《灵枢·五色》。

王宫（wáng gōng） **royal palace** Also called the deepest point，which is located in the midst of the eyes，and is the site for facial color inspection for heart disease. The heart is the monarch organ，therefore this site is called the royal palace. See *Ling Shu* chapter 49.

开鬼门 鬼门，即汗孔。开鬼门，指解表发汗的治疗方法。出《素问·汤液醪醴论》。

开鬼门（kāi guǐ mén） **to open the demon gates** Demon gates refer to sweat pores. Open the demon gates is a therapeutic method，that is used to resolve the exterior and induce sweating. See *Su Wen* chapter 14.

井 五腧穴之一。位于四肢末端，为十二经之"根"。脉气之起始。十二经各有一个井穴，对病邪在脏者，有特殊的治疗作用。出《灵枢·九针十二原》。

井（jǐng） **well** One of the five transport acupoints，located at the ends of the four limbs. They are the root of the twelve channels，and the origin of channel qi. Each of the twelve channels has a well，which is especially useful for treating disease with pathogenic qi in the viscera. See *Ling Shu* chapter 1.

井木 井，井穴，五腧穴之一。十二经均有井穴，在手足指趾端。五脏阴经的井穴在五行属木。

出《灵枢·本输》。

井木（jǐng mù）　**well wood** The well acupoint is one of the five transport acupoints. Each of the twelve channels has a well acupoint，which is located at the end of the fingers and toes. The well acupoints of the five visceral yin channels pertain to wood among the five elements. See *Ling Shu* chapter 2.

井金　井，井穴，五腧穴之一。十二经均有井穴，在手足指趾端。六腑阳经的井穴在五行属金。出《灵枢·本输》。

井金（jǐng jīn）　**well metal** The well point is one of the five transport acupoints. Each of the twelve channels has a well acupoint，which is located at the end of the fingers and toes. The well acupoints of the yang channels of the six bowels pertains to metal in the five elements. See *Ling Shu* chapter 2.

井疽　病名。发于胸窝之疽初起如豆。形容疽深脓水淋漓难尽如井。故名。后世又名穿心冷瘘、心漏疽、穿心毒等，难治。出《灵枢·病疽》。

井疽（jǐng jū）　**well-like carbuncle（heart-penetrating carbuncle）** Disease name of a carbuncle which occurs in the chest and is similar to a soy bean in its early stages. The carbuncle is deep in the muscle with dripping pus，and is also called cold heart-penetrating fistula, heart-dripping carbuncle and heart-penetrating toxin etc.，a disease difficult to cure. See *Ling Shu* chapter 81.

天之常数　天，即自然。此指自然赋予人体经脉气血的正常数量。出《素问·血气形志》。

天之常数（tiān zhī cháng shù）　**regular numbers of heaven** Heaven refers to nature，whereas regular numbers refer to the normal number of channels, collaterals, qi and blood in the body given by nature. See *Su Wen* chapter 24.

天子　指掌握自然规律的人。出《素问·宝命全形论》。

天子（tiān zǐ）　**son of heaven** Refers to the people who know well the laws of nature. See *Su Wen* chapter 25.

天井　经穴名。手少阳三焦经之合穴。在肘外大骨之后，肘尖上一寸，两筋之间陷者中。出《灵枢·本输》。

天井（tiān jǐng）　**Tian Jing (SJ 10)** Acupoint name for the *he-*

sea point of the triple *jiao* meridian of hand *shaoyang*. It is located in the indentation between the two sinews，one *cun* above the tip of the elbow，behind the massive bone at the exterior aspect of the elbow. See *Ling Shu* chapter 2.

天元 天之本原。出《素问·本病论》。

天元(tiān yuán) *tian yuan* The origin of heaven. See *Su Wen* chapter 73.

天元册 书名，即《太始天元册》。出《素问·六微旨大论》。

天元册(tiān yuán cè) *Principal Qi of Heaven* Name of the book *Principal Qi of Heaven*. See *Su Wen* chapter 68.

天元纪大论 《素问》篇名。此篇通过论述五运主岁，六气司天等一些基本法则及自然气候变化的原因和规律，揭示了自然界事物变化的根源和规律。

天元纪大论(tiān yuán jì dà lùn) **Major Discussion on the Law of Motions and Changes in Nature** Chapter title in *Su Wen*. In this chapter，some of the basic rules including "five circuits governing the year" and "six-qi governing the heaven" as well as the causes and rules of climate changes are discussed，and the origin and laws of changes in nature are revealed.

天气 ① 指司天之气。出《素问·六元正纪大论》。② 指五运。出《素问·六微旨大论》。③ 指清气。出《素问·阴阳应象大论》。④ 指六气。出《素问·六微旨大论》。

天气(tiān qì) ① Refers to qi of heaven. See *Su Wen* chapter 71. ② Refers to five circuits. See *Su Wen* chapter 68. ③ Refers to clear qi. See *Su Wen* chapter 5. ④ Refers to six kinds of qi. See *Su Wen* chapter 68.

天气通于肺 指肺主呼吸，经口鼻与自然界清气相通。出《素问·阴阳应象大论》。

天气通于肺(tiān qì tōng yú fèi) **The qi of heaven communicates with lung.** Refers to lung governing respiration，by entering through the mouth and nose，it communicates with clear qi in nature. See *Su Wen* chapter 5.

天化 言临床用药之寒热轻重多少。如气候热而症候亦热，是谓同热，则治疗须多用感受清凉的司天之气而化生的偏凉性药物，故曰天化。出《素问·六元正纪大论》。

天化(tiān huà) **Movement of qi**

that dominates the heavens. In terms of clinical practice and how drugs are used, depending on the light or heavy presence of cold and heat, more or less restraint is used. When there is agreement in terms of heat, more heaven qi is employed to cause transformation, and drugs that are cool in nature may be used. See *Su Wen* chapter 71.

天刑 运气术语。根据值年司天之气与中运的五行生克关系, 凡阳年中气克运的年份, 称为天刑之年。该年气候和病候变化特别剧烈, 六十年中庚子、庚午、庚寅、庚申、戊辰、戊戌年属天刑年。出《素问·本病论》。

天刑(tiān xíng) **heaven inhibition** Terminology of circuits and qi. According to the promoting and restraining relationship among the five elements of the current qi of heaven and the middle movement, when qi inhibits movement in a yang year, it is called a year of heaven inhibition. In this year, there are drastic changes in climate and pathology. In a sixty year period (one cycle), the years of *geng zi*, *geng wu*, *geng yin*, *geng shen*, *wu chen* and *wu xu* are years of heaven inhibition. See *Su Wen* chapter 73.

天师 黄帝对岐伯的尊称。出《素问·上古天真论》。

天师(tiān shī) **heavenly teacher** The respectful title given by Huang Di to Qi Bo. See *Su Wen* chapter 1.

天岁 指司天之气。出《素问·本病论》。

天岁(tiān suì) **qi that dominates the heavens in a year.** Refers to the qi of the heaven. See *Su Wen* chapter 73.

天年 ① 人的自然寿命, 即天寿。出《素问·上古天真论》。②《灵枢》篇名。该篇讨论了人体的生长、发育、衰老、死亡各个阶段的主要生理特点和血气之盛衰, 脏器之强弱与寿夭的关系。因文中主要围绕寿夭问题进行研究, 故名。

天年(tiān nián) ① Natural lifespan of humans, or called the life span allotted by heaven. See *Su Wen* chapter 1. ② Chapter title in *Ling Shu*. In this chapter, the main physiological features of growth, development, aging and death as well as abundance and scarcity of qi and blood are discussed, and the relationship between strength and weakness of the organs and lifespan are investigated. The chapter was given this title since it mainly discusses lifespan, thus its name.

天牝 鼻。出《素问·刺法论》。

天牝（tiān pìn） *tian pin* Nose. See *Su Wen* chapter 72.

天冲 木星位置居天时之称谓。出《素问·刺法论》。

天冲（tiān chōng） **Tian Chong** Jupiter's appellation when it dominates heaven. See *Su Wen* chapter 72.

天池 经穴名。属手厥阴心包经。在腋下三寸,乳头旁一寸。出《灵枢·本输》。

天池（tiān chí） **Tian Chi (PC 1)** Acupoint name belonging to the pericardium meridian of hand *jueyin*. It is three *cun* below the axilla and one *cun* from the nipple. See *Ling Shu* chapter 2.

天寿 指自然赋予人的寿命。出《素问·上古天真论》。

天寿（tiān shòu） **life span allotted by heaven** Natural lifespan of humans. See *Su Wen* chapter 1.

天芮 土星位置居天时之称谓。出《素问·刺法论》。

天芮（tiān ruì） **Tian Rui** Saturn's appellation when it dominates heaven. See *Su Wen* chapter 72.

天忌 即天时的宜忌。人与自然相应,四时气候的变化对人体有一定影响,因此调养身体、医治疾病都要随四时气候的变化而采取不同的方法。出《素问·八正神明论》。

天忌（tiān jì） **prohibitions of heaven** Refers to the taboos of climate. The relevance between humans and nature is that climatic changes during the four seasons influence the human body, thus health preservation and treatment of disease should be done according to the different climatic changes. See *Su Wen* chapter 26.

天忌日 人体各部位与天地八方九宫之位相应,故有相应的时日,若某部位患有痈肿,不可在其相应之时日用溃破法治疗,因其时正是该部得天时之助,正气充实之时,若使溃破,反伤正气,是为禁忌。以其日有忌于天,故称。出《灵枢·征四失论》。

天忌日（tiān jì rì） **days of heavenly prohibitions** All parts of the body are in unity with the Eight Directions and Nine Palaces of heaven and earth, therefore on some days, abscesses on any part of the body

四画

cannot be treated by bursting it, because at that particular time the body is strengthened and vital qi is in abundance. If the abscess were to be bursted, the vital qi would instead be damaged, thus bursting it at that time would be forbidden. This is called the day of heavenly prohibitions as it is in disagreement with the heaven. See *Ling Shu* chapter 78.

天纲　指天体运行的规律。出《素问·五运行大论》。

天纲（tiān gāng）　**mainstay of heaven** The law of celestial motion. See *Su Wen* chapter 67.

天英　火星位置居天时之称谓。出《素问·刺法论》。

天英（tiān yīng）　**Tian Ying** Mars' appellation when it dominates the heaven. See *Su Wen* chapter 72.

天枢　穴位名。在脐旁二寸，属足阳明胃经。出《素问·至真要大论》。

天枢（tiān shū）　**Tian Shu（ST 25）** Acupoint name, located two *cun* away from the umbilicus, and belonging to the stomach meridian of foot *yangming*. See *Su Wen* chapter 74.

天命　即天寿，人的自然寿命。

出《素问·生气通天论》。

天命（tiān mìng）　**life span allotted by heaven** Lifespan, that is the natural lifespan of humans. See *Su Wen* chapter 3.

天周　绕天一周的意思，当即指整个天地间。出《灵枢·卫气行》。

天周（tiān zhōu）　**celestial circle** Rotate around the heaven in a cycle, that is, refers to the whole universe. See *Ling Shu* chapter 76.

天府　经穴名。属手太阴肺经。在腋下三寸，臂臑内廉动脉陷中。出《灵枢·本输》。

天府（tiān fǔ）　**Tian Fu（LU 3）** Acupoint name belonging on the lung meridian of hand *taiyin*, and is located three *cun* below the axilla in the arterial depression of the brachial diaphragm. See *Ling Shu* chapter 2.

天政　司天之气发挥作用。出《素问·六元正纪大论》。

天政（tiān zhèng）　**policy of heaven** The effect of the exertion of Celestial qi. See *Su Wen* chapter 71.

天柱　① 金星位置居天时之称谓。出《素问·刺法论》。② 经穴名。属足太阳膀胱经，在挟项后发际大筋外廉凹陷中。出《素问·气穴论》。

天柱（tiān zhù） ① Venus' appellation when it dominates the heaven. See *Su Wen* chapter 72. ② Acupoint name（BL 10）belonging to the bladder meridian of foot *taiyang* and located in the depression on the neck beside the midline. See *Su Wen* chapter 58.

天度 划分天体运行的单位。古人将周天分为三百六十五度，以校正日月的运行。出《素问·六节藏象论》。

天度（tiān dù） **degrees of heaven** Unit of celestial motion. In ancient China，the universe was made of 365 degrees to determine the passage of the sun and the moon. See *Su Wen* chapter 9.

天宦 天，先天；宦，太监，即被阉割男性生殖器的内宫侍者。天宦，指先天性的男性生殖器发育不全者。主要是先天冲任之脉不充盛之缘故。出《灵枢·标本病传论》。

天宦（tiān huàn） **congenital eunuch** Congenital agenesis of the male genitalia，mainly due to congenital inadequacy of the thoroughfare vessel and the conception vessel. See *Ling Shu* chapter 65.

天宫 指九宫中的离宫。出《灵枢·九宫八风》。

天宫（tiān gōng） *tian gong* Refers to *li gong* in the Nine Palaces. See *Ling Shu* chapter 77.

天突 经穴名。属任脉，在喉结下四寸，胸骨上窝正中处。出《素问·气穴论》。

天突（tiān tū） **Tian Tu（CV 22）** Acupoint name belonging on the conception vessel and located four *cun* below the Adam's apple，right in the middle of the superior sternal fossa. See *Su Wen* chapter 58.

天癸 在肾气充盛到一定阶段产生的一种与人体生长发育及生殖机能有密切关系的物质。出《素问·上古天真论》。

天癸（tiān guǐ） *tian gui* A substance produced at a certain stage of kidney qi sufficiency and closely related to human growth，development and reproductive function. See *Su Wen* chapter 1.

天真 出《素问·上古天真论》。（1）自然纯真，质朴无邪的天性。见《素问直解》。（2）先天真元之气。见《素问集注》。

天真（tiān zhēn） **true qi endowed by heaven** See *Su Wen* chapter 1.（1）Simple and innocent na-

四画

ture. See *Su Wen Zhi Jie* (*Direct Interpretation on Su Wen*). (2) Congenital true vital qi. See *Su Wen Ji Zhu* (*Collected Annotation of Su Wen*).

天息 天,指自然。息,指呼吸。天息,人之呼吸与自然相通。出《素问·刺法论》。

天息(tiān xī) ***tian xi*** Tiān refers to the natural world. xī refers to respiration. Natural respiration, meaning that humans communicate with nature through respiration. See *Su Wen* chapter 72.

天容 经穴名。属手太阳小肠经穴名。在耳下曲颊后。出《灵枢·本输》。

天容(tiān róng) **Tian Rong (SI 17)** Acupoint name, belonging to the small intestine meridian of hand *taiyang*, and located below the ear behind the angle of the jaw. See *Ling Shu* chapter 2.

天符 运气术语。凡是值年中运与司天之气的五行属性相同之年,称为天符。六十年中己丑、己未、戊寅、戊申、戊子、戊午、乙卯、乙酉、丁巳、丁亥、丙辰、丙戌十二年为天符年。如乙酉年,乙年为金运,酉年阳明燥金司天,中运和司天之气均属金,运和气相同,即是天符。出《素问·天元纪大论》。

天符(tiān fú) ***tian fu* (heavenly complements)** Terminology of circuits and qi. Heavenly complements refer to the years when the attributes of the five elements of the middle movement are the same with that of the qi of heaven. In sixty years (one cycle), the twelve years of *ji chou*, *ji wei*, *wu yin*, *wu shen*, *wu zi*, *wu wu*, *yi mao*, *yi you*, *ding si*, *ding hai*, *bing chen*, and *bing xu* are years of heaven complements. For instance, in the year of *yi you*, the year of *yi* has metal movement, the year of *you* has *yangming* metal in heaven, and both the middle movement and the qi of heaven correspond to metal in the five elements, thus this would be a year of tian fu (heavenly complement). See *Su Wen* chapter 66.

天窗 经穴名。属手太阳小肠经。别名窗笼。在曲颊下扶突后,动脉应手陷者中。出《素问·气穴论》。

天窗(tiān chuāng) **Tian Chuang (SI 16)** Acupoint name belonging to the small intestine meridian of hand *taiyang*, and located below the angle of the jaw behind the acupoint Fu Tu (LI 18) at the arterial depression. It is also called Chuang Long (SI 19). See *Su Wen* chapter 58.

天蓬　水星位置居天时之称谓。出《素问·刺法论》。

天蓬（tiān péng）　**Tian Peng** Mercury's appellation when it dominates the heaven. See *Su Wen* chapter 72.

天数　① 即天寿,人的自然寿数。出《素问·上古天真论》。② 六气交司的时刻。出《素问·六微旨大论》。③ 指司天之气。出《素问·本病论》。

天数（tiān shù）　① The lifespan allotted by heaven, refers to the natural lifespan of humans. See *Su Wen* chapter 1. ② The moment when two of the six qi connect. See *Su Wen* chapter 68. ③ Refers to Celestial qi. See *Su Wen* chapter 73.

天牖　经穴名。属手少阳三焦经,在乳突后下方,胸锁乳突肌后缘,约平下颌角处。出《素问·气穴论》。

天牖（tiān yǒu）　**Tian You**（TE 16）Acupoint name, belonging to the triple *jiao* meridian of hand *shaoyang*, and located

posteriorly and inferiorly to the mastoid process, at the posterior margin of the sternocleidomastoid muscle, at approximately the same level as the mandibular angle. See *Su Wen* chapter 58.

夫子　对老师的尊称。这里指岐伯。出《素问·离合真邪论》。

夫子（fū zǐ）　**Sir** Respectful term for teachers, and here refers to Qi Bo. See *Su Wen* chapter 27.

云门　经穴名。属手太阴肺经,在巨骨下,气户两旁各 2 寸陷者中。出《素问·水热穴论》。

云门（yún mén）　**Yun Men**（LU 2）An acupoint on the lung meridian of hand *taiyin* located in the indentation two *cun* from each side of Qi Hu (ST 13) below Ju Gu（LI 16）acupoint. See *Su Wen* chapter 61.

专阴　专,独的意思。专阴,即独阴无阳。出《素问·阴阳类论》。

专阴（zhuān yīn）　**only yin** *Zhuān* refers to only, unique. Thus, yin only with no yang. See *Su Wen* chapter 79.

木　五行之一。由自然界"草木"抽象而来。其特性是曲直,即树木的生长形态,是枝干曲直,向上向外舒展,引申为具有生长、升发、条达舒畅等作用性质的事物。根据五行归类的方法,归属于木的,在五脏为肝,在气候为风,在季节为春,在方位为东,在五味为酸,在五色为青等。出《素问·阴阳应象大论》。

木(mù)　**wood** One of the five elements. It is derived from grass and trees in nature. It has the characteristics of being curved or straight, refers to the growth pattern of trees that stretch up and out. Thus wood is used to indicate all things that grow, ascend and stretch. According to the categorization of the five elements, anything that corresponds to wood pertains to the liver in the five viscera, wind in climates, spring in seasons, east in directions, sourness in tastes, and green in colors. See *Su Wen* chapter 5.

木曰发生　木运太过曰发生,是木气有余,未至其时而生长发育。出《素问·五常政大论》。

木曰发生(mù yuē fā shēng)　**Wood is known as growth in advance.** Excessive wood movement leads to effusive generation, which means that abundant wood qi causes growth and development before its due time.

See *Su Wen* chapter 70.

木曰委和　木运不及曰委和。木气不足,不能敷布阳和,则生发之机萎弱不和,故称。出《素问·五常政大论》。

木曰委和(mù yuē wěi hé)　**Wood is known as loss of harmony.** Weak wood circuit leads to discarded harmony as insufficient wood qi cannot spread yang harmony, leading to a loss of harmony in germinal power. See *Su Wen* chapter 70.

木曰敷和　木运平和曰敷和。以能敷布阳和而生万物,故称。出《素问·五常政大论》。

木曰敷和(mù yuē fū hé)　**Wood is known as distribution and harmony.** Placid wood movement is called extended harmony, and occurs when yang harmony is spread so as to engender all things. See *Su Wen* chapter 70.

木气　运气学说的六气之一,为厥阴风木所主之气。出《素问·六微旨大论》。

木气(mù qì)　**wood qi** One of the six qi in the circuits and qi theory, which is governed by *jueyin* wind-wood. See *Su Wen* chapter 68.

木形之人　体质名,又称上角,阴阳二十五人之一。出《灵枢·

阴阳二十五人》。木形之人在五音属角，角音之中有正、偏、太、少的区别，分为上角，大角，左角，钛角，判角，以此类比木形人中的五种体质类型。上角得木气之全者，大角、左角、钛角、判角得木气之偏者，故上角之人为标准木形人，其体形多头小，面长，两肩广阔，背部挺直，身体小弱，手足灵活，肤青。其禀性是：有才能，常劳心，体力不强，多忧善虑，做事勤劳。该体质大多能耐于春夏，不耐于秋冬，故秋冬易生病。

木形之人（mù xíng zhī rén）
people pertaining to the wood element Name of constitution, and also called upper *jue*. It is one of the twenty-five types of people divided according to yin and yang. See *Ling Shu* chapter 64. People of wood constitution pertain to the *jue* tone in the five tones, and are classified into positive, partial, more and lesser *jue*, including upper *jue*, *da jue*, *zuo jue*, *di jue and pan jue* in order to illustrate the five types of body constitutions pertaining to people of wood constitution. People of upper *jue* have complete wood qi, and those of *da jue*, *zuo jue*, *di jue* and *pan jue* have partial wood qi, therefore those of *shang jue* are the standard people of wood constitution. These people tend to have a small head, long face, broad shoulders, straight back, small and weak trunk, agile hands and feet, and greenish skin. They are talented people that work with their minds, have poor physical strength, worry a lot and are hardworking. They mostly tolerate the spring and summer weather, but cannot tolerate the weather in autumn and winter, and thus tend to get ill in the latter.

木运　五运之一。根据天干化五运之理，凡逢丁、逢壬的年时，由木运主事。其时，气候偏湿，多风，风湿之气流行；物候表现为万物开始萌芽生发，一派生机勃勃之景象。疾病多见伤肝的症候。出《素问·天元纪大论》。

木运（mù yùn）　**wood movement** One of the five circuits. According to the theory that the Heavenly Stems transform the five circuits, the wood movement predominates in the years of *ding* and *ren* when the climate is wet, there is much wind, and qi of wind and dampness prevails. All things start to grow and there is a scene of vitality. In most cases of disease, the liver is damaged. See *Su Wen* chapter 66.

木郁　木运之气被郁遏。运气学说中，按五行相克规律，由于一方太盛或所克一方太弱而使受克一方被抑制，不能正常发挥作用的现象，称为郁。五行中，金能克木，若金太过或木不及时则会发生金偏旺而使木气被郁。出《素问·六元正纪大论》。

木郁（mù yù）　**stagnation of wood** The qi of wood circuit is oppressed. In the circuits and qi theory, according to the rule of restrain of the five elements, the inhibited element is oppressed if the inhibiting element is too strong, or the inhibited element is too weak to function normally. In the five elements, metal restrains wood, and if metal is too strong or wood is too weak, wood qi will be oppressed. See *Su Wen* chapter 71.

木郁达之　木郁，即木气被郁。从自然气候变化言，春应温而反凉，春应生而不生；从人体言，肝气失于疏泄，气血郁结不畅，皆称为"木郁"。达，即通条

畅达。凡木气抑郁为病，应当治之以疏通条达。出《素问·六元正纪大论》。

木郁达之（mù yù dá zhī）　**When wood [qi] is oppressed, unblock it.** Wood oppression, refers to wood qi being oppressed. According to climate changes in nature, spring should be warm and engendering all things. However, when wood qi is oppressed, the climate is cool and things are not engendered as they should in this season. As for the human body, liver qi does not function normally, leading to the obstructed flow of qi and blood. Dá refers to regulate and disperse qi. To treat diseases due to oppressed wood qi, the oppression should be unblocked and the qi dispersed. See *Su Wen* chapter 71.

五十九刺　指治疗热病的五十九穴。出《灵枢·热病》。其所载与《素问·水热穴论》"热病五十九俞"不同。

五十九刺（wǔ shí jiǔ cì）　**fifty-nine piercings** Refers to the fifty-nine acupoints for treating febrile disease. See *Ling Shu* chapter 23. These points are different from the "fifty-nine transporters" in *Su Wen* chapter 61.

五十营　《灵枢》篇名。营：营运、运周。此篇主要讨论经脉元气在人体内循环营运一昼夜为五十周次的道理。故名。

五十营（wǔ shí yíng）　**Fifty Ying** Chapter title in *Ling Shu*. Yíng refers to transport and circulate. In this chapter，there is a discussion of how the original qi in the channels circulates in the body for fifty cycles，thus its name.

五入　入，归走之意。饮食五味入胃后，各归走其所相应之脏腑。出《素问·宣明五气》。

五入（wǔ rù）　**five entries** *Rù* refers to entry，or going into. Foods of the five flavors go into the stomach and enter the corresponding viscera and bowels. See *Su Wen* chapter 23.

五久劳　同"五劳"。出《灵枢·九针论》。

五久劳（wǔ jiǔ láo）　**five exhaustions** As the same as"五劳". See *Ling Shu* chapter 78.

五尸鬼　指木、火、土、金、水五种疫邪。出《素问·本病论》。

五尸鬼（wǔ shī guǐ）　**five cadaveric ghosts** The five epidemic evils of wood，fire，earth，metal

and water. See *Su Wen* chapter 73.

五中　指五脏。出《素问·方盛衰论》。

五中（wǔ zhōng）　**five insides** Refers to the five viscera. See *Su Wen* chapter 80.

五气　① 五脏之气。出《素问·阴阳应象大论》。② 五运之气。出《素问·六节藏象论》。③ 臊、焦、香、腥、腐。出《素问·五藏别论》。④ （脾）土之气。出《素问·奇病论》。⑤ 五脏逆气。出《素问·宣明五气》。⑥ 应作天气，即司天之气。出《素问·六元正纪大论》。

五气（wǔ qì）　① Qi of the five viscera. See *Su Wen* chapter 5. ② Qi of the five circuits. See *Su Wen* chapter 9. ③ The smells of urine，burnt，fragrant，fishy and rotten. See *Su Wen* chapter 11. ④ Qi of the （spleen）earth. See *Su Wen* chapter 47. ⑤ Inverse qi of the five viscera. See *Su Wen* chapter 23. ⑥ It should be the qi of heaven，namely Celestial qi. See *Su Wen* chapter 71.

五气之发　指木、火、土、金、水五气，受所不胜之气的克制达到一定限度，郁极而发。出《素问·六元正纪大论》。

五气之发（wǔ qì zhī fā）　**outbreak of the five qi** Refers to within the five qi of wood，fire，earth，metal and water，one qi breaks out when it is restrained to an extreme degree by its un-restricted qi. See *Su Wen* chapter 71.

五气更立　五气，指木、火、土、金、水五运之气。更立，更迭主时。五运之气更迭主时，互有胜克，从而有盛衰的变化。出《素问·六节藏象论》。

五气更立（wǔ qì gēng lì）　**Five qi take their positions one after another.** The five qi refers to the qi of the five circuits of wood，fire，earth，metal and water. *Gēng lì*，refers to that each of the five qi dominates a season one after another. They restrict and are restricted，resulting in changes between periods of abundance and depletion. See *Su Wen* chapter 9.

五风　八风邪气入侵五脏之经而发之病证。出《素问·金匮真言论》。

五风（wǔ fēng）　**five winds** The disease which is caused by the pathogenic qi of the eight winds invading the channels of the five viscera. See *Su Wen* chapter 4.

五火　五脏偏亢的阳气。出《素问·解精微论》。

五火（wǔ huǒ）　**five fires** Yang qi that is too exuberant in the five viscera. See *Su Wen* chapter 81.

五节　① 指振埃、发蒙、去爪、彻衣、解惑五种针刺方法。出《灵枢·刺节真邪》。② 指五时。出《灵枢·本藏》。

五节（wǔ jié）　① Five types of acupuncture methods，referred to as shaking off dust，redeeming out of ignorance，trimming the finger or toe or nails，undressing and resolving the doubts. See *Ling Shu* chapter 75. ② Five phases corresponding to the four seasons. See *Ling Shu* chapter 47.

五主　主，主持、掌握之意。五脏之所主。即心主脉，肺主皮，肝主筋，脾主肉，肾主骨。出《素问·宣明五气》。

五主（wǔ zhǔ）　**five governances** *Zhǔ* means to govern，or dominate，which is the governance of the body parts by the five viscera. The following are the body parts governed by the five viscera：The heart governs the channels；the lung governs the skin; the liver governs the sinews; the spleen governs the muscles; and the kidney governs the bones. See *Su Wen* chapter 23.

五发 又名"五病所发"。见《素问·宣明五气》《灵枢·九针论》。

五发(wǔ fā) **five outbreaks** Also called the outbreak of five kinds of diseases. See *Su Wen* chapter 23. See *Ling Shu* chapter 78.

五过 ① 指针刺补泻过度。出《灵枢·五禁》。② 指诊治疾病时医生易犯的五种过错。内容包括不了解病人社会生活的变迁,贵贱贫富的变化,饮食居处的优劣,精神状态的好坏以及疾病的始末过程等。出《素问·疏五过论》。

五过(wǔ guò) ① Refers to excessive supplementing or draining while needling in acupuncture. See *Ling Shu* chapter 61. ② Refers to the five kinds of mistakes doctors are prone to make in diagnosing and treating diseases, as doctors are not aware of the ups and downs in the patients' social life, the changes in social status and wealth, the good and the bad of the patient's diet and dwelling conditions, the patient's mental state and the whole course of the disease. See *Su Wen* chapter 77.

五夺 夺,失去,耗损。五夺指脱形肉,亡血,大汗亡阳,大泄亡阴,产后暴崩等五种元气大虚的病情。凡遇此五种情况,针刺不能用泻法。出《灵枢·五禁》。

五夺(wǔ duó) **five pillages** *Duó* refers to depletion, or exhaustion. The five pillages refer to the five conditions of insufficient vital qi triggering disease, namely pillages of flesh, blood, sweat or yang, fluid or yin, and postpartum collapse. These five conditions cannot be treated using the drainage method in acupuncture. See *Ling Shu* chapter 61.

五邪 ① 邪入于人体阴阳的五种病状。出《灵枢·九针论》。② 五种邪气,即痈邪,盛大之邪,微弱之邪,热邪,寒邪,合称五邪。出《灵枢·刺节真邪》。③ 邪气侵入五脏所致的病证。出《灵枢·五邪》。邪气在肺,皮肤疼痛,恶寒发热,咳喘引肩背痛,汗出;邪气在肝,两胁作痛,筋脉抽掣,木旺土虚,则中焦虚寒;邪气在脾,肌肉痛,热中,善饥,或寒中,肠鸣腹痛;邪气在肾,骨痛,阴痹,腹胀,腰痛,肩背颈项强痛,时眩,大便难;邪气在心,心痛喜悲,时眩仆。④《灵枢》篇名。该篇主要论述邪气入侵五脏所引起的病证及治疗时应取的经穴。⑤ 五种邪脉。出《素问·宣明五气》。

五邪（wǔ xié） ① Five conditions of disease when evil qi enters the yin and yang of the body. See *Ling Shu* chapter 78. ② The five evil qi, namely, obstruction-illnesses evil, the evil qi in large quantities, the evil qi in minimal quantities, heat qi and cold qi. See *Ling Shu* chapter 75. ③ Diseases and syndromes caused by the invasion of evil qi into the five viscera. See *Ling Shu* chapter 20. With evil qi in the lung, there are skin pains, chills and fever, cough and asthma leading to pains in the shoulders and back, and sweating; with evil qi in the liver, there are aches in the two flanks and twitching in muscles and sinews, as well as deficiency cold of the middle *jiao* when the wood is flourishing and the soil is deficient; with evil qi in the spleen, there are muscle pains, heat strokes, rapid hungering, or cold stroke, bowel tingling and abdominal pains; with evil qi in the kidney, there are bone pains, yin impediment, abdominal distention, low back pains, strong pains in the shoulders, back and neck, dizziness now and then, and difficulty in defecation; with evil qi in the heart, there are heartaches, sorrow, and vertigo now and then. ④ Chapter title in *Ling Shu*. In this chapter, the diseases and syndromes due to the invasion of evil qi into the five viscera, and points in the channels for treatment are discussed. ⑤ Five evil pulse conditions. See *Su Wen* chapter 23.

五行 ① 指金、木、水、火、土五种物质。出《素问·藏气法时论》。古代哲学家在朴素的唯物论和自发的辩证法思想指导下,认为自然界万物都是由上述五种物质构成的,并以五行生克制化的原理,来说明事物在运动变化过程中的相互关系,形成了五行学说。五行学说运用于医学,作为阐述人体生理、病理、诊断、治疗各个方面的理论工具,尤其是结合阴阳学说,创立了以"四时五脏阴阳"理论为核心的外应五时、五气,内系五脏(六腑)、五体、五官、五华等以五脏为主体的功能活动系统,奠定了中医学理论的基础。② 指五运。出《素问·五运行大论》。

五行(wǔ xíng)　① Refers to the five substances of metal, wood, water, fire and earth. See *Su Wen* chapter 22. Under the guidance of simple materialism and spontaneous dialectics, ancient philosophers believed that all things in nature were composed of the above five kinds of substances, and explained the mutual relationship of things in the process of movement and change by the principle of engendering and restraining of the five elements, forming the five elements theory. The five elements theory is applied in medicine as a theoretical tool to expound human physiology, pathology, diagnosis and treatment, especially in combination with the theory of yin and yang. It has established a functional activity system with the five viscera as the main body, corresponding to the five seasons and five qi outside the body and connected to the five viscera (six bowels), five body constituents, five sense organs and five outward manifestations inside the body, which takes the theory of "four seasons, five viscera, yin and yang" as its core and lays the foundation for other theories in traditional Chinese medicine. ② Refers to the five circuits. See *Su Wen* chapter 67.

五色　① 即青、赤、黄、白、黑五种颜色。或泛指人体面部的色泽。出《灵枢·五色》。古人认为不同的色泽,反映不同性质的病变,如"青黑为痛,黄赤为热,白为寒"。而五色与五脏是以五行关系相配合的,即心主赤、肝主青、脾主黄、肺主白、肾主黑。人体脏腑肢节在面部各有具体的分属部位。所以中医可以通过色诊来诊断疾病、判断生死。②《内经》引用的古医籍名,已佚。③《灵枢》篇名,篇内专论颜面部五色的变化与脏腑之间的相应关系。故名。

五色(wǔ sè)　① The five colors, namely green, red, yellow, white and black, or the facial complexion of humans. See *Ling Shu* chapter 49. The ancient Chinese believed that different colors reflected different pathological changes, such as "green and black for pain, yellow and red for heat, and white for cold". The five colors and five viscera are coordinated by the five elements, namely, the heart corresponds to red, liver to green, spleen to yellow, lung to white and kidney to black. There are specific parts of the body's viscera and limbs in the face, so in traditional Chinese medicine, diagnosis and prognosis of disease can be clarified through the examination of the complexion. ② An ancient medical book lost in history that was quoted in *Nei Jing* (*Internal Classic*). ③ Chapter title in *Ling Shu*. In this chapter, changes of facial complexions and their relationship with the viscera and bowels are discussed, thus its name.

五色各有藏部　青黑为痛,黄赤为热,白为寒,青、黄、赤、白、黑五色各有所主之病。五脏六腑在面部亦有相应的部位,如五脏次于中央,六腑挟其两侧。诊察这些部位的色泽,可以判断五脏六腑的病变。出《灵枢·五色》。

五色各有藏部（wǔ sè gè yǒu zàng bù）　**Each of the five complexions has its specific location where one of the viscera reveals its condition.** Green and black stands for pain, yellow and red for heat and white for cold. Each of the five colors, i.e. green, yellow, red, white and black, indicates a specific disease. Five viscera and six bowels also have their corresponding parts on the face, that is, the five viscera are located inferior to the center, and the six bowels are located at both sides of the face. Examining the color of these parts helps to judge the pathological changes of the five viscera and six bowels. See *Ling Shu* chapter 49.

五色命藏　以体表五色之诊命名其五脏之病。出《灵枢·五色》。

五色命藏（wǔ sè mìng zàng）　**Five complexions serve to identify the viscera.** Diseases of the five viscera are named by examining the five colors on the surface of the body. See *Ling Shu* chapter 49.

五决　即五脉,为五脏之脉,如心脉钩,肺脉毛,肝脉弦,脾脉代,肾脉石。出《素问·五藏生成》。

五决（wǔ jué）　**five decisive criteria** The five pulses or the pulses of the five viscera，that is，the heart pulse as *gou* (strong or hook-like)；the lung pulse as *mao*（mild）；the liver pulse as *xian*（taut or wiry）；the spleen pulse as *dai*（slow irregular and intermittent）；and the kidney pulse as *shi* (deep or sinking). See *Su Wen* chapter 10.

五并　并，合并，聚合之意。指五脏精气相乘，偏盛于一脏为病，可出现情志异常变化。出《素问·宣明五气》。

五并（wǔ bìng）　**five accumulations** *Bìng* refers to accumulation, or combination. In the over-restriction of essence qi of the five viscera，abnormal exuberance of essence qi of one viscera leads to disease，causing abnormal changes of emotions. See *Su Wen* chapter 23.

五阳　出《素问·汤液醪醴论》。(1) 五脏之阳气。见《素问》王冰注。(2) 五脏之胃气。见《类经·论治十五》。

五阳（wǔ yáng）　**five yang** See *Su Wen* chapter 14. (1) Yang qi of the five viscera. See *Su Wen* annotated by Wang Bing. (2) Stomach qi of the five viscera. See *Lei Jing*（*Classified Classic*）"On Treatment Chapter 15".

五阴　五脏之精气。出《灵枢·经脉》。

五阴（wǔ yīn）　**five yin** Essence qi of the five viscera. See *Ling Shu* chapter 10.

五形　即五形之人。出《灵枢·阴阳二十五人》。

五形（wǔ xíng）　**five physical appearances** Five constitution types of people. See *Ling Shu* chapter 64.

五形之人　体质分类名。古人按五行学说，结合人体肤色、体形、禀性以及对自然界变化的适应能力等方面的特征，归纳总结出五种不同的体质类型，即金型之人、木型之人、水型之人、火型之人、土型之人。出《灵枢·阴阳二十五人》。

五形之人（wǔ xíng zhī rén）　**five types of people** Categorization of body constitution. According to the theory of the five elements，the ancients in China summed up five different types of constitutions according to the characteristics of human skin color，body shape，tem-

四画

perament and adaptability to changes of nature, including metal, wood, water, fire and earth type people. See *Ling Shu* chapter 64.

五形志　形,形体;志,指精神情志。五形志,指因形体、情志苦乐不同而产生的五种病变情况。出《素问·血气形志》。

五形志(wǔ xíng zhì)　**Five combinations of physical and mental appearances** *Xíng* refers to the body's constitution. *Zhì* refers to the mind and spirit. Thus five combinations of physical and mental appearances refers to five kinds of pathological changes caused by various physical and mental appearances. See *Su Wen* chapter 24.

五运　运气术语。即木运、火运、土运、金运、水运。是木、火、土、金、水五方五行之气的运动。其以五行配天干,如土主甲乙,金主乙庚,水主丙辛,木主丁壬,火主戊癸,以推演逐年季节的气候变化。既用以说明形成气候变化的地面因素,也用以解释宇宙运动的变化规律,又有大运(中运、岁运)、主运、客运之分。大运:统主一岁全年之运气,因其以一运统治一年,也称"岁运"。又因其居

天地上下升降运动之中,亦称中运。主运:是五运之气,分别主治一年五时的正常气候变化,每运主一时,依五行相生的顺序,始于木运,终于水运,年年不变。客运:与主运相对而言。因其十年内年年不同,如客之来去,故称。客运虽同主运一样,以五运分主一年之五时,且亦依循五行太少相生的顺序,分作五步推运,但其是随每年的大运而变,以中运为初运,逐年变迁,十年一周期,而不同于主运的初木,二火,三土,四金,终水年年不变。见"五运客运图"。出《素问·天元纪大论》。

五运(wǔ yùn)　**five circuits** Terminology of circuits and qi, and the five circuits including the circuits of wood, fire, earth, metal and water. These are the circuits and qi of the five elements. In relation of the five elements to the Heavenly Stems, earth corresponds to *jia* and *yi*, metal to *yi* and *geng*, water to *bing* and *xin*, wood to *ding* and *ren*, and fire to *wu* and *gui*, so as to deduce the seasonal climatic changes year by year. This can be used to explain the ground factors that cause climatic changes, and also to explain the changing laws of the universe's movement. It can be divided into overall circuit (central circuit or annual circuit), host circuit, and guest circuit. Overall circuit dominates the circuit of qi in the whole year, and also called annual circuit. It is in the center of ascending and descending circuit of the universe, hence also called central circuit. Host circuit refers to the qi of the five elements, governing normal climatic changes in the five seasons of the year. Each circuit dominates a season in the order of the generation of the five elements, starting from the wood circuit and ending in the water circuit, and this order is unchanged year by year. In contrast, the guest circuit is different year by year in the period of a decade, just like a guest coming and going. As is the case with the host circuit, for the guest circuit, each of the five circuits govern one of the five seasons and the circuits are deduced in five steps in the order of generation. However, guest circuit changes with the overall circuit of each year, with the central circuit as the primary circuit, and change annually in cycles of ten years. This is different from that of the host circuit, in which the order of first wood, second fire, third earth, fourth metal and fifth water remains the same year by year. Refer to "diagrams of host and guest circuits" below. See *Su Wen* chapter 66.

五运六气 五运，是指木、火、土、金、水五行五方之气的运动，它既是用以说明形成气候变化的地面因素，同时也是古代用以解释宇宙运动规律的一个哲学概念。六气，是指风、寒、暑、湿、燥、火六种气候变化要素。五运六气作为一种学说，是以五行、六气，三阴三阳等理论为基础，运用天干、地支等作为演绎工具符号，来推论气候变化、生物的生化和疾病流行规律，是我国古代的医学气象学。即它是以自然界的气候变化，以及生物体对这些变化所产生的相应反映作为基础，从而把自然气候现象和生物的生命现象统一起来，把自然气候变化和人体发病规律统一起来，从宇宙的节律上来探讨气象变化对人体健康与疾病发生的关系。出《素问·六元正纪大论》。

五运六气（wǔ yùn liù qì）　**five circuits and six qi** The five circuits refer to the circuits and qi of the five elements, such as wood, fire, earth, metal and water. The term "five circuits" is not only a ground factor to explain the formation of climatic changes, but also a philosophical concept to explain the laws of the universe's circuits in ancient times. Six qi refers to the six elements of climatic change: wind, cold, summerheat, dampness, dryness and fire. The five circuits and six qi theory is based on the theories of the five elements, six qi, three yin and three yang, using the Heavenly Stems and Earthly Branches as deductive tool symbols to infer the patterns of climate change, engenderment and transformation of living creatures as well as disease prevalence, hence the existence of medical meteorology in ancient China. It is based on climatic changes in nature and the corresponding response of organisms to these changes, so as to unify the natural climatic phenomenon and the biological life phenomenon, the natural climatic changes and the patterns of disease occurrence, and explore the relationship between meteorological changes and human health and disease by considering the rhythm of the universe. See *Su Wen* chapter 71.

五运行大论　《素问》篇名。五运行,指天之五气、地之五行的变化运行。该篇主要论述五行六气的变化运行规律及其对人体及万物生化的影响。

五运行大论（wǔ yùn xíng dà lùn）　**Major Discussion on the Changes of the Five Circuits** Chapter title in *Su Wen*. The five movements refer to the changes in circuits of the five qi of heaven, and the five circuits of earth. In this chapter, patterns of changes and movements of the five elements and the six qi, as well as their impact on engenderment and transformation of the human body and all things, are discussed.

五运相袭　运气术语。袭,承袭。五运所立之年时,随五行之相生相互承袭而轮转,往来不息。

出《素问·六节藏象论》。

五运相袭(wǔ yùn xiāng xí) **five periods succeed each other** A term of circuits and qi. *Xí* refers to following in an orderly manner. In periods of one year governed by the five circuits, the five periods succeed each other in the order of generation of the five elements. See *Su Wen* chapter 9.

五走 五，食物或药物之五种性味。走，归向。言五味入胃后，按其属性各有不同走向，此为五味理论，即后世药物归经的理论之滥觞。出《灵枢·九针论》《灵枢·五味》。

五走(wǔ zǒu) **five accesses** *Wǔ* here means the five flavors of food or medicine. *Zǒu* here means to proceed to. When medicines of the five flavors enter the stomach, they proceed to different directions according to their attributes. This is the origin of the theory of five flavors and the theory of channel tropism in later generations. See *Ling Shu* chapter 78 and *Ling Shu* chapter 56.

五声 泛指人发出的各种声调。出《素问·针解》。

五声(wǔ shēng) **five pitches of voice** General refers to various voice pitches made by people. See *Su Wen* chapter 54.

五劳 即五劳所伤：久视伤血，久卧伤气，久坐伤肉，久立伤骨，久行伤筋。其中久立、久行、久视则是过劳，久卧、久坐是过逸。过劳与过逸均是影响人体产生疾病的因素。出《素问·宣明五气》《灵枢·九针论》。

五劳(wǔ láo) **five exhaustions** Injuries due to the five exhaustions：Straining the eyes for a long time impairs the blood；sleeping for a long time impairs qi；sitting for a long time impairs the muscles；standing for a long time impairs the bones；and walking for a long time impairs the sinews. Among them, standing, walking and straining the eyes for a long time are excessive laboring, while sleeping and sitting for a long time are inadequacy. Overstain and indulgence in easy life are both pathogenic factors. See *Su Wen* chapter 23 and *Ling Shu* chapter 78.

五时 指春、夏、长夏、秋、冬五季。出《灵枢·经别》。

五时(wǔ shí) **five seasons** Refers to spring, summer, late sum-

四画

mer, autumn and winter. See *Ling Shu* chapter 11.

五里 ① 经穴名。今称手五里，属手阳明大肠经。在曲池穴直上三寸处。出《灵枢·本输》。② 里，通"理"。即五方五行之理。出《素问·阴阳应象大论》。

五里（wǔ lǐ） ① Wu Li（LI 13） acupoint, called Shou Wu Li nowadays, belongs to the large intestine meridian of hand *yangming*. It is located three *cun* above Qu Chi（LI 11）. See *Ling Shu* chapter 2. ② 里 is the same as 理. Namely, the arrangements of the five directions and the five elements. See *Su Wen* chapter 5.

五乱 ① 即"五邪所乱"。邪犯五脏引起阴阳气血逆乱的五种病证。出《素问·宣明五气》。② 邪气伤犯心、肺、肠胃、臂胫、头所发生的五种病证。出《灵枢·五乱》。③《灵枢》篇名。该篇主要讨论了五种气机逆乱的病证及治疗。

五乱（wǔ luàn） ① Disorders caused by the five evil qi, or the five kinds of diseases and syndromes due to chaotic counterflow of yin, yang, qi and blood caused by the invasion of evil qi into the five viscera. See *Su Wen* chapter 23. ② Five kinds of diseases and syndromes due to the invasion of evil qi into the heart, lung, intestines, stomach, arms, legs, and head. See *Ling Shu* chapter 34. ③ Chapter title in *Ling Shu*. In this chapter, diseases and syndromes caused by disordered circuits and qi are discussed and the treatment is explored.

五兵 指五种兵器。出《灵枢·玉版》。

五兵（wǔ bīng） **five weapons** Refers to five kinds of weapons in ancient times. See *Ling Shu* chapter 60.

五体 ① 五种体质类型的人。出《灵枢·根结》。②《素问·阴阳应象大论》有"在体为筋""在体为脉""在体为肉""在体为皮毛""在体为骨"的记载，后世将皮、肉、筋、骨、脉合称五体。

五体（wǔ tǐ） ① Classification of five body constitutions among people. See *Ling Shu* chapter 5. ② Five body parts. In *Su Wen* chapter 5, refers to the five elements, "in the body it（wood）is the sinews", "in the body it（fire）is the vessels", "in the body it（earth）is the flesh", "in the body it（metal） is the skin and its hair" and "in the body it (water) is the bones". The skin, flesh, muscle, bone and meridian are called five constituents by the later generations.

五位　即东南西北中五方之位。出《素问·天元纪大论》。

五位（wǔ wèi）　**five positions** The five positions, namely the east, south, west, north and center. See *Su Wen* chapter 66.

五谷　五种谷物。具体所指不一。① 秔米、麻、大豆、麦、黄黍。出《灵枢·五味》。② 粳米、小豆、麦、大豆、黄黍。出《素问·藏气法时论》。③ 麦、黍、稷、稻、豆。出《素问·金匮真言论》。④ 泛指饮食物。出《灵枢·本输》。

五谷（wǔ gǔ）　**five grains** Five types of grains of different species. ① Non-glutinous rice, sesame, large beans, wheat and yellow millet. See *Ling Shu* chapter 56. ② Non-glutinous rice, red beans, wheat, soy beans and yellow millet. See *Su Wen* chapter 22. ③ Wheat, glutinous millet, paniceled millet, rice and beans. See *Su Wen* chapter 4. ④ Generally refers to food in general. See *Ling Shu* chapter 2.

五谷之府　指胃。胃为水谷之海，受纳五谷，故称。府，聚物之处。出《灵枢·本输》。

五谷之府（wǔ gǔ zhī fǔ）　**repository of five grains** Refers to the stomach, which is the reservoir of water and grains and receives the five grains, thus its name. *Fǔ* is the site where things accumulate. See *Ling Shu* chapter 2.

五诊　五脏病的外在征象。出《素问·方盛衰论》。

五诊（wǔ zhěn）　**five diagnostic indicators** The outer signs of disease of the five viscera. See *Su Wen* chapter 80.

五态之人　体质名。为太阴之人，少阴之人，太阳之人，少阳之人，阴阳和平之人的合称。又称"五人"。其中太阴之人多阴而无阳，少阴之人多阴少阳，太阳之人多阳无阴，少阳之人多阳少阴，阴阳和平之人阴阳平和，提示临床应视人五态气血筋骨的差异而治之。出《灵枢·通天》。

五态之人（wǔ tài zhī rén）　**five types of people** Name of constitution. The general term for people of *taiyin* type, people of *shaoyin* type, people of *taiyang* type, people of *shaoy-*

四画

ang type and people of balanced yin and yang type. Among them, the people of *taiyin* type are characterized by superabundance of yin and absence of yang, those of *shaoyin* type by superabundant yin and scanty yang, those of *taiyang* type by excessive yang and no yin, those of *shaoyang* type by excessive yang and lesser yin, and those of balanced yin and yang type by harmony between yin and yang, suggesting that in clinical practice, disease should be treated by considering the differences in physical build, qi, blood, muscles, sinews and bones. See *Ling Shu* chapter 72.

五味 ① 即酸、苦、甘、辛、咸,泛指饮食物。出《素问·五藏别论》。②《灵枢》篇名。此篇主要论述五味与五脏在生理、病理上的相互关系,强调了五味入胃,须经胃气的作用,才能成为营气、卫气、宗气,故名。

五味(wǔ wèi) ① Sour, bitter, sweet, acrid or pungent and salty flavors. Refers to food in general. See *Su Wen* chapter 11. ② Chapter title in *Ling Shu*. In this chapter, the relationship between the five flavors and the five viscera physiologically and pathologically is discussed, paying attention to the fact that food of the five flavors enters the stomach and can only engender the nutrient qi, defensive qi and pectoral qi with the help of the stomach qi, thus its name.

五味各走其所喜 根据五行之理,药、食物各有酸、苦、甘、辛、咸五种性味,摄入后,各有其选择性的归属。如酸味先归于肝,苦味先归于心,甘味先归于脾,辛味先归于肺,咸味先归于肾。此乃后世药物归经理论的基础,提示人们应注意药、食物对五脏疾病的宜忌。出《灵枢·五味》。

五味各走其所喜(wǔ wèi gè zǒu qí suǒ xǐ) **Each of the five flavors proceeds to its preferred zang organ.** According to the theory of the five elements, drugs and food both have five flavors, namely sour, bitter, sweet, pungent and salty. After ingestion, they proceed to their corresponding organs. For instance, the sour flavor first proceeds to the liver; the bitter flavor first proceeds to the heart; the sweet flavor first proceeds to the spleen; the pungent flavor first proceeds to the lung; the salty flavor first proceeds to the kidney. This is the basis of the channel tropism theory of drugs, and suggests that attention should be paid to indications and contraindications of drugs and food. See *Ling Shu* chapter 56.

五味论 《灵枢》篇名。五味。指酸、苦、甘、辛、咸五种滋味,泛指饮食物。此篇专论五味和五脏五体的关系,指出五味能养五脏,也能损伤五脏,引起病变,故名。

五味论(wǔ wèi lùn) **Discussion on Five Flavors** Chapter title in *Ling Shu*. The five flavors refer to the sour, bitter, sweet, pungent and salty tastes, or food in general. In this chapter, the relationship of the five flavors with the five viscera and the five body parts is discussed, and that the five flavors can not only nourish the five viscera, but also damage them resulting in pathological changes is pointed out, thus its name.

五果 指桃、李、杏、栗、枣五种果实。古人将它们分别与肾、心、肺、脾、肝五脏相配,认为五果

对五脏精气有帮助作用。出《素问·藏气法时论》。

五果(wǔ guǒ) **five fruits** Refers to peaches, plums, apricots, chestnuts and dates. In ancient China, these fruits were believed to correspond respectively to the kidney, heart, lung, spleen and liver and be good for the essence qi of the five viscera. See *Su Wen* chapter 22.

五变 ①《灵枢》篇名。五变,指风厥、消瘅、寒热、痹、积聚五种病变。此篇主要列举五种不同的病变,阐述外邪致病过程中,五脏的强弱是疾病发生与否的关键,并指出同时受病,不同的体质,会发生不同疾病的道理。故名。② 五脏的五种病理变化。出《灵枢·顺气一日分为四时》。

五变(wǔ biàn) ① Chapter title in *Ling Shu*. The five changes refer to the five pathological changes including wind syncope, consumptive disease, cold-heat, obstruction disorder and abdominal mass. In this chapter, five different kinds of pathological changes are described, and the condition of the five viscera is believed to decide whether the occurrence or the no occurrence of the disease is to take place when exogenous pathogenic factors attack the body. The idea specifies that people with different body constitutions develop different diseases despite being attacked by the same pathogenic factor, thus its name. ② Five pathological changes of the five viscera. See *Ling Shu* chapter 44.

五法　言治病应掌握的五种方法,包括医生在自身精神专注的同时,把握好患者神气的变化;知晓养生之道;了解药性;选用大小适宜的砭石,以及审察脏腑气血的各种病理变化等。出《素问·宝命全形论》。

五法（wǔ fǎ）　**five methods** The five well-known treatment methods. In the treatment of disease, physicians should concentrate on and pay attention to changes in the patients' spirit, know the way to preserve health, understand the properties of drugs, select the treatment tools of appropriate size, and examine the various pathological changes of the viscera, qi and blood, etc. See *Su Wen* chapter 25.

五治　出《素问·六节藏象论》。

（1）五运所主之时气。见《素问》王冰注。（2）根据五脏主时所取相应之治法。见《素问经注节解》。

五治（wǔ zhì）　**five treatments** See *Su Wen* chapter 9. (1) The seasonal qi that is dominated by the five movements. See *Su Wen* annotated by Wang Bing. (2) The corresponding treatment methods according to the governing qi of the five viscera. See *Su Wen Jing Zhu Jie Jie* (*Annotation and Explanation of Su Wen*).

五宜　① 言五脏患病时应该选用相适宜的饮食五味。出《灵枢·五味》。② 指毛、羽、倮、介、鳞五类动物的生长繁殖随气候而变化,故对五气、五色、五味也各有所宜。出《素问·五常政大论》。

五宜（wǔ yí）　① It is said that food of specific flavors are appropriate for specific diseases of the five viscera. See *Ling Shu* chapter 56. ② Refers to the growth and reproduction of the five classes of animals, i.e. those with and without hair, those with feathers, those with shells and those with scales, changes with the climate, and these are always dependant on what is appropriate for the respective qi，color and taste. See *Su Wen* chapter 70.

五官　① 指耳、目、口、鼻、舌。其与五脏在生理功能上相通。出《灵枢·五阅五使》。② 指五色所主的证候，即青黑为痛，黄赤为热，白为寒。出《灵枢·五色》。

五官（wǔ guān）　① Refers to the five administrative organs，namely the ears，eyes，mouth，nose and tongue，all interconnected with the five viscera physiologically. See *Ling Shu* chapter 37. ② The syndromes indicated by the five colors，that is，greenish and black are associated with pain，yellow and red are associated with heat，and white is associated with cold. See *Ling Shu* chapter 49.

五实　① 指五种属实症状，即脉盛、皮热、腹胀、前后不通、闷瞀。出《素问·玉机真藏论》。② 指五体之实证。出《素问·宝命全形论》。

五实（wǔ shí）　① Refers to the five symptoms of repletion，including an abounding pulse in the vessels，hot skin，abdominal distension，blockages in front and behind，and mental and physical pressure. See *Su Wen*

chapter 19. ② Refers to the repletion syndrome of the five body parts. See *Su Wen* chapter 25.

五经　五脏之经络。出《素问·经脉别论》。

五经（wǔ jīng）　**five conduits** The meridians and collaterals of the five viscera. See *Su Wen* chapter 21.

五星　指岁星、荧惑星、镇星、太白星、辰星。出《素问·气交变大论》。

五星（wǔ xīng）　**five stars** Refers to Jupiter，Mars，Saturn，Venus and Mercury. See *Su Wen* chapter 69.

五胠俞　出《素问·刺疟》。(1) 指背部足太阳膀胱经第二旁线的五个穴名。见《类经·疾病五十》。(2) 谓谚语穴。见《素问》王冰注。

五胠俞（wǔ qū shū）　**five upper flank transporters on the back** See *Su Wen* chapter 36. (1) Refers to the five acupoints along the second sideline of the bladder meridian of foot *taiyang* on the back. See *Lei Jing*（*Classified Classic*）"On Diseases Chapter 50". (2) The Yi Xi acupoint. See *Su Wen* annotated by Wang Bing.

五胜更立 五行之气相胜，谓之五胜。其气盛胜旺，各有其主时，而随五行规律不断更替出现，从而有胜亦有制，化生万物。出《素问·宝命全形论》。

五胜更立（wǔ shèng gēng lì）**Five dominations take their positions one after another.** Alternative dominations among the five elements. The qi of each element dominates in alternative order the five elements, leading to the conditions of dominating and being inhibited, engendering and transforming all creatures. See *Su Wen* chapter 25.

五脉 ① 五脏之经脉。出《素问·五藏生成》。② 五脏所主之脉象。见《类经·疾病十四》。③ 五脏之腧。出《灵枢·小针解》。

五脉（wǔ mài） ① Vessels of the five viscera. See *Su Wen* chapter 10. ② Pulse manifestations dominated by the five viscera. See *Lei Jing*（*Classified Classic*）"On Diseases Chapter 14". ③ Transporters of the five viscera. See *Ling Shu* chapter 3.

五度 脉度、藏度、肉度、筋度、俞度的总称。出《素问·方盛衰论》。

五度（wǔ dù）**five measurements** An general term for pulse, vis-

cera, muscles, sinew and acupoint measurements. See *Su Wen* chapter 80.

五疫 即木疫、火疫、土疫、金疫、水疫五种温疫。出《素问·刺法论》。

五疫（wǔ yì）**five kinds of pestilence** Namely, wood，fire，earth，metal and water pestilence. See *Su Wen* chapter 72.

五音 ① 古代五声音阶中的角、徵、宫、商、羽五个音级。《内经》中把五音与五行五脏等相配来说明医学道理。出《素问·脉要精微论》。② 泛指声音。出《灵枢·脉度》。

五音（wǔ yīn） ① The five sound levels of *jue*，*zhi*，*gong*，*shang* and *yu* in the musical scales of ancient China. In *Nei Jing*（*Internal Classic*），the matching of the five tones with the five elements and the five viscera is used to explain medical theories. See *Su Wen* chapter 17. ② Refers to voices in general. See *Ling Shu* chapter 17.

五音五味 《灵枢》篇名。五音，即角、徵、宫、商、羽，在此指五音所属的各种类型的人。五味，指酸、苦、甘、辛、咸饮食五味。该篇承接《灵枢·阴阳二十五人》的内容进一步阐述二十五种人经脉气血相异的理论,并把五谷、五畜、五果依五行归类,说明其治疗作用,故名。另外,揭示了女性和宦者不能生胡须的道理,以及六经气血多少的一般规律。

五音五味(wǔ yīn wǔ wèi) **Five Musical Notes and Five Flavors** Chapter title in *Ling Shu*. The five tones, including *jue*, *zhi*, *gong*, *shang* and *yu*, are used here to indicate various types of people corresponding to the five tones. The five flavors of food are sour, bitter, sweet, pungent and salty. Following *Ling Shu* chapter 64, the theory that there are twenty-five types of people all different in channels, qi and blood is further explained, and the five grains, the five domestic animals and the five fruits are classified according to the five elements to specify their therapeutic effects, thus its name. In addition, the reason why females and eunuchs do not have beards is explained, and the regular pattern of the amount of qi and blood in the six pairs of channels is revealed.

五逆 ① 五种脉证相逆之证。出《灵枢·五禁》。② 五种逆而不顺之证的组合。出《灵枢·玉版》。

五逆(wǔ nì) ① Five syndromes with opposing pulses and symptoms. See *Ling Shu* chapter 61. ② Five combinations of opposing symptoms. See *Ling Shu* chapter 60.

五宫 即五脏。古称房屋为宫。五脏为蓄藏精气之处,故称五宫。出《素问·生气通天论》。

五宫(wǔ gōng) **five palaces** Namely the five viscera. In ancient China, houses were called palaces. The five viscera are the sites where essence qi is stored, thus called the five palaces. See *Su Wen* chapter 3.

五神 指五脏之神。出《素问·本病论》。

五神(wǔ shén) **five spirits** Refers to the spirit of the five viscera. See *Su Wen* chapter 73.

五恶 恶(wù 误),厌憎,不喜欢。五脏各有所恶,即心恶热,肺恶寒,肝恶风,脾恶湿,肾恶燥。出《素问·宣明五气》。

五恶(wǔ wù) **five aversions** *Wù* refers to hate, or dislike. The aversions of the five viscera, that is, the heart is averse to heat, the lung is averse to cold, the liver is averse to wind, the spleen is averse to

四画

dampness and the kidney is averse to dryness. See *Su Wen* chapter 23.

五病 ① 即五气所病，指脏腑之气失调所致的病变。即心为噫、肺为咳、肝为语、脾为吞、肾为欠，为嚏，胃为气逆为哕，为恐，大肠小肠为泄，下焦溢为水，膀胱不利为癃，不约为遗溺，胆为怒。出《素问·宣明五气》。② 五病所发。为五脏阴阳之发病部位、季节。阴病发于骨，阳病发于血，阴病发于肉，阳病发于冬，阴病发于夏。出《素问·宣明五气》。③ 指身热、咽喉痹阻、人迎躁盛、喘息、气逆五种病气有余之证。出《素问·奇病论》。

五病(wǔ bìng) ① Namely, diseases due to disorder of the five qi of the viscera and bowels. The disorder of heart qi causes eructation; the disorder of lung qi causes cough; the disorder of liver qi causes polylogia; the disorder of spleen qi causes acid regurgitation; the disorder of kidney qi causes yawning and sneezing; the disorder of stomach qi causes reverse flow of qi, hiccup and fear; the disorder of large intestine and small intestine qi causes diarrhea; the extravasation of lower *jiao* qi causes edema; the unsmooth transformation of bladder qi causes retention of urine; the loss of control of bladder qi causes enuresis; disorder of gallbladder qi causes frequent anger. See *Su Wen* chapter 23. ② Location of disease and seasons when disease occurs. That is, yin disease occurs in the bones; yang disease occurs in the blood; yin disease occurs in the muscles; yang disease occurs in winter while yin disease occurs in summer. See *Su Wen* chapter 23. ③ Refers to the five kinds of diseases due to exuberant pathogenic qi: scorching fever, obstruction of the throat, rapid pulsation of *ren ying* pulse, panting and the reverse flow of qi. See *Su Wen* chapter 47.

五病所发 又名"五发"。五脏阴阳之病发生的部位和季节。阴病发于骨，阳病发于血，阴病发于肉，阳病发于冬，阴病发于夏。出《素问·宣明五气》。

五病所发(wǔ bìng suǒ fā) **outbreak of five diseases** Also named "five onsets". The location and season of the occurrence of the diseases of the five viscera and yin-yang. That is，yin diseases occurs in the bones；yang diseases occurs in the blood；yin diseases occurs in the muscles；yang diseases occurs in the winter while yin diseases occurs in summer. See *Su Wen* chapter 23.

五部　① 五脏系于外部的五个部位：伏兔、腓、背、五脏之俞、项。出《灵枢·寒热病》。② 五脏所在的部位。出《素问·方盛衰论》。

五部（wǔ bù）　① The five parts on the exterior that are connected with the five viscera：*fu tu* region，calf，back，transport openings of the five viscera and nape. See *Ling Shu* chapter 21. ② Locations of the five viscera. See *Su Wen* chapter 80.

五畜　指牛、羊、豕、犬、鸡五种动物。古人将它们分别与肝、肺、脾、心、肾五脏相配，认为五畜有益于五脏的精气。出《素问·藏气法时论》。

五畜（wǔ chù）　**five domestic animals** Refers to cows，sheep，pigs，dogs and chickens. In ancient China，these animals were believed to correspond to the liver，lung，spleen，heart and kidney，respectively and supplement the essence qi of the five viscera. See *Su Wen* chapter 22.

五阅五使　《灵枢》篇名。五阅，五脏之外候。五使，体表五色的变化，为五脏之气所指使。此篇主要讨论五脏与五官、五色内外相应关系以及观察五官、五色的变化以测候五脏的正常与否。故名。

五阅五使（wǔ yuè wǔ shǐ）　**Five Observations and Five Manifestations** Chapter title in *Ling Shu*. "Five observations" refer to the external signs of the five viscera. "Five manifestations" refer to the changes in the five complexions of the face that are caused by qi of the five viscera. In this chapter，correspondence of the five viscera in the interior to the five sensing organs and the five colors at the exterior is discussed，and advice is given to observe changes in the sense organs and colors to determine whether the viscera is working normally or not，thus its name.

五窍　见"胃之五窍"条。出《灵枢·胀论》。

五窍（wǔ qiào）　**five openings** See "胃之五窍". See *Ling Shu* chapter 35.

五菜 指葵、藿、薤、葱、韭五种蔬菜。古人将它们分别与肝、脾、肺、肾、心五脏相配,认为五菜对五脏精气有充养作用。出《素问·藏气法时论》。

五菜(wǔ cài) **five vegetables** Refers to cluster mallow, bean leaves, leeks, scallions and Chinese chives. In ancient China, they were believed to correspond to the liver, spleen, lung, kidney and heart, respectively, and to supplement and nourish the essence qi of the five viscera. See *Su Wen* chapter 22.

五虚 ① 指五种属虚症状。即脉细、皮寒、气少、泄利前后、饮食不入。出《素问·玉机真藏论》。② 指皮、肉、筋、脉、骨五体之虚证。出《素问·宝命全形论》。

五虚(wǔ xū) ① Refers to the five symptoms of deficiency, including a thin pulse, cold skin, being short of qi, an unimpeded outflow coming from the front and back, unable to ingest beverages or food. See *Su Wen* chapter 19. ② Deficiency syndrome of the five body parts, including the skin, flesh, sinews, meridians and bones. See *Su Wen* chapter 25.

五常 木、火、土、金、水五运变化之常理。一般有平气、太过、不及等常规。出《素问·五运行大论》。

五常(wǔ cháng) **five constants** The constant pattern of changes of the five movements, i.e. the movements of wood, fire, earth, metal and water. Usually the constants include balanced, excessive and insufficient qi. See *Su Wen* chapter 67.

五常政大论 《素问》篇名。此篇通过分析五运之平气、太过不及,以及六气五类相互制约而岁有胎孕不育和在泉六化五味有薄厚之异等,论述了五运在其运行变化中的常规以及外在表现,故名。

五常政大论(wǔ cháng zhèng dà lùn) **Major Discussion on the Administration of the Five Movements** Chapter title in *Su Wen*. See *Su Wen* chapter 70. In this chapter, by having analyzed the balanced, excessive and insufficient qi of the five movements, mutual restriction of the six qi and five kinds of relative age inhibitions, including infertility and sterility, transformation of the six qi and the five flavors in the spring, the regular and external manifestations in changes of the five circuits, are all discussed, thus its name.

五液 指津液所化生的汗、泪、涕、唾、涎等五种分泌物。心为汗,肺为涕,肝为泪,脾为涎,肾为唾。出《素问·宣明五气》。

五液（wǔ yè） **five fluids** Refers to the five secretions produced from body fluid, namely sweat, tears, snivel, spittle and saliva. The heart fluid transforms into sweat; the lung fluid transforms into snivel; the liver fluid transforms into tears; the spleen fluid transforms into saliva; and the kidney fluid transforms into spittle. See *Su Wen* chapter 23.

五裁 饮食的五种节制。裁,节制之意。如筋病不宜多食酸,气病不宜多食辛,骨病不宜多食咸,血病不宜多食苦,肉病不宜多食甘。因五味分走五脏,气血筋骨肉,分属五脏,五味太过,必然有害,故须节制。出《灵枢·九针论》。

五裁（wǔ cái） **to avoid certain kinds of food after the contraction of five kinds of diseases** Five kinds of diet control. *Cái*

refers to control. For instance, sour foods are restricted after contracting diseases of the sinews, acrid foods are limited after contracting diseases of qi, salty foods are reduced after contracting disease of the bones, bitter foods are restricted after contracting diseases of the blood, and sweet foods are avoided after contracting diseases of the flesh. Since the essence of the the five flavors enters their respective zang organ, and the qi, blood, sinews, bones and flesh pertain to their respective zang organ, eating too much of a certain flavor is harmful and should be avoided. See *Ling Shu* chapter 78.

五焦 即第五胸椎。焦,椎。出《灵枢·背腧》。

五焦（wǔ jiāo） **the fifth vertebra** Namely the fifth thoracic vertebra. *Jiāo* refers to vertebra. See *Ling Shu* chapter 51.

五禁 ① 五脏之病对药食五味的禁忌。即肝病禁辛,心病禁咸,脾病禁酸,肾病禁甘,肺病禁苦。出《灵枢·五味》。② 气、血、骨、肉、筋疾病对药食五味的禁忌。如气病不多食辛,血病不多食咸,骨病不多食苦,肉病不多食甘,筋病不多食酸。出《素问·宣明五气》。③五种针刺禁忌的时日及部位。出《灵枢·五禁》。④《灵枢》篇名。该篇以针刺宜忌为中心,重点介绍针刺的五禁、五夺、五过、五逆等,提示人们在治疗时应当知所避忌。

flesh diseases should avoid eating excessive sweet flavors, and patients with sinew diseases should avoid eating excessive sour flavors. See *Su Wen* chapter 23. ③ Time and locations to be avoided in acupuncture for treating disease. See *Ling Shu* chapter 61. ④ Chapter title in *Ling Shu*. This chapter deals with the indications and contraindications of acupuncture; the five contraindications, the five exhaustions, the five errors and the five contrary phenomena, are highlighted to remind practitioners of the things to be avoided during acupuncture. See *Ling Shu* chapter 61.

五禁(wǔ jìn)　① Ingesting drugs and food of one of the five flavors is prohibited in diseases of the five viscera. Drugs and food with acrid flavor are prohibited in liver disease, those with salty flavor are prohibited in heart disease, those with sour flavor are prohibited in spleen disease, those with sweet flavor are prohibited in kidney disease, and those with bitter flavor are prohibited in lung disease. See *Ling Shu* chapter 56. ② Drugs and food of one of the five flavors are prohibited in diseases of the qi, blood, bones, flesh and sinews. Patients with qi diseases should avoid eating excessive pungent flavors, patients with blood diseases should avoid eating excessive salty flavors, patients with bone diseases should avoid eating excessive bitter flavors, patients with

五腧　即井、荥、输、经、合五腧穴。是十二经脉在肘膝关节以下的五个特定穴位。此以水流的大小来比喻经脉之气由小而大,由浅入深,由远到近的特点。脉气起始如泉水初出谓井,其穴多在四肢末端;脉气稍大,如水成小流谓荥,其穴多在指(趾)掌(蹠)附近;脉气较盛,如水流由浅及深灌注,谓输,其穴在腕、踝关节附近;脉气流注如水之长流谓经,其穴多在前臂及小腿部;脉气汇集,如水流汇入江河,谓合,其穴在肘、膝关节附近。出《灵枢·九针十二原》。

五腧（wǔ shū） **transport points of the five viscera** Namely, the well, brook, stream, river and sea acupoints. They are the five special acupoints of the twelve channels below the elbows or knees. The size of the water flow is used to describe the characteristics of channel qi, that is, from small to big, shallow to deep, and far to near. The well acupoints are generally located at the ends of the limbs, as channel qi originates like spring water going out of a well; the brook acupoints are mostly located near the palms and the soles since channel qi is bigger and flows like a brook; the stream acupoints are generally located at the wrists and ankles since channel qi is quite vigorous, like a stream flowing from shallow to deep; the river acupoints are mostly located at the forearm and lower leg, since channel qi moves like the long flow of water; the sea acupoints are generally located near the elbows and knees, since channel qi comes together and moves like water flowing to the sea. See *Ling Shu* chapter 1.

五痹 五种痹证。出《素问·移精变气论》。（1）指皮、肉、筋、脉、骨五体痹。见《素问》王冰注。（2）指心、肝、脾、肺、肾五脏痹。见《素问集注》。

五痹（wǔ bì） **five blockages** Five kinds of blockage syndromes. See *Su Wen* chapter 13. (1) Refers to skin, flesh, sinews, meridians, and bones, the five body parts blockages. See *Su Wen* annotated by Wang Bing. (2) Refers to blockages of the heart, liver, spleen, lung and kidney, the five viscera blockages syndromes. See *Su Wen Ji Zhu*（*Collected Annotation of Su Wen*）.

五精 五脏精气。出《素问·宣明五气》。

五精（wǔ jīng） **five essences** Essence qi of the five viscera. See *Su Wen* chapter 23.

五精所并 见"五并"条。出《素问·宣明五气》。

五精所并（wǔ jīng suǒ bìng） **accumulation of five essences** See "五并". See *Su Wen* chapter 23.

五癃津液别 《灵枢》篇名。五，指汗、溺、唾、泪、髓五种体液。

癃，即癃闭。别，分别、区别。五谷所化生的津液可分别转变为汗、溺、唾、泪、髓等五种产物，在病理情况下，津液逆行，水停下焦而为癃闭。故名。

五癃津液别（wǔ lóng jīn yè bié）**Differentiation Among the Retention of Five Kinds of Fluid** Chapter title in *Ling Shu*. "Five kinds of fluid" include sweat, urine, saliva, tears and marrow. *Lóng* refers to the retention of fluids; *bié* refers to separating, or distinguishing. Fluids generated from food can be transformed into the above five products. In pathological conditions, fluids flow in the wrong direction, and water accumulates in the lower *jiao*, leading to the retention of fluids, thus its name.

五藏　心、肺、脾、肝、肾五个脏器的总称，具有藏精气的作用，并与精神情志活动有关。出《素问·五藏别论》。《内经》藏象理论，以五脏为人体生命活动中心，分别与六腑及其他组织器官相联系，构成一个统一整体。五脏各有其生理活动特点，但又相互联系，相互影响。

五藏（wǔ zàng）　**five viscera** Namely, the heart, lung, spleen,

liver and kidney. They store essence qi and are also related to mental activity. See *Su Wen* chapter 11. According to the theory of the manifestations of the viscera in *Nei Jing*（*Internal Classic*），as the center of human activities，the five viscera are connected with the six bowels and other tissues and organs to form a unified whole. Each of the five viscera has its own characteristics of physiological activities，but they also are related to and influence each other.

五藏气　指五脏之气失调，所引起的病证。出《灵枢·九针论》。

五藏气（wǔ zàng qì）　**qi of the five viscera** Diseases influenced by the disorder of the five visceral qi. See *Ling Shu* chapter 78.

五藏六府之海　指胃。出《灵枢·五味》。

五藏六府之海（wǔ zàng liù fǔ zhī hǎi）　**sea of the five viscera and the six bowels**. Refers to the stomach. See *Ling Shu* chapter 56.

五藏六府之盖　指肺。出《灵枢·九针论》。

五藏六府之盖（wǔ zàng liù fǔ zhī gài）　**canopy covering the five**

viscera and the six bowels Refers to the lung. See *Ling Shu* chapter 78.

五藏生成 《素问》篇名。五藏，心肝脾肺肾；生成，相生相成。此篇从生理、病理、诊断三方面论述了五脏相生相成的道理，故名。

五藏生成(wǔ zàng shēng chéng) **Discussion on Various Relationships Concerning the Five Viscera** Chapter title in *Su Wen*. The five viscera are the heart, liver, spleen, lung and kidney. *Shēng chéng* refers to mutual-generation. In this chapter, the various relationships concerning the five viscera are discussed, e. g. physiology, pathology and diagnostics, thus its name. See *Su Wen* chapter 10.

五藏阳以竭 为水肿病的病机。以，同"已"。出《素问·汤液醪醴论》。(1)五脏阳气已经竭绝。见《素问》王冰注。(2)五脏之气内伤而衰竭。见《新校正》。(3)五脏阳气阻遏，阳气不能气化和运行水液，水气停聚。竭，释义为阻遏。

五藏阳以竭(wǔ zàng yáng yǐ jié) **Yang qi is exhausted in the five viscera.** The pathogenesis of edema. See *Su Wen* chapter 14.

(1) The yang qi of the five viscera is depleted. See *Su Wen* annotated by Wang Bing. (2) The qi of the five viscera is damaged in the interior and is weakened. See *Xin Jiao Zheng* (*New Revisions of Su Wen*). (3) The yang qi of the five viscera is blocked and can not transport or transform fluids, causing retention of fluids in the body. *Jié* means obstrustion.

五藏别论 《素问》篇名。五藏，此处泛指人体脏腑。别，区别。此篇主要论述五脏、六腑、奇恒之腑的功能及其区别，故称别论。

五藏别论 (wǔ zàng bié lùn) **Different Discussion on the Five Viscera** Chapter title in *Su Wen*. "The five viscera" here refers to viscera in general. Bié refers to difference. In this chapter, the functions and differences of the five viscera, the six bowels and the extraordinary fu organs are discussed.

五藏俞 指五脏的背俞穴，即肺俞、心俞、肝俞、脾俞、肾俞。均属足太阳经。出《素问·水热穴论》。

五藏俞(wǔ zàng shū) **transport acupoints of the five viscera**

四画

Refers to the transport acupoints on the back belonging to the meridian of the foot *taiyang*, namely the lung, heart, liver, spleen and kidney transport acupoints. See *Su Wen* chapter 61.

五藏常内阅于上七窍　阅,经历之意,引申作相通。五脏在内,精气分别与上七窍(双目、双耳、鼻、口、舌)相通。上七窍常能反映相关内脏的功能状况。出《灵枢·脉度》。

五藏常内阅于上七窍(wǔ zàng cháng nèi yuè yú shàng qī qiào)　**The five viscera regularly communicate with the seven orifices internally.** *Yuè* means to experience, or to extend in order to connect. The essence qi of the five viscera in the interior communicates respectively with the upper seven orifices (eyes, ears, nose, mouth and tongue). These orifices can often reflect the condition of the functions of the related viscera. See *Ling Shu* chapter 17.

支正　经穴名。手太阳小肠经之络穴。在腕背横纹尺侧端上五寸处。出《灵枢·经脉》。

支正(zhī zhèng)　**Zhi Zheng (SI 7)** Acupoint name of a connecting acupoint on the small

intestine meridian of hand *taiyang*. It is located at five *cun* above the ulnar side of the transverse crease on the dorsal carpus. See *Ling Shu* chapter 10.

支节　四肢骨节。支,同肢。出《灵枢·海论》。

支节(zhī jié)　**limbs and joints** The four limbs and joints. See *Ling Shu* chapter 33.

支沟　经穴名。手少阳三焦经之经穴。在腕后三寸,两骨之间陷者中。出《灵枢·本输》。

支沟(zhī gōu)　**Zhi Gou (SJ 6)** An acupoint on the triple *jiao* meridian of hand *shaoyang* located in the indentation between the two bones three *cun* above the wrist. See *Ling Shu* chapter 2.

不仁　① 指感觉障碍。出《素问·风论》。② 指神志障碍。出《素问·诊要经终论》。

不仁(bù rén)　① Refers to a sensory disturbance. See *Su Wen* chapter 42. ② Refers to a mental disorder. See *Su Wen* chapter 16.

不月　即闭经。出《素问·阴阳别论》。

不月(bù yuè)　**without menstruation** Amenorrhoea. See *Su Wen* chapter 7.

不当位　① 客主加临中,位置逆

而不顺之谓。出《素问·五运行大论》。（1）君火为上，相火为下。若客气相火（即下）反加于主气君火（即上）之上为不当位。见《素问集注》。（2）下为子，上为母，若以子临母，如土临火，火临木之类，是下临之不当位。②胜复之气，先时而至之谓。出《素问·至真要大论》。

不当位（bù dàng wèi）　① The wrangling guest robs the place of the host. See *Su Wen* chapter 67. (1) The monarch fire is at the upper position，and the minister fire is at the lower position. If the minister fire（lower）comes up on the monarch fire（upper），it does not occupy its proper position. See *Su Wen Ji Zhu*（*Collected Annotation of Su Wen*）. (2) The lower is son and the upper is mother. If the son comes up on the mother，e.g. earth up on fire and fire on wood，the former does not occupy its proper position. ② The dominating qi or the revenge qi that arrives before due. See *Su Wen* chapter 74.

不时卧　言不能按时而卧。出《素问·太阴阳明论》。

不时卧（bù shí wò）　**unable to lie down at an appropriate time** Meaning difficult to lie down when the time is appropriate. See *Su Wen* chapter 29.

不足补之　治法。虚损不足之病，当用补益之法以培补之。出《素问·至真要大论》。

不足补之（bù zú bǔ zhī）　**to supplement the insufficient** A therapeutic method used to treat disease due to deficiency，the supplementing method. See *Su Wen* chapter 74.

不间藏　五脏病变按五行相克规律传变。如心病传肺，肺病传肝等。出《素问·平人气象论》。

不间藏（bù jiān zàng）　**not to skip a zang organ** Diseases of the five viscera are subject to transmission and change，and they follow the rule of inhibition of the five elements. For instance，diseases of the heart may be transmitted to the lung and diseases of the lung to the liver etc. See *Su Wen* chapter 18.

不得卧　① 失眠。出《灵枢·大惑论》。② 不得平卧。出《素问·逆调论》。

不得卧（bù dé wò）　① Insomnia. See *Ling Shu* chapter 80. ② Unable to lie flat. See *Su Wen* chapter 34.

不得前后　前谓小便，后谓大便。不得前后，即大小便不通。出《素问·缪刺论》。

不得前后（bù dé qián hòu）　**front and back inability** "Front" refers to urination and "back" refers to defecation. This expression means that a person cannot urinate from the front or defecate from the back. See *Su Wen* chapter 63.

太一天符　运气术语。凡主岁的中运，司天之气与年支三者的五行属性相同，即称太一天符之年。因其三者相合，故又称三合。此年既是天符年，又是岁会年。出《素问·六微旨大论》。

太一天符（tài yī tiān fú）　*tai yi tian fu*（**heavenly complement**）Circuits and qi terminology. In the year of the *tai yi tian fu*（heavenly complement），the middle movement conforms to the qi that governs the heavens and the element in the five elements that dominates in that year. This is called triple combination，and is a year both of *tian fu*（heavenly complements）and *sui hui*（peace）. See *Su Wen* chapter 68.

太乙　太，至尊之谓。乙，即一，万数之始。言宇宙万物之主宰。出《灵枢·九宫八风》。

太乙（tài yǐ）　*tai yi Tài* means the supreme and *yǐ* refers to one，the beginning of everything. It refers to the master of all things in the universe. See *Ling Shu* chapter 77.

太乙帝君　言众神之领。出《素问·本病论》。

太乙帝君（tài yǐ dì jūn）　**Emperor Tai Yi** Leader of the gods. See *Su Wen* chapter 73.

太乙游宫　北斗所指的月令。出《素问·本病论》。

太乙游宫（tài yǐ yóu gōng）　**State of Polaris** Monthly climate referred to by the Big Dipper. See *Su Wen* chapter 73.

太仓　① 胃。其为贮存水谷的仓廪，故称。出《灵枢·胀论》。② 经穴名，即中脘穴之别名。属任脉，为胃之募穴。出《灵枢·根结》。

太仓（tài cāng）　① The stomach which stores water and grains. See *Ling Shu* chapter 35. ② Acupoint name，Zhong Wan（CV12），belonging to the conception vessel. It is front-mu acupoint of the stomach. See *Ling Shu* chapter 5.

太白　① 经穴名。足太阴脾经的俞穴、原穴，位于足内侧核骨下陷者中,当赤白肉际处。出《灵枢·九针十二原》。② 五大行星之一。见"太白星"。出《素问·气交变大论》。

太白（tài bái） ① Acupoint name，Tai Bai (SP 3)，located on the spleen meridian of foot *taiyin* in the depression of the nucleus bone inside the foot，between the white and red flesh. It is also a transport and source acupoint. See *Ling Shu* chapter 1. ② One of the five planets (the metal，wood，water，fire and earth planets，or Venus，Jupiter，Mercury，Mars and Saturn)，i.e. the planet of metal，or Venus. See *Su Wen* chapter 69.

太白星 金星,为五大行星之一,与五行中的金,五脏中的肺相通应。出《素问·金匮真言论》。

太白星（tài bái xīng） **Taibai planet** Venus，one of the five planets corresponding to metal in the five elements and to the lung in the five viscera. See *Su Wen* chapter 4.

太冲 ① 太冲脉,即冲脉。出《素问·阴阳离合论》。② 冲脉与肾脉合而盛大之义。出《素问·水热穴论》。③ 经穴名。属足厥阴肝经,在足背第一、二趾骨结

合部前方凹陷处。出《灵枢·本输》。

太冲（tài chōng） ① Taichong vessel，or the thoroughfare vessel. See *Su Wen* chapter 6. ② It means that the thoroughfare vessel and the kidney vessel converge，and qi is exuberant. See *Su Wen* chapter 61. ③ Acupoint name，Tai Chong (LR 3)，belonging to the liver meridian of foot *jueyin*，and located in the indentation in front of the joint of the first and second phalanges on the dorsum of the foot. See *Ling Shu* chapter 2.

太冲脉 指冲脉。出《素问·上古天真论》。

太冲脉（tài chōng mài） **Taichong vessel** Refers to the thoroughfare vessel. See *Su Wen* chapter 1.

太阳 ① 指三阳。出《素问·阴阳类论》。② 指心。出《灵枢·九针十二原》。③ 指手之阳面外侧。出《灵枢·阴阳系日月》。④ 单指或统指手足太阳小肠、膀胱及其经脉。出《素问·六节藏象论》。⑤ 指夏季阳气隆盛之时。出《素问·四气调神大论》。⑥ 指六气中之寒气,主水。出《素问·五常政大论》。

四画

太阳（tài yang） ① Refers to the third yang. See *Su Wen* chapter 79. ② Refers to the heart. See *Ling Shu* chapter 1. ③ Refers to the lateral dorsal aspect of the hand. See *Ling Shu* chapter 41. ④ Solely or in conjunction refers to the small intestine and bladder meridians of hand and foot *taiyang*. See *Su Wen* chapter 9. ⑤ Refers to the time when yang qi is exuberant in summer. See *Su Wen* chapter 2. ⑥ Refers to cold qi in the six qi that governs water. See *Su Wen* chapter 70.

太阳之人 体质名,属五态之人中多阳无阴者。其人无能自负,好高骛远,处事不顾是非后果,外表常挺胸凸肚,趾高气扬。故治疗时应谨慎调节,以泻阳护阴为原则。否则,易发生阳脱、阴阳皆脱而引起发狂、暴死不知人等重证。出《素问·刺法论》。

太阳之人（tài yáng zhī rén） *taiyang*-type people Name of constitution of people characterized by excessive yang without yin. The people of *taiyang* type are incompetent and conceited, they aim too high and act carelessly. They are often proud as a peacock, squaring their shoulders and having a large stomach that sticks out. To treat such people, the doctor must be very careful to prevent the loss of yin and only concentrate on reducing the yang. Otherwise, yang collapse or the collapse of yin and yang might occur, leading to severe syndromes such as mania, loss of consciousness and sudden death. See *Su Wen* chapter 72.

太阳之政 即太阳司天之政。出《素问·六元正纪大论》。

太阳之政（tài yáng zhī zhèng） *taiyang* in domination Namely, *taiyang* dominating the heavens. See *Su Wen* chapter 71.

太阳之复 运气术语。复,即六气偏胜情况下而产生的复气。此指少阳相火、少阴君火之气偏胜至一定程度,太阳寒水之气来复,气候由热变冷,人体多见寒气偏胜之心、胃、膀胱等寒病。出《素问·至真要大论》。

太阳之复（tài yáng zhī fù） **retaliation of *taiyang*** Terminology of circuits and qi. Retaliation refers to the revenging qi emerging when one of the six qi is in unilateral dominance. Here, it means that when the qi of the *shaoyang* ministerial fire and the qi of the *shaoyin* monarch fire are so exuberant that qi of the *taiyang* cold water takes revenge，the climate changes from hot to cold，and the human body is prone to getting cold diseases in the heart，stomach and bladder etc. See *Su Wen* chapter 74.

太阳之胜　运气术语。指太阳寒水偏胜之气。如太阳司天在泉之时，寒气偏盛，气候寒冷，人体多见寒气偏胜之肾病。出《素问·至真要大论》。

太阳之胜(tài yáng zhī shèng) **predominant *taiyang*** Terminology of circuits and qi，refers to the predominant qi of *taiyang* cold water. When *taiyang* dominates the heavens and it is in spring，the cold qi is exuberant with a cold climate and invades the human body to cause disease of the kidney. See *Su Wen* chapter 74.

太阳为开　出《灵枢·根结》。

太阳为开(tài yáng wéi kāi) ***Taiyang* is responsible for opening.** See *Ling Shu* chapter 5.

太阳正经　指足太阳经腧穴。出《素问·刺腰痛》。(1)指委中穴。见《素问直解》。(2)指昆仑穴。见《素问注证发微》。

太阳正经(tài yáng zhèng jīng) **regular *taiyang* channel** Refers to the transport acupoints of the bladder meridian of foot *taiyang*. See *Su Wen* chapter 41. (1) Refers to Wei Zhong (BL 40) acupoint. See *Su Wen Zhi Jie*（*Direct Interpretation on Su Wen*）. (2) Refers to Kun Lun (BL 60) acupoint. See *Su Wen Zhu Zheng Fa Wei*（*Annotation and Elaboration on Su Wen*）.

太阳主外　卫气的运行，起始于足太阳经而复会于足太阳经，故曰太阳主外。出《灵枢·营卫生会》。

太阳主外(tài yáng zhǔ wài) ***Taiyang* controls the exterior.** The circulation of defensive qi starts and also ends at the bladder meridian of foot *taiyang*，thus it is said that *taiyang* controls the exterior. See *Ling Shu* chapter 18.

太阳司天　运气术语。指上半年由太阳寒水之气主事时的气候病候等情况。凡纪年地支逢辰、戌之年，均属太阳寒水司天。该年上半年气候寒冷。水能制火，临床多见心病。出《素问·五常政大论》。

太阳司天（tài yáng sī tiān）
Taiyang **governs the heavens.** Terminology of circuits and qi. Refers to the climate，diseases and syndromes appearing when the qi of *taiyang* cold water is in domination in the first half of a year. In years with Earthly Branches such as *chen* and *xu*，it is the qi of *taiyang* cold water that governs the heavens. In the first half of the year，the climate is cold. Since water restrains fire，diseases of the heart are commonly seen clinically. See *Su Wen* chapter 70.

太阳司天之政　指太阳寒水司天的气候、物候及疾病流行情况，凡逢纪年地支是辰、戌的年份为太阳寒水司天，其特点是：太阳主寒，该年上半年气候寒冷。物候以豆、稷类谷物生长良好。鳞虫、倮虫生育良好，羽虫生育不利。临床多见心病、肾病及心肾同病等疾患。出《素问·六元正纪大论》。

太阳司天之政（tài yáng sī tiān zhī zhèng）　*Taiyang* **dominates the heavens.** Refers to the climate，phenology and epidemics of disease when the qi of the *taiyang* cold water governs the heavens. In years with Earthly Branches such as *chen* and *xu*，it is the qi of *taiyang* cold water that governs the heavens. It is cold in the first half of the year. In phenology，grains like beans and millets grow well；creatures with scales and those without hair develop well，while those with feathers do not. Clinically，diseases of the heart and kidney and concomitant diseases of these two organs are commonly seen. See *Su Wen* chapter 71.

太阳在泉　运气术语。指下半年由太阳寒水之气主事时的气候物候等情况。凡纪年地支逢丑、未之年均属太阳寒水在泉。该年下半年气候偏于寒冷，其所生长的药物或食物，在性味上也偏于寒凉，而具有温热作用的药食物则生长不良。出《素问·五常政大论》。

太阳在泉（tài yáng zài quán）　*Taiyang* **is in spring.** Terminology of circuits and qi. Refers to the climate and phenology when the qi of *taiyang* cold water is in domination in the second half of a year. In years with earthly branches such as *chou* and *wei*，it is the qi of *taiyang* cold water that is in spring. In the second half of the year, the climate is cold, and consequently, the drugs and food are cool or cold in property, and those that are warm or hot in property do not grow well. See *Su Wen* chapter 70.

太阳厥逆 十二经厥之一,为足太阳膀胱经气厥乱所致。症见仆倒、僵卧、呕血、衄血等。出《素问·厥论》。

太阳厥逆(tài yáng jué nì) *jue ni* (**syncope or cold limbs**) **of** *taiyang* One kind of *Jue ni* (syncope or cold limbs) of the twelve channels due to the reverse flow of qi. It is caused by adverse flow of qi of the bladder meridian of foot *taiyang*. Symptoms include falling down, lying stiff and motionless, vomiting blood and nosebleeds etc. See *Su Wen* chapter 45.

太阳寒化 运气术语。化,制化,制其生化之意。根据五行生克之理,太阳寒水之气,所以制约火热之气,不使过于偏胜,从而维持自然气候的正常,有利于万物的生长化成。出《素问·六元正纪大论》。

太阳寒化(tài yáng hán huà) **cold transformation of** *taiyang* Terminology of circuits and qi. Transformation means restriction and generation. According to the relationship of promoting and restraining of the five elements, the qi of *taiyang* cold water restrains the qi of fire heat, so that the latter cannot be in unilateral dominance and normality of climate in nature can be maintained, allowing for generation, growth, transformation and maturity of all things. See *Su Wen* chapter 71.

太阳藏 指太阳经脉。藏,指脏腑。脏腑与经脉相连属,言太阳经脉,必赅括其所属脏腑。出《素问·经脉别论》。

太阳藏(tài yáng zàng) *taiyang zang* **organ** Refers to the *taiyang* channel. *Zàng* refers to the viscera and bowels. Since the viscera and bowels are connected with their meridians, when talking about the *taiyang* meridian, mention of the connected viscera and bowels must also be mentioned. See *Su Wen* chapter 21.

太阴 ① 单指或统指手足太阴经脉及所属脏(脾、肺)。出《素问·太阴阳明论》。② 指肾。出《灵枢·九针十二原》。③ 指足之阴面内侧。出《灵枢·阴阳

四画

系日月》。④ 指六气中的湿气，主土。出《素问·五常政大论》。

太阴(tài yīn)　① Solely or generally refers to the *taiyin* meridians of the foot and hand and their respective viscera (spleen and lung). See *Su Wen* chapter 29. ② Refers to the kidney. See *Ling Shu* chapter 1. ③ Refers to the medial dorsal aspect of the foot. See *Ling Shu* chapter 41. ④ Refers to one of the six qi, the damp qi that belongs to earth in the five elements. See *Su Wen* chapter 70.

太阴之人　体质名，属五态之人中多阴无阳者。其人阴血混浊，卫气涩滞，阴阳不和，筋脉弛缓，皮肤厚，贪得无厌，看风使舵，藏而不露，外表色黑无泽，身材高大但不曲偻，故以疾泻为治疗原则。出《灵枢·通天》。

太阴之人(tài yīn zhī rén)　*taiyin-type people* Name of constitution, for those people characterized by the superabundance of yin and the absence of yang among the five types of people. These people have turbid yin blood, unsmooth defensive qi, an imbalance between yin and yang, loose tendons and thick skin. They are greedy, change their course for convenience and never show their true feelings. In appearance, they are characterized by a black and gloomy complexion, and are tall and straight stature. The disease of such people can be treated by needling with drastic reducing techniques. See *Ling Shu* chapter 72.

太阴之政　即太阴司天之政。出《素问·六元正纪大论》。

太阴之政(tài yīn zhī zhèng)　*taiyin in domination* Namely, *taiyin* dominating the heavens. See *Su Wen* chapter 71.

太阴之复　运气术语。复，即六气偏胜情况下而产生的复气。此指太阳寒水之气偏胜至一定程度，太阴湿土之气来复，气候变为暖湿、多雨。人体多见湿气偏盛之脾胃病。出《素问·至真要大论》。

太阴之复(tài yīn zhī fù)　*retaliation of taiyin* Terminology of circuits and qi. Retaliation refers to the revenging qi emerging when one of the six qi is in unilateral dominance. Here, it refers to when the qi of *taiyang* cold water is so exuberant that the qi of *taiyin* damp earth takes revenge，the climate changes to warm and damp with lots of rain，and the human body is prone to getting diseases of the spleen and stomach due to excessive damp qi. See *Su Wen* chapter 74.

太阴之胜　运气术语。指太阴湿土偏胜之气。如太阴司天、在泉之时,湿气偏盛,气候潮湿,降雨量多,人体多见湿病及脾胃病。出《素问·至真要大论》。

太阴之胜（tài yīn zhī shèng）**predominant taiyin** Terminology of circuits and qi. Refers to the predominant qi of *taiyin* damp earth. When *taiyin* dominates the heavens and it is in spring，the damp qi is exuberant with a wet climate and lots of rain，and people are prone to getting dampness diseases of the spleen and stomach. See *Su Wen* chapter 74.

太阴之厥　六经厥之一。为脾气不运,足太阴经气逆乱所致。症见腹满,纳少,食则呕,大便不利等。出《素问·厥论》。

太阴之厥（tài yīn zhī jué）*jue* **syndrome of taiyin** One kind of *jue* syndrome due to the reverse flow of qi of the six foot channels. It is caused by the impaired circulation of spleen qi due to adverse flow of qi of the spleen meridian of foot *taiyin*. Symptoms include abdominal distention，poor appetite，vomiting while eating and difficult defecation etc. See *Su Wen* chapter 45.

太阴司天　运气术语。指上半年由太阴湿土之气主事时的气候病候等情况。凡纪年地支逢丑、未之年,均属太阴湿土司天。该年上半年气候偏于潮湿,雨水较多。土能制水,临床多见肾病。出《素问·五常政大论》。

太阴司天（tài yīn sī tiān）*Taiyin* **governs the heavens.** Terminology of circuits and qi. Refers to the climate，diseases and syndromes of when the qi of *taiyin* damp earth is in domination in the first half of a year. In years with Earthly Branches such as *chou* and *wei*，it is the qi of *taiyin* damp earth that governs the heavens. In the first half of the year，the climate is wet with lots of rain，and as earth restrains water，diseases of the kidney are commonly seen clinically. See *Su Wen* chapter 70.

四画

太阴司天之政　指太阴湿土司天的气候、物候及疾病流行情况。凡逢纪年地支是丑、未的年份为太阴湿土司天,其特点是太阴主湿。该年上半年气候偏于潮湿,雨水较多。物候以稷、豆类谷物生长良好,倮虫、鳞虫生育良好,羽虫生育不利。临床多见脾湿之病及湿胜伤肾之病。政,主事,施政之意。出《素问·六元正纪大论》。

太阴司天之政(tài yīn sī tiān zhī zhèng) *Taiyin* dominates the heavens. Refers to the climate, phenology and epidemics of disease when the qi of *taiyin* damp earth governs the heavens. In years with Earthly Branches such as *chou* and *wei*, it is the qi of *taiyin* damp earth that governs the heavens and the first half of the year is wet with lots of rain. In phenology, grains like millet and beans grow well; creatures without hair and those with scales develop well, while those with feathers do not. Clinically speaking, diseases of the spleen and kidney are commonly seen due to the excess dampness. *Zhèng* refers to being in charge, or administration. See *Su Wen*

chapter 71.

太阴在泉　运气术语。指下半年由太阴湿土之气主事时的气候物候等情况。凡纪年地支逢辰、戌之年均属太阴湿土在泉。该年下半年气候偏湿、偏热,其所生食物、药物在性味上偏湿、偏温,而具有滋润作用的药食物则生长不良。出《素问·五常政大论》。

太阴在泉(tài yīn zài quán) *Taiyin* is in spring. Terminology of circuits and qi. Refers to the climate and phenology when the qi of *taiyin* damp earth is in domination in the second half of a year. In years with Earthly Branches such as *chen* and *xu*, it is the qi of *taiyin* damp earth that is in spring. In the second half of the year, the climate is damp and hot, and consequently, those drugs and foods that are damp or warm in property prosper, and those with nourishing properties do not grow well. See *Su Wen* chapter 70.

太阴阳明论　《素问》篇名。太阴,足太阴脾经;阳明,足阳明胃经。此篇专论脾胃两经在生理上以膜相连、表里相合,在病理上互相影响。故名。其内容侧重论脾,讨论了脾的主时,主四肢,为胃行其津液等问题。

太阴阳明论(tài yīn yáng míng lùn) **Discussion on *Taiyin* and *Yangming*** Chapter title in *Su Wen*. *Taiyin* refers to the spleen meridian of foot *taiyin*, and *yangming* refers to the stomach meridian of foot *yangming*. In this chapter, channels of the spleen and stomach are specifically discussed. The two organs are connected with a membrane physiologically, correlated on the interior and exterior, and pathologically influenced by each other. The spleen is paid special attention to, and the season and the limbs that it corresponds to are explored. Furthermore, it clearly details the promoting of the movement of fluids for the stomach.

太阴雨化 运气术语。雨,同湿义。化,制化,制则生化之意。根据五行生克原理,太阴湿土之气,可以制约寒水之气,不使过于偏胜,从而维持自然气候之正常,有利于万物生长化成。出《素问·六元正纪大论》。

太阴雨化(tài yīn yǔ huà) **rain transformation of *taiyin*** Terminology of circuits and qi. Rain means humidity, and transformation means restriction and generation. According to the relationship of promoting and restraining of the five elements, the qi of *taiyin* damp earth restrains the qi of cold water, therefore the latter can not be in unilateral dominance, and the climate can be maintained as normal. This is beneficial to the generation, growth, transformation and maturity of all living things. See *Su Wen* chapter 71.

太阴厥逆 十二经厥之一。为足太阴脾经气厥逆之证。症见下肢挛急,心痛,引腹等。出《素问·厥论》。

太阴厥逆(tài yīn jué nì) ***jueni*(syncope or cold limbs) of *taiyin*** One kind of *jueni*(syncope or cold limbs) due to reverse flow of qi in the twelve meridians. It is caused by the adverse flow of qi of the spleen meridian of foot *taiyin*. Symptoms include spasms in the lower limbs and heart pain involving the abdomen. See *Su Wen* chapter 45.

太阴藏 指太阴经脉。藏,指脏腑。脏腑与经脉相连属,言太阴经脉，必赅括其所属脏腑。出《素问·经脉别论》。

太阴藏（tài yīn zàng） *taiyin viscera* Refers to the *taiyin* meridian. *Zàng* refers to the viscera and bowels，and as the viscera and bowels are connected to their respective meridians，when speaking of the *taiyin* meridian，their connected viscera and bowels are naturally mentioned as well. See *Su Wen* chapter 21.

太羽 运气术语。水运太过之谓。羽，代表水运。太，太过。出《素问·六元正纪大论》。

太羽（tài yǔ） *tai yu* Terminology of circuits and qi indicating excessive water movement. *Yǔ* stands for water movement and *tài* means excessive. See *Su Wen* chapter 71.

太角 运气术语。木运太过之谓。角，木运；太，太过。出《素问·六元正纪大论》。

太角（tài jué） *tai jue* Terminology of circuits and qi indicating excessive wood movement. *Jué* stands for wood movement and *tài* means excessive. See *Su Wen* chapter 71.

太始天元册 古经名。出《素问·天元纪大论》。可能是一部古代的天象学的典籍。

太始天元册（tài shǐ tiān yuán cè） *Tai shi Tian Yuan Ce* An ancient classic. See *Su Wen* chapter 66. Perhaps an ancient classic on astronomy.

太宫 运气术语。土运太过之谓。宫，土运；太，太过。出《素问·六元正纪大论》。

太宫（tài gōng） *tai gong* Terminology of circuits and qi indicating excessive earth movement. *Gōng* stands for earth movement and *tài* means excessive. See *Su Wen* chapter 71.

太息 较为深长的呼吸。多因忧愤或胸脘不畅而作。出《灵枢·口问》。

太息（tài xī） *sigh* Taking a rather deep breath，mainly due to worry and indignation，or chest tightness，or stuffiness in the stomach. See *Ling Shu* chapter 28.

太虚 指天空。出《素问·天元纪大论》。

太虚（tài xū） *great void* Refers to the sky. See *Su Wen* chapter 66.

太商 运气术语。金运太过之谓。商，金运；太，太过。出《素问·六元正纪大论》。

太商（tài shāng） *tai shang* Terminology of circuits and qi indicating excessive metal movement. *Shāng* stands for metal movement and *tài* means excessive. See *Su Wen* chapter 71.

太渊 经穴名。手太阴肺经之腧穴，原穴，又名大泉，在鱼际后一寸陷中。出《灵枢·本输》。

太渊（tài yuān） **Tai Yuan（LU 9）** Acupoint name，belonging to the lung meridian of hand *taiyin*，and located in the depression one *cun* behind the thenar. It is a transport acupoint and a source acupoint，and is also called Da Quan. See *Ling Shu* chapter 2.

太溪 ① 经穴名。足少阴肾经之腧穴，原穴。别名吕细，内昆仑。在足内踝后侧跟骨之上，动脉陷者中。出《灵枢·本输》。② 指位于太溪穴处的肾经动脉，可诊察肾气的盛衰。出《素问·气交变大论》。

太溪（tài xī） ① Acupoint name，Tai Xi（KI 3）belongs to the kidney meridian of foot *shaoyin*. It is a transport acupoint and a source acupoint，and is also called Lü Xi or Nei Kun Lun. It is located above the calcaneus behind the medial malleolus，in the depression of the pulsating vessel. See *Ling Shu* chapter 2.

② Refers to the Tài Xī acupoint of the pulsating vessel of the kidney meridian of foot *shaoyin*，which can be used to determine either the exuberance or debilitation of kidney qi. See *Su Wen* chapter 69.

太徵 运气术语。火运太过之谓。徵，火运；太，太过。出《素问·六元正纪大论》。

太徵（tài zhǐ） *tai zhi* Terminology of circuits and qi indicating excessive fire movement. Zhǐ stands for fire circuit and *tài* means excessive. See *Su Wen* chapter 71.

太簇 阳六律之一，为羽音，即水音。出《素问·本病论》。

太簇（tài cù） *tai cu* One of the six yang pitch-pipes，or the *yu* sound，namely the sound of water. See *Su Wen* chapter 73.

巨气 大气，即人体正气。出《素问·汤液醪醴论》。

巨气（jù qì） **great qi** Major qi or vital qi of the human body. See *Su Wen* chapter 14.

巨分 上下牙床分合处，色诊上与大腿内侧相应。出《灵枢·五色》。

巨分（jù fēn） **grand section** Major crease on the angle of the mouth that corresponds to the medial sides of the thighs in the examination of complexions. See *Ling Shu* chapter 49.

巨阳 即太阳。巨，大也。"大"与"太"通。指手、足太阳经脉。出《素问·热论》。

巨阳（jù yáng） *juyang* Namely *taiyang*. *Jù* means "大"（great）. "大" is the same as "太", and refers to the *taiyang* channels of the foot and hand. See *Su Wen* chapter 31.

巨阳之厥 六经厥之一。巨阳，即太阳。太阳经气逆乱所致。症见头肿、头重、眩晕欲仆等。出《素问·厥论》。

巨阳之厥（jù yáng zhī jué） *jue syndrome of juyang* One kind of *jue* syndrome due to reverse flow of qi of the six foot channels. *Juyang* is namely *taiyang*. This syndorme is caused by the adverse flow of qi of the bladder meridian of foot *taiyang*. Symptoms include swelling and heaviness of the head, and dizziness and shaking as if about to fall. See *Su Wen* chapter 45.

巨针 古代针具之一，即九针中之大针。出《灵枢·热病》。

巨针（jù zhēn） **large needle** One of the needles in ancient China, that is the big needle among the nine needles. See *Ling Shu* chapter 23.

巨刺 九刺法之一种，左病取右，右病取左而刺其大经的交叉刺法。与缪刺之左右交叉刺而刺其络者不同。出《灵枢·官针》。

巨刺（jù cì） *ju needling* One of the nine needling methods. That is, to treat a disease in the left part of the body by needling the acupoints on main channels located on the right part of the body, and to treat a disease in the right part of the body by needling the acupoints on main channels located on the left part of the body. This is different from *miuci*（contralateral collateral needling）characterized by the needling of acupoints on collaterals at the right side to treat diseases on the left side, and needling the acupoints on collaterals on the left side for treating diseases on the right side. See *Ling Shu* chapter 7.

巨屈 颊下曲骨处，相当颊车穴部位。面部色诊用以测候膝部的状况。出《灵枢·五色》。

巨屈（jù qū） **grand curvature** Curved bones below the cheeks （at the *Jia Che* acupoint）that correspond to the knees in the examination of complexions. See *Ling Shu* chapter 49.

巨骨　手阳明大肠经穴名，在肩端肩胛骨与锁骨间之凹陷处。出《素问·气府论》。

巨骨（jù gǔ）　**Ju Gu (LI 16)** The name of an acupoint belonging to the large intestine meridian of hand *yangming*. It is located in the depression at the shoulder end between the shoulder blade and the collarbone. See *Su Wen* chapter 59.

巨虚　小腿胫骨外侧筋骨间凹陷处均可称巨虚。出《素问·针解》。

巨虚（jù xū）　*ju xu* The depression at the lateral muscles and bones of the tibia. See *Su Wen* chapter 54.

巨虚下廉　经穴名。属足阳明胃经，又称下巨虚。为小肠之下合穴。在足三里直下六寸处，胫骨外侧。出《灵枢·本输》。

巨虚下廉（jù xū xià lián）　**Ju Xu Xia Lian (ST 39)** Acupoint name, belonging to the stomach meridian of foot *yangming*, and also called Xia Ju Xu (ST 39). It is related to the small intestine and is located six *cun* directly below Zu San Li (ST

36) at the lateral aspect of the tibia. See *Ling Shu* chapter 2.

巨虚上下廉　即巨虚上廉、巨虚下廉。出《素问·气穴论》。

巨虚上下廉（jù xū shàng xià lián）　**the upper and lower borders of Ju Xu** The upper border and the lower border of Ju Xu. See *Ling Shu* chapter 58.

巨虚上廉　经穴名。属足阳明胃经，又称上巨虚。与大肠之下合穴。在足三里下三寸。出《灵枢·本输》。

巨虚上廉（jù xū shàng lián）　**Ju Xu Shang Lian (ST 37)** Acupoint name, belonging to the stomach meridian of foot *yangming*, which is also called Shang Ju Xu (ST 37). It is related to the large intestine and located three *cun* below Zu San Li (ST 36). See *Ling Shu* chapter 2.

牙车　下颚骨，俗称下牙床。出《灵枢·五色》。

牙车（yá chē）　**gums** The lower jaw, or the lower gum. See *Ling Shu* chapter 49.

切而散之　言针刺虚证应用补法的辅助手法，是用手抚摸穴位后，指头切撤其穴，使经气布散。出《素问·离合真邪论》。

切而散之（qiē ér sàn zhī）　**feeling the acupoint to disperse**

qi Auxiliary maneuvers used in tonifying acupuncture therapy to treat deficiency syndrome, in which the hand palpates to locate the acupoint, then squeezes it and disperses the channel qi from it. See *Su Wen* chapter 27.

切痛 痛如刀切。出《灵枢·邪气藏府病形》。

切痛（qiē tòng） **cutting pain** Pain as if being cut with a knife. See *Ling Shu* chapter 4.

少 ①（哨 shào）年轻人。出《灵枢·卫气失常》。②（嫂 sǎo）不足。出《素问·评热病论》。③ 指运气不及。出《素问·六元正纪大论》。

少（shào） ① When it is pronounced *shào*, it refers to young people. See *Ling Shu* chapter 59. ②（sǎo）When it is pronounced *shǎo*, it means lack. See *Su Wen* chapter 33. ③（shǎo）Refers to not enough circuits and qi. See *Su Wen* chapter 71.

少水 少,不足之意。水属阴,肾为水脏。少水。指肾阴虚。出《素问·逆调论》。

少水（shào shuǐ） **deficient water** *Shào* refers to insufficient, or deficiency. Water belongs to yin, and the kidney is the viscera belongs to water. Deficient water refers to kidney yin deficiency. See *Su Wen* chapter 34.

少气 ① 气虚衰少。出《素问·平人气象论》。② 呼吸气短。出《素问·三部九候论》。

少气（shǎo qì） ① Insufficiency of qi. See *Su Wen* chapter 18. ② Shortness of breath. See *Su Wen* chapter 20.

少火 出《素问·阴阳应象大论》。(1) 药食气味温和者为少火。见《素问注证发微》。(2) 平和的阳气,属生理之火。见《类经·阴阳一》。

少火（shào huǒ） **mild fire** See *Su Wen* chapter 5. (1) Herbs and food that are mild in property belong to mild fire. See *Su Wen Zhu Zheng Fa Wei* (*Annotation and Elaboration on Su Wen*). (2) Peaceful yang qi, belongs to physiological fire. See *Lei Jing* (*Classified Classic*) "Yin and Yang Chapter 1".

少火之气壮 气味温和的药食属少火,食之能使正气壮盛。出《素问·阴阳应象大论》。

少火之气壮（shào huǒ zhī qì zhuàng） **Mild fire strengthens the qi.** Herbs with a mild flavor belong to mild fire. Healthy qi can be strengthened by ingesting mild herbs. See *Su Wen* chapter 5.

少火生气 义同"少火之气壮"。出《素问·阴阳应象大论》。

少火生气(shào huǒ shēng qì) **Mild fire supplements the qi.** The same meaning as 少火之气壮. See *Su Wen* chapter 5.

少师 传说中上古时代的医家,为黄帝之臣。出《灵枢·寿夭刚柔》。

少师(shào shī) **Shao Shi** A legendary physician in ancient China and one of the ministers of the Yellow Emperor. See *Ling Shu* chapter 6.

少阳 ① 指肝。出《灵枢·九针十二原》。② 指一阳。出《素问·阴阳类论》。③ 指足少阳胆、手少阳三焦。出《素问·经脉别论》。④ 指之阳面外侧。出《灵枢·阴阳系日月》。⑤ 指六气中之相火。出《素问·六元正纪大论》。

少阳(shào yáng) ① Refers to the liver. See *Ling Shu* chapter 1. ② Refers to the first yang. See *Su Wen* chapter 79. ③ Refers to the gallbladder meridian of foot *shaoyang* and the triple *jiao* meridian of hand *shaoyang*. See *Su Wen* chapter 21. ④ Refers to the lateral dorsal aspect of the foot. See *Ling Shu* chapter 41. ⑤ Refers to the ministerial fire in the six qi. See *Su Wen* chapter 71.

少阳之人 体质名,属五态之人中多阳少阴者。其人善于观察,企攀权贵,自高自大,乐于交际,外表站立时好仰头,行走时身体摇摆,两臂常反背在身后。故治疗以实阴泻阳为原则,但注意不可单独泻阳太过,以避免阳气耗脱,中气不足。出《灵枢·通天》。

少阳之人(shào yáng zhī rén) *shaoyang*-type people Name of constitution, of those people characterized by excessive yang and insufficient yin among the five types of people. These people are observant, tufthunting, arrogant and sociable. In appearance, they like to raise their head high when standing, and sway their body when walking, with their hands clasped behind their back. To treat such people, the doctor reinforces the yin and reduces the yang. However, the yang qi in the collaterals is not to be over reduced, so as to avoid the exhaustion of yang qi and the insufficiency of middle qi. See *Ling Shu* chapter 72.

少阳之政 即少阳司天之政。出《素问·六元正纪大论》。

少阳之政（shào yáng zhī zhèng）*shaoyang* in domination Namely, *shaoyang* dominating the heavens. See *Su Wen* chapter 71.

少阳之复 运气术语。复，即六气偏胜情况下而产生的复气。此指阳明燥金之气偏胜至一定程度，少阳相火之气来复，气温由凉转热，人体多见热气偏胜，五脏内热之病。出《素问·至真要大论》。

少阳之复（shào yáng zhī fù）**retaliation of *shaoyang*** Terminology of circuits and qi, in which "retaliation" refers to the revenging qi emerging, when one of the six qi is in unilateral dominance. Here, it refers to when the qi of the *yangming* dry metal is so exuberant that the qi of the *shaoyang* ministerial fire takes revenge, and the climate changes from cool to hot, causing the body to becoming prone to diseases of internal heat of the five viscera due to exuberant heat qi. See *Su Wen* chapter 74.

少阳之胜 运气术语。指少阳相火偏胜之气。如少阳司天在泉之时，火气偏盛，气候炎热，人体多见火热之气偏盛之心、胃病变。出《素问·至真要大论》。

少阳之胜（shào yáng zhī shèng）**predominance of *shaoyang*** Terminology of circuits and qi. Refers to the predominance of *shaoyang* ministerial fire qi. When *shaoyang* dominates the heavens and it is in spring, the fire qi is exuberant with a hot climate which invades the human body causing diseases of the heart and stomach. See *Su Wen* chapter 74.

少阳之维 维，络也。少阳之维，即足少阳胆经之络穴光明。出《素问·骨空论》。

少阳之维（shào yáng zhī wéi）**collaterals of *shaoyang*** *Wéi* means connection and refers to the connecting acupoint Guang Ming（GB 37）on the gallbladder meridian of foot *shaoyang*. See *Su Wen* chapter 60.

少阳之厥 六经厥之一。为足少阳胆经气逆乱。症见耳聋、颊肿、胁痛等。出《素问·厥论》。

少阳之厥（shào yáng zhī jué）***jue* syndrome of *shaoyang*** One of *jue* syndromes due to the reverse flow of qi of the six foot meridians. This syndrome is caused by the adverse flow of qi of the gallbladder meridian of foot *shaoyang*, and the symptoms include deafness, buccal swelling and hypochondriac pain etc. See *Su Wen* chapter 45.

少阳为枢　少阳在表里之间,转输阳气,犹枢轴之作用。出《灵枢·根结》。

少阳为枢(shào yáng wéi shū) ***Shaoyang* is responsible for pivoting.** *Shaoyang* is located between the exterior and the interior, and transfers yang qi, thus acting as a pivot. See *Ling Shu* chapter 5.

少阳主胆　足少阳经属胆络肝,故云。出《素问·热论》。

少阳主胆(shào yáng zhǔ dǎn) ***Shaoyang* governs the gallbladder.** The gallbladder meridian of foot *shaoyang* pertains to the gallbladder and connects with the liver. See *Su Wen* chapter 31.

少阳司天　运气术语。指上半年由少阳相火之气主事时的气候病候等情况。凡纪年地支逢寅、申之年,均属少阳相火司天。该年上半年气候偏热,火气偏胜。火盛刑金,临床多见肺病热证。出《素问·五常政大论》。

少阳司天(shào yáng sī tiān) ***Shaoyang* governs the heavens.** Terminology of circuits and qi. Refers to climate, diseases and syndromes occurs when the qi of the *shaoyang* ministerial fire is in domination in the first half of a year. In years with Earthly Branches such as *yin* and *shen*, the qi of the *shaoyang* ministerial fire governs the heavens. In the first half of the year, fire qi is exuberant and the climate is hot. As fire restrains metal, diseases of the lung are commonly seen clinically, due to heat. See *Su Wen* chapter 70.

少阳司天之政　政,主事,施政之意。指少阳相火司天的气候、物候及疾病流行情况。凡逢纪年地支是寅、申的年份为少阳相火司天。其特点是少阳主火,气候是火气偏胜。该年上半年气候偏热。物候上是以麦、麻类植物生长良好,羽虫、毛虫生育良好,倮虫生育不利。临床多见心肺热病和肺脾失调等疾病。出《素问·六元正纪大论》。

少阳司天之政(shào yáng sī tiān zhī zhèng) ***Shaoyang* dominates the heavens.** *Zhèng* refers to being in charge, or administration. It refers to the climate, phenology and epidemics of disease when the qi of the *shaoyang* ministerial fire governs the heavens. In years with Earthly Branches such as *yin* and *shen*, the qi of the *shaoyang* ministerial fire governs the heavens, the climate with full of fire qi, and it is hot in the first half of the year. In phenology, grains like wheat, hemp and flax grow well; creatures with feathers and those with hair develop well, while those without hair do not. Clinically speaking, heat diseases of the heart and lung, and disorders of the lung and spleen are commonly seen. See *Su Wen* chapter 71.

少阳在泉 运气术语。指下半年由少阳相火之气主事时的气候物候等情况。凡纪年地支逢巳、亥之年,均属少阳相火在泉。该年下半年气候偏热。其所生成的食物或药物,在气味上也偏于湿热。而具有寒凉作用的药食物则生长不良。出《素问·五常政大论》。

少阳在泉(shào yáng zài quán) *Shaoyang* is in spring. Terminology of circuits and qi. Refers to climate and phenology when the qi of the *shaoyang* ministerial fire is in domination in the second half of a year. In years with Earthly Branches such as *si* and *hai*, the qi of the *shaoyang* ministerial fire is in spring. In the second half of the year, the climate is hot, and consequently, drugs and foods are damp and hot in property, whereas those that are cold or cool in property do not grow well. See *Su Wen* chapter 70.

少阳厥 病名。由手足少阳经气上逆而见耳鸣的病证。出《素问·经脉别论》。

少阳厥(shào yáng jué) *shaoyang jue* A disease or syndrome manifesting with tinnitus due to the adverse flow of qi of the *shaoyang* meridian of the foot and hand. See *Su Wen* chapter 21.

少阳厥逆 十二经厥之一。为足少阳经气厥逆之证。出《素问·厥论》。

少阳厥逆(shào yáng jué nì) *jue ni* (syncope or cold limbs) of *shaoyang* meridian One of the kinds of *Jue ni* (syncope or cold limbs) due to the reverse flow of qi of the twelve channels. It is caused by the adverse flow of the qi of the meridian of foot *shaoyang*. See *Su Wen* chapter 45.

少阳藏 指少阳经脉。藏,指脏腑,脏腑与经脉相连属,说到少阳经脉,必赅括其所属脏腑。出《素问·经脉别论》。

少阳藏（shào yáng zàng）
shaoyang zang **organ** Refers to the *shaoyang* meridian. *Zàng* refers to the viscera and bowels. Since the viscera and bowels are connected with their respective channels, when speaking of *shaoyang*, the connected viscera and bowels must also be mentioned. See *Su Wen* chapter 21.

少阴 ① 指手、足少阴心肾及其经脉。出《素问·诊要经终论》。② 指肺。出《灵枢·九针十二原》。③ 指手之阴面内侧。出《灵枢·阴阳系日月》。④ 指六气中君火之气,主热。出《素问·五常政大论》。

少阴（shào yīn） ① Refers to the foot and hand *shaoyin* meridian and their connected viscera（heart and kidney）. See *Su Wen* chapter 16. ② Refers to the lung. See *Ling Shu* chapter 1. ③ Refers to the medial palmar aspect of the hand. See

Ling Shu chapter 41. ④ Refers to one of the six qi, the monarch fire that governs heat. See *Su Wen* chapter 70.

少阴之人 体质名,属五态之人中多阴少阳者。其人小胃而大肠,六腑不调,阳明脉小,太阳脉大,心胸狭窄,无同情心,好嫉妒,急躁贪心,外表清高,但行动诡秘,出没无常。其气血易败脱,故治疗必须仔细审察而调摄之。出《灵枢·通天》。

少阴之人（shào yīn zhī rén）
shaoyin-**type people** Name of constitution, of those people characterized by superabundant yin and less yang among the five types of people. These people have small stomachs and large intestines, an imbalance of the six bowels, a weakness of the channel qi of foot *yangming* and forcefulness of the channel qi of hand *taiyang*. They are narrow-minded, unsympathetic, jealous, impatient and greedy. They look aloof but behave furtively. To treat such people, the doctor must be careful in diagnosis and treatment. These kinds of people suffer easily from loss of blood and consumption of qi. See *Ling Shu*

四画

chapter 72.

少阴之政 即少阴司天之政。出《素问·六元正纪大论》。

少阴之政（shào yīn zhī zhèng） *shaoyin in domination Shaoyin* dominates the heavens. See *Su Wen* chapter 71.

少阴之复 运气术语。复，即六气偏胜情况下而产生的复气。此指阳明燥金凉气偏胜至一定程度，少阴君火之气来复，气温由凉转热。人体临床多见热气偏胜，五脏内热，疮疡类疾患。出《素问·至真要大论》。

少阴之复（shào yīn zhī fù） **retaliation of shaoyin** Terminology of circuits and qi, in which "retaliation" refers to the revenging qi emerging when one of the six qi is in unilateral dominance. Here, it means when the qi of the *yangming* dry metal is so exuberant that the qi of the *shaoyin* monarch fire takes revenge, the climate changes from cool to hot, and the human body is prone to getting sores and ulcer diseases caused by the internal heat of the five viscera due to exuberant heat qi. See *Su Wen* chapter 74.

少阴之胜 运气术语。指少阴君火偏胜之气。如少阴君火司天、在泉之时，热气偏盛，气候偏热，人体多见心气偏胜之心病。出《素问·至真要大论》。

少阴之胜（shào yīn zhī shèng） **predominant shaoyin** Terminology of circuits and qi. Refers to the predominant qi of the *shaoyin* monarch fire. When the *shaoyin* monarch fire dominates the heavens and it is in spring, the heat qi is exuberant with a hot climate, and people are prone to getting diseases of the heart due to exuberant heart fire. See *Su Wen* chapter 74.

少阴之厥 六经厥之一。为足少阴经气机逆乱所致。症见口干、尿赤、腹满、心痛等。出《素问·厥论》。

少阴之厥（shào yīn zhī jué） **jue syndrome of shaoyin** One kind of *jue* syndrome due to reverse flow of qi of the six foot channels. It is caused by the adverse flow of qi of the kidney meridian of foot *shaoyin*. The symptoms include dry mouth, reddish urine, abdominal fullness and heart pain. See *Su Wen* chapter 45.

少阴为枢 三阴中，太阴主阴之表，厥阴主阴之里，少阴居阴分之中，为出入之枢纽。出《灵枢·根结》。

少阴为枢（shào yīn wéi shū）
Shaoyin is responsible for pivoting. Among the three yin meridians, *taiyin* governs the exterior of yin, *jueyin* governs the interior of yin, and *shaoyin* is located between both *taiyin* and *jueyin*, acting as a pivot. See *Ling Shu* chapter 5.

少阴司天 运气术语。指上半年由少阴君火之气主事时的气候病候等情况。凡纪年地支逢子、午之年，均属少阴君火司天。该年上半年气候偏热。火能刑金，临床多见肺病热证。出《素问·五常政大论》。

少阴司天（shào yīn sī tiān）
Shaoyin governs the heavens. Terminology of circuits and qi. Refers to the climate, diseases and syndromes when the qi of the *shaoyin* monarch fire is in domination in the first half of a year. In years with Earthly Branches such as *zi* and *wu*, it is the qi of the *shaoyin* monarch fire that governs the heavens. In the first half of the year, the climate is hot. Since fire restrains metal, lung diseases due to excess heat is commonly seen clinically. See *Su Wen* chapter 70.

少阴司天之政 政，主事，施政之意。指少阴君火司天的气候、物候及疾病流行情况。凡逢纪年地支子、午的年份为少阴君火司天，其特点是少阴主热，气候是热气偏胜，该年上半年偏热。物候以麦、稻谷类植物生长良好，羽虫、介虫生育良好，毛虫生育不利。临床多见心火亢盛，乘金伤肺等症状。出《素问·六元正纪大论》。

少阴司天之政（shào yīn sī tiān zhī zhèng）
Shaoyin dominates the heavens. *Zhèng* refers to being in charge, or administration. It refers to the climate, phenology and epidemics of disease when the qi of the *shaoyin* monarch fire governs the heavens. In years with Earthly Branches such as *zi* and *wu*, it is the qi of the *shaoyin* monarch fire that governs the heavens. *Shaoyin* governs heat, therefore the heat qi is exuberant, and the climate is hot in the first half of the year. In phenology, grains like wheat and rice grow well; creatures with feathers and those with shells grow well, while caterpillars do not. Clinically speaking, diseases due to

the impairment of the lung by exuberant heart fire that restrains metal is commonly seen. See *Su Wen* chapter 71.

少阴在泉　运气术语。指下半年由少阴君火之气主事时的气候物候等情况。凡纪年地支逢卯、酉之年均属少阴君火在泉。该年下半年气候偏热，其所生的食物、药物，在性味上偏热，而具有寒凉作用的药食物则生长不良。出《素问·五常政大论》。

少阴在泉（shào yīn zài quán）*Shaoyin* is in spring. Terminology of circuits and qi. Refers to climate and phenology when the qi of the *shaoyin* monarch fire is in domination in the second half of a year. In years with Earthly Branches such as *mao* and *you*, it is the qi of the *shaoyin* monarch fire that is in spring. In the second half of the year, the climate is hot, and consequently, drugs and foods hot in property prosper, whereas those which are cooling in property do not grow well. See *Su Wen* chapter 70.

少阴脉　足少阴肾经，其脉从肾上贯膈，入肺中，循喉咙，挟舌本。出《素问·热论》。

少阴脉（shào yīn mài）　*Shaoyin* **Meridian** Namely, the kidney meridian of foot *shaoyin*. It ascends and passes through the diaphragm from above the kidney. Then it enters the lung, runs upwards to the throat and terminates at the root of the tongue. See *Su Wen* chapter 31.

少阴独无腧　指《灵枢·本输》记载了十一经的五输穴，独手少阴心经未列出，故曰。出《灵枢·邪客》。

少阴独无腧（shào yīn dú wú shū）**Heart meridian of hand** *shaoyin* **is without transport acupoints.** Refers to *Ling Shu* chapter 2, the five transport acupoints of the eleven meridians are recorded, but those of the heart meridian of hand *shaoyin* are not mentioned. See *Ling Shu* chapter 71.

少阴热化　运气术语。化，制化，制则生化之意。根据五行生克之理，少阴君火之气可以制约凉燥之金气，不使过于偏胜，从而维持自然气候的正常，有利于万物的生长化成。出《素问·六元正纪大论》。

少阴热化（shào yīn rè huà）**heat transformation of** *shaoyin* Terminology of circuits and qi, in which "transformation" means restriction and generation. According to the relationship of promoting and restraining of the five elements，the qi of the *shaoyin* monarch fire restrains the qi of the cool and dry metal，thus the latter cannot be in unilateral dominance and normality of climate in nature can be maintained，allowing for generation，growth，transformation and the maturity of all things. See *Su Wen* chapter 71.

少阴厥逆 十二经厥之一。因足少阴肾经气厥逆所致。症见呕吐泄利等。出《素问·厥论》。

少阴厥逆（shào yīn jué nì） *jue ni*（**syncope or cold limbs**）**of** *shaoyin* One kind of *jue ni*（syncope or cold limbs）which arises due to the reverse flow of qi of the twelve channels. It is caused by the adverse flow of qi of the kidney meridian of foot *shaoyin*，and symptoms include vomiting and diarrhea. See *Su Wen* chapter 45.

少羽 ① 体质名。阴阳二十五人中水形人之一种。出《灵枢·五音五味》。② 运气名。指水运不及之年。出《素问·五常政大论》。③ 运气中五步推运之运步。出《素问·六元正纪大论》。

少羽（shào yǔ） ① Name of constitution，for people with a water type constitution out of the twenty-five types of people divided according to yin and yang. See *Ling Shu* chapter 65. ② Terminology of circuits and qi，and refers to a year with insufficient water movement. See *Su Wen* chapter 70. ③ The five step calculation of the steps in movement within the circuits and qi theory. See *Su Wen* chapter 71.

少羽之人 体质名。羽，五音之一，五行属水。少羽，羽音之一，此代表阴阳二十五人中水形人之一种，其特征是心情郁闷不舒。出《灵枢·阴阳二十五人》。

少羽之人（shào yǔ zhī rén） *shaoyu*-type people Name of constitution. *Yǔ* is one of the five sounds and pertains to water in the five elements. *Shào yǔ* is one of the *yu* sounds，and people belonging to the water type constitution，of the twenty-five types of people divided according to yin and yang，are characterized by a depressed mood. See *Ling Shu* chapter 64.

四画

少角　① 运气术语。谓木运不及。角,木运。少,不及。见《素问·五常政大论》。② 五音所属人的体质类型之一。属木形体质。出《灵枢·五音五味》。

少角(shào jué)　*shao jue* Terminology of circuits and qi. Refers to deficient wood movement. *Jué* stands for wood movement, and *shào* means deficient. See *Su Wen* chapter 71. ② One of the body constitutions categorized by the five sounds. People with this constitution belong to the wood type. See *Ling Shu* chapter 65.

少泽　经穴名。手太阳小肠经之井穴。在手小指外侧端。出《灵枢·本输》。

少泽(shào zé)　**Shao Ze（SI 1）** Acupoint name of the well acupoint on the small intestine meridian of hand *taiyang*. It is located laterally at the tip of the little finger. See *Ling Shu* chapter 2.

少俞　传说中上古时代的医家,黄帝之臣。出《灵枢·五变》。

少俞(shào shū)　**Shao Shu** A legendary physician in ancient China and one of the ministers of the Yellow Emperor. See *Ling Shu* chapter 46.

少宫　① 体质名。阴阳二十五人中土形人之一种。出《灵枢·五音五味》。② 运气名。指土运不及之年。出《素问·五常政大论》。③ 运气五步推运中土运不及之运步。出《素问·六元正纪大论》。

少宫(shào gōng)　① Name of constitution. People with this constitution belong to the earth type of people among the twenty-five types of people divided according to yin and yang. See *Ling Shu* chapter 65. ② Terminology of circuits and qi. Refers to the year with insufficiency of earth movement. See *Su Wen* chapter 70. ③ The five step calculation of the steps in movement within the circuits and qi theory indicating insufficient earth movement. See *Su Wen* chapter 71.

少宫之人　体质名。宫,五音之一,五行属土。少宫,宫音之一,此代表阴阳二十五人中土形人之一种,其特征是比较圆滑。出《灵枢·阴阳二十五人》。

少宫之人(shào gōng zhī rén)　*shaogong*-type people Name of constitution. *Gong* is one of the five sounds and pertains to earth in the five elements. *Shao* *gong* is one of the *gong* sounds. *Shao gong* people belong to the earth type of people among the twenty-five types of people divided according to yin and yang, and are tactful. See *Ling Shu* chapter 64.

少海　经穴名。手少阴心经之合穴,别名曲节,在肘内廉节后陷者中。出《灵枢·根结》。

少海(shào hǎi)　**Shao Hai（HT 3）** Acupoint name. Refers to the *he*-sea acupoint on the heart meridian of hand *shaoyin*, and also called Qu Jie. It is located in the depression behind the elbow at the inner side of the upper arm. See *Ling Shu* chapter 5.

少商　① 经穴名。属于太阴肺经,为本经井穴。在拇指桡侧指甲角旁约 0.1 寸处。出《灵枢·本输》。② 运气名。指金运不及之年。出《素问·五常政大论》。③ 运气五步推运中的运步,表示金运不及。出《素问·六元正纪大论》。④ 体质名。阴阳二十五人中金形人之一种。出《灵枢·五音五味》。

少商(shào shāng)　① Acupoint name, Shao Shang（LU 11）, which is the well acupoint of the lung meridian of hand *taiyin*. It is located approximately 0.1

cun next to the corner of the thumbnail at the radial aspect. See *Ling Shu* chapter 2. ② Terminology of circuits and qi. Refers to a year with insufficient of metal movement. See *Su Wen* chapter 70. ③ The five step calculation of the steps in movement within the circuits and qi theory indicating insufficiency of metal circuit. See *Su Wen* chapter 71. ④ Name of constitution. The metal-type people among the twenty-five types of people divided according to yin and yang. See *Ling Shu* chapter 65.

少商之人　体质名。商,五音之一,五行属金。少商,商音之一,此代表阴阳二十五人中金形人之一种,其特征是威严而庄重。出《灵枢·阴阳二十五人》。

少商之人(shào shāng zhī rén) *shaoshang*-type people Name of constitution. *Shāng* is one of the five sounds and pertains to metal in the five elements. *Shao shang* is one of the *shang* sounds. *Shaoshang*-type people belong to the metal-type people among the twenty-five types of people divided according to yin and yang, and are dignified and solemn. See *Ling Shu* chapter 64.

少腹 又称小腹，腹部脐下部分。出《素问·举痛论》。

少腹（shào fù）　**lower abdomen** Also known as the lower abdomen, the part of the abdomen below the umbilicus. See *Su Wen* chapter 39.

少瞑 不想睡眠。出《灵枢·大惑论》。

少瞑（shào míng）　**sleeplessness** No desire to go to bed. See *Ling Shu* chapter 80.

少徵 ① 体质名。阴阳二十五人中火形人之一种。出《灵枢·五音五味》。② 运气名。指火运不及之年。出《素问·六元正纪大论》。③ 运气五步推运中的运步，表示火运不及。出《素问·六元正纪大论》。

少徵（shào zhǐ）　① Name of constitution. Refers to the fire-type people among the twenty-five types of people divided according to yin and yang. See *Ling Shu* chapter 65. ② Terminology of circuits and qi and refers to the year with insufficient fire movement. See *Su Wen* chapter 71. ③ The five step calculation of the steps in movement within the circuits and qi theory indicating insufficient fire movement. See *Su Wen* chapter 71.

少徵之人 体质名。徵（zhǐ 指），五音之一，五行属火。少徵，徵音之一，此代表阴阳二十五人中火形人之一种，其特征是多疑。出《灵枢·阴阳二十五人》。

少徵之人（shào zhǐ zhī rén）　*shaozhi*-type people Name of constitution. *Zhǐ* is one of the five sounds and pertains to fire in the five elements. *Shào zhǐ* is one of the *zhi* sounds. *Shao-zhi*-type people belong to the fire type among the twenty-five types of people divided according to yin and yang, and they are of suspicious nature. See *Ling Shu* chapter 64.

日华气 日初出之精气。出《素问·刺法论》。

日华气（rì huá qì）　**solar essence** Essence qi at sunrise. See *Su Wen* chapter 72.

日昳 午后未时，为土旺之时。出《素问·藏气法时论》。

日昳（rì dié）　**afternoon** *Wei* period in the afternoon, i.e. 1 p.m. to 3 p.m., when earth qi is vigorous. See *Su Wen* chapter 22.

中工 指医术中等的医生。其只能将察色、辨脉、诊尺肤三法中的二法结合起来,治愈率是十分之七。出《灵枢·邪气藏府病形》。

中工（zhōng gōng）**mediocre practitioner** Doctors with mediocre medical skills who only practice two of the three methods（examination of complexion, pulse differentiation and examination of cubital skin）in diagnosing disease, and who treat patients with a cure rate of 70%. See *Ling Shu* chapter 4.

中气 ① 指中焦脾胃之气。出《灵枢·口问》。② 运气术语。又称中见之气。是在本气之中可以见到的气,即六气变化至一定程度时向相反方面转化的气。如太阳与少阴,其气表里互通,可以相互转化而互为中气。出《素问·至真要大论》。③ 肠胃之气。出《素问·痹论》。

中气（zhōng qì） ① Refers to the qi of the spleen and stomach in the middle *jiao*. See *Ling Shu* chapter 28. ② Terminology of circuits and qi, and also named the qi of *zhong jian*. It is the qi that can be seen in one of the six qi, which transforms to the opposite direction when changing to a certain extent. For instance, the qi of *taiyang* and *shaoyin* are connected in the exterior and the interior, and the two kinds of qi are in the middle qi of each other. See *Su Wen* chapter 74. ③ Qi of the intestine and stomach. See *Su Wen* chapter 43.

中风 为风邪所伤害。中,伤也。出《灵枢·邪气藏府病形》。

中风（zhòng fēng） **wind attack** Attack by pathogenic wind. *Zhòng* refers to being attacked by something. See *Ling Shu* chapter 4.

中正之官 指胆。出《素问·灵兰秘典论》。

中正之官（zhōng zhèng zhī guān） **official of justice** Refers to the gallbladder. See *Su Wen* chapter 8.

中古 《内经》将时代划分为上古、中古、今世。中古为上古与今世之间者。出《素问·移精变气论》。

中古（zhōng gǔ） **middle antiquity** In *Nei Jing*（*Internal Classic*）, time is divided into remote antiquity, middle antiquity and the modern time. Middle antiquity is between remote antiquity and the modern time. See *Su Wen* chapter 13.

中冲 经穴名。手厥阴心包经之

井穴。在手中指的尖端。出《灵枢·本输》。

中冲（zhōng chōng）　**Zhong Chong (PC 9)** Acupoint name and is the well acupoint of the pericardium meridian of hand *jueyin*. It is located at the tip of the middle finger. See *Ling Shu* chapter 2.

中运　运气术语。统主一年的五运之气，又称岁运、大运。凡逢甲、己之年为土运所统，逢乙、庚之年为金运所统，逢丙、辛之年为水运所统，逢丁、壬之年为木运所统，逢戊、癸之年为火运所统。出《素问·刺法论》。

中运（zhōng yùn）　**central motion** Terminology of circuits and qi and refers to the qi of the five circuits that governs the whole year. It is also called annual or overall circuit. Years with Heavenly Stems such as *jia* and *ji* are governed by the earth circuit, those with Heavenly Stems such as *yi* and *geng* are governed by the metal circuit, those with Heavenly Stems such as *bing* and *xin* are governed by the water circuit, those with Heavenly Stems such as *ding* and *ren* are governed by the wood circuit, and those with Heavenly Stems such as *wu* and *gui* are governed by the fire circuit. See *Su Wen* chapter 72.

中极　经穴名。属任脉，为膀胱之募穴，在腹正中线当脐下四寸处。出《素问·骨空论》。

中极（zhōng jí）　**Zhong Ji (CV 3)** Acupoint name belonging to the conception vessel，and is the front-mu acupoint of the bladder. It is located at four *cun* below the umbilicus along the midline of abdomen. See *Su Wen* chapter 60.

中府　指胃。出《素问·离合真邪论》。

中府（zhōng fǔ）　*zhong fu* Refers to the stomach. See *Su Wen* chapter 27.

中封　经穴名。足厥阴肝经之经穴。别名悬泉。在内踝前一寸半陷中，取穴时摇动其足，将足上仰，则穴处出现凹陷，可得其穴。出《灵枢·本输》。

中封（zhōng fēng）　**Zhong Feng (LR 4)** Acupoint name belonging on the liver meridian of foot *jueyin*，also called Xuan Quan. It is located in an indentation 1.5 *cun* anterior to the medial malleolus. It can be identified by actively moving the foot and lifting it up until the indentation is spotted. See *Ling Shu* chapter 2.

中宫　九宫中的中央招摇宫，居土位。出《灵枢·九宫八风》。

中宫（zhōng gōng）　**central palace** Refers to the Zhaoyao Palace within the center of the nine palaces and holds the place of earth. See *Ling Shu* chapter 77.

中根　出《素问·五常政大论》。（1）指生命的根本。见《素问》王冰注。（2）指人体五脏神气。见《类经·运气十五》。（3）指天之五运。见《素问直解》。

中根（zhōng gēn）　**inner root** See *Su Wen* chapter 70. (1) Refers to the root of life. See *Su Wen* annotated by Wang Bing. (2) Refers to the spirit qi of the five viscera in the human body. See *Lei Jing*（*Classified Classic*）"Circuits and Qi Chapter 15". (3) Refers to the five motions of the heavens. See *Su Wen Zhi Jie*（*Direct Interpretation on Su Wen*）.

中䯏　即中段脊椎骨，两旁对应五脏俞穴。䯏同膂。出《素问·气穴论》。

中䯏（zhōng lǚ）　**Zhong Lv** The middle part of spine, of which are located the transport acupoints of the five viscera on both sides. "䯏" is the same as

"膂". See *Su Wen* chapter 58.

中渚　经穴名。手少阳三焦经之输穴。在小指与环指本节后的凹陷中。出《灵枢·本输》。

中渚（zhōng zhǔ）　**Zhong Zhu（SJ 3）** An acupoint name belonging to the transport acupoint of the triple *jiao* meridian of hand *shaoyang*. It is located in the indentation proximal to the metacarpal bones of the little finger and the ring finger. See *Ling Shu* chapter 2.

中渎之府　指三焦，其为水液流布之道，犹如水液流行于沟渠之中。渎，沟渠之谓。出《灵枢·本输》。

中渎之府（zhōng dú zhī fǔ）　**water-regulating fu-organ** Refers to the triple *jiao* which is the way along which water flows, just like water runs in irrigation canals and ditches. *Dú* refers to canals or ditches. See *Ling Shu* chapter 2.

中焦　三焦之一，位于躯体之中段，是脾胃所居之处，与腐熟消化水谷有密切关系。出《灵枢·营卫生会》。

中焦（zhōng jiāo）　**middle *jiao*** The middle *jiao* is one of the triple *jiao* which is located at the middle of the trunk, where the spleen and stomach are situated. It is closely related to the function of the digestion and decomposition of water and grains. See *Ling Shu* chapter 18.

中焦如沤　言中焦的功能。出《灵枢·营卫生会》。形容中焦脾胃腐熟水谷,吸收精微,进而将营养物质上输转送到全身的功能。

中焦如沤（zhōng jiāo rú òu）**Middle *jiao* is like a froth of bubbles.** Refers to the function of the middle *jiao*. See *Ling Shu* chapter 18. It means that the spleen and the stomach of the middle *jiao* are responsible for the digestion and decomposition of water and grains, the absorption of essence, and the transporting of nutrients upwards and distributing them all over the body.

中寒　亦称内寒。为寒留于中,阳气受损,经脉气血凝涩之证。出《素问·调经论》。

中寒（zhōng hán）**direct cold attack** Also called internal cold, it is the syndrome of cold qi accumulating in the middle, causing damage to yang qi and resulting in the unsmooth circulation of the blood and stagnation in the channels. See *Su Wen* chapter 62.

中满　胃腹胀满。出《素问·阴阳应象大论》。

中满（zhōng mǎn）**abdominal fullness** Abdominal distention and stomach fullness. See *Ling Shu* chapter 5.

中膂　经穴名。又名中膂俞。属足太阳膀胱经,在平第三骶后孔,当骶部中线旁开 1.5 寸处。出《灵枢·刺节真邪》。

中膂（zhōng lǚ）**Zhong Lü（BL 29）Acupoint name**, also called the Zhong Lv transport acupoint. It belongs to the bladder meridian of foot *taiyang* and is on the same level with the third posterior sacral foramen, 1.5 *cun* beside the midline of the sacral region. See *Ling Shu* chapter 75.

中精之府　指胆。中精,受精汁之意。出《灵枢·本输》。

中精之府（zhōng jīng）**viscera containing essence** Refers to the gallbladder that receives and contains essence. See *Ling Shu* chapter 2.

内风　病证名。由入房汗出,精气内耗,腠理外泄,感受风邪的风证。出《素问·风论》。

内风（nèi fēng）**interior-wind**

四画

syndrome Disease name. Refers to the wind syndrome caused by wind attack following sweating after sexual intercourse when the essence qi is consumed and the muscular interstice is open. See *Su Wen* chapter 42.

内关 ① 三阴之气闭于内,与三阳之气隔绝,而见寸口脉大而且数,盛于人迎四倍的脉象。为阴阳隔绝,不易治疗的死症,预后极差。又称"溢阴""关阴"。出《灵枢·禁服》。② 经穴名。属手厥阴心包经,为本经络穴。在前臂掌侧,腕横纹上二寸,于两筋之间。出《灵枢·经脉》。

内关(nèi guān) ① Meaning internal closure, a pulse manifestation when the qi of the three yin (*jueyin*, *shaoyin* and *taiyin*) is closed internally and isolated from the qi of the three yang (*taiyang*, *shaoyang* and *yangming*), and the *cun kou* pulse is four times greater and faster than that of the *ren ying*. It is a fatal sign that indicates a disease with isolation of yin from yang, which is difficult to treat and has a poor prognosis. It is also called the overflow of yin or closure of yin. See *Ling Shu*

chapter 48. ② Acupoint name, Nei Guan (PC 6), belonging to the pericardium meridian of hand *jueyin* and is the connecting acupoint of the main channel. It is located between two sinews, two *cun* above the transverse crease of the wrist on the palmar side of the forearm. See *Ling Shu* chapter 10.

内针 进针。内,通纳。即在病人正吸气之时进针。出《素问·八正神明论》。

内针(nèi zhēn) **needle insertion** "内" is the same as "纳" in ancient Chinese. Namely, inserting the needle simultaneously while the patient is inhaling. See *Su Wen* chapter 26.

内治经 治疗内部疾病的方法。出《素问·至真要大论》。

内治经(nèi zhì jīng) **When a disease is in the interior, treat it in the interior.** A method to treat disease in the interior. See *Su Wen* chapter 74.

内经 即《黄帝内经》。

内经(nèi jīng) *Nei Jing* (*Internal Classic*) That is, the *Huang Di Nei Jing* (*Yellow Emperor's Internal Classic*).

内庭 经穴名。足阳明胃经之荥穴。在第二足趾外侧本节前陷者中。出《灵枢·本输》。

内庭（nèi tíng）　**Nei Ting（ST 44）** Acupoint name of the brook acupoint on the stomach meridian of foot *yangming*. It is located in the indentation distal and lateral to the second metatarsophalangeal joint. See *Ling Shu* chapter 2.

内热　① 指中焦郁热之证。出《素问·调经论》。由于劳倦伤脾,谷气不盛,形气衰少,运化乏权,上下不通,致胃气郁热,热气熏中。因形气衰少,形属阴,故曰阴虚生内热。当与后世所谓阴虚内热之证有殊。② 体内热感。出《素问·厥论》。③ 刺法,即温针法,或药熨法。出《灵枢·寿夭刚柔》。

内热（nèi rè）　① Refers to the syndrome of heat being suppressed in the middle *jiao*. See *Su Wen* chapter 62. Overstrain impairs the spleen, leading to the inadequacy of grain qi, weakness of physical qi, disorder of transportation and transformation, obstruction between the upper and the lower, all causing the heat qi of the stomach to be suppressed resulting in impairment of the middle *jiao*. Since the physical qi is insufficient and physique pertains to yin, internal heat is generated by yin deficiency. This syndrome should be differentiated from the syndrome of yin deficiency with internal heat in later generations. ② Heaty sensation in the human body. See *Su Wen* chapter 45. ③ Acupuncture technique for inducing heat inside, by warm needling, or with hot medicinal compresses. See *Ling Shu* chapter 6.

内格　① 人体不能顺应四时阴阳而产生的疾病。出《素问·四气调神大论》。② 指火热之气格拒于内所产生的病理现象。出《素问·六元正纪大论》。

内格（nèi gé）　① The physiological functions of the body fail to adapt to the changes of yin and yang in the four seasons. See *Su Wen* chapter 2. ② Pathology caused by fire qi being retaining inside. See *Su Wen* chapter 71.

内眦　指内侧眼角,也指眼眶下边。出《灵枢·癫狂病》。

内眦（nèi zì）　**inner corner** Refers to the inner corner of the eyes, or the parts below the orbit. See *Ling Shu* chapter 22.

内温　温,同蕴。内温,谓血气蕴

蓄于内。出《灵枢·九针十二原》。

内温(nèi wēn)　**internal stagnation** "温" is the same as "蕴". The condition in which the blood is unable to dissipate and the qi has difficulty dispersing. See *Ling Shu* chapter 1.

内寒　又称"中寒",指阴寒内盛,阳气不足,血气凝涩的病机。出《素问·调经论》。

内寒(nèi hán)　**internal cold** Also called direct cold attack. It is the pathogenesis with abundant yin coldness in the interior and insufficient yang qi, leading to blood stasis and qi stagnation. See *Su Wen* chapter 62.

内漏　出《素问·刺禁论》。(1)指脉破而漏。见《素问》王冰注。(2)指耳底脓生。见《类经·针刺六十四》。(3)指脉气外泄。见《素问》吴崑注。

内漏(nèi lòu)　**internal leaking** See *Su Wen* chapter 52. (1) Refers to leaking due to broken channels. See *Su Wen* annotated by Wang Bing. (2) Refers to suppuration in the eardrum. See *Lei Jing*(*Classified Classic*) "Needling Chapter 64". (3) Refers to leaking of qi out of the channels. See *Su Wen* annotated by Wu Kun.

内癀　即肠内癀烂,下脓血之病。出《灵枢·邪气藏府病形》。

内癀(nèi kuì)　**interior abscess** That is, intestinal ulceration with pus and bloody stools. See *Ling Shu* chapter 4.

水　① 五行之一。由自然界的"水"抽象而来。其特性是润下。即具有滋润和向下的特点。引申为具有寒凉、滋润、向下等作用或性质的事物。根据五行归类的方法,归属于水的,在五脏为肾,在气候为寒,在季节为冬,在方位为北,在五味为咸,在五色为黑等。出《素问·阴阳应象大论》。② 病名。水肿病之总称。出《素问·阴阳别论》。③ 主肾及阴精、水液。出《素问·上古天真论》。④ 自然界的水。出《素问·四气调神大论》。⑤ 运气术语,指水运,或太阳寒水之气。出《素问·五常政大论》。⑥ 病理性渗出物。出《素问·六元正纪大论》。

水(shuǐ)　① One of the five elements, which is abstracted from water in nature and characterized by moistening and descending. Furthermore, its meaning is widened to refer to everything that is cold, moistens and descends. According to the five elements, anything in the category of water pertains to the kidney in the five viscera，cold in climate，winter in seasons，the north in directions，salty in the five flavors and black in the five colors. See *Su Wen* chapter 5. ② Disease name. Refers to edema in general. See *Su Wen* chapter 7. ③ It governs the kidney，yin essence and fluids in the body. See *Su Wen* chapter 1. ④ Water in nature. See *Su Wen* chapter 2. ⑤ Terminology of circuits and qi. Refers to water circuits，or *taiyang* cold water qi. See *Su Wen* chapter 70. ⑥ Pathological exudate. See *Su Wen* chapter 71.

水曰流衍 衍，满溢之意。水运太过，其流衍溢，故称。出《素问·五常政大论》。

水曰流衍（shuǐ yuē liú yǎn）

Water excess is known as *liu yan* (overflow). *Yǎn* refers to excess，or overflow of water. An excess of water movement results in an overflow of water. See *Su Wen* chapter 70.

水曰涸流 水运不及曰涸流，涸流，水流干涸之意。出《素问·五常政大论》。

水曰涸流（shuǐ yuē hé liú）

Water insufficiency is known as

dryness. *Hé liú* refers to dryness. Insufficient water movement results in dryness. See *Su Wen* chapter 70.

水曰静顺 水运平和曰静顺，以水性清净柔顺，故称。出《素问·五常政大论》。

水曰静顺（shuǐ yuē jìng shùn）

Balance of water is known as *jing shun* (quietness and smoothness). Placid water movement results in quietness and smoothness，as the nature of water is quiet and gentle. See *Su Wen* chapter 70.

水气 ① 六气之一。又称太阳寒水之气，是运气学说中主气之终之气，司大雪至小寒四个节气。出《素问·六微旨大论》。② 水饮，肺肾功能失调而产生的病理性产物。出《素问·气厥论》。③ 水邪。出《素问·疟论》。

水气（shuǐ qì） ① One of the six qi，and also called *taiyang* cold water qi. It is the final governing qi in the circuits and qi theory. It governs the four solar terms from Da Xue (Greater Snow) to Xiao Han (Slight Cold). See *Su Wen* chapter 68. ② Water and fluids，which are the pathological products of lung and kidney dysfunction. See *Su Wen* chapter 37. ③ Pathogenic water. See *Su Wen* chapter 35.

水闭 小便不通。出《素问·六元正纪大论》。

水闭（shuǐ bì）**retention of water** Dysuria. See *Su Wen* chapter 71.

水形之人 体质名。又称上羽，阴阳二十五人之一。水形之人在五音属羽，羽音之中有正、偏、太、少的区别，分为上羽、众羽、桎羽、少羽、大羽，以此类比水形人中的五种体质类型。上羽得水气之全者，众羽、桎羽、少羽，大羽得水气之偏者，故上羽之人为标准水形人，其体形特征：面部粗糙，肤黑，头大，颊腮清瘦，两肩狭小，腹大，手足好动，行路时身摇，尻骨和脊背很长。其禀性无所畏惧，善于欺骗人，以致常因杀戮致死。该体质大多能耐于秋冬，不耐于春夏，故春夏多发病。出《灵枢·阴阳二十五人》。

水形之人（shuǐ xíng zhī rén）**people pertaining to the water element** Name of constitution, also called *shang yu*, out of the twenty-five types of people divided according to of yin and yang. Water type people pertain to *yu* in the five tones, which is classified into positive, partial, more, and less *yu*, including *shang yu*, *zhong yu*, *zhi yu*, *shao yu* and *da yu*, in order to illustrate the five types of body constitutions of water type of people. People of *shang yu* have complete water qi, and those of *zhong yu*, *zhi yu*, *shao yu* and *da yu* have partial water qi, therefore those of *shang yu* are the standard water type of people, who have unsmooth facial skin, a black complexion, a big head, broad cheeks, small shoulders, a big abdomen, active hands and feet, a long coccyx bone and a long back. They also sway their bodies when walking, and have no respect for or fear of others, thus they frequently cheat and bully others, and often get massacred. These type of people can easily tolerate the weather in autumn and winter, but cannot tolerate the weather in spring and summer, therefore they tend to get ill in the spring and summer. See *Ling Shu* chapter 64.

水运 五运之一。根据天干化五运之理，凡逢丙、逢辛的年时，由水运主事。其时气候偏寒、偏冷,寒冷之气流行;物候表现为万物封藏;疾病多见骨节疼痛,伤肾的症候等。出《素问·天元纪大论》。

水运（shuǐ yùn）　**water circuit** One of the five circuits. According to the theory that the Heavenly Stems transforms the five circuits, the water circuit predominates in the years of *bing* and *xin* when there is cold climate and prevailing cold qi. In phenology, all things are in storage. Commonly seen, are diseases with pain in the bones and joints, and syndromes due to kidney damage. See *Su Wen* chapter 66.

水位　即太阳寒水旺盛所主的时令。出《素问·六微旨大论》。

水位（shuǐ wèi）　**water domination** The season dominated by exuberant *taiyang* cold water qi. See *Su Wen* chapter 68.

水谷之海　海,汇聚之处。四海之一,指胃。胃为仓禀之官,受纳饮食五谷,为水谷聚集之处,故名。出《素问·五藏别论》。

水谷之海（shuǐ gǔ zhī hǎi）　**sea of water and grains** *Hǎi* means a place for confluence, and is one of the four seas in traditional Chinese medicine refers to the stomach. The stomach is the granary official that receives water and grains, and is the place where water and grains collect, thus its name. See *Su Wen* chapter 11.

水谷之悍气　水谷精气中性质慓悍、滑利的部分,可以形成卫气。出《素问·痹论》。

水谷之悍气（shuǐ gǔ zhī hàn qì）　*han* qi（**Swift-qi**）**of water and grains** A part of the essence qi from water and grains that is quick and fierce. It forms the defensive qi. See *Su Wen* chapter 43.

水谷之精气　水谷,泛指饮食物。水谷经过脾胃所化生的精微物质统称水谷精气,是维持生命活动的基本物质,也是化生人体营卫气血津液的原始物质。出《素问·痹论》。

水谷之精气（shuǐ gǔ zhī jīng qì）　**essence qi from water and grains** Water and grains refer to water and food in general. Essence qi from water and grains is the essential substance that is generated by the spleen and stomach through transformation. It is the basic substance for maintaining life activities, and also the raw material for generating nutrient qi, defensive qi, qi in general, and the blood and fluids in the body. See *Su Wen* chapter 43.

水饮 水湿之邪。出《素问·五常政大论》。

水饮（shuǐ yǐn） **water and fluids** Pathogenic water-dampness. See *Su Wen* chapter 70.

水郁 水运之气被郁遏。运气学说中,按五行相克规律,由于一方太盛或所克一方太弱而使受克一方被抑制,不能正常发挥作用的现象,称为郁。五行中,土能克水,若土太过或水不及时则会发生土偏旺而使水气被郁。出《素问·六元正纪大论》。

水郁（shuǐ yù） **stagnation of water** Oppression of the water movement qi. In the circuits and qi theory, according to the restraining rule of the five elements, the inhibited element is oppressed if the inhibiting element is too strong, or the inhibited element is too weak to function normally. In the five elements, earth restrains water, and if earth is too strong or water is too weak, the water qi will be oppressed. See *Su Wen* chapter 71.

水郁折之 水郁,水气被郁。从自然气候变化言,冬应寒而不寒,冬应藏而不藏;从人体言,肾失气化,水气潴留或上逆等病理变化,皆称水郁。折,断其所由而止之,言水气抑郁的应该用各种方法调制其水气。如益气、培土、壮火、补肾、泄水等法。出《素问·六元正纪大论》。

水郁折之（shuǐ yù zhé zhī） **Water stagnation should be treated by inhibiting.** "Stagnation of water" means that the water qi is oppressed. In terms of the climatic changes in nature, instead of being cold, it is not cold, and instead of being in storage in winter, nothing is in storage. In the human body, stagnation of water refers to the pathological changes caused by the retention or reverse upward flow of water qi, due to the kidney failing in transforming qi. "Inhibiting" means to check its generation from the source. For people with stagnation of water, various methods should be used to regulate water qi, including tonifying qi, banking up earth, invigorating fire, supplementing the kidney and discharging water. See *Su Wen* chapter 71.

四画

四画

水胀　①《灵枢》篇名。水胀,是因水液代谢障碍导致水液停留的一种病证。此篇讨论了水胀、肤胀、鼓胀、肠覃、石瘕诸病证的病因、病机、症候的鉴别与治疗等问题。② 病名。即水肿。出《灵枢·五癃津液别》。

水胀(shuǐ zhàng)　**water distention** ① Chapter title in *Ling Shu*. Water distention is a syndrome caused by fluid retention due to a disturbance of the water metabolism. In this chapter, differentiation of etiology, pathogenesis and symptoms of diseases and syndromes including water distention, cutaneous distension, drum distension, lower abdominal mass in woman, and stony uterine mass, are discussed and treatment is explored. ② Disease name, that is edema. See *Ling Shu* chapter 36.

水宗　水之源。指肾,肾主水,主持全身水液的代谢。出《素问·解精微论》。

水宗(shuǐ zōng)　**basis of water** Source of water. Refers to the kidney which governs the metabolism of fluids in the body. See *Su Wen* chapter 81.

水泉　① 小便。出《素问·脉要精微论》。膀胱气化失司,令小便失禁。② 河水。出《素问·气交变大论》。火运太过之年,火热流行,河水干涸。

水泉(shuǐ quán)　① Urine. See *Su Wen* chapter 17. Failure of the bladder's domination of qi transformation leads to urinary incontinence. ② Water in the river. See *Su Wen* chapter 69. In years with excessive fire movement, heat prevails and water in the river dries up.

水俞　治疗水病的穴位。出《素问·骨空论》。

水俞(shuǐ shū)　**water transport points** Acupoints used to treat water disease. See *Su Wen* chapter 60.

水俞五十七处　治疗水病的五十七处穴位。出《素问·水热穴论》。

水俞五十七处(shuǐ shū wǔ shí qī chù)　**fifty-seven water transport openings** The fifty-seven water transport acupoints to treat water disease. See *Su Wen* chapter 61.

水俞五十七穴　指治疗水病的五十七穴。据王冰注,包括腰骶部二十五穴:脊中、悬枢、命门、腰俞、长强;大肠俞、小肠俞、膀胱俞、中膂内俞、白环俞;胃仓、肓门、志室、胞肓、秩边。下腹部二十六：中注、四满、气穴、大赫、横骨；外陵、大巨、水道、归来、气街（冲）。膝以下十二穴：太冲、复溜、阴谷；照海、交信、筑宾。在正中者为单穴，两侧者为双穴。出《素问·骨空论》。

水俞五十七穴(shuǐ shū wǔ shí qī xuè) **fifty-seven water transport acupoints** Fifty-seven acupoints used to treat water disease. According to Wang Bing's annotation, a medical expert in the Tang dynasty, who was dedicated to *Su Wen*, the acupoints include twenty-five acupoints in the lumbosacral region: Ji Zhong (DU 6), Xuan Shu (DU 5), Ming Men (DU 4), Yao Shu (DU 2), Chang Qiang (DU 1), Da Chang Shu (BL 25), Xiao Chang Shu (BL 27), Pang Guang Shu (BL 28), Zhong Lv Nei Shu (BL 29), Bai Huan Shu (BL 30), Wei Chan (BL 50), Huang Men (BL 51), Zhi Shi (BL 52), Bao Huang (BL 53) and Zhi Bian (Bl 54); twenty points in the lower abdomen: Zhong Zhu (KI 15), Si Man (KI 14), Qi Xue (KI 13), Da He (KI 12), Heng Gu (KI 11), Wai Ling (ST 26), Da Ju (ST 27), Shui Dao (ST 28), Gui Lai (ST 29) and Qi Jie (or Qi Chong, ST 30); twelve points below the knee: Tai Chong (LR 3), Fu Liu (KI 7), Yin Gu (KI 10), Zhao Hai (KI 6), Jiao Xin (KI 8) and Zhu Bin (KI 9). The acupoints in the center are single acupoints and those on both sides are double acupoints. See *Su Wen* chapter 60.

水热穴论 《素问》篇名。水，指水病。热，指热病。穴，俞穴。此篇主要论述水病热病的发病机理，并介绍了治疗水病热病的俞穴以及四时的取穴部位，故名。

水热穴论(shuǐ rè xuè lùn) **Discussion on Water and Heat Diseases** Chapter title in *Su Wen*. *Shuǐ* refers to water diseases. *Rè* refers to heat diseases. *Xuè* refers to acupoints. In this chapter, the pathogenesis of water and heat diseases is discussed, as well as the transport acupoints used to treat the diseases and those to be used during the four seasons, are introduced. Hence the name.

水液 ① 体内的津液。出《素问·水热穴论》。② 人体代谢过程中产生的液体,如汗、尿、涎等。出《素问·至真要大论》。

水液(shuǐ yè)　① Body fluids. See *Su Wen* chapter 61. ② The liquids produced by the processes of metabolism, such as sweat, urine, saliva, etc. See *Su Wen* chapter 74.

水道　① 水液通行的道路。出《素问·灵兰秘典论》。② 河道。出《灵枢·痈疽》。

水道(shuǐ dào)　① The way for watery fluids to flow. See *Su Wen* chapter 8. ② River course. See *Ling Shu* chapter 81.

水溺　溺(niào 尿),同尿。水溺,即小便。出《素问·腹中论》。

水溺(shuǐ niào)　**urination** The pronunciation and meaning of "溺" is the same as "尿". The discharge of urine. See *Su Wen* chapter 40.

水瘕　由水湿潴留所致的病变。出《灵枢·邪气藏府病形》。

水瘕(shuǐ jiǎ)　**watery abdominal mass** Diseases caused by the retention of water-dampness. See *Ling Shu* chapter 4.

水精　指津液。由水谷经脾胃化生,内含精微物质,故称。出《素问·经脉别论》。

水精(shuǐ jīng)　**essence of water** Refers to the body fluids, which are generated by the spleen and stomach through transformation, and contain essential substances. See *Su Wen* chapter 21.

水藏　肾。肾五行属水,主水而藏精,精亦水之类。出《素问·逆调论》。

水藏(shuǐ zàng)　**organ of water** Refers to the kidney, which pertains to water in the five elements. It governs water and stores essence that is also watery. See *Su Wen* chapter 34.

手太阳　十二经脉之一。即手太阳小肠经。出《素问·气府论》。

手太阳(shǒu tài yáng)　**hand *taiyang*** One of the twelve channels. That is, the small intestine meridian of hand *taiyang*. See *Su Wen* chapter 59.

手太阳之正　手太阳列出之正经,又称手太阳经别,为十二经别之一,与手少阴经别相合。其从肩关节部分出,进入腋内,走向心,联系小肠。出《灵枢·经别》。

手太阳之正(shǒu tài yáng zhī zhèng)　**regular meridian of hand *taiyang*** The meridian divergence of the small intestine meridian of hand *taiyang*, which is one of the twelve channel divergences. It conflows with the channel divergence of the heart channel of hand *shaoyin*, and diverges at the shoulder division, entering the axilla, extending to the heart and connecting with the small intestine. See *Ling Shu* chapter 11.

手太阳之别 十五别络之一,穴名支正。其络于腕上五寸处流注手少阴;分支上走肘部,散络肩髃。出《灵枢·经脉》。

手太阳之别(shǒu tài yáng zhī bié) **collateral stemming from the Hand *Taiyang* Meridian** One of the fifteen connecting collaterals, of which the connecting acupoint is called Zhi Zheng (SI 7). The collateral ascends five *cun* from the wrist and pours into the heart meridian of hand *shaoyin*. Its branch continues to ascend up to the elbow and wraps around the shoulder bones. See *Ling Shu* chapter 10.

手太阳之筋 即手太阳经筋,为十二经筋之一。起于手小指上边,结于腕背,向上沿前臂内侧缘,结于肘内锐骨(肱骨内上踝)的后面,进入并结于腋下。其分支向后走腋后侧缘,向上绕肩胛,沿颈旁出走足太阳经筋的前方,结于耳后乳突;分支进入

耳中;直行者,出耳上,向下结于下颌,上方连属目外眦。还有一条支筋从颌部分出,上下颌角部,沿耳前,连属目外眦,上额,结于额角。出《灵枢·经筋》。

手太阳之筋(shǒu tài yáng zhī jīn) **sinew of the hand *taiyang* meridian** One of the twelve channel sinews which starts from the tip of the little finger, connects to the dorsal aspect of the wrist, ascends along the inner edge of the forearm, connects in the elbow (medial epicondyle of the humerus) behind the capitulum ulnae, and enters to connect at the axillary. One of the branches goes along the posterolateral margin of the axillary, ascends around the scapula, along the side of the neck, anterior to the sinew of the bladder meridian of foot *taiyang*, and connects to the mastoid process behind the ear; another branch enters the ear; the third branch runs straight, goes above the ear, descends to the lower jaw, and connects to the outer canthus of the eye. There is also a branch from the jaw at the maxillary angle and the man-

四画

dibular angle，running anterior to the ear，connecting with the outer canthus of the eye and the upper forehead at the frontal angle. See *Ling Shu* chapter 13.

手太阴　十二经脉之一。即手太阴肺经。出《灵枢·经脉》。

手太阴（shǒu tài yīn）　**hand *taiyin*** One of the twelve meridians，that is the lung meridian of hand *taiyin*. See *Ling Shu* chapter 10.

手太阴之正　手太阴别出之正经，又称手太阴经别，为十二经别之一，与手阳明经别相合。其从手太阴经渊腋处分出，行手少阴经之前，进入胸腔走向肺，散布于大肠；上行出缺盆，沿喉咙与手阳明经相合。出《灵枢·经别》。

手太阴之正（shǒu tài yīn zhī zhèng）　**regular meridian of hand *taiyin*** The meridian divergence of the lung meridian of hand *taiyin*，which is one of the twelve channel divergences. It conflows with the channel divergence of the large intestine meridian of hand *yangming*. It originates from the lung meridian of hand *taiyin* at Yuan Ye (GB 22)，runs in front of the heart meridian of hand *shaoyin*，enters the chest，extends to the lung，spreads over the large intestine，goes upward out of Que Pen (ST 12)，along the throat，and connects with the large intestine meridian of hand *yangming*. See *Ling Shu* chapter 11.

手太阴之别　十五别络之一，穴名列缺。其络起于腕上一寸半，分肉间，同手太阴经直入掌中，散布鱼际；分支走向手阳明经。出《灵枢·经脉》。

手太阴之别（shǒu tài yīn zhī bié）　**collateral stemming from the hand *taiyin* meridian** One of the fifteen connecting collaterals with the connecting acupoint called Lie Que (LU 7). The collateral originates 1.5 *cun* above the wrist and extends along the meridian of hand *taiyin*. It enters straight into the palm，where it dissipates and enters the Yu Ji (LU 10). Its branch runs toward the meridian of hand *yangming*. See *Ling Shu* chapter 10.

手太阴之筋　即手太阴经筋，为十二经筋之一。起于手大拇指上，沿指上行，结于鱼际后，行于寸口动脉外侧。上沿前臂，结于肘中；再向上沿上臂内侧，进入腋下，出缺盆，结于肩髃前方，上面结于缺盆,下面结于胸里,分散通过膈部,会合于膈下,到达季胁。出《灵枢·经筋》。

手太阴之筋(shǒu tài yīn zhī jīn) **sinew of the meridian of hand *taiyin*** One of the twelve channel sinews which starts from the top of the thumb, runs along the finger, connects at the back of Yu Ji (LU 10), and goes laterally along the pulsating vessel at *cun kou*. It goes upward along the forearm, and connects to the transverse line of elbow; it then runs upward along the inner side of the upper arm, enters the axilla, leaves from the acupoint Que Pen (ST 12), and connects in front of the acupoint Jian Yu (LI 15). At the top, it connects to the acupoint Que Pen (ST 12) and at the bottom, it connects at the chest. It spreads and passes through the diaphragm. The branches conflow below the diaphragm until arriving at the free rib. See *Ling Shu* chapter 13.

手少阳 十二经脉之一。即手少阳三焦经。出《素问·气府论》。

手少阳(shǒu shào yáng) **hand *shaoyang*** One of the twelve

channels, namely the triple *jiao* meridian of hand *shaoyang*. See *Su Wen* chapter 59.

手少阳之正 手少阳别出之正经,又称手少阳经别,为十二经别之一,与手厥阴经别相合,其从头顶部分出,向下进入缺盆,经上、中、下三焦,散布于胸中。出《灵枢·经别》。

手少阳之正(shǒu shào yáng zhī zhèng) **regular meridian of hand *shaoyang*** The meridian divergence of the triple *jiao* meridian of hand *shaoyang*, and one of the twelve channel divergences. It conflows with the channel divergence of the pericardium meridian of hand *jueyin*. It originates from the top of the head, runs downward, enters Que Pen (ST 12), and spreads in the chest through the upper, middle and lower *jiao*. See *Ling Shu* chapter 11.

手少阳之别 十五别络之一,穴名外关。其络从腕上二寸处外绕臂部,流注心中,会合于厥阴。出《灵枢·经脉》。

手少阳之别(shǒu shào yáng zhī bié) **collateral stemming from the meridian of hand *shaoyang*** One of the fifteen connecting collaterals with the connecting

四画

acupoint called Wai Guan（SJ 5）. The collateral starts at two *cun* from the wrist，winds around the exterior of the arm and pours into the chest where it links up with the pericardium meridian of hand *jueyin*. See *Ling Shu* chapter 10.

手少阳之筋　即手少阳经筋，为十二经筋之一。起于环指末端，结于腕背，向上沿前臂结于肘部，上绕上臂外侧缘上肩，走向颈部，合于手太阳经筋。其分支当下颌角处进入，联系舌根；另一支从下颌角上行，沿耳前，连属目外眦，上经额部，结于额角。出《灵枢·经筋》。

手少阳之筋（shǒu shào yáng zhī jīn）　**sinew of the hand *shaoyang* meridian** One of the twelve channel sinews，that is the meridian of hand *shaoyang*. It starts at the end of the ring finger，connects to the back of the wrist，connects to the elbow along the forearm，wraps around the upper shoulder at the outer edge of the upper arm，goes to the neck，and conflows with the sinew of the small intestine meridian of hand *taiyang*. One of the branches enters at the mandibular angle，and connects with the root of the tongue; the other branch runs upward from the mandibular angle，goes in front of the ear，connects with the outer canthus，passes the forehead and connects at the frontal angle. See *Ling Shu* chapter 13.

手少阴　十二经脉之一。即手少阴心经。出《灵枢·经脉》。

手少阴（shǒu shào yīn）　**hand shaoyin** One of the twelve meridians，namely the heart meridian of hand *shaoyin*. See *Ling Shu* chapter 10.

手少阴之正　手少阴别出之正经，又称手少阴经别，为十二经别之一，与手太阳经别相合。其经别出后走入腋下渊腋穴处两筋之间，进入胸腔，归属于心，上走喉咙，出于面部，在目内眦处与手太阳经相合。出《灵枢·经别》。

手少阴之正（shǒu shào yīn zhī zhèng）　**regular channel of the hand shaoyin meridian** The meridian divergence of the heart meridian of hand *shaoyin*，and one of the twelve meridian divergences. It conflows with the channel divergence of the small intestine meridian of hand *taiyang*. It diverges from the heart meridian of hand *shaoyin*, enters between the two sinews at the acupoint Yuan Ye (GB 22) under the axilla, goes into the thoracic cavity, returns to the heart, goes upward along the throat and out of the face, and conflows with the small intestine meridian of hand *taiyang* at the inner canthus. See *Ling Shu* chapter 11.

手少阴之别 十五别络之一,穴名通里。其络于腕上一寸分出上行,沿经脉进入心中,联系舌本,属于目系;分支走向手太阳经。出《灵枢·经脉》。

手少阴之别(shǒu shào yīn zhī bié) **collateral stemming from the meridian of hand *shaoyin*** One of the fifteen connecting collaterals with the connecting acupoint called Tong Li (HT 5). It starts at one *cun* from the wrist and extends separately upward. It follows the heart meridian of hand *shaoyin* and enters the heart. It connects with the root of the tongue and links up with the eye. Its branch runs towards the small intestine meridian of hand *taiyang*. See *Ling Shu* chapter 10.

手少阴之筋 即手少阴经筋。为十二经筋之一。起于手小指内侧,结于腕后锐骨,向上结于肘内侧,再向上进入腋内,交手太阴经筋,行于乳里,结于胸中,沿膈向下,系于脐部。出《灵枢·经筋》。

手少阴之筋(shǒu shào yīn zhī jīn) **sinew of the hand *shaoyin* meridian** One of the twelve channel sinews which starts from the inner side of the little finger, connects to the capitulum ulnae at the back of the wrist, joins at the inner side of the elbow, goes upward and then enters the axilla meeting the lung meridian of hand *taiyin*, goes into the breast and connects to the chest, goes down along the diaphragm, and links up with the navel. See *Ling Shu* chapter 13.

手心主 即手厥阴心包经。出《灵枢·经脉》。

手心主(shǒu xīn zhǔ) **hand heart ruler** That is, the pericardium meridian of hand *jueyin*. See *Ling Shu* chapter 10.

手心主之正 手厥阴别出之正经,又称手厥阴经别,为十二经别之一,与手少阳经别相合。其从腋下三寸处别出进入胸中,分别归属于上、中、下三焦;

向上沿喉咙出于耳后,当完骨部,与手少阳经相合。出《灵枢·经别》。

手心主之正（shǒu xīn zhǔ zhī zhèng）**regular channel of the hand heart ruler** The meridian divergence of the pericardium meridian of hand *jueyin* which is one of the twelve channel divergences. It conflows with the channel divergence of the triple *jiao* meridian of hand *shaoyang*. It diverges from the pericardium meridian of hand *jueyin* at three *cun* under the axilla, enters the chest, and returns to the upper, middle and lower *jiao*, respectively; it goes upward around the throat, exits behind the ear and conflows with the triple *jiao* meridian of hand *shaoyang* at the mastoid process of the temporal bone. See *Ling Shu* chapter 11.

手心主之别　十五别络之一,穴名内关。其络于腕上二寸处,出两筋之间,沿经向上联系于心包,散络心系。出《灵枢·经脉》。

手心主之别（shǒu xīn zhǔ zhī bié）**collateral stemming from the hand heart ruler** One of the fifteen connecting collaterals with the connecting acupoint called Nei Guan （PC 6）. It starts at two *cun* above the wrist and exits between the two sinews. It extends along the pericardium meridian of hand *jueyin* upward and links up with the pericardium. See *Ling Shu* chapter 10.

手心主之筋　即手厥阴经筋,为十二经筋之一。起于手中指,与手太阴经筋并行,结于肘内侧,上经上臂内侧,结于腋下,向下散布于胁肋的前后,其分支进入腋内,散布于胸中,结于膈。出《灵枢·经筋》。

手心主之筋（shǒu xīn zhǔ zhī jīn）**sinew of the hand heart ruler** One of the twelve channel sinews, that is the sinew of the pericardium meridian of hand *jueyin*. It starts from the middle finger, runs in parallel with sinew of the lung meridian of hand *taiyin*, connects at the medial side of the elbow, runs along the medial side of the upper arm, connects under the axilla, and spreads downward to the front and back of the rib flank. Its branch enters the axilla, scatters into the chest, and connects at the diaphragm. See *Ling Shu* chapter 13.

手阳明　十二经脉之一。即手阳

明大肠经。出《灵枢·九针论》。

手阳明（shǒu yáng míng） **hand yangming** One of the twelve meridians. Refers to the large intestine meridian of hand *yangming*. See *Ling Shu* chapter 78.

手阳明之正 手阳明别出之正经，又称手阳明经别，为十二经别之一，与手太阴经别相合。其从手上行，当肩髃部分出，进入项后柱骨，下走大肠，联属于肺；向上者，沿喉咙，出缺盆，与手阳明本经相合。出《灵枢·经别》。

手阳明之正（shǒu yáng míng zhī zhèng） **regular channel of the meridian of hand yangming** The meridian divergence of the large intestine meridian of hand *yangming*, and one of the twelve channel divergences. It conflows with channel divergence of the lung meridian of hand *taiyin*. It runs upward from the hand, diverges at the acupoint Jian Yu（LI 15）, enters the spine, descends to the large intestine and links up with the lung; it ascends along the throat up to the acupoint Que Pen (ST 12), and links up with the large intestine meridian of hand *yangming*. See *Ling Shu* chapter 11.

手阳明之别 十五别络之一，穴名偏历。其络于腕上三寸处分出，一支走向手太阴经；一支上沿臂部，络肩髃，上向下颌角，分布牙齿；另一支入耳会合宗脉。出《灵枢·经脉》。

手阳明之别（shǒu yáng míng zhī bié） **collateral stemming from the meridian of hand yangming** One of the fifteen connecting collaterals with the connecting acupoint called Pian Li (LI 6). It sets out at three *cun* above the wrist with one branch running toward the lung meridian of hand *taiyin*. Another branch ascends along the arms, wraps around the acupoint Jian Yu (LI 15), runs upward to the mandibular angle and travels into the teeth. The third branch enters the ear and conflows with the ancestral vessel. See *Ling Shu* chapter 10.

手阳明之筋 即手阳明经筋，为十二经筋之一。起于示指末端，结于腕背，向上沿前臂结于肘外侧，上经上臂外侧，结于肩髃；其分支，绕肩胛，挟脊旁；直行者，从肩髃部上颈，分支上面颊，结于鼻旁；直行的上出手太阳经筋的前方，上额角，络头

四画

部,向下至右下颌。出《灵枢·经筋》。

手阳明之筋(shǒu yáng míng zhī jīn) **sinew of the meridian of hand yangming** One of the twelve channel sinews, namely the sinew of the large intestine meridian of hand *yangming*. It starts at the tip of the index finger, connects at the back of wrist, runs along the forearm and joins at the lateral side of the elbow, going along the lateral side of the upper arm, and connects at the acupoint Jian Yu (LI 15). One of its branches circles around the scapula and on both sides of the spine; another branch runs to the neck from the shoulder tip, one of the subbranches runs upward to the face, and connects beside the nose; the other sub-branch runs straight out in front of the sinew of the small intestine of hand *taiyang*, goes upward to the frontal angle, wraps around the head, and runs downward to the right lower jaw. See *Ling Shu* chapter 13.

手鱼 指手掌拇指本节后半满突起如鱼状的肌肉。又称"鱼际"。出《素问·刺禁论》。

手鱼(shǒu yú) **thenar** Refers to the muscles, like a fish in appearance, at the back of the basic joint of the thumb in the palm. Also called *yu ji*. See *Su Wen* chapter 52.

手鱼之络 手鱼际部位之脉络。出《灵枢·经脉》。

手鱼之络(shǒu yú zhī luò) **thenar collateral** Collateral of the thenar. See *Ling Shu* chapter 10.

手鱼腹 指手鱼的中央部分。出《素问·刺禁论》。

手鱼腹(shǒu yú fù) **belly of the thenar** The middle part of the thenar. See *Su Wen* chapter 52.

手厥阴 十二经脉之一。即手厥阴心包经。出《素问·五常政大论》。

手厥阴(shǒu jué yīn) **hand jueyin** One of the twelve meridians, that is the pericardium meridian of hand *jueyin*. See *Su Wen* chapter 70.

气 ① 指一种极细微的物质,是构成世界万物的本原。出《素问·宝命全形论》。② 地球周围的大气。出《素问·五运行大论》。③ 节气。十五天为一气。出《素问·六节藏象论》。④ 气候。出《灵枢·五乱》。⑤ 气势。出《灵枢·逆顺》。⑥ 呼吸之气。出《灵枢·口问》。⑦ 气质。出《灵枢·阴阳二十五人》。⑧ 病邪。出《灵枢·百病始生》。⑨ 药性。出《素问·至真要大论》。⑩ 针刺的得气感。出《灵枢·九针十二原》。⑪ 正气，与邪气相对而言。出《素问·评热病论》。⑫ 水谷精气。出《灵枢·营卫生会》。⑬ 元气。出《素问·阴阳应象大论》。⑭ 卫气。出《灵枢·痈疽》。⑮ 营气。出《灵枢·痈疽》。⑯ 宗气。出《灵枢·决气》。⑰ 五脏之气。出《素问·阴阳应象大论》。⑱ 脉气，寓有脉象之义。出《灵枢·五色》。⑲ 矢气。出《素问·脉解》。⑳ 神气。出《灵枢·大惑论》。㉑ 运气。出《素问·五运行大论》。

气(qì) ① Qi. Refers to an extremely fine substance that is the origin of all things in the world. See *Su Wen* chapter 25. ② The atmosphere around the earth. See *Su Wen* chapter 67. ③ Solar term. One qi or solar term lasts fifteen days. See *Su Wen* chapter 9. ④ Climate. See *Ling Shu* chapter 34. ⑤ An imposing manner. See *Ling Shu* chapter 55. ⑥ Air that people breathe. See *Ling Shu* chapter 28. ⑦ Temperament. See *Ling Shu* chapter 64. ⑧ Pathogenic factors. See *Ling Shu* chapter 66. ⑨ Drug property. See *Su Wen* chapter 74. ⑩ Sensation of obtaining qi in acupuncture. See *Ling Shu* chapter 1. ⑪ Healthy qi that is opposite to pathogenic qi. See *Su Wen* chapter 33. ⑫ Essence qi of water and grains. See *Ling Shu* chapter 18. ⑬ Orginal qi. See *Su Wen* chapter 5. ⑭ Defensive qi. See *Ling Shu* chapter 81. ⑮ Nutrient qi. See *Ling Shu* chapter 81. ⑯ Pectoral qi. See *Ling Shu* chapter 30. ⑰ Qi of the five viscera. See *Su Wen* chapter 5. ⑱ Meridian qi，implying pulse manifestation. See *Ling Shu* chapter 49. ⑲ Flatus. See *Su Wen* chapter 49. ⑳ Spirit qi. See *Ling Shu* chapter 80. ㉑ Circuits and qi. See *Su Wen* chapter 67.

气口　即寸口。又名脉口，是切脉的主要部位，在桡动脉搏动明显处。出《素问·经脉别论》。

气口 (qì kǒu)　*qi kou* That is, *cun kou*，also called *mai kou* and it is the main pulse-taking section located at the site with the palpable pulsation of the radial artery. See *Su Wen*

四画

chapter 21.

气门　① 即汗孔,又名玄府。出《素问·生气通天论》。② 出《灵枢·官能》。〈1〉气街,气脉门户。见《类经·针刺十》。〈2〉气穴,即俞穴。见《灵枢注证发微》。

气门（qì mén）　① The sweat pores, also called the mysterious house. See *Su Wen* chapter 3. ② See *Ling Shu* chapter 73. 〈1〉 The qi pathway that is the gate of the qi and the pulse. See *Lei Jing*（*Classified Classic*）"Needling Chapter 10".〈2〉Qi acupoints, refers to acupuncture points. See *Su Wen Zhu Zheng Fa Wei*（*Annotation and Elaboration on Su Wen*）.

气之精为白眼　肺主气,气之精即肺之精。白眼即眼白部分,能反映肺之生理病理状态。出《灵枢·大惑论》。

气之精为白眼（qì zhī jīng wéi bái yǎn）　**Essence of qi infusing into the white part of the eye.** The lung governs qi and the essence of qi is the essence of the lung. The white part of the eye reflects the physiological and pathological conditions of the lung. See *Ling Shu* chapter 80.

气化　① 指自然界风寒暑湿燥火六气的变化及春生、夏长、长夏化、秋收、冬藏的物化现象。出《素问·气交变大论》。② 指人体在气的作用下,精、血、津液、组织器官等进行的变化。出《素问·灵兰秘典论》。

气化（qì huà）　① Qi transformation. Refers to the natural changes in the six qi（wind, cold, summerheat, dampness, dryness and fire）and the phenomena of generation in spring, growth in summer, transformation in late summer, harvest in autumn and storage in winter. See *Su Wen* chapter 69. ② Refers to changes in the essence, blood, body fluids, tissues and organs that occur under the effect of qi in the human body. See *Su Wen* chapter 8.

气立　生命体因外界之气而立。出《素问·五常政大论》。(1) 泛指生命体与自然环境之间的交换气化运动,其升降出入,因化而立,为生命之本。见《素问直解》《素问集注》。(2) 具体指植物与外界之间的气化运动及完成生长化收藏的过程。见《类经·运气十五》。

气立（qì lì）　**origin of qi** Living things originate from qi in nature. See *Su Wen* chapter 70.

(1) In a general sense, it refers to exchanges and movements of qi between living things and nature. The ascending, descending, exiting and entering of qi are motivated by qi transformation and are the root of life. See *Su Wen Zhi Jie* (*Direct Interpretation on Su Wen*) and *Su Wen Ji Zhu* (*Collected Annotation of Su Wen*). (2) Specifically, it refers to the transformation of qi between plants and nature, and the processes of generation, growth, transformation, harvest and storage. See *Lei Jing* (*Classified Classic*) "Circuits and Qi Chapter 15".

气穴　泛指腧穴。经气输注出入之处,故名。出《素问·阴阳应象大论》。另,《针灸甲乙经》有气穴穴,在脐下三寸,关元穴旁半寸处,属足少阴肾经。

气穴 (qì xué) **acupoints** The points where the qi of the channels enters and departs. See *Su Wen* chapter 5. In addition, there is an acupoint called *Qi Xue* (KI 13) in *Zhen Jiu Jia Yi Jing* (*A - B Classic of Acupuncture and Moxibustion*) that is located three *cun* below the umbilicus, 0.5 *cun* beside the acupoint *Guan Yuan* (CV 4). The acupoint Qi Xue (KI 13) belongs to the kidney meridian of foot *shaoyin*.

气穴论　《素问》篇名。此篇内容主要论述三百六十五个气穴的分部以及孙络、溪谷、经脉、脏腑之间的联系。故名。

气穴论 (qì xué lùn) **Discussion on Acupoints** Chapter title in *Su Wen*. This chapter discusses the locations of 365 acupoints and the connections among the tertiary collateral vessels, muscle interspaces, channels, vessels and the viscera and bowels.

气交　运气术语。谓天地之气上下相交之处,为人们赖以生存的空间。出《素问·六微旨大论》。

气交 (qì jiāo) **Qi from the upper and lower communicate with each other** Terminology of the circuits and qi. Refers to the region where qi from the upper and the lower communicate with each other, the place where people live. See *Su Wen* chapter 68.

气交变大论　《素问》篇名。气交变,指天地之气相交而产生的自然界反常变化。该篇主要论述由于气交变引起的五运六气的太过不及,对自然界引起的变化,以及五方五气的德、化、政、令、灾、变以及对人体发病的关系,故名。

气交变大论(qì jiāo biàn dà lùn) **Major Discussion on the Changes of Qi Convergence** Chapter title in *Su Wen*. "Changes of qi convergence" refers to abnormal changes in nature caused by the confluence of qi of the heavens and earth. Discussions in this chapter include, excessive and deficient conditions of the five circuits and six qi caused by the confluence of qi, the corresponding changes, as well as the functions and transformations, administration and order, changes and harm of the five qi in the five directions, and their relationship with diseases of the human body. See *Su Wen* chapter 69.

气并 ① 阴阳之气交通。出《素问·腹中论》。② 气偏盛。并,偏盛之意。气血阴阳应相对平衡,故气偏盛则血虚。出《素问·调经论》。

气并(qì bìng) ① Communication between the qi of the yin and yang. See *Su Wen* chapter 40. ② Exuberance of qi. *Bìng* here means exuberance. There needs to exist a relative balance between the qi and blood, the yin and yang, therefore an exuberance of qi leads to a deficiency of blood. See *Su Wen* chapter 62.

气忤 忤(wǔ 五),违逆。气忤,即气逆。出《素问·离合真邪论》。

气忤(qì wǔ) **qi revolt** *Wǔ* means to reverse, or the reverse flow of qi. See *Su Wen* chapter 27.

气味 ① 指水谷精微。出《素问·五藏别论》。② 指药、食的性味。出《素问·阴阳应象大论》。

气味(qì wèi) ① Refers to the essence of water and grains. See *Su Wen* chapter 11. ② Refers to the properties of medicines and food. See *Su Wen* chapter 5.

气迫 运气术语。迫,逼迫伤害之意,时令已到而气候未到,为气之不及,则为所不胜之气侵迫,而所胜之气因缺乏制约亦妄行反迫。出《素问·六节藏象论》。

气迫(qì pò) **qi threatening** Terminology of circuits and qi, in which *pò* refers to force or to harm. Deficiency of qi means that the seasonal qi arrives but the climate does not, consequently the qi cannot dominate and is threatened due to lack of inhibition. See *Su Wen* chapter 9.

气府论 《素问》篇名。气府，指俞穴。又，专指六府脉气所发之穴。此篇主要论述手足之阳脉及督、任、冲诸脉之脉气所发之穴经，故名。

气府论（qì fǔ lùn） **Discussion on Acupoints（Qi Palaces）**Chapter title in *Su Wen*. Qi palaces refer to the acupoints in general，or the acupoints where the qi of the vessels of the six bowels originates. In this chapter, the acupoints and channels where the qi of the yang vessels of foot and hand，the governor vessel，the conception vessel，and the thoroughfare vessel，originates are described. See *Su Wen* chapter 59.

气泄 即矢气，俗称放屁。出《素问·玉机真藏论》。

气泄（qì xiè） **qi outflow** Namely flatulence，and is commonly known as farting. See *Su Wen* chapter 19.

气食少火 义同"少火之气壮"，参见该条。出《素问·阴阳应象大论》。

气食少火（qì shí shào huǒ） **Mild fire warms qi.** See "少火之气壮". See *Su Wen* chapter 5.

气逆 即气机逆乱。凡气之升降出入反常运动，概称气逆。出《素问·通评虚实论》。

气逆（qì nì） **adverse flow of qi** That is，a disorder in circuits and qi. Abnormal movements in the ascending，descending，exiting and entering of qi is called adverse flow of qi. See *Su Wen* chapter 28.

气索 索，消、乏之义。气索，气乏、气短之状。出《灵枢·癫狂》。

气索（qì suǒ） **qi shortness** *Suǒ* refers to consumption，or exhaustion. Qi shortness refers to shortness of breath. See *Ling Shu* chapter 22.

气海 宗气汇聚之所，位于胸部膻中处。海，百川汇聚之处。出《灵枢·海论》。

气海（qì hǎi） **sea of qi** It is the site where the pectoral qi conflows，and is located at the center of the chest. *Hǎi* refers to where all rivers converge. See *Ling Shu* chapter 33.

气虚宜掣引之 治法。出《素问·阴阳应象大论》。（1）掣，音义如"导"。气虚者，宜用导引之法使之流畅而充实。见《素问》王冰注。（2）抽取之意。气虚者当引取挽回其气，使之复常。含补之义。见《类经·论治八》。

四画

四画

气虚宜掣引之（qì xū yí dǎo yǐn zhī）　**Qi deficiency syndrome or asthenia should be treated by lifting therapy**. A treatment method. See *Su Wen* chapter 5. (1) The pronunciation and meaning of 掣 are the same as 导. To treat a syndrome of qi deficiency, conduction exercises should be adopted for qi to be replenished and flow smoothly. See *Su Wen* annotated by Wang Bing. (2) Meaning to extract. For patients with qi deficiency, lifting therapy should be used to retrieve the qi in order for it to return to normal. It also includes the meaning of supplementing the qi. See *Lei Jing* (*Classified Classic*)"On Treatment Chapter 8".

气脱　气的突然亡失。出《灵枢·决气》。

气脱（qì tuō）　**exhaustion of qi** Sudden loss of qi. See *Ling Shu* chapter 30.

气淫　① 运气学说中时令未到而气候先到，则为太过，以致侵犯己所不胜而又欺凌己之所胜，称谓气淫。出《素问·六节藏象论》。② 邪气侵淫脏腑。出《灵枢·邪气藏府病形》。

气淫（qì yín）　① Refers to the excess of qi. In the circuits and qi theory, if a climate precedes a season, it is called excess. Excess usually damages the qi that it normally is inferior to and over-restricts the qi that it usually dominates. See *Su Wen* chapter 9. ② It refers to the invasion of the viscera by pathogenic qi. See *Ling Shu* chapter 4.

气厥　义同"气逆"，见该条。出《素问·气厥论》。

气厥（qì jué）　*qi jue* The meaning of "气厥" is the same as "气逆". See *Su Wen* chapter 37.

气厥论　《素问》篇名。厥，逆也。气厥，指脏腑气机逆而不顺。此篇主要论述由于脏腑气机逆乱，寒热相移而引起的各种疾病。

气厥论（qì jué lùn）　**Discussion on the Reverse Flow of qi** Chapter title in *Su Wen*. *Jué* refers to reversal. *Qì jué* means that the qi movement of the viscera is unsmooth. In this chapter, various diseases caused by cold and heat transfer due to disordered qi movement of the viscera and bowels are discussed. See *Su Wen* chapter 37.

气街　① 气行往来的道路，又称四街。出《灵枢·卫气》。② 腹股沟经脉搏动处。出《素问·气府论》。③ 穴位名。气冲穴别名。属足阳明胃经。出《素问·气府论》。

气街（qì jiē）　① Ways for qi to flow，and also called the four streets. See *Ling Shu* chapter 52. ② The sites where vessels pulsate in the groin. See *Su Wen* chapter 59. ③ Acupoint name，Qi Jie (ST 30). Another name for the Qi Chong acupoint belonging to the stomach meridian of foot *yangming*. See *Su Wen* chapter 59.

气道　① 营卫之气通行的道路，包括肌肉腠理之间隙。出《灵枢·营卫生会》。② 呼吸之气的通道。出《灵枢·口问》。

气道（qì dào）　① The way for the nutrient qi and the defensive qi to flow，including the muscular interspaces. See *Ling Shu* chapter 18. ② The passage of breath. See *Ling Shu* chapter 28.

气数　指二十四节气的常数，为纪万物生化的节律。出《素问·六节藏象论》。

气数（qì shù）　**number of qi** Refers to a constant number of 24 solar terms in order to record the pattern of growth and changes of all things in nature.

See *Su Wen* chapter 9.

气鞕　鞕，同硬。气鞕指喉舌部强硬。出《灵枢·寒热病》。

气鞕（qì biān）　**stiffness of the tongue** The meaning of "鞕" is the same as "硬". It refers to the rigidity of the throat and the tongue. See *Ling Shu* chapter 21.

气癃　由气滞而致的小便不利。出《灵枢·胀论》。

气癃（qì lóng）　**difficulty urinating** Inhibited urination due to qi stagnation. See *Ling Shu* chapter 35.

毛　① 指毛脉。脉来轻虚以浮，如按在毛上的一种脉象，属于肺，为秋季应时之正常脉。若过于轻浮则说明胃气冲和已少，为肺有病变的脉象；若如风吹毛，散乱无绪，全无胃气冲和之象，则为肺的脏真之气败露，属危候。出《素问·宣明五气》。② 指皮毛。出《灵枢·本神》。③ 指阴毛。出《灵枢·经脉》。④ 指毛虫。出《素问·五常政大论》。

毛（máo）　① Refers to a messy pulse，which is rather a light pulse that feels like pressing on hairs. It pertains to the lung and is the normal seasonal pulse in autumn. A pulse that feels too light indicates diminished stomach qi, suggesting diseases of the lung. A messy pulse that feels as if the wind is blowing hairs indicates the absence of stomach qi, suggesting that the lung qi has genuinely become be exhausted and exposed, which is a fatal symptom. See *Su Wen* chapter 23. ② Refers to skin and hair. See *Ling Shu* chapter 8. ③ Refers to pubic hair. See *Ling Shu* chapter 10. ④ Refers to animals with fur. See *Su Wen* chapter 70.

毛折　毛发枯焦断折,是气血败绝之象。出《素问·玉机真藏论》。

毛折(máo zhé)　**hair breaking off** Hair that is scorched and broken reflects the withering and exhaustion of qi and blood. See *Su Wen* chapter 19.

毛际　阴毛丛生之处。出《素问·骨空论》。

毛际(máo jì)　**pubes** The areas with pubic hair. See *Su Wen* chapter 60.

毛刺　九刺法之一。即浅刺皮毛,用以治疗皮肤表层的痹症。现在临床上所用皮肤针、滚刺筒之类的针具,即受此启发而来,治疗范围也有所扩大。出《灵枢·官针》。

毛刺(máo cì)　*mao needling* One of the nine needling methods, in which superficial skin is needled to treat impediments on the skin's surface. Nowadays, instruments like skin needles and roller needles used clinically were designed by drawing inspiration from this method, and these needles are used to treat a greater range of diseases. See *Ling Shu* chapter 7.

毛悴色夭　皮毛憔悴,肤色枯暗而夭然不泽。出《灵枢·本神》。

毛悴色夭(máo cuì sè yāo)　**brittle hair and haggardness** Haggard and dark skin that has no luster. See *Ling Shu* chapter 8.

升降不前　运气术语。升降被抑,欲升不升,欲降不降之谓,是反常情况。运气学说中,岁气的左、右间气,随年支的变动而变动,即旧岁在泉之右间升为新岁司天之左间,为升;旧岁司天之右间,降为新岁在泉之左间,为降。如辰年,旧岁卯年在泉之右间厥阴风木,当升为新岁司天之左间;旧岁卯年司天之右间少阳相火,当降为新岁在泉之左间。出《素问·刺法论》。

升降不前(shēng jiàng bù qián)　**failure to ascend and descend** Terminology of circuits and qi, in which the ascending and descending of qi is inhibited abnormally. In the circuits and qi theory, the intermediate qi of the yearly qi on both right and left sides moves and changes with the earthly branches. Ascending refers to the fact that the intermediate qi is on the right side and that it is in Spring, if the intermediate qi is on the left side then it will dominate the heavens in the new year; the intermediate qi on the right side, that dominates the heavens in the last year, descends to be the intermediate qi on the left side in the Spring of the new year. For instance, in the year of *chen*, the qi of *jueyin* wind wood, the intermediate qi on the right side that is in the Spring of the year of *mao* should rise to be the intermediate qi in the left side that dominates the heavens in the new year; the qi of the *shaoyang* ministerial fire, the intermediate qi in the right side that dominates the heavens in the year of *mao*, should descend to be the intermediate qi on the left side that is in the Spring of the new year. See *Su Wen* chapter 72.

升降出入　升降出入,是气的基本运动形式。一切物质的变化离不开气的升降出入运动。故非出入,则无以生、长、壮、老、已;非升降,则无以生、长、化、收、藏。出《素问·六微旨大论》。

升降出入(shēng jiàng chū rù) **ascending, descending, exiting and entering** Ascending, descending, exiting and entering is the basic pattern of the movement of qi. Changes of all things are dependent on the movement of qi. Failure of qi to exit and enter leads to no generation, growth, development, aging or death; and failure of qi to ascend and descend results in no engenderment, growth, transformation, harvest or storage. See *Su Wen* chapter 68.

夭　① 夭折,短命。出《灵枢·寿夭刚柔》。② 没有光泽。出《灵枢·决气》。

夭(yāo)　① Early death. See *Ling Shu* chapter 6. ② Lusterless. See *Ling Shu* chapter 30.

夭疽　病名。发于颈部,凶险难治之疽,故名。出《灵枢·痈疽》。

夭疽(yāo jū)　**incurable carbuncle**

Disease name of one that occurs in the neck and is difficult to cure. See *Ling Shu* chapter 81.

长 ①（cháng 怅），长脉。脉应指部位长，从寸至关，搏然指下；又指应指时间长。长而柔和，提示气血充盈，畅达，多见于正常人。若长而弦硬，则为病脉，多见于肝病。出《素问·脉要精微论》。②（zhǎng 掌），谓青年成长时期。出《素问·上古天真论》。③（zhǎng 掌）长大，生的进一步。出《素问·四气调神大论》。④（zhǎng 掌）首，居第一的。出《素问·风论》。⑤（zhǎng 掌）年岁高。出《素问·示从容论》。⑥（zhǎng 掌）长养。出《素问·太阴阳明论》。⑦（zhǎng 掌）主。出《素问·热论》。

长(cháng) ① When it is pronounced *cháng*, it means a long pulse, extending from *cun* to *guan*, pulsating under the fingers; or a pulse that lasts for a long time. A long and gentle pulse indicates plentiful qi, and blood that flows smoothly, which is usually seen in healthy people. A long and taut pulse indicates disease, usually of the liver. See *Su Wen* chapter 17. ② (zhǎng) When pronounced *zhǎng*, it may refer to the growth period in youth. See *Su Wen* chapter 1. ③ （zhǎng) When pronounced *zhǎng*, it may refer to growth, or the phase following engenderment. See *Su Wen* chapter 2. ④ (zhǎng) When pronounced *zhǎng*, it may mean the first, or chief. See *Su Wen* chapter 42. ⑤ （zhǎng) When pronounced *zhǎng*, it may refer to old age. See *Su Wen* chapter 76. ⑥ （zhǎng) When pronounced *zhǎng*, it may mean growing and nourishing. See *Su Wen* chapter 29. ⑦ （zhǎng) When pronounced *zhǎng*, it may refer to leader. See *Su Wen* chapter 31.

长气 促使万物生长的气候，在五行属火。出《素问·五常政大论》。

长气(zhǎng qì) **growing qi** The climate that promotes all things to grow. It pertains to fire in the five elements. See *Su Wen* chapter 70.

长虫 即蛔虫。出《素问·咳论》。

长虫(cháng chóng) **long worm** Refers to roundworms. See *Su Wen* chapter 38.

长则气治 长，指脉形长，过于本位。治，正常之意。为气血充盈畅达之象,故属正常脉象。出《素问·脉要精微论》。

长则气治 (cháng zé qì zhì)
Long pulse indicates peaceful flow of qi. *Cháng* refers to a pulse extending beyond its position. *Zhì* means normal. This term means a smooth flow of qi and blood, and is one of the normal pulse manifestations. See *Su Wen* chapter 17.

长针 九针之一。长七寸,针锋锐利,针身薄而长,后人称为"环跳针",近人又发展为芒针,用于肌肉肥厚处,治邪深病久之痹。出《灵枢·九针十二原》。

长针 (cháng zhēn) **long needle** One of the nine needles, which is 7 *cun* long, sharp and thin. It is called *huantiao* needle by later generations and was further developed into elongated needles, which were used to pierce thick muscles in treating impediments from deep invasion by pathogenic factors and prolonged diseases. See *Ling Shu* chapter 1.

长刺节论 《素问》篇名。长,扩大。刺节,针刺的方法。长刺节,即扩大五节、十二节的内容,此篇主要论述了头痛、寒热、痛肿、少腹有积、寒疝、筋痹、骨痹、癫狂、大风等病证的针刺方法,故名。

长刺节论 (cháng cì jié lùn)
Further Elucidation of Needling Therapy Chapter title in *Su Wen*. *Cháng* meaning to extend, and *cì jié* a needling method. *Cháng cì jié* means to extend the contents on the five and twelve methods of needling. Discussed in this chapter are, needling therapies for diseases and syndromes like headaches, syndromes of cold and heat, carbuncles and swelling, distension in the lower abdomen, cold hernia, tendon and bone impediments, mania and syndromes of great wind. See *Su Wen* chapter 55.

长命 人类生长的寿命。出《素问·五常政大论》。

长命 (cháng mìng) **longevity** Life span of humans. See *Su Wen* chapter 70.

长政 指万物生长的气候。政,施政。长政,也即火政。出《素问·气交变大论》。

长政 (cháng zhèng) **growth policy** The climate that promotes all things to grow. *Zhèng* refers to administration. *Cháng zhèng* is also named the fire administration. See *Su Wen* chapter 69.

长夏　指农历六月,为脾所主的季节。出《素问·藏气法时论》。

长夏(cháng xià)　**late summer** Refers to June in the lunar calendar, and is the season governed by the spleen. See *Su Wen* chapter 22.

长强　经穴名。属督脉经。在脊骶端,尾骨尖下半寸处。出《灵枢·经脉》。

长强(cháng qiáng)　**Chang Qiang (DU 1)** Acupoint name belonging to the governor vessel. It is located 0.5 *cun* below the apex of the coccyx. See *Ling Shu* chapter 10.

反阳　指水运不及之年,寒气不足,阳热之气反盛。出《素问·五常政大论》。

反阳(fǎn yáng)　**rebelling yang** Refers to the years with insufficient water movement leading to insufficient cold qi, and causing a rebellious exuberance of yang heat qi. See *Su Wen* chapter 70.

反折　角弓反张。出《素问·诊要经终论》。

反折(fǎn zhé)　**bent backward** Opisthotonus. See *Su Wen* chapter 16.

反佐　言方剂中佐药药性与主药相反的治疗方法,即寒药方中佐以热药,热药方中佐以寒药。如《伤寒论》中白通加猪胆汁汤,引用猪胆汁即为反佐法。另有汤药内服的反佐法,即热药冷服、寒药温服,以避免格拒现象的出现。出《素问·至真要大论》。

反佐(fǎn zuǒ)　**using corrigent** It refers to a therapeutic method in which the medicine properties of the assistant drugs are contrary to those of the principal drugs in a prescription. That is, having hot natured drugs in a prescription of cold natured drugs, and vice versa. For instance, in the medical classic *Shang Han Lun* (*On Cold Damage*) by Zhang Zhongjing, for Bai Tong Jia Zhu Dan Zhi Decoction (Bai Tong with Pig's Bile Decoction), the inclusion of pig's bile to the Bai Tong Decoction is an example of using corrigent. In addition, there is a similar practice with using corrigent in taking decoctions, that is, for a prescription hot in property, the decoction is taken when cold, and for a prescription cold in property, the decoction is taken when warm，so as to avoid repulsion. See *Su Wen* chapter 74.

反者反治　出《素问·至真要大论》。（1）脉证不相应者用反治。见《素问》吴崑注。（2）运气不及则反佐治之。见《素问集注》。

反者反治（fǎn zhě fǎn zhì）　**Diseases contrary to the rule are treated contrary to the rule.** See *Su Wen* chapter 74. (1) Treatments contrary to the rule are used for diseases with pulses contrary to the symptoms. See *Su Wen* annotated by Wu Kun. (2) Treatments contrary to the rule are adopted for diseases due to insufficient circuits and qi. See *Su Wen Ji Zhu* (*Collected Annotation of Su Wen*).

反治　与正治相对，又称从治。当疾病出现假象时，用药顺从病之假象，如热因热用，塞因塞用等。出《素问·至真要大论》。

反治（fǎn zhì）　**contrary treatment** Opposite to normal treatment，and also called conforming treatment. To treat diseases with pseudo-symptoms，the property of drugs used conforms to the symptoms. For instance，to treat heat with heat（or to treat false-heat syndrome with

drugs hot in property），and to treat the obstructed by obstructing（or to treat obstructive syndrome with tonics）. See *Su Wen* chapter 74.

反戾　反，角弓反张。反戾，即肢体反屈之谓。出《素问·至真要大论》。

反戾（fǎn lì）　**contortion** Opisthotonus，or limbs and trunk bent backwards. See *Su Wen* chapter 74.

反僵　角弓反张，肢体僵硬。出《灵枢·癫狂病》。

反僵（fǎn jiāng）　**bent backwards and stiff** Opisthotonus with stiffness of the limbs and trunk. See *Ling Shu* chapter 22.

父母　① 喻指阴阳，是万物变化的根本。出《素问·阴阳应象大论》。② 喻指生命活动的重要脏器。出《素问·刺禁论》。（1）指心肺。见《类经·针刺六十四》。（2）指心肾。见《素问集注》。（3）指气海。见《素问》王冰注。（4）指肺脾。见《素问直解》。

父母（fù mǔ）　① Signifying yin and yang，or the root of changes in all things. See *Su Wen* chapter 5. ② Refers to the vital organs for life activities. See *Su Wen* chapter 52.

（1）Refers to the heart and lung. See *Lei Jing* (*Classified Classic*) "Needling Chapter 64". (2) Refers to the heart and kidney. *See Su Wen Ji Zhu* (*Collected Annotation of Su Wen*). (3) Refers to the sea of qi. See *Su Wen* annotated by Wang Bing. (4) Refers to the lung and spleen. See *Su Wen Zhi Jie* (*Direct Interpretation on Su Wen*).

从革 指运气中金运不及之年。从,顺从;革,变革。从革,指代五行中金的特性因火而变革。出《素问·五常政大论》。

从革(cóng gé) **accepted change** Refers to years with deficient metal movement in the circuits and qi theory. *Cóng* refers to obey. *Gé* refers to transformation. The properties of metal can be changed because of fire in the five elements. See *Su Wen* chapter 70.

从容 ① 古医籍名。已佚。出《素问·阴阳类论》。《素问·示从容论》主要是讲辨证问题,故《从容》可能是一部关于辨证的古经。② 举动。出《素问·著至教论》。③ 和缓镇定的态度。出《素问·示从容论》。

从容(cóng róng) ① *Cong Rong* (*Leisureliness*). An ancient Chinese medical book that was lost in history. See *Su Wen* chapter 79. This chapter is mainly about syndrome differentiation, thus it is likely that Cong Rong (*Leisureliness*) is an ancient classic on syndrome differentiation. ② Solitary behavior. See *Su Wen* chapter 75. ③ Calm attitude. See *Su Wen* chapter 76.

凶风 八风之一,指由东北方刮来的风。出《灵枢·九宫八风》。

凶风(xiōng fēng) ***xiong* wind** One of the eight winds, and refers to the wind from the northeast. See *Ling Shu* chapter 77.

分气 ① 分肉间的邪气。出《灵枢·九针十二原》。② 分出于口鼻的呼吸之气。出《灵枢·忧恚无言》。

分气(fēn qì) ① Pathogenic qi in the muscular interstices. See *Ling Shu* chapter 1. ② Respiratory air from the mouth and the nose. See *Ling Shu* chapter 69.

分肉 ① 肌肉。出《灵枢·官针》。(1) 内层的肌肉。前人将肌肉分为内外二层,外层为白肉(皮下脂肪),内层为赤肉(肌肉组织),赤白相分,故云。见

《灵枢注证发微》。(2) 有分理之肌肉，现代称为骨骼肌。见《类经·针刺六》。② 阳辅别名。出《素问·气穴论》。

分肉(fēn ròu) ① The flesh or muscles. See *Ling Shu* chapter 7. (1) Inner muscles. In ancient China, the muscles were divided into two layers: the white flesh (subcutaneous fat) on the outer layer and the red flesh (muscular tissue) on the inner layer. The white and red flesh is mentioned separately. See *Su Wen Zhu Zheng Fa Wei* (*Annotation and Elaboration on Su Wen*). (2) Skeletal muscles, or the striated muscles. See *Lei Jing* (*Classified Classic*) "Needling Chapter 6". ② Another name for the acupoint Yang Fu (GB 38). See *Su Wen* chapter 58.

分纪 指分野纪度，即天体所划分的区域和度数。出《素问·六节藏象论》。

分纪(fēn jì) **regions and orders** Refers to regions and degrees divided by celestial bodies. See *Su Wen* chapter 9.

分刺 九刺法之一，是针刺直达肌肉间隙的一种刺法，用治肌肉痹证。出《灵枢·官针》。

分刺(fēn cì) *fen* **needling** One of the nine needling methods, in which the muscular interstices are pierced directly. It is used to treat impediment of the muscles or flesh. See *Ling Shu* chapter 7.

分注 大小便俱下。出《素问·至真要大论》。

分注(fēn zhù) **simultaneous urination and defecation** Urination and defecation at the same time. See *Su Wen* chapter 74.

分部 指皮部。出《素问·阴阳应象大论》。

分部(fēn bù) **skin divisions** See *Su Wen* chapter 5.

分理 ① 分，分肉；理，纹理、腠理。谓肌肉间之界畔纹理。出《素问·诊要经终论》。② 划分节气的规律。出《灵枢·卫气行》。

分理(fēn lǐ) ① *Fēn* means muscles. *Lǐ* means tissues, or interstices. *It* refers to the borders and textures between muscles. See *Su Wen* chapter 16. ② The law by which the solar terms are differentiated. See *Ling Shu* chapter 76.

分腠 指分肉、腠理。出《灵枢·寒热病》。

分腠(fēn còu) **muscular interstices** Refers to the partings of the flesh. See *Ling Shu* chapter 21.

公孙 经穴名。足太阴脾经络穴。又是八脉交会穴之一,通冲脉。在足大指本节后一寸。出《灵枢·经脉》。

公孙(gōng sūn) **Gong Sun**(**SP 4**) Acupoint name, which is the connecting acupoint of the spleen meridian of foot *taiyin*, and one of the acupoints where the eight extraordinary meridians conflow. It leads to the thoroughfare vessel and is located one *cun* behind the metatarsal bone of the big toe. See *Ling Shu* chapter 10.

仓门 九宫之一。又名震宫,居东方,主春令。出《灵枢·九宫八风》。

仓门(cāng mén) *cang men* **palace** One of the nine palaces, which is also called *Zhen* palace. It is located in the east and governs Spring. See *Ling Shu* chapter 77.

仓果 九宫之一。又名兑宫,居西方,主秋令。出《灵枢·九宫八风》。

仓果(cāng guǒ) *Cang guo* **palace** One of the nine palaces, which is also called *Dui* palace. It is located in the west and governs Autumn. See *Ling Shu* chapter 77.

仓廪之本 义同"仓廪之官"。出《素问·六节藏象论》。

仓廪之本(cāng lǐn zhī běn) **roots of the granary** Same meaning as "仓廪之官". See *Su Wen* chapter 9.

仓廪之官 指脾胃。脾胃有受纳水谷,运化精微的功能,犹如主管仓储的官吏,故名。出《素问·灵兰秘典论》。

仓廪之官(cāng lǐn zhī guān) **granary official** Refers to the spleen and stomach. These two organs receive water and grains, and transport and transform the essence, just as an official in charge of a granary would do. See *Su Wen* chapter 8.

月事 即月经,是胞宫周期性出血的生理现象。通常女子十四岁左右开始出现,四十九岁左右停止,其间除妊娠、哺乳期外,一般每月按时来潮一次。出《素问·上古天真论》。

月事(yuè shì) **monthly affair** Namely menstruation, which is a physiological condition with periodic bleeding of the uterus. Generally speaking, females have the first occurrence of menstruation at approximately the age of 14 and the last at about the age of 49. Menstruation occurs cyclically once a month during a female's lifetime except during pregnancy and lactation. See *Su Wen* chapter 1.

欠　① 俗称呵欠。张口呵吸，或伸臂展腰之状。常于卫气将循行于阴分，人在欲寐未寐时所作，为生理现象。出《灵枢·口问》。此外欠亦可作为症状而见于脏腑经脉的病变。出《素问·宣明五气》《素问·阴阳别论》。② 合口之谓。出《灵枢·本输》。

欠(qiàn)　① Yawning, or meaning to breathe with an open mouth，or with stretching of the arms and waist. It often occurs when the defensive qi is about to enter the yin aspect and a person is about to sleep, which is a physiological phenomenon. See *Ling Shu* chapter 28. In addition，yawning can also be a symptom seen in diseases of the viscera and channels. See *Su Wen* chapter 7 and chapter 23. ② Closing the mouth. See *Ling Shu* chapter 2.

欠欤　张口打呵欠。出《灵枢·经脉》。

欠欤(qiàn qù)　**yawning with wide open mouth** Yawning with mouth open. See *Ling Shu* chapter 10.

风　① 由空气的流动所形成的气候现象。为六气之一，是春季所主的气候，五行属木。出《素问·阴阳应象大论》。② 病因名。即风邪，为六淫之一，属阳邪，为外感疾病的先导。出《素问·骨空论》。③ 病机名。临床见肢体痉挛、抽搐、角弓反张等症候，其病机大多属于风。出《素问·至真要大论》。④ 风水病。症见面目、下肢，乃至全身突然浮肿的病。出《素问·平人气象论》。⑤ 一种与疟相似的病证。症见身热、汗出、恶风等。出《素问·评热病论》。⑥ 肢体振摇、头目眩晕的病证。出《素问·至真要大论》。⑦ 指风邪伤犯阳经或阳分的病证。出《灵枢·寿夭刚柔》。⑧ 指风气。出《素问·天元纪大论》。⑨ 指耳鸣声。出《素问·缪刺论》。

风(fēng)　① A climatic phenomenon caused by the flow of air. One of the six qi. It is predominant in spring and pertains to wood in the five elements. See *Su Wen* chapter 5. ② A cause of disease. It is also called pathogenic wind，one of the six exogenous pathogenic factors which leads to diseases. It pertains to yang and is the forerunner in causing exogenous diseases. See *Su Wen* chapter 60. ③ Pathogenesis. Clinically speaking，the pathogenesis of symptoms including limb spasms，convulsions and opisthotonos are all related to wind. See *Su Wen* chapter 74. ④ Wind water or wind edema，with sudden swelling in the face and lower limbs，or all over the body. See *Su Wen* chapter 18. ⑤ A disease similar to malaria，with symptoms such as general fever，sweating and aversion to wind etc. See *Su Wen* chapter 33. ⑥ Diseases and syndromes with symptoms of a shaking body and dizziness. See *Su Wen* chapter 74. ⑦ Diseases and syndromes due to the invasion of the yang channel or the yang aspect by pathogenic wind. See *Ling Shu* chapter 6. ⑧ Wind qi. See *Su Wen* chapter 66. ⑨ Tinnitus. See *Su Wen* chapter 63.

风无常府 言风邪善行而数变，其侵犯人体无所不到。出《素问·疟论》。

风无常府（fēng wú cháng fǔ） **Wind does not invade the body through a fixed region.** Meaning that pathogenic wind is active and changeable，and it can in-

vade every part of the body. See *Su Wen* chapter 35.

风水 病证名。感受风邪而见全身浮肿的病证，为肾风的进一步发展。出《素问·水热穴论》。

风水（fēng shuǐ） **wind water** Disease name of the syndrome with general swelling due to pathogenic wind，which is a further development of kidney wind. See *Su Wen* chapter 61.

风气 ① 春天的自然气候，主生发，与肝胆相应。出《素问·阴阳应象大论》。② 风邪。出《素问·痹论》。③ 运气概念中六气之一，厥阴为标，风气为本，风化厥阴。出《素问·天元纪大论》。

风气（fēng qì） ① Normal climate in Spring，which governs generation and corresponds to the liver and gallbladder. See *Su Wen* chapter 5. ② Pathogenic wind. See *Su Wen* chapter 43. ③ One of the six qi in the movement of qi theory. *Jueyin* is *biao*（branch）and wind qi is *ben*（root），thus wind transforms *jueyin*. See *Su Wen* chapter 66.

风以动之 见"燥以干之……火以温之"条。出《素问·五运行大论》。

风以动之（fēng yǐ dòng zhī）
wind shakes it See "燥以干
之……火以温之". See *Su Wen*
chapter 67.

风伤肝　风气通于肝,风气盛则伤
肝。出《素问·五运行大论》。

风伤肝（fēng shāng gān）**wind
harms the liver** Wind qi transpasses the liver, and its predominance damages the liver.
See *Su Wen* chapter 67.

风伤筋　风气通于肝,肝主筋,故
风邪易于伤筋,出现拘挛、抽
搐、角弓反张等筋脉为病。出
《素问·阴阳应象大论》。

风伤筋（fēng shāng jīn）**wind
harms the sinews** Wind qi
transpasses the liver, and the
liver governs the sinews, thus
pathogenic wind often damages
the sinews, and diseases occur
with symptoms including spasms,
convulsions and opisthotonos.
See *Su Wen* chapter 5.

风池　经穴名。属足少阳胆经,
在乳突后方,胸锁乳突肌与斜
方肌之间,平风府处。出《灵
枢·热病》。

风池（fēng chí）**Feng Chi（GB
20）** Acupoint name belonging
to the gallbladder meridian of
foot *shaoyang*. It is located behind the mastoid process, be-

tween the sternocleidomastoid
and trapezius muscles, at the
same level with the acupoint
Feng Fu（Du 16）. See *Ling Shu*
chapter 23.

风论　《素问》篇名。此篇重点论
述了风邪侵入人体后所引起的
各种疾病的病机、症状和诊察
方法。故名。

风论（fēng lùn）**Discussion on
Wind** Chapter title in *Su Wen*.
This chapter focuses on the
pathogenesis, symptoms and
diagnostic methods of various
diseases due to invasion of the
human body by pathogenic
wind. Hence the name.

风位　即厥阴风木旺盛所主之时
令。出《素问·六微旨大论》。

风位（fēng wèi）**wind position**
The season dominated by exu-
berant *jueyin* wind wood. See
Su Wen chapter 68.

风者百病之长也　长,首也。风
为六淫之首,常为外邪致病的
先导,故称百病之长。出《素
问·玉机真藏论》。

风者百病之长也（fēng zhě bǎi
bìng zhī zhǎng yě）**Wind is the
leading factor responsible for all
diseases.** *Zhǎng* refers to head.
Wind is the first of the six exogenous pathogenic qi and is

often the forerunner of exogenous pathogens causing disease. See *Su Wen* chapter 19.

风者百病之始也 风为六淫之首,是外感疾病的首要病因。出《素问·生气通天论》。

风者百病之始也(fēng zhě bǎi bìng zhī shǐ yě) **Wind is the origin of all diseases.** Wind is the first of the six exogenous pathogenic qi and is the leading factor causing exogenous diseases. See *Su Wen* chapter 3.

风者善行而数变 善行,流动不居。数,多。数变,变化多端。风性主动,致病急,变化快,病位不定。出《素问·风论》。

风者善行而数变(fēng zhě shàn xíng ér shuò biàn) **Wind tends to move and change.** *Shàn xíng* means the tendency to move freely. *Shuò* means more. *Shuò biàn* refers to changeable. Wind is active and can rapidly lead to disease. It is changeable and can cause diseases in any part of the body. See *Su Wen* chapter 42.

风肿 病证名。由风邪所引起的肿胀。出《灵枢·五变》。

风肿(fēng zhǒng) **wind swelling** Disease name in which swelling is caused by pathogenic wind. See *Ling Shu* chapter 46.

风府 经穴名。属督脉经。在项后正中入发际一寸处。太阳经脉上连于风府,诸阳之气总会于风府。出《灵枢·本输》。

风府(fēng fǔ) **Feng Fu (DU 16)** Acupoint name belonging to the governor vessel, and located one *cun* inside the hairline, midline on the back of the neck. The *taiyang* channels connect to, and qi of all of the yang channels converge at Feng Fu acupoint. See *Ling Shu* chapter 2.

风疟 病名。疟疾之一种。由风邪入侵而引起的汗出恶风,先寒后热,寒少热多的病证。出《素问·刺疟》。

风疟(fēng nüè) **wind malaria** Disease name of one kind of malaria, of which the cause is invasion by pathogenic wind leading to sweating, aversion to wind, chills first and fever afterwards, with fever being more tangible than the chills. See *Su Wen* chapter 36.

风胜乃摇 摇,摇动。义见"风胜则动"条。出《素问·六元正纪大论》。

风胜乃摇(fēng shèng nǎi yáo) **Wind dominates and causes shaking.** *Yáo* refers to shake.

See "风胜则动". See *Su Wen* chapter 71.

风胜则动 动，指肢体振摇，抽搐。风气通于肝，肝主筋脉，风气胜则肝与筋脉受病，出现筋脉拘挛、抽搐、摇动等症。出《素问·阴阳应象大论》。

风胜则动（fēng shèng zé dòng）
Predominance of wind causes restlessness. Restlessness means shaking and convulsions of the body. Wind qi transpasses the liver, and the liver governs the sinews, thus predominance of wind qi leads to diseases of the liver and sinews, resulting in symptoms such as spasms of the sinews, convulsions and tremors. See *Su Wen* chapter 5.

风胜湿 风属木，湿属土，木能克土，故风能胜湿。临床有湿侵经络脏腑，可用祛风以除湿的治疗方法。出《素问·阴阳应象大论》。

风胜湿（fēng shèng shī） **Wind dominates over dampness.** Wind pertains to wood, dampness pertains to earth, and wood restrains earth, therefore wind dominates over dampness. Clinically speaking, diseases due to the invasion of the channels, collaterals and the viscera by dampness can be treated by dispelling wind to remove the dampness. See *Su Wen* chapter 5.

风逆 风感于外，厥气内逆的病证。主症有突然四肢肿胀，汗出淋漓，身冷颤栗，口出唏嘘之声，饥饿时感到心烦，饱食后动扰不宁。出《灵枢·癫狂病》。

风逆（fēng nì） **adverse wind** Diseases caused by the invasion of pathogenic wind and the adverse flow of qi. Syndromes resulting from the attack by exogenous pathogenic factors and internal adverse flow of qi. Symptoms include sudden swelling of the limbs, heavy sweating, chills, sighing, vexation when hungry and restlessness after repletion. See *Ling Shu* chapter 22.

风根 出《素问·腹中论》。（1）以风邪为病因之本。见《太素·杂病》。（2）指风毒根于中。见《素问》吴崑注。（3）指寒气。见《类经·疾病七十三》。

风根（fēng gēn） **wind root** See *Su Wen* chapter 40.（1）With pathogenic wind as the root cause of disease. See *Tai Su (Grand Plain)* "Miscellaneous Diseases".（2）Refers to wind toxins with roots in the umbilicus. See *Su Wen* annotated by

Wu Kun. (3) Refers to cold qi. See *Lei Jing*（*Classified Classic*）"On Diseases Chapter 73".

风痉　病证名。由风邪侵犯经络所引起的颈项强直、角弓反张的病证。出《灵枢·热病》。

风痉（fēng jīng）　**wind convulsion** Disease name of the syndrome with neck stiffness and opisthotonos, caused by the invasion of pathogenic wind into the channels and collaterals. See *Ling Shu* chapter 23.

风消　病证名。出《素问·阴阳别论》。（1）因风热、风木之邪而导致肌肉消瘦。见《类经·疾病六》。（2）津液消竭。见《素问集注》。（3）上消证。见《素问识》。

风消（fēng xiāo）　**wind consumption** Disease name. See *Su Wen* chapter 7.（1）Emaciation of muscles due to pathogenic wind heat and wind wood. See *Lei Jing*（*Classified Classic*）"On Diseases Chapter 6".（2）Depletion of body fluids. See *Su Wen Ji Zhu*（*Collected Annotation of Su Wen*）.（3）Upper consumptive thirst syndrome. See *Su Wen Zhi*（*Understanding Su Wen*）.

风厥　① 病名。因肝经风木之气,贼犯阳明,致气机逆乱,故名。症见惊骇、背痛、善噫、善呵欠等。出《素问·阴阳别论》。② 为太阳感受风邪,引动少阴之气厥而上逆之证。症见发热、汗出、烦满等。出《素问·评热病论》。③ 由腠理疏松,风邪入侵,厥逆于内,致漉漉汗出之证。出《灵枢·五变》。

风厥（fēng jué）　① Disease name, which is caused by the reverse movement of qi due to the invasion of the stomach by the qi of the liver channel's wind wood. Symptoms include panicking, back pain, and frequent sighing and yawning. See *Su Wen* chapter 7. ② A syndrome caused by the reverse movement of qi of the kidney meridian of foot *shaoyin* due to the attack of the bladder meridian of foot *taiyang* by pathogenic wind. Symptoms include fever, sweating, vexation and fullness. See *Su Wen* chapter 33. ③ A disease with heavy sweating caused by the reverse flow of qi in the interior due to the invasion by pathogenic wind when the muscular interstices are loose. See *Ling Shu* chapter 46.

四画

风痹　① 指由血虚失于濡养而引起的皮肤枯涩麻木一类病证。出《灵枢·论疾诊》。② 风与痹之合称。指既有皮肤表证，又有筋骨酸痛麻重的病证。出《灵枢·寿夭刚柔》。

风痹（fēng bì）　① Refers to the syndrome with dry，rough and numb skin caused by the failure of being nourished due to blood insufficiency. See *Ling Shu* chapter 74. ② A collective term for wind and impediment. It refers to exterior syndromes of the skin as well as severe syndromes with aches，numbness and heaviness of the sinews and bones. See *Ling Shu* chapter 6.

风痿　病证名。因脾弱生风，致使四肢痿弱不用之证。出《灵枢·邪气藏府病形》。

风痿（fēng wěi）　**wind flaccidity** Disease name of the syndrome with flaccidity of the four limbs due to wind generated by deficient spleen qi. See *Ling Shu* chapter 4.

丹天之气　古代望气家在西北方位牛、女、奎、壁星宿之间看到的红色天象，主火运。出《素问·五运行大论》。

丹天之气（dān tiān zhī qì）　**qi of a vermilion heaven** A red celestial phenomenon，observed by scholars in ancient China，who read the future from clouds among the constellations *niu*，*nü*，*kui* and *bi* in the northwest. It dominates the fire movement. See *Su Wen* chapter 67.

丹胗　胗，同疹。丹胗，红色的瘾疹。出《素问·至真要大论》。

丹胗（dān zhěn）　**vermilion papules** "胗" is the same as "疹". Reddish eruptions. See *Su Wen* chapter 74.

丹熛　熛，火焰。丹熛，指局部红肿焮热丹毒一类外科疾患。出《素问·至真要大论》。

丹熛（dān biāo）　**vermilion gangrene** *Biāo* refers to flames. Vermilion gangrene refers to a class of surgical diseases such as erysipelas with local redness，swelling and thermal sensation. See *Su Wen* chapter 74.

乌鲗骨　药名，即乌贼骨，又名海螵蛸。气味咸温微涩，入肝肾经。主治女子赤白漏下及血枯经闭。出《素问·腹中论》。

乌鲗骨（wū zéi gǔ）　**cuttlefish bone** Name of a medicine, that is cuttlebone, salty in taste, warm in property and slightly astringent. It enters the liver and kidney, and is used to treat metrostaxis with red and white vaginal discharge, and amenorrhoea due to blood desiccation in women. See *Su Wen* chapter 40.

六元　运气术语。指六气,即风、火、湿、热、燥、寒为气候变化之本元。出《素问·六元正纪大论》。

六元(liù yuán)　**six principal qi** Terminology of circuits and qi which refers to the six qi, and the origin of climatic changes, including wind, fire, dampness, heat, dryness and cold. See *Su Wen* chapter 71.

六元正纪大论　《素问》篇名。六元,即风、热、火、湿、燥、寒六气;正纪,即正常的规律;大论,内容宏富之论。此篇主要论述六气司天于上,在泉于下,左右间气纪步,运气相合而三十年为一纪,六十年为一周,其中有化有变,有胜有复,体现了六气的正常变化规律与宇宙万物变化的关系。

六元正纪大论(liù yuán zhèng jì dà lùn)　**Major Discussion on the Normal Rule of the Six Principal Qi** Chapter title in *Su Wen*. The six principal qi refers to wind, heat, fire, dampness, dryness and cold. *Zhèng jì* refers to the normal rule. *Dà lùn* refers to a discussion with abundant contents. In this chapter, discussion on the six qi dominating the heavens as well as being in spring is expounded on elaborately. It numbers the six steps of a year with the middle qi on the left and right, and when the movement conforms to the qi, thirty years constitute a *ji* and sixty years a cycle. There are transformation and changes, and domination and retaliation of qi, both reflecting the relationships between the patterns of normal changes of the six qi and changes of all things in the universe.

六气　① 指风、热、火、湿、燥、寒。又称六元。出《素问·六元正纪大论》。② 指配主气六步的六气。六气配主气六步,即为初之气配厥阴风木,二之气配少阴君火,三之气配少阳相火,四之气配太阴湿土,五之气配阳明燥金,终之气配太阳寒水。出《素问·六微旨大论》。③ 指人体精、气、津、液、血、脉。出《灵枢·决气》。④ 指六个节气,为一时。出《素问·六节藏象论》。

六气(liù qì) ① Refers to wind, heat, fire, dampness, dryness and cold, and also called the six principal qi. See *Su Wen* chapter 71. ② Refers to the six qi that correspond to the six steps of a year. The initial qi corresponds to *jueyin* wind wood, the second qi to *shaoyin* monarch fire, the third qi to *shaoyang* ministerial fire, the fourth qi to *taiyin* damp earth, the fifth qi to *yangming* dry metal and the final qi to *taiyang* cold water. See *Su Wen* chapter 68. ③ Refers to essence, qi, thin and thick body fluids, blood and vessels. See *Ling Shu* chapter 30. ④ Refers to the six solar terms, which constitute a season. See *Su Wen* chapter 9.

六气标本　标,指三阴三阳。本,指风热燥湿火寒六气。六气有标有本,如风为本,厥阴为标;热为本,少阴为标;火为本,少阳为标;湿为本,太阴为标;燥为本,阳明为标;寒为本,太阳为标。出《素问·至真要大论》。

六气标本(liù qì biāo běn)　**Six qi following biao (branch) and ben (root).** *Biao* (branch) refers to three yin and three yang; *Ben* (root) refers to the six qi, namely wind, heat, dryness, dampness, fire and cold. In the six qi, some correspond to *biao* (branch), and other correspond to *ben* (root). For instance, wind is *ben* (root) and *jueyin* is *biao* (branch); heat is *ben* and *shaoyin* is *biao*; fire is *ben* and *shaoyang* is *biao*; dampness is *ben* and *taiyin* is *biao*; dryness is *ben* and *yangming* is *biao*; cold is *ben* and *taiyang* is *biao*. See *Su Wen* chapter 74.

六气相胜　运气术语。六气有太过不及盛衰之异,其相互间可因偏盛而乘胜之。具体有厥阴风木之胜,少阴君火之胜,太阴湿土之胜,少阳相火之胜,阳明燥金之胜,太阳寒水之胜。出《素问·至真要大论》。

六气相胜(liù qì xiāng shèng)　**mutual domination of the six qi** Terminology of circuits and qi, in which the six qi may be either in excess or insufficient. One qi may restrict or over-restrict (dominate) another qi when it is in excess. Specifically, there is *jueyin* wind wood, *shaoyin* monarch fire, *taiyin* damp earth, *shaoyang* ministerial fire, *yangming* dry metal and *taiyang* cold water domination. See *Su Wen* chapter 74.

六化 风、寒、暑、湿、燥、火六气的正常生化。出《素问·六元正纪大论》。

六化(liù huà) **transformation of the six qi** The normal generation and transformation of the six qi，namely wind，cold，summerheat，dampness，dryness and fire. See *Su Wen* chapter 71.

六六之节 运气术语。节，节段。① 干支相配,六十日甲子一周为一节,六个甲子日,三百六十日为一年,以合周天之数。出《素问·六节藏象论》。② 六六,指三阴三阳与天之六气。一年中六气变化情况可以根据阴阳多少特点用三阴三阳划分为六个节段。出《素问·六微旨大论》。

六六之节(liù liù zhī jié) **six-six system** Terminology of circuits and qi，and *jié* refers to segments. ① In combination of the heavenly stems with the earthly branches，sixty days constitute one *jia zi* day or one term，and six *jia zi* days or three hundred and sixty days complete a year，thus corresponding to a complete circle of three hundred and sixty degrees. See *Su Wen* chapter 9.

② "Six-six" refers to three yin and three yang and the six qi of the heavens. Changes of the six qi in a year can be categorized into six sections using three yin and three yang based on the amount of yin and yang existing. See *Su Wen* chapter 68.

六节藏象论 《素问》篇名。六节,古人以干支纪年,六十日为一甲子日,称一节,六节为一年。藏,内脏。象,征象。六节藏象,天以六六之节以成岁,人之藏象与之相应。此篇讨论了天体运动和四季气候变化的规律与人体生理、病理的关系;人体十二脏腑的主要功能及其与外环境的关系。

六节藏象论(liù jié zàng xiàng lùn) **Discussion on the Six-six System and the Manifestations in the Viscera** Chapter title in *Su Wen*. In ancient China，the years were numbered by the heavenly stems and the earthly branches. Sixty days constituted one *jia zi* day or one term，and six terms completed a year. *Zàng* refers to the internal organs. *Xiàng* refers to the manifestation in the internal organs. The viscera and their manifestations in the human body correspond to the six-six system of the heavens. In this chapter, the relationships of the law of changes in celestial movement and climate in the four seasons along with the physiology and pathology of the human body are discussed; the main functions of the twelve viscera and bowels and their relationships with the external environment are explored.

六合 ① 指东、南、西、北四方及上下。出《素问·生气通天论》。② 十二经别根据十二经脉的表里关系，分为六对，每一对互为表里的脏腑为一合，共称为六合。出《灵枢·经别》。③ 专指第六合，即手阳明与手太阴经经别表里相合。出《灵枢·经别》。

六合（liù hé） ① Refers to the east, south, west, north, upper and lower directions. See *Su Wen* chapter 3. ② Six pairs of meridians, as the meridian divergences are divided into six pairs according to the relationship of the interior and exterior. A pair consists of two channels with a viscera and its corresponding fu organ in the interior and exterior, respectively. There are six pairs in total. See *Ling*

Shu chapter 11. ③ Specifically refers to the sixth pair, that is, the large intestine meridian of hand *yangming* in the exterior and the lung meridian of hand *taiyin* in the interior. See *Ling Shu* chapter 11.

六阳 指手足三阳经脉。出《灵枢·脉度》。

六阳（liù yáng） **six yang** Refers to the three yang meridians of the hand and the foot. See *Ling Shu* chapter 17.

六变 ① 风、寒、暑、湿、燥、火六气太过、不及的异常变化。出《素问·六元正纪大论》。② 指阴阳气血寒热的六种病理变化。出《灵枢·邪气藏府病形》。

六变（liù biàn） ① Abnormal changes due to the excess or insufficiency of the six qi, namely wind, cold, summerheat, dampness, dryness and fire. See *Su Wen* chapter 71. ② Refers to the six kinds of pathological changes with abnormalities in yin, yang, qi, blood, cold and heat. See *Ling Shu* chapter 4.

六府 府，通腑。胆、胃、大肠、小肠、三焦、膀胱六个器官的总称。具有传化物的功能，受纳水谷，消化吸收，传送排出，共同完成食物在体内消化排泄的过程。六个器官各自有其生理活动的特点，而又相互协作，密切联系。出《素问·上古天真论》。

六府(liù fǔ) **six bowels** "府" is the same as "腑". The general name for the gallbladder, stomach，large intestine，small intestine，triple *jiao* and bladder. They transport and transform food. They receive and digest water and grains，absorb the essence，transfer and remove the dregs，and complete the process of digestion and excretion in the body. Although each of the six bowels is unique in its physiological activity，they also work together and are closely related to each other. See *Su Wen* chapter 1.

六府之咳 为胃、胆、大肠、小肠、膀胱、三焦咳之总称。由五脏咳不愈传变而成。其特点为由实转虚，可概括为"上逆"与"下泄"。皆由咳久所致。出《素问·咳论》。

六府之咳(liù fǔ zhī ké) **cough of the six bowels** General name for coughs of the stomach, gallbladder，large intestine，small intestine，bladder and triple *jiao*，and is transmitted from the five viscera with lingering coughs. It is characterized by a change from excess to deficiency，summarized as the "upward reversal of lung qi" and "purgation". It is caused by a prolonged cough. See *Su Wen* chapter 38.

六府之俞 指六府的背俞穴，即胃俞，三焦俞，胆俞，大肠俞，小肠俞，膀胱俞。均属足太阳经。出《素问·气府论》。

六府之俞(liù fǔ zhī shū) **transport acupoints of the six bowels** Refers to the transport acupoints of the six bowels located on the back，including the stomach transport（BL 21），the triple *jiao* transport（BL 22），the gallbladder transport（BL 19），the large intestine transport（BL 25），the small intestine transport（BL 27）and the bladder transport（BL 28）. They all belong to the bladder meridian of foot *taiyang*. See *Su Wen* chapter 59.

六府气 指六府之气失调所引起的病证。出《灵枢·九针论》。

六府气(liù fǔ qì) **qi of the six bowels** Refers to the diseases and syndromes caused by the disorder of the qi of the six bowels. See *Ling Shu* chapter 78.

六府胀 病证名。为胃、大肠、小肠、膀胱、三焦、胆胀之总称。出《灵枢·胀论》。

六府胀(liù fǔ zhàng) **distension of the six bowels** Disease name of the syndrome manifesting with distension of the stomach, large intestine, small intestine, bladder, triple *jiao* and gallbladder. See *Ling Shu* chapter 35.

六经 三阴三阳经脉之合称，即太阳、阳明、少阳、太阴、少阴、厥阴经脉。六经各有手足之分，故又称十二经脉。出《素问·阴阳应象大论》。

六经(liù jīng) **six meridians** A combined term for three yin meridians and three yang meridians, namely the meridians of *taiyang*, *yangming*, *shaoyang*, *taiyin*, *shaoyin* and *jueyin*. Each of these six meridians has meridians of foot and hand, thus twelve meridians in total. See *Su Wen* chapter 5.

六律 我国古代音乐的律制。相传伶伦截竹为管，以管之长短，分别声音的清浊高下，分为十二律，由低至高分别为黄钟、大吕、太簇、夹钟、姑洗、仲吕、蕤宾、林钟、夷则、南吕、无射和应钟。十二律分阴阳，阳六为律，阴六为吕，故浑称六律。出《素问·针解》。

六律(liù lǜ) **six pitch-pipes** A tuning system in ancient China. Legend has it that Linglun made pipes out of bamboo, the tone was distinguished by the length of the pipes. There were 12 notes in total, including *huang zhong*, *da lyu*, *tai cu*, *jia zhong*, *gu xi*, *zhong lyu*, *rui bin*, *lin zhong*, *yi ze*, *nan lv*, *wu she* and *ying zhong*. The 12 notes pertained to yin and yang, with six pertaining to yang, and six pertaining to yin. Therefore, they are also called the six notes. See *Su Wen* chapter 54.

六期 六年。一年为一期。出《素问·天元纪大论》。

六期(liù qī) **six stages** Six years. One stage is one year. See *Su Wen* chapter 66.

六输 ① 六腑经脉的井、荥、输、原、经、合六类穴。出《灵枢·顺气一日分为四时》。② 泛指三阴三阳六经之输脉。出《灵枢·百病始生》。

六输(liù shū) ① Six kinds of acupoints of the channels of the six bowels, i.e. the well, brook, stream, source, river and sea points. See *Ling Shu* chapter 44. ② The channels, including the six pairs of yin and yang channels. See *Ling Shu* chapter 66.

六微旨大论　《素问》篇名。六，即风、热、火、湿、燥、寒六气；微，精微；旨，要旨，要领。此篇主要论述天道六六之节，上应天气，下应地理，以及六气主岁、主时和客主加临等运气理论。

六微旨大论(liù wēi zhǐ dà lùn) **Major Discussion on the Abstruseness of the Six Kinds of Qi** Chapter title in *Su Wen*. *Liù* refers to the six kinds of qi including wind, heat, fire, dampness, dryness and cold. *Wēi* refers to essence; *Zhǐ* refers to the essential points, or main points. This chapter focuses on the circuits and qi theory, including the six-plus-six system, the qi of the heavens and structures of the earth, the governance of years by six qi, the governance of seasons by qi, the host qi, the guest qi and their governance etc.

方士　指通晓方术的人，此指医生。出《素问·五藏别论》。

方士(fāng shì) ***fang shi*** People who have a good knowledge of medicine, divination, and similar arts. Here, it refers to doctors. See *Su Wen* chapter 11.

方上　鼻准头两侧的鼻翼部位。面部色诊用以测候胃的状况。出《灵枢·五色》。

方上(fāng shàng) **regions lateral to the nose apex** The alar regions on both sides of the nose. In examining the complexion of the face, these regions reflect the condition of the stomach. See *Ling Shu* chapter 49.

方盛衰论　《素问》篇名。方，比方，比较；盛衰，指阴阳形气之盛衰。此篇着重讨论如何才能了解阴阳形气盛衰的问题。

方盛衰论(fāng shèng shuāi lùn) **Discussion on Superabundance and Decline of Yin and Yang** Chapter title in *Su Wen*. *Fāng* means analogy, or take something for instance, or compare to; *Shèng shuāi* refers to the waxing and waning movement of yin and yang qi. This chapter focuses on how to understand the waxing and waning movement of yin and yang qi.

火　① 五行之一，由自然界之"火"抽象而来，其特性是炎上，具有温热、上升之性，引申为具有温热升腾作用性质的事物。

根据五行属性归类的方法，归属于火的，在五脏为心，在气候为热，在季节为夏，在方位为南，在五味为苦，在五色为赤等。出《素问·阴阳应象大论》。② 病因，指火邪，为六淫之一。出《素问·至真要大论》。③ 病机。为病机十九条之一。出《素问·至真要大论》。④ 阳气。出《素问·阴阳应象大论》。⑤ 艾火，亦称火焫。出《灵枢·论痛》。⑥ 指心。出《灵枢·热病》。⑦ 火热的气候。出《素问·水热穴论》。

火（huǒ） ① Fire. One of the five elements. It is abstracted from fire in nature and characterized by flaring up. It warms and rises, and its meaning is widened, refers to everything that warms and rises. According to the categorization of the five elements, anything in the category of fire pertains to the heart in the five viscera, heat in climate, summer in seasons, the south in directions, bitter in five flavors and red in the five colors. See *Su Wen* chapter 5. ② A cause of disease, and refers to pathogenic fire, one of the six exogenous pathogenic factors. See *Su Wen* chapter 74. ③ Pathogenesis. One of the nineteen items of pathogenesis. See *Su Wen* chapter 74. ④ Yang qi. See *Su Wen* chapter 5. ⑤ Moxa fire. See *Ling Shu* chapter 53. ⑥ Refers to the heart. See *Ling Shu* chapter 23. ⑦ Hot climate. See *Su Wen* chapter 61.

火曰升明 火运平和曰升明，以火性上升而明显之故。出《素问·五常政大论》。

火曰升明（huǒ yuē shēng míng） **Balance of fire is known as Shengming (elevation and brightness).** The balance of fire movement gives rise to elevation and brightness, since fire rises and is bright. See *Su Wen* chapter 70.

火曰伏明 火运不及曰伏明。火气不足，则光明之气伏而不升，故称。出《素问·五常政大论》。

火曰伏明（huǒ yuē fú míng） **Insufficiency of fire is known as *fu ming* (loss of brightness).** The insufficiency of fire movement leads to loss of brightness. A shortage of fire qi causes qi brightness to descend instead of rising. See *Su Wen* chapter 70.

火曰赫曦 赫曦，火热旺盛之意。火运太过，火热炎盛，故称。出《素问·五常政大论》。

火曰赫曦（huǒ yuē hè xī）
Excess of fire is known as *he xi* (flaming). *Hè xī* refers to the excessive fire. Excessive fire movement leads to exuberant fire with high temperatures. See *Su Wen* chapter 70.

火气 ① 运气术语，六气之一。为少阳相火或少阴君火所主之气。出《素问·六微旨大论》。② 火热之邪。出《素问·解精微论》。③ 人体阳气。出《灵枢·刺节真邪》。

火气（huǒ qì） ① Terminology of circuits and qi and one of the six qi. It is the qi governed by *shaoyang* ministerial fire or *shaoyin* monarch fire. See *Su Wen* chapter 68. ② Pathogenic fire or heat. See *Su Wen* chapter 81. ③ Yang qi of the human body. See *Ling Shu* chapter 75.

火以温之 见"燥以干之……火以温之"条。出《素问·五运行大论》。

火以温之（huǒ yǐ wēn zhī） **warmed by fire** See "燥以干之……火以温之". See *Su Wen* chapter 67.

火形之人 体质名。又称上徵，阴阳二十五人之一。出《灵枢·阴阳二十五人》。火形之

人在五音属徵（zhǐ 指），徵音之中有正、偏、太、少的区别，分为上徵、质徵、少徵、右徵、判徵，以此类比火形人中的五种体质类型。上徵得火气之全者，质徵、少徵、右徵、判徵得火气之偏者，故上徵之人为标准火形人。其体形特征：脊背肌肉宽厚，肤红，脸形瘦尖，头小，肩背髀腹匀称，手足小，步履稳重。其禀性是：多气、轻财、缺乏信心，多虑，认识事物敏捷清楚，爱好漂亮，性情急，该体质大多耐于春夏，不耐于秋冬，故秋冬易发病。

火形之人（huǒ xíng zhī rén）
people pertaining to the fire element Name of constitution, also called *shang zhi*, which is one of the twenty-five types of people divided according to yin and yang. See *Ling Shu* chapter 64. Fire type of people pertain to *zhi* in the five tones, and are classified into positive, partial, more and less *zhi*, including *shang zhi*, *zhi zhi*, *shao zhi*, *you zhi* and *pan zhi* to illustrate the five types of body constitutions of the fire type of people. People of *shang zhi* have all the fire qi, and those of *zhi zhi*, *shao zhi*,

you zhi and *pan zhi* have partial fire qi, thus those of *shang zhi* are standard fire type of people, who have broad and thick back muscles, red skin, a thin and pointed face, a small head, well-proportioned shoulders, back, thighs and abdomen and small hands and feet. They walk steadily. They are brave, generous, diffident, suspicious, quick in comprehension, fond of looking smart and hasty. These type of people can mostly tolerate the weather in spring and summer, but cannot tolerate the weather in autumn and winter, and therefore they tend to get ill in autumn and winter.

火运 五运之一。根据天干化五运之理,凡逢戊、逢癸的年时,由火运主事。其时气候炎热,万物茂盛,欣欣向荣,病多伤心。出《素问·天元纪大论》。

火运(huǒ yùn) **fire circuit** One of the five circuits, which is in accordance with the idea of Heavenly Stems transforming into five movements, and in years with Heavenly Stems such as *wu* and *gui*, the fire circuit is dominant. In those years, the climate is hot with scenes of flourishing life, and diseases of the heart are mostly seen clinically. See *Su Wen* chapter 66.

火郁 火运之气被郁遏。运气学说中,按五行相克规律,由于一方太盛或所克一方太弱而使受克一方被抑制,不能正常发挥作用的现象,称为郁。五行中,水能克火,若水太过或火不及则会发生水偏旺而使火气被郁。出《素问·六元正纪大论》。

火郁(huǒ yù) **stagnation of fire** The qi of fire circuit is oppressed. In the circuits and qi theory, according to the rule of restraining in the five elements, the inhibited element is oppressed if the inhibiting element is too strong, or the inhibited element is too weak to function normally. In the five elements, water restrains fire, and if water is too strong or fire is too weak, fire qi will be oppressed. See *Su Wen* chapter 71.

火郁发之 火郁,即火气被郁于里。从自然气候变化言,夏应热反寒,应长而不长;从人体言,火热被其他外邪遏郁于里的病理变化,皆称火郁。发,发越,凡火气抑郁者应以发散法治之,如发汗等。出《素问・六元正纪大论》。

火郁发之(huǒ yù fā zhī) **Stagnation of fire should be treated by dispersing.** Stagnation of fire means that fire qi is oppressed in the interior. In terms of changes of climate in nature, the climate is cold instead of being hot and all things stagnate instead of growing in summer. In the human body, stagnation of fire refers to the pathological changes with fire heat oppressed in the interior by other exogenous pathogenic factors. For people with stagnation of fire, dispersing methods should be used in the treatment, such as promoting sweating. See *Su Wen* chapter 71.

火府　火热之气聚合的节气。府,会聚。出《素问・六元正纪大论》。

火府(huǒ fǔ)　**fire palace** It refers to the solar terms with accumulation of fire heat qi. *Fǔ* refers to accumulation. See *Su Wen* chapter 71.

火政　指火热的气候流行。政,施政。出《素问・五常政大论》。

火政(huǒ zhèng)　**policy of fire** It refers to the domination of hot climate. *zhèng* refers to administration. See *Su Wen* chapter 70.

火焫　艾火。出《灵枢・论痛》。

火焫(huǒ ruò)　**burning Moxa fire.** See *Ling Shu* chapter 53.

火淫　火热偏胜的气候。出《素问・至真要大论》。

火淫(huǒ yín)　**excess of fire** Climate with an abundance of fire heat. See *Su Wen* chapter 74.

心　① 五脏之一。位居上焦,是五脏中最重要的器官。出《灵枢・邪客》。为君主之官,总司人体生命及精神意识思维活动,并有推动血液在脉内运行的作用。其经脉为手少阴心经,与手太阳小肠经相表里,五行配属为火,主时于夏。其在体为脉,在志为喜,在液为汗,在窍为舌,在味为苦,病理特征为热。② 心的脉象。出《素问・阴阳别论》。③ 心窝部。出《素问・咳论》。④ 心宿。二十八宿之一。出《素问・五运行大论》。⑤ 心在面部的望诊部位(两眦之间)。出《灵枢・五色》。

心(xīn)　① One of the five and most important viscera located at the upper *jiao*. See *Ling Shu* chapter 71. The heart is the monarch organ in charge of life activities, and promotes blood to flow in the vessels. The channel of the heart is the heart meridian of hand *shaoyin*, which has an interior-exterior relationship with the small intestine meridian of hand *taiyang*. It pertains to fire in the five elements and to summer in the four seasons. It governs vessels in the five body constituents, joy in the five emotions, sweat in the five kinds of fluid, tongue in the five orifices and bitter in five flavors. Its pathological characteristic is fever. ② Pulse manifestation of the heart. See *Su Wen* chapter 7. ③ The precordial region. See *Su Wen* chapter 38. ④ The stellar division of *xin*, one of the 28 stellar divisions. See *Su Wen* chapter 67. ⑤ The site for complexion examination in the face that reflects the condition of the heart（between two canthus）. See *Ling Shu* chapter 49.

心下否痛　指心下胃脘部位痞塞疼痛的症状，否，通"痞"。出《素问·五常政大论》。

心下否痛（xīn xià pǐ tòng）**blockage and pain below the heart** A symptom, i.e. blockage and pain in the stomach below the heart. "否" is the same as "痞". See *Su Wen* chapter 70.

心手少阴之脉　即手少阴心经，为十二经脉之一。其循行路线从心中开始，出属心系，穿过横膈，络于小肠。一支从心系上挟咽喉，连系到"目系"。再一支从心系上行于肺部，再向下走腋窝下，沿上臂内侧后缘，下行肘内，沿着前臂内侧后缘，直达掌后小指侧高骨的尖端（锐骨），入掌内后方，沿小指内侧至指尖（接手太阳小肠经）。出《灵枢·经脉》。

心手少阴之脉（xīn shǒu shào yīn zhī mài）**heart meridian of hand *shaoyin*** That is, the heart meridian of hand *shaoyin* which is one of the twelve channels. It originates from the heart. Emerging, it spreads over the heart system. It passes through the diaphragm to connect with the small intestine. One branch runs alongside from the heart to the throat to connect with the eye system. The other branch from the heart system goes upward to the lung. Then it turns downward and emerges from the axilla. From there it goes along the posterior border of the medial side of the upper arm and runs down to the cubital fossa. From there it descends along the posterior border of the medial side of the forearm to the pisiform region proximal to the palm and enters the palm. Then it follows the medial side of the little finger to its tip where it links with the small intestine meridian of hand *taiyang*. See *Ling Shu* chapter 10.

心气　① 指心的精气与心主血脉,心主神明等功能有关。出《灵枢·脉度》。② 心的病气。出《素问·玉机真藏论》。③ 指心。出《素问·痿论》。

心气（xīn qì）　① Refers to essence qi of the heart and its related functions, e.g. the heart governs the blood vessels and the spirit brilliance. See *Ling Shu* chapter 17. ② Pathogenic qi of the heart. See *Su Wen* chapter 19. ③ The heart. See *Su Wen* chapter 44.

心气内洞　即心气内虚,夏令属火,逆之则心阳中空而虚。出《素问·四气调神大论》。

心气内洞（xīn qì nèi dòng）　**deficiency of heart qi** Summer pertains to fire, and violation of summer qi prevents the heart yang from developing, resulting in deficiency of heart qi. See *Su Wen* chapter 2.

心风　病名,五脏风之一。病起于心之穴被风邪所中。症候所见与心的病理特点有关,故名。出《素问·风论》。

心风（xīn fēng）　**heart wind** Disease name, and one kind of wind of the five viscera. It is caused by the attack of pathogenic wind to the heart. The symptoms and signs are related to pathological characteristics of the heart, thus its name. See *Su Wen* chapter 42.

心风疝　病证名。因阳明邪盛犯心所致的病证,以脉滑为特征。出《素问·四时刺逆从论》。

心风疝（xīn fēng shàn）　**heart wind hernia** The syndrome due to the attack by surplus qi in the *yangming* meridian on the heart, characterized by a slippery pulse. See *Su Wen* chapter 64.

心火　指心藏。心在五行属火,故称心火。出《素问·气交变大论》。

心火（xīn huǒ）　**heart fire** It refers to the heart, which pertains to fire in the five elements，hence the name heart fire. See *Su Wen* chapter 69.

心为汗 汗为五液之一。心主血，血中津液可渗于脉外，随卫气外泄为汗。出《素问·宣明五气》。

心为汗（xīn wéi hàn） **Heart governs sweat.** Sweat is one of the five fluids. The heart governs blood，and fluids in the blood can exude from the vessels，circulate with the defensive qi and be expelled from the body. See *Su Wen* chapter 23.

心为阳中之太阳 根据阴阳五行原理，阴阳之中又有阴阳可分。出《灵枢·顺气一日分为四时》。心属阳，位居膈上，亦属阳，心气通于夏，阳气最盛，故为阳中之太阳。出《灵枢·阴阳系日月》。

心为阳中之太阳（xīn wéi yáng zhōng zhī tài yáng） **Heart pertains to *taiyang* within yang.** According to the theories of yin and yang，and the five elements，yin and yang are infinitely divisible. See *Ling Shu* chapter 44. The heart pertains to yang and its location above the diaphragm also pertains to yang. Heart qi corresponds to summer with the most exuberant yang qi，thus the heart pertains to *taiyang* within the yang. See *Ling Shu* chapter 41.

心生血 血赖心之神气而化成。出《素问·阴阳应象大论》。

心生血（xīn shēng xiě） **Heart generates blood.** Blood is formed by the spirit qi of the heart. See *Su Wen* chapter 5.

心包 即心之包络。出《灵枢·经脉》。

心包（xīn bāo） **pericardium** The heart enclosure or pericardiac network. See *Ling Shu* chapter 10.

心包络 简称心包，又称心主。出《灵枢·经脉》。是心的外围组织。包为心之包膜，络为膜内之脉络，流行血气，有裹护心脏，代心受邪的作用。其经脉为手厥阴心包经，与手少阳三焦经相表里。

心包络（xīn bāo luò） **pericardiac network** The pericardium，in short，is also called the heart ruler. See *Ling Shu* chapter 10. It is the tissues surrounding the heart. The pericardium is the enclosure of the heart and inside is a network of vessels，in which blood and qi flows. It envelopes and protects the heart and is attacked by pathogenic factors that would have otherwise attacked the heart directly. Its channel is the heart meridian of hand *jueyin*, which has an interior-exterior relationship with the triple *jiao* meridian of hand *shaoyang*.

心包络脉 即手厥阴心包经脉。出《素问·刺法论》。

心包络脉（xīn bāo luò mài）**channel of the pericardium network** That is, the pericardium meridian of hand *jueyin*. See *Su Wen* chapter 72.

心主 指心包络。包络为心之外卫,代心行令,代心受邪,为心所主。出《灵枢·经脉》。

心主（xīn zhǔ）**heart ruler** The pericardium network. It surrounds and acts on behalf of the heart. It is attacked by pathogenic factors that otherwise would attack the heart. It is governed by the heart. See *Ling Shu* chapter 10.

心主手厥阴心包络之脉 即手厥阴心包经,为十二经脉之一。其循行路线从胸中开始,出属心包络,穿过横膈,依次络于上、中、下三焦。一支从胸出胁部,在腋下三寸处,向上抵腋窝,沿上臂内侧,行于手太阴手少阴两经中间,入肘中,下行前臂掌侧两筋之间,入掌内,沿中指桡侧,直达中指桡侧端(中冲穴)。再一支从掌中心沿环指,直达指尖(接手少阳三焦经),出《灵枢·经脉》。

心主手厥阴心包络之脉（xīn zhǔ shǒu jué yīn xīn bāo luò zhī mài）**heart ruler-pericardium meridian of hand *jueyin*** Namely, the pericardium meridian of hand *jueyin*, one of the twelve meridians. It starts from the chest and enters the pericardium to which it pertains to. Then it ascends through the diaphragm to connect with the upper *jiao*, middle *jiao* and lower *jiao* respectively. Its branch runs around the chest and emerges from the intercostal region. From the region three *cun* below the axilla, it ascends to the axilla. Along the medial side of the upper arm, it runs downward between the lung meridian of hand *taiyin* and the heart meridian of hand *shaoyin* to the cubital fossa, descends along the arm and runs between the two tendons of the long extensor muscle and short extensor muscle to the palm. Then it passes along the middle finger to its tip（the acupoint Zhong Chong，PC 9）. The other branch forks from the palm and runs along the ring finger to its tip to link with the triple *jiao* meridian of hand *shaoyang*. See *Ling Shu* chapter 10.

心主舌　舌为人体官窍之一，与心气相通，是心功能活动反映于体表的重要部位。出《素问·阴阳应象大论》。

心主舌(xīn zhǔ shé)　**Heart governs the tongue.** The tongue is one of the sense organs in the human body. It communicates with qi of the heart，and is an important site where functional activities of the heart are reflected on the body's surface. See *Su Wen* chapter 5.

心主汗　义同"心为汗"，参该条。出《灵枢·九针论》。

心主汗(xīn zhǔ hàn)　**Heart governs sweat.** See"心为汗". See *Ling Shu* chapter 78.

心主身之血脉　心有推动脉内血液流行周身的作用。出《素问·痿论》。

心主身之血脉(xīn zhǔ shēn zhī xuè mài)　**Heart governs the blood vessels in the body.** The heart has the function of pro-

moting blood to circulate in the vessels all over the body. See *Su Wen* chapter 44.

心主脉　心主血，血行脉中，故心所主之外合为脉。出《素问·宣明五气》。

心主脉(xīn zhǔ mài)　**Heart governs the vessels.** The heart governs the blood which flows in the vessels，thus it is externally related to the vessels. See *Su Wen* chapter 23.

心主夏　此以五行学说归纳脏腑与季节时日的关系及治法。夏季主火属南方。手少阴心是火脏，为丁火、阴火；手太阳小肠与心相表里，为丙火、阳火，故治法相同。出《素问·藏气法时论》。

心主夏(xīn zhǔ xià)　**Heart governs summer.** According to the theory of the five elements，the relationships of the viscera with the seasons，days and times of day are summarized，and corresponding treatment methods are discussed. Summer is governed by fire and pertains to the south. The heart of hand *shaoyin* is the fire viscera，such as the *ding* fire or yin fire. The small intestine meridian of hand *taiyang* has an exterior-interior relationship with the heart meridian of hand *shaoyin*. The small intestine pertains to *bing* fire, or yang fire. Therefore, the methods for treating diseases related to the heart and small intestine are the same. See *Su Wen* chapter 22.

心主噫 噫,嗳气之谓,本属脾胃病,由太阴经阳明上走于心而为。出《灵枢·九针论》。

心主噫（xīn zhǔ yì） **Heart controls sighing.** Yì refers to sighing. Sighing is a symptom of spleen and stomach diseases, and is controlled by the heart as the heart meridian of hand *taiyin* passes the stomach meridian of foot *yangming* and proceeds to the heart. See *Ling Shu* chapter 78.

心合小肠 合,配合之意。手太阳小肠经与手少阴心经相为表里,心与小肠在功能上具有相应关系。出《灵枢·本藏》。

心合小肠（xīn hé xiǎo cháng） **Heart coordinates with the small intestine.** *Hé* refers to coordinate. The small intestine meridian of hand *taiyang* has an exterior-interior relationship with the heart meridian of hand

shaoyin. The heart and the small intestine are functionally related. See *Ling Shu* chapter 47.

心合脉 合,配合之意。出《灵枢·五色》。

心合脉（xīn hé mài） **Heart coordinates with the vessels.** *Hé* refers to coordinate. See *Ling Shu* chapter 49.

心肝澼 为心肝之病而致的肠澼。出《素问·大奇论》。

心肝澼（xīn gān pì） **dysentery related to the heart and liver** Dysentery caused by heart and liver disease. See *Su Wen* chapter 48.

心肠痛 表现为心腹疼痛而烦闷难忍,腹部有上下移动的肿块,时痛时止,伴有腹热,口渴流涎等。是有蛔虫的表现。出《灵枢·厥病》。

心肠痛（xīn cháng tòng） **pain in the heart and small intestine** Displaying intolerable pain in the heart and abdomen, and unbearable vexation, with lumps moving up and down in the abdomen and intermittent pain, accompanied with heatiness in the abdomen, thirst and drooling. These are the manifestations of having roundworms in the body. See *Ling Shu*

chapter 24.

心系　系，联属之意。指心脏与其他脏器相联系的脉络。出《素问·举痛论》。

心系（xīn xì）　**heart system** *Xì* means to connect. It refers to the network connecting the heart with the other viscera. See *Su Wen* chapter 39.

心应脉　应，应合之意。出《灵枢·本藏》。

心应脉（xīn yìng mài）　**Heart corresponds to the vessels.** *Yìng* means to coordinate. See *Ling Shu* chapter 47.

心胀　病证名。五脏胀之一。症见心烦、短气、卧不安。出《灵枢·胀论》。

心胀（xīn zhàng）　**distension of the heart** Syndrome name, and one kind of distension of the five viscera. Symptoms include vexation，shortness of breath and sleeplessness. See *Ling Shu* chapter 35.

心疟　五脏疟之一。症见心烦、喜冷水，恶寒重，发热轻等。出《素问·刺疟》。

心疟（xīn nüè）　**heart malaria** One kind of malaria of the five viscera, with manifestations of vexation，preference for cold water，chills and mild fever.

See *Su Wen* chapter 36.

心疝　病名。疝之一种，特征为少腹肿大有形，心脉急促滑大而搏指。出《素问·脉要精微论》。

心疝（xīn shàn）　**heart hernia** Disease name of one kind of hernia characterized by visible distension of the lower abdomen，and with a rapid，full，and slippery palpable pulse. See *Su Wen* chapter 17.

心咳　五脏咳之一。证候特点为咳而心胸部疼痛，故称心咳。出《素问·咳论》。

心咳（xīn ké）　**heart cough** One kind of cough of the five viscera characterized by painful coughing in the thoracic region around the heart. See *Su Wen* chapter 38.

心俞　经穴名。属足太阳膀胱经。在第五椎下两旁各一寸五分处。出《灵枢·背腧》。

心俞（xīn shū）　**Xin Shu (BL 15)** Acupoint name belonging on the bladder meridian of foot *taiyang*, located 1.5 *cun* inferior and lateral to the fifth thoracic vertebra. See *Ling Shu* chapter 51.

心脉　① 心病时的脉象。出《素问·脉要精微论》。② 心所主的脉象。出《素问·宣明五气》。③ 指手少阴心脉。出《灵枢·邪客》。

心脉（xīn mài）　① Pulse manifestations in diseases of the heart. See *Su Wen* chapter 17. ② Pulse manifestations governed by the heart. See *Su Wen* chapter 23. ③ Refers to the heart meridian of hand *shaoyin*. See *Ling Shu* chapter 71.

心脉钩　指脉来应指充盈，去势似较衰，其状如钩的脉象，是心的正常脉。出《素问·宣明五气》。

心脉钩（xīn mài gōu）　**Heart pulse appears *gou* (strong or hook-like)**. Refers to a vessel that feels full and descends slowly, just like a hook. It is the normal pulse of the heart. See *Su Wen* chapter 23.

心恶热　恶，厌憎之意。心属火，热本心脏之主气，太过则病，故恶热。此言心脏之病理。出《素问·宣明五气》。

心恶热（xīn wù rè）　**Heart detests heat**. Wù means hate, or dislike. The heart pertains to fire, and heat is its dominating qi. However, excessive heat leads to disease, therefore the heart detests heat. This is related to the pathology of the heart. See *Su Wen* chapter 23.

心部于表　部，分部之意。表，浅表。表属阳，心亦属阳，居于膈上而主火，火性炎散，故心气分部于表。出《素问·刺禁论》。

心部于表（xīn bù yú biǎo）　**Heart governs the surface**. *Bù* means to distribute. *Biǎo* means surface. The surface pertains to yang. The heart also pertains to yang, and is located above the diaphragm. As it governs fire, which warms and rises, the heart qi governs the surface. See *Su Wen* chapter 52.

心悗　悗，（mēn）音义同闷。心悗，心气不舒而觉烦闷。出《灵枢·口问》。

心悗（xīn mēn）　**chest oppression** The pronunciation and meaning of "悗" are the same as "闷". It refers to vexation due to the unsmooth flow of heart qi. See *Ling Shu* chapter 28.

心悬　形容饥饿时心窝部空虚心慌之感觉。出《素问·玉机真藏论》。

心悬（xīn xuán）　**precordial pain radiating upwards** Describes the feeling of emptiness and nervousness in the precordium when hungry. See *Su Wen* chapter 19.

心掣　出《素问·阴阳别论》。（1）掣，牵引，谓心动不宁，如有所引。见《类经・疾病六》。
（2）谓心虚寒而掣痛。见《素问
直解》。（3）即怔忡。见《素问
识》引《锦囊秘录》。

心掣（xīn chè）　**dragging pain of the heart and chest** See *Su Wen* chapter 7.（1）*Chè* refers to drag，and means the heart is beating restlessly as if its being dragged. See *Lei Jing*（*Classified Classic*）"On Diseases Chapter 6".（2）Dragging pain due to deficient cold of the heart. See *Su Wen Zhi Jie*（*Direct Interpretation on Su Wen*）.（3）Severe palpitations. See *Su Wen Zhi*（*Understanding Su Wen*）cited from *Jin Nang Mi Lu*（*Secret Record of Silk Bag*）.

心痛　①指胸部疼痛，为剧咳所致。出《素问・咳论》。②心区疼痛，为厥心痛与真心痛之主症。出《灵枢・厥病》。③胃脘部痛。出《灵枢・杂病》。

心痛（xīn tòng）　① Refers to chest pain caused by a racking cough. See *Su Wen* chapter 38. ② Pain in the cardiac region. It is the main symptom of reversal heartache and genuine heartache. See *Ling Shu* chapter 24. ③ Stomachache. See *Ling Shu* chapter 26.

心痹　病证名。五脏痹之一。由肌痹日久，反复感受风寒湿邪，发展而成。所见诸症与心的经脉痹阻不通有关。出《素问・痹论》。

心痹（xīn bì）　**heart impediment** Syndrome name and one of the impediment syndromes of the five viscera. It arises from prolonged muscular impediment and recurrent attacks by pathogenic wind，cold and dampness. The symptoms are related to the blockage of the heart channel. See *Su Wen* chapter 43.

心藏神　神指精神情志、思维意识、智慧聪明；分述之，则为神、魂、魄、意、志，各属其相应之心、肝、肺、脾、肾五脏，合之则为神，归藏于心，而能主宰生命，明了万事。心藏神的生理功能失常，可出现神志不宁，健忘、谵妄等精神情志异常的征象或全身脏腑功能失调等病状。出《素问・调经论》。

心藏神（xīn cáng shén）　**Heart stores *shen*.** *Shen* refers to the spirit or the mind. Specifically，it refers to *shen*（spirit），*hun*（ethereal soul），*po*（corporeal soul），*yi*（thinking）and *zhi*（emotions），which pertains to the heart，liver，lung，spleen and kidney, respectively. Collectively they are called *shen* (spirit) which is stored in the heart. *Shen* (spirit) dominates life and determines everything. Abnormal physiological functions of *shen* stored in the heart leads to signs of mental disorder including restlessness, forgetfulness and delirium as well as dysfunction of the viscera in the body. See *Su Wen* chapter 62.

四画

尺　即尺肤。出《素问·平人气象论》。

尺（chǐ）　**Chi** That is, *chi fu* (cubital skin). See *Su Wen* chapter 18.

尺肤　前臂内侧自肘关节至腕关节的皮肤,长约一尺许,故谓尺肤。出《灵枢·论疾诊尺》。

尺肤（chǐ fū）　*chi fu* (**cubital skin**) It is the skin on the medial side of the forearm between the elbow and the wrist, approximately one *chi* in length, hence named *chi fu*. See *Ling Shu* chapter 74.

尺泽　经穴名。属手太阴肺经,为本经合穴。在肘窝横纹上,当肱二头肌腱桡侧缘处。出《灵枢·本输》。

尺泽（chǐ zé）　**Chi Ze** (**LU 5**) Acupoint name belonging to the lung meridian of hand *taiyin*, and the *he*-sea acupoint of this channel. It is located above the transverse striation of the elbow fossa, at the radial border of the biceps tendon. See *Ling Shu* chapter 2.

尺脉　即尺肤与脉。出《素问·平人气象论》。

尺脉（chǐ mài）　*Chi mai* Namely, *chi fu* (cubital skin) and pulse. See *Su Wen* chapter 18.

引针　拔出针体。出《素问·八正神明论》。

引针（yǐn zhēn）　**withdrawal of the needle** To remove the needle. See *Su Wen* chapter 26.

丑未之纪　指纪年地支是丑、未之年,为太阴湿土司天,纪,纪年。出《素问·六元正纪大论》。

丑未之纪（chǒu wèi zhī jì）　**years of *chou* and *wei*** Refers to the years with the Earthly Branches of *chou* and *wei*, when the damp earth of *taiyin* governs the heavens. *Jì* refers to the year. See *Su Wen* chapter 71.

以平为期　平,平调。期,限度。言一切治疗均以人体气血阴阳及脏腑功能恢复协调平衡为限。出《素问·三部九候论》。

以平为期（yǐ píng wéi qī）　**Treatment is continued until a**

balance of qi and blood is reached. *Píng*, or balance, and *qī*, or limitation. Meaning that no matter what the disease, treatment can be only be stopped when there is a balance of yin and yang, qi and blood in the body, and the restored harmony of visceral functions. See *Su Wen* chapter 20.

以痛为输　在痛处取穴,即所谓天应穴,阿是穴。出《灵枢·经筋》。

以痛为输(yǐ tòng wéi shū)　**The pain site is taken as the acupoint.** The acupoints used at the exact location of pain. These kind of acupoints are Tian Yin acupoints or A Shi acupoints. See *Ling Shu* chapter 13.

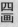

四画

五　画

玉机　古医籍篇名。出《素问·玉版论要》。

玉机（yù jī）　**The Jade Palate** Chapter title in an ancient classic. See *Su Wen* chapter 15.

玉机真藏论　《素问》篇名。玉机，表示珍重之意。真藏，指真脏脉。此篇主要论述四时五脏的平脉、病脉，并阐述了五脏疾病的传变规律以及五脏虚实的生与死，篇中认为真脏脉能别生死，故当特别注重，故名。

玉机真藏论（yù jī zhēn zàng lùn）　**Discussion on Genuine-Zang Pulses** Chapter title in *Su Wen*. *Yù jī* means to value, or to treasure; *Zhēn zàng* means genuine-zang pulses. This chapter mainly talks about normal pulses and abnormal pulses among the five organs in the four seasons, disease transformation between these organs, and the relationship between an organ's condition and its corresponding pulse. This chapter believes that genuine-zang pulses can be used to judge a patient's condition,

thus it was so named.

玉英　经穴名。又名玉堂，属任脉经，位于胸骨中线平第三肋间处。为足厥阴肝经经气所结之处。出《灵枢·根结》《灵枢·胀论》。

玉英（yù yīng）　**Yu Ying（CV 18）** Acupoint name on the conception vessel located in the midline of the sternum, and parallel to the third intercostal where the liver qi converges. It is also called *Yu Tang*. See *Ling Shu* chapter 5 and *Ling Shu* chapter 35.

玉版　① 版，指简牍。以玉石作简牍，以示所刻文章的珍贵。出《素问·玉版论要》。②《灵枢》篇名。本篇以痈疽为例说明病是积微之所生，如治不及时可导致五逆的症候，揭示早期诊断、早期治疗的重要性。另从针具虽小，可以活人，也可以杀人，来告诫人们在临床应用时必须审慎从事。因内容重要，"著之玉版"，故名。

玉版（yù bǎn）　① *Bǎn* refers to bamboo or wooden slips. The

contents of important articles were inscribed on jade instead of bamboo, or wood, to show their preciousness. See *Su Wen* chapter 15. ② Chapter title in *Ling Shu*. This chapter expounds, using the obstruction- and impediment-illness as the example, that diseases emerge from minimal accumulations. If left untreated, the symptoms of the five movements against the norms will occur, which demonstrates the significance of early diagnosis and treatment. In addition, this chapter signals out the dangers of the clinical application of needles, as acupuncture not only saves people, it can also kill.

玉版论要　《素问》篇名。此篇论述了运用揆度奇恒的方法，测度色脉的逆顺，以判断疾病的预后。为显示其重要，将其大要，刻写在玉版上，故名。

玉版论要（yù bǎn lùn yào）　**Discussion on the Jade Inscription** Chapter title in *Su Wen*. This chapter discusses the methods of using *qi heng* (extraordinary) to measure and analyze pulses and complexions, which are used to evaluate the prognosis of a disease. The main points were inscribed on jade to show their preciousness, hence the name.

未至而至　前一"至"指时令之到来；后一"至"，指气候之到来。时令未到而气候先至，是应至之气太过的表现。出《素问·六微旨大论》。

未至而至（wèi zhì ér zhì）　**arrival of climate but non-arrival of the concerned season** The former *zhì* refers to the arrival of the concerned season, and the latter one refers to the arrival of normal climate. Therefore, when the climate arrives before the season, the expected qi is excessive. See *Su Wen* chapter 68.

示从容论　《素问》篇名。示，示范；《从容》，《内经》引用的古医书。此篇内容主要讨论诊断时应根据《从容》来分析病情，并列举肝、脾、肾、肺病进行示范，故名。

示从容论（shì cóng róng lùn）　**Discussion on How to Diagnose Diseases** Chapter title in *Su Wen*. *Shì* means demonstration. *Cóng róng* is an ancient medical work quoted in *Nei Jing* (*Internal Classic*). This chapter mainly puts forward the idea that di-

五画

agnosis should be based on *cóng róng*, which is expounded, using the examples of liver, spleen, kidney and lung disease. Hence the name.

正　① 指经别。出《灵枢·经别》。② 正常。出《素问·六微旨大论》。③ 校正。出《素问·六节藏象论》。④ 正气。出《素问·六元正纪大论》。⑤ 稳健。出《素问·上古天真论》。⑥ 直刺。出《素问·针解》。⑦ 专注。出《素问·针解》。⑧ 合于常规的。出《素问·至真要大论》。⑨ 察。出《素问·阴阳类论》。

正（zhèng）　① Refers to separate meridians. See *Ling Shu* chapter 11. ② Healthy. See *Su Wen* chapter 68. ③ Adjust. See *Su Wen* chapter 9. ④ Healthy qi. See *Su Wen* chapter 71. ⑤ Steady. See *Su Wen* chapter 1. ⑥ Perpendicular needling. See *Su Wen* chapter 54. ⑦ Concentration. See *Su Wen* chapter 54. ⑧ Normal. See *Su Wen* chapter 74. ⑨ Observe. See *Su Wen* chapter 79.

正气　① 又称真气,是人体生命活动的动力,并具有抗病能力。② 指正风,即四时正常的气候,与邪气相对而言。参"正风"条。

正气（zhèng qì）　① Healthy qi, and also called genuine qi, which is the engine of human life able to prevent disease. ② Refers to normal wind, or normal climate in the four seasons, which is opposite to evil qi. See "正风".

正气存内　正气充实于内,邪气就不能侵犯,同时还必须避免接触疫毒之气。此言疫病发生的机理,体现了以外因为发病条件,以内因为发病关键的发病学观点。出《素问·刺法论》。

正气存内（zhèng qì cún nèi）**healthy qi inside the body** To keep healthy qi sufficiently stored inside the body, and so as to avoid evil qi（pathogenic factors） from invading the body, one should keep away from pestilence. This term indicates both external and internal factors working together leading to diseases. See *Su Wen* chapter 72.

正化　运气术语。指四时正常之变化。出《素问·六元正纪大论》。

正化（zhèng huà）　*zheng hua* Terminology in the circuits and qi, refers to the normal changes of qi in the four seasons. See *Su Wen* chapter 71.

正月太阳寅　正月为一年之首，万物开始发芽生长，寅为东方木，主春，故十二月建以正月建寅；太阳为三阳之首。出《素问·脉解》。

正月太阳寅(zhēng yuè tài yáng yín)　*Zhēng yuè* is the first month of the lunar year，when all living things begin to grow. *Yín* refers to the earth of the east，and dominates spring. Thus *zhēng yuè* corresponds to yín according to the twelve months，of which *taiyang* is the first of the three yang. See *Su Wen* chapter 49.

正风　又名正气，指适时而至的风，如春季的东风，夏季的南风等。出《灵枢·刺节真邪》。

正风(zhèng fēng)　**healthy wind** Also named healthy qi，and refers to seasonal winds，such as the east wind in spring，and the south wind in summer. See *Ling Shu* chapter 75.

正邪　① 正邪为一种无法察觉，常乘人体虚弱侵入，而发病较轻的致病因子。也指八方之正风，如春之东风，夏之南风等。出《素问·八正神明论》。② 能够刺激和干扰正常身心活动的各种因素，如饥饱劳逸，精神情志等。出《灵枢·淫邪发梦》。

③ 指正气和邪气。出《灵枢·小针解》。

正邪(zhèng xié)　① A pathogenic factor that invades the body during weakness and causes mild disease. It also refers to healthy wind from the eight directions，such as the east wind in spring，and the south wind in summer. See *Su Wen* chapter 26. ② Factors that can disturb normal physical and mental conditions，such as hunger，overeating，and emotional disturbances etc. See *Ling Shu* chapter 43. ③ Refers to healthy qi and pathogenic qi. See *Ling Shu* chapter 3.

正岁　运气术语。指正常平和之年。即无太过、不及的平气之年，其气与时令节候相偕而至。出《素问·六元正纪大论》。

正岁(zhèng suì)　*zheng sui* Terminology of the circuits and qi，also named an even year. Namely，it is a year in which the normal qi is neither excessive nor insufficient，and arrives just at the right time. See *Su Wen* chapter 71.

正阳　① 正午时间。出《灵枢·禁服》。② 正当阳位，主南方之火。出《素问·五常政大论》。

正阳（zhèng yáng）　① Noon. See *Ling Su* chapter 48. ② Proper yang position，governing the south fire. See *Su Wen* chapter 70.

正位之司　正位行司其令，即岁气按时而临。出《素问·本病论》。

正位之司（zhèng wèi zhī sī）**governor in its corresponding position** The corresponding qi takes its position in its corresponding season on time. See *Su Wen* chapter 73.

正角　运气术语。角，木运。正，正常。谓木运平气之年。出《素问·五常政大论》。

正角（zhèng jué）　*zheng jue* Terminology of circuits and qi. *Jué* refers to wood movement，and *zhèng* means proper，or normal. Thus，it refers to normal wood-circuits and qi. See *Su Wen* chapter 70.

正治　① 正确治疗。出《素问·生气通天论》。② 针对病机、症状，从正面治疗的常规治法，如以热治寒之类。出《素问·至真要大论》。

正治（zhèng zhì）　① Proper treatment. See *Su Wen* chapter 3. ② In response to the pathogenesis and symptoms, patients can be treated with routine treatment，such as treating cold with heat. See *Su Wen* chapter 74.

正宫　运气术语。宫，土运。正，正常。谓土运平气之年。出《素问·五常政大论》。

正宫（zhèng gōng）　*zheng gong* Terminology of circuits and qi. *Gong* refers to earth circuit，and *zheng* means proper，or normal. *Zheng gong* refers to the normal circuit of earth qi. See *Su Wen* chapter 70.

正商　运气术语。商，金运。正，正常。谓金运平气之年。出《素问·五常政大论》。

正商（zhèng shāng）　*zheng shang* Terminology of circuits and qi. *Shang* refers to metal circuit and *zheng* means proper，or normal. *Zheng shang* refers to the normal circuit of metal-qi. See *Su Wen* chapter 70.

正徵　运气术语。徵，火运。正，正常。谓火运平气之年。出《素问·五常政大论》。

正徵（zhèng zhǐ）　*zheng zhi* Terminology of circuits and qi. *Zhi* refers to fire circuit and *zheng* means proper，or normal. *Zheng zhi* refers to the normal circuit of fire-qi. See *Su Wen* chapter 70.

去爪　刺五节法之一。用于关节肢络四肢的病变，以及阴囊水肿。应取铍针或砭石以出其水，其效好像修掉多余的指甲一样，故名。出《灵枢·刺节真邪》。

去爪（qù zhuǎ）　One of the needling in five sections methods applied for joint or limb diseases, and edema of scrotum. It uses sword-shaped needles or *bian* stones to treat, as if cutting off nails, hence the name. See *Ling Shu* chapter 75.

去宛陈莝　宛，通郁，郁积。陈，陈旧。莝（cuò 错）铡草。去除陈久之积草。以喻驱除郁积体内的病理产物，如恶血、水液等。出《素问·汤液醪醴论》。

去宛陈莝（qù wǎn chén cuò）　宛 is the same as 郁, which means retention, *Chén* means old, and *cuò* means cut grass. This metaphor refers to removing retention inside the body, such blood stasis, or stagnant turbid fluids. See *Su Wen* chapter 14.

甘入脾　与"甘生脾"同理，见该条。出《素问·宣明五气》。

甘入脾（gān rù pí）　Sweet flavor enters the spleen. See the term "甘生脾". See *Su Wen* chapter 23.

甘生脾　甘为五味之一，根据五行理论，甘与脾同属土行，故甘味入口，先入脾而滋养脾土。出《素问·至真要大论》。

甘生脾（gān shēng pí）　Sweet flavor generates the spleen. Sweetness is one of five flavors, and according to the five-element theory, the nature of sweetness and the spleen both belong to earth. Sweetness enters the spleen first and then, supplements spleen-earth. See *Su Wen* chapter 74.

甘伤肉　甘入脾，脾与肉相合，甘味固能滋养脾土，但若太过，则伤肌肉。出《素问·阴阳应象大论》。

甘伤肉（gān shāng ròu）　Excessive sweetness may be harmful to the muscles. Sweetness enters the spleen, but excessive sweetness may harm the muscles. See *Su Wen* chapter 5.

甘伤脾　甘味入脾而养脾，太过则伤脾。出《素问·五运行大论》。

甘伤脾（gān shāng pí）　Excessive sweetness harms the spleen. Sweetness enters the spleen, but excessive sweetness may harm the spleen. See *Su Wen* chapter 67.

甘走肉　五禁之一。甘入脾，脾主肌肉，故甘味走肉。甘助湿，过于甘则湿阻脾土而伤肉。出《素问·宣明五气》《灵枢·五味论》。

甘走肉（gān zǒu ròu） **Sweet flavor enters the muscles.** One of the five contraindications, for as sweetness enters the muscles, and the spleen governs the muscles, this sweetness may lead to excessive dampness, and and thus be harmful to the muscles. See *Su Wen* chapter 23 and *Ling Shu* chapter 63.

甘者令人中满 五行甘味属土，过食甘味可使人脾气壅滞而脘腹胀闷，是导致脾瘅的一个原因，出《素问·奇病论》。

甘者令人中满（gān zhě lìng rén zhōng mǎn） **Sweet food may cause abdominal distention in people.** The nature of sweetness belongs to earth. Excessively ingesting sweet food may cause spleen-qi retention, leading to abdominal distention. See *Su Wen* chapter 47.

甘疽 病名。发于胸部两侧的疽。色青，常发寒热，病势缠绵。因其位属阳明，阳明为土，土味甘，故名。出《灵枢·痈疽》。

甘疽（gān jū） ***gan ju*** Disease name. The onset of gangrene at the chest bilaterally. The color of this kind of gangrene is deep green, and the patient may present with fever and aversion to cold. The location of the gangrene is in the *yangming* meridian, which in nature belongs to earth, and the corresponding flavor of earth is sweet, thus it is called *gan ju*. See *Ling Shu* chapter 81.

艾 药名。有温气血、散寒湿的作用。灸法常以艾作炷灸患处，以达到温通经络、调理气血的作用。出《素问·汤液醪醴论》。

艾（ài） **moxa** A medicinal herb indicated for warming qi and blood, and dispelling cold and dampness. Moxibustion usually uses moxa sticks applied over the skin to warm meridians and regulate the qi and blood. See *Su Wen* chapter 14.

节 ① 骨节。出《素问·五藏生成篇》。② 穴俞。出《灵枢·九针十二原》。③ 节制。出《素问·阴阳应象大论》。④ 关键，原由。出《素问·阴阳应象大论》。⑤ 节度。出《素问·六节藏象论》《素问集注》。⑥ 调节。出《灵枢·本神》。

节（jié） ① Bone joint. See *Su Wen* chapter 10. ② Acupuncture point. See *Ling Shu* chapter 1.

③ Regulation. See *Su Wen* chapter 5. ④ Crux. See *Su Wen* chapter 5. ⑤ Measurement. See *Su Wen* chapter 9 and *Su Wen Ji Zhu*（*Collected Annotation of Su Wen*）. ⑥ Adjustment. See *Ling Shu* chapter 8.

节解　关节间隙。出《灵枢·九针论》。

节解（jié jiě）　**crevice of bones** See *Ling Shu* chapter 78.

本标　指六气标本。出《素问·六微旨大论》。

本标（běn biāo）　**root and branch** Refers to the root and branch of the six qi. See *Su Wen* chapter 68.

本神　《灵枢》篇名。本，根本，根据；神，泛指精、神、魂、魄、意、志、思、智、虑等精神意识思维活动。该篇主要论述了神的概念，神与五脏在生理、病理上的联系。指出在诊治疾病时就要根据病人"神"的变化，施以相应的治法，故名。

本神（běn shén）　**Basic state of spirit** Chapter title in *Ling Shu*. *Běn* refers to basic state，and *shén* means mental condition. This chapter mainly talks about the concept of *shén* and its relationships with the five organs physiologically as well

as pathologically，and also points out that it is important to focus on a patient's mental condition and give proper treatment based on it.

本病论　《素问》遗篇名。唐王冰注《素问》时已佚，仅目录中存有篇名，并注明"亡"。至宋代林亿等校正《素问》时发现有流传本。刘温舒著《素问入式运气论奥》，又将该篇附列书后，但学术界普遍认为非《素问》原著。遗篇主要论述了天地气交的反常变化，使"四时失序，万化不安"，以致变生疾病或引起疫疬流行。但是，疾病发生的根本原因在于"人气不足，天气如虚，人神失守"。故以名篇。

本病论（běn bìng lùn）　**Discussion on the Diseases Caused by Abnormal Changes of Qi-Motion** Chapter title in *Su Wen*. The original contents of this chapter have been lost in history when Wang Bing annotated *Su Wen* in the Tang dynasty. In the Song dynasty, Lin Yi found a copy of the chapter when he corrected *Su Wen*. The contents of this chapter have been included in *Su Wen Ru Shi Yun Qi Lun Ao* written by Liu Wenshu, but some scholars be-

五画

lieved that they were not the original contents. This chapter mainly discusses that an "abnormal qi convergence may lead to diseases and epidemics，but the root causes of diseases are deficiencies of qi inside the human body，abnormal heaven qi，and mental disturbances."

本输 ①《灵枢》篇名。本，推求本源；输，古通腧、俞，即井、荥、输、经、合五俞穴。《灵枢注证发微》："本篇输字，是言推本各经之有腧穴也，故名篇。"其内容主要论述五俞穴的部位，五行属性及取穴方法；手足六阳经及任、督脉的分布和经脉阴阳表里的配合关系。② 各经在四肢的输穴。出《灵枢·邪客》。

本输(běn shū) ① Chapter title in *Ling Shu*. *Běn* means seek for the root and origin，and "输" is the same as "腧" or "俞"，which refers to the five *shu* acupoints. *Su Wen Zhu Zheng Fa Wei* (*Annotation and Elaboration on Su Wen*) states，"Here，*shū* means to discuss *shu*-points on meridians." This chapter is mainly about the location，nature and locating method of the five *shu*-acupoints，the

distribution of the six yang meridians，conception vessel，and governor vessel，and the relationships between the yin meridians and the yang meridians. ② *Shu*-acupoints of the meridians on the four limbs. See *Ling Shu* chapter 71.

本藏　《灵枢》篇名，本，根本；藏，脏腑。本藏，即脏腑是人体的根本。此篇主要论述从人体外部征象推求脏腑功能的常与变。

本藏(běn zàng) **The Viscera as the Foundation of Human Beings** Chapter title in *Ling Shu*. *Běn* means root；*Zàng* means organs. *Běn zàng* refers to the organs being the root of the human body. This chapter is mainly about judging the function of the organs according to their external manifestations in the human body.

术　① 药名。指白术，味甘苦，性温，燥湿止汗，健脾胃。与泽泻麋衔组合成方，治疗酒后中风者。出《素问·病能论》。② 医术。出《素问·示从容论》。③ 方法。出《素问·上古天真论》。

术(zhú) ① Bai Zhu (*Rhizoma Atractylodis Macrocephalae*). Drug name. Refers to Bai Zhu (*Rhizoma Atractylodis Macro-*

cephalae）, which is bitter in taste, warm in nature, and has the function of drying dampness, stopping sweating and supplementing the spleen and stomach. The formula consisting of Bai Zhu（*Rhizoma Atractylodis Macrocephalae*）, Ze Xie（*Rhizoma Alismatis*）and Mi Xian（*Herba Pyrolae*）can be taken for stroke after inebriation. See *Su Wen* chapter 46. ②（*shù*）Medical skills. See *Su Wen* chapter 76. ③（*shù*）Method. See *Su Wen* chapter 1.

左角 ① 体质名。阴阳二十五人中木形人之一。出《灵枢·五音五味》。见"左角之人"。② 左侧额角。出《素问·缪刺论》。③ 背俞取穴法中，所用三角形的左底角。出《素问·血气形志》。

左角（zuǒ jué） ① Name of constitution. It refers to the wood-type people, out of the twenty-five types of people according to yin and yang. See the *Ling Shu* chapter 65. See the term "左角之人". ② The left corner of the forehead. See *Su Wen* chapter 63. ③ The bottom left corners of triangles in the method for locating the back-*shu* acupoints. See *Su Wen* chapter 24.

左角之人 体质名。角，五音之一，五行属木。左角，角音之一，此代表阴阳二十五人中木形之一种，其特征是随和顺从。出《灵枢·阴阳二十五人》。

左角之人（zuǒ jué zhī rén） *zuo-jue*-type people Name of constitution. *Jue*, one of the five musical notes, belongs to wood in the five elements. *Zuo jue*, one of the *jue* notes, refers to a type of wood constitution manifesting calmness and friendliness. See *Ling Shu* chapter 64.

左角宫 体质名。阴阳二十五人中土形人之一种。出《灵枢·五音五味》。见"左宫之人"。

左角宫（zuǒ jué gōng） Name of constitution. It refers to the earth-type people, out of the twenty-five types of people divided according to yin and yang. See *Ling Shu* chapter 65. See the term "左宫之人".

左间 运气术语。即左间气。凡客气中位于司天之气左侧（主气的四之气）及在泉之气的左侧（主气的初之气）的间气，称左间。出《素问·本病论》。参"间气"条。

左间（zuǒ jiān） **the left interme-**

diate qi Terminology of circuits and qi, namely, the intermediate qi located on the left side of the qi controlling heaven (the fourth qi of dominant qi) and the qi with terrestrial effect (the initial qi of dominant qi). See *Su Wen* chapter 73. See the term "间气".

左宫之人　体质名。宫,五音之一,五行属土。左宫,宫音之一,此代表阴阳二十五人中土形人之一种,其特征是神情表现兀兀然而独立不动。出《灵枢·阴阳二十五人》。参"土形之人"。

左宫之人(zuǒ gōng zhī rén) ***zuogong*-type people** Name of constitution. *Gong* is one of the five musical notes, and belongs to earth. *Zuo gong*, one of the *gong* notes, refers to a type of earth constitution with enterprising and self-determination characteristics. See *Ling Shu* chapter 64. See the term "土形之人."

左商　体质名。阴阳二十五人中金形人之一种。出《灵枢·五音五味》。参"金形之人"条。

左商(zuǒ shāng)　Name of constitution. It refers to the metal-type people, out of the twenty-five types of people divided according to yin and yang. See *Ling Shu* chapter 65. See the term "金形之人".

厉　疫疠之病。出《素问·至真要大论》。

厉(lì)　**epidemics** Epidemic diseases. See *Su Wen* chapter 74.

厉兑　经穴名。是阳明胃经之井穴,在足第二趾外侧,甲根角旁十分之一寸处。出《灵枢·本输》。

厉兑(lì duì)　**Li Dui（ST 45）** Acupoint name, which is the well acupoint of the stomach meridian, and located at the lateral side of the second toe. See *Ling Shu* chapter 2.

厉痈　病名。发于足旁之痈肿。初起如小指大,呈黑色,宜急治,以去其黑色,否则可致不治。出《灵枢·痈疽》。

厉痈(lì yōng)　**carbuncle** Disease name of a carbuncle at the side of the foot. At onset, the size of the carbuncle is as small as the little finger, and it is black. The color will fade if the patient receives timely treatment; otherwise it is difficult to treat. See *Ling Shu* chapter 81.

石　① 肾所主脉象,其脉来沉滑如石,应于冬,冬季有胃气的肾脉应微微沉坚而石。如脉来紧急如夺绳索，如指弹石辟辟然，是肾的藏真之气显露的真藏脉，属危候。出《素问·宣明五气》《素问·平人气象论》。② 指用砭石针刺。出《素问·腹中论》。③ 砭石。出《素问·病能论》。

石（shí）　① A state of kidney pulse in winter. The kidney dominates the pulse，and its pulse is as heavy and smooth as a stone. In winter，the kidney pulse with stomach qi should be slightly heavy and firm. If the pulse is taken in an emergency，it is like grabbing a rope；if the pulse feels as if the finger is hitting a stone，it is the true hidden pulse，which is dangerous. See *Su Wen* chapter 23 and *Su Wen* chapter 18. ② Needling by using a *Bian*-stone. See *Su Wen* chapter 40. ③ *Bian*-stone. See *Su Wen* chapter 46.

石水　① 病名。水病之一种。症见下至小腹，上至胃脘皆胀满重垂。病机为阳衰阴盛，阳不化水，水邪在下如石之沉，故名。出《素问·阴阳别论》。② 指时令，即冬月水冰如石之时。出《素问·阴阳类论》。

石水（shí shuǐ）　① Disease name of one of the water diseases. Symptoms are distention around the stomach and lower abdomen，as the yang is unable to transform the water due to yang deficiency，thus leading to water retention around the lower *jiao*. See *Su Wen* chapter 7. ② The period that water is frozen like a stone in winter. See *Su Wen* chapter 79.

石药　金石类药物。出《素问·腹中论》。

石药（shí yào）　**mineral medicine** Mineral-type medicine. See *Su Wen* chapter 40.

石瘕　病名。为胞宫内之肿物。主症腹大如怀孕之状，按之坚硬，月经不能按时来行。此病仅见于女子。出《灵枢·水胀》。

石瘕（shí jiǎ）　**uterine mass** Disease name of a uterine mass that is hard when pressed and makes the patient look as if pregnant. It also manifests with irregular menstruation，and this disease only occurs in women. See *Ling Shu* chapter 57.

右迁　运气术语。木火土金水五行之气主岁，每年向右退行一步即自东向西迁移。出《素问·天元纪大论》。

右迁（yòu qiān）　**Terminology of** circuits and qi. The qi of the five elements moves one step, from the east to the west, every year. See *Su Wen* chapter 66.

右角 ① 体质名。阴阳二十五人中木形人之一种。出《灵枢·五音五味》。② 背俞取穴法中，所用三角形的右底角。出《素问·血气形志》。③ 右侧额角。出《灵枢·经筋》。

右角（yòu jué） ① Name of constitution. It refers to wood-type people, out of the twenty-five types of people divided according to yin and yang. See *Ling Shu* chapter 65. ② A method for locating back-shu acupoints at the bottom right corners of triangles. See *Su Wen* chapter 24. ③ Right corner of the forehead. See *Ling Shu* chapter 13.

右间 运气术语。即右间气。凡客气中位于司天之气右侧（主气的二之气）及在泉之气右侧（主气的五之气）的间气，称右间。出《素问·本病论》。参"间气"条。

右间（yòu jiān） **Right Interval** Terminology of circuits and qi, that is right interval qi. It refers to the interval qi located at the right side of the qi governing heaven (second qi of the host climatic qi) and on the right side of the qi in the spring (fifth qi of the host climatic qi). See *Su Wen* chapter 73. See the term "间气".

右商 体质名。阴阳二十五人中金形人之一种。出《灵枢·五音五味》。见"右商之人"。

右商（yòu shāng） Name of constitution. It refers to metal-type people, out of the twenty-five types of people divided according to yin and yang. See *Ling Shu* chapter 65. See the term "右商之人".

右商之人 体质名。商，五音之一，五行属金。右商，商音之一，此代表阴阳二十五人中金形人之一种，其特征是美俊潇洒。出《灵枢·阴阳二十五人》。

右商之人（yòu shāng zhī rén） *youshang*-**type people** Name of constitution. *Shāng* is one of the five musical notes, and belongs to metal. *Yòu shāng*, one of the *shang* notes, refers to metal-type people out of the twenty-five types of people divided according to yin and yang, whom with the manifestation of beauty. See *Ling Shu* chapter 64.

右徵 体质名。阴阳二十五人中火形人之一种。出《灵枢·五音五味》。见"右徵之人"。

右徵（yòu zhǐ）　Name of constitution. It refers to the fire-type people，out of the twenty-five types of people divided according to yin and yang. See *Ling Shu* chapter 65. See the term "右徵之人".

右徵之人　体质名。徵（zhǐ 指），五音之一，五行属火。右徵，徵音之一，此代表阴阳二十五人中火形人之一种，其特征是勇猛而不甘落后。出《灵枢·阴阳二十五人》。参"火形之人"条。

右徵之人（yòu zhǐ zhī rén）　*youzhi*-type people　Name of constitution. It refers to the fire-type people，out of the twenty-five types of people divided according to yin and yang. *Zhi*，one of the musical notes，belongs to fire. *You zhi*，one of *zhi* notes，refers to fire type constitutions manifestating bravery. See *Ling Shu* chapter 64. See the term "火形之人".

平人　即阴阳协调、气血平和、健康无病的正常人。出《素问·平人气象论》《灵枢·终始》《素问·调经论》。

平人（píng rén）　normal people　Healthy people with harmonious yin and yang and normal movement of qi and blood. See *Su Wen* chapter 18，*Ling Shu* chapter 9 and *Su Wen* chapter 62.

平人气象论　《素问》篇名。平人，正常人；气，脉气；象，脉象。此篇主要论述正常人脉息动数变化，以及四时五脏的平脉、病脉、死脉的形象；提出了脉之胃气多寡、有无是鉴别平、病、死脉的关键，强调胃气的重要性。因篇中以正常人的脉象来衡量病人的脉象，故以名篇。

平人气象论（píng rén qì xiàng lùn）　Discussion on the Pulse Conditions of Healthy People　Chapter title in *Su Wen*. *Píng rén* refers to healthy people，*qì* refers to pulse qi，and *xiàng* refers to pulse condition. This chapter mainly explains the normal pulse of healthy people，changes of abnormal pulses and failure pulses in different seasons. It also emphasizes the importance of stomach-qi in terms of differentiating between these three kinds of pulses. The chapter was named after its main content.

平人绝谷　《灵枢》篇名。平人，健康的正常人；绝谷，不进饮食。此篇论述了正常人七日不

五画

进食则死的机理,《灵枢集注》曰:"人之脏腑形骸,精神气血,皆藉水谷之所资生,水谷绝则形与气俱绝矣。"故名。

平人绝谷(píng rén jué gǔ) **Normal Patients Have no Desire to Eat** Chapter title in *Ling Shu*. *Píng rén* refers to healthy people, and *jué gǔ* refers to patients who have no desire to eat. This chapter discusses why people die if they do not eat for seven days. *Ling Shu Ji Zhu*（*Collected Annotation of Ling Shu*）states, "People need water and food to keep a good physical and mental condition. Without a desire to eat for a long time may cause exhaustion of qi and body", thus its name.

平气　① 运气术语。谓无太过不及之岁气。五运值年时,凡运太过而被抑,或运不及而得助,就成为平气。如戊辰年,戊属阳火,辰是太阳寒水司天,火运虽太过,但被客气司天的太阳寒水之抑制,则由太过而变为平气。出《素问·六节藏象论》。② 平和之气。出《素问·至真要大论》。

平气(píng qì)　① Terminology of the circuits and qi, in which a year has neither excessive nor deficient qi. When excessive qi is inhibited and deficient qi supported, normal circuits and qi is obtained. For instance, in the year of *wu chen*, although the fire movement is excessive, as *wu* pertains to yang fire, it is inhibited by *chen*, pertaining to *taiyang* cold water, and when the guest qi governs the heavens it turns into normal circuits and qi. See *Su Wen* chapter 9. ② Moderate qi. See *Su Wen* chapter 74.

平心脉　心的正常脉象。脉来柔滑,势如连珠。出《素问·平人气象论》。

平心脉(píng xīn mài)　**normal heart pulse** A pulse soft and smooth as pearls. See *Su Wen* chapter 18.

平旦　清晨卯时。出《素问·生气通天论》。

平旦(píng dàn)　*ping dan* It refers to the early hours of 5a.m.-7a.m. See *Su Wen* chapter 3.

平肝脉　有胃气的正常肝脉。其来柔软而有弹性,如举起之长竿之末梢,具冲和之象,与春季相应。出《素问·平人气象论》。

平肝脉(píng gān mài)　**normal liver pulse** A normal liver pulse with stomach qi. It is soft and elastic，as the end of a long raised bamboo pole，with a harmonious appearance，and corresponding to spring. See *Su Wen* chapter 18.

平肾脉　有胃气的正常肾脉，其来圆滑连贯而有冲和之象，与冬季相应。出《素问·平人气象论》。

平肾脉（píng shèn mài）　**normal kidney pulse** A normal kidney pulse with stomach qi. It is smooth and continuous, harmonious in appearance, and corresponding to winter. See *Su Wen* chapter 18.

平肺脉　正常的肺脉，其来如榆荚落下时那样轻浮和缓而流利，是有胃气的脉象。出《素问·平人气象论》。

平肺脉（píng fèi mài）　**normal lung pulse** A normal lung pulse, which beats in a light floating way, as the drop of an elm leaf. See *Su Wen* chapter 18.

平治于权衡　权，秤锤。衡，秤杆。权衡，调节之意。言治疗时应根据阴阳虚实，偏胜偏衰的情况加以调节，使其达到动态的平衡。出《素问·汤液醪醴论》。

平治于权衡（píng zhì yú quán héng）　**to restore the balanced order of weight and beam** *Quán* refers to weight，and héng refers to the scale beam. *Quán héng* means to adjust. Treatment of disease should focus on restoring harmony according to the deficiency and excess of yin and yang，and the rising and declining conditions，so as to achieve dynamic balance. See *Su Wen* chapter 14.

平息　正常调匀之呼吸。出《素问·平人气象论》。

平息（píng xī）　**normal breath** Even and normal breathing. See *Su Wen* chapter 18.

平脾脉　脾的正常脉象。脉来和缓柔利，从容不迫，脉律分明。出《素问·平人气象论》。

平脾脉（píng pǐ mài）　**normal spleen pulse** A normal spleen pulse beats smoothly, softly and regularly. See *Su Wen* chapter 18.

北政　出《素问·至真要大论》。见"视岁南北"条。

北政（běi zhèng）　**the northern policy** See *Su Wen* chapter 74. See "视岁南北".

目　① 五官之一，主视觉。为肝之窍，与肝有密切联系。五脏的精气亦皆上注于目，故目不仅反映肝的功能状况，还反映五脏精气之盛衰。出《灵枢·脉度》

五画

《灵枢·大惑论》。② 指代眼睑。出《素问·至真要大论》。

目（mù）　① The eyes. One of the five sense organs，governing vision. Eyes are closely connected with the liver as its orifice. In addition，the essence qi of the five viscera all flow upwards into the eyes. Therefore，eyes reflect the condition of the liver's function as well as the exuberance and debilitation of the essence qi of the five viscera. See *Ling Shu* chapter 17 and chapter 80. ② The eyelids. See *Su Wen* chapter 74.

目下网　足阳明的细筋在下眼睑中的网络，与目上网协同司眼睑之开合。出《灵枢·经筋》。

目下网（mù xià wǎng）　**net below the eyes** The net below the eyes，which is formed by the foot *yangming* conduit，and located at the bottom eyelids，serving to manage the opening or closing of the eyelids. See *Ling Shu* chapter 13.

目下果　即下眼睑。果，通裹。出《灵枢·师传》。

目下果（mù xià guǒ）　**lower eyelids** The lacrimal sacs，i.e. the lower eyelids. "果" is the same as "裹" in ancient Chinese.

See *Ling Shu* chapter 29.

目上网　足太阳的细筋在上眼睑中的网络，有维系眼睑，约束开合的作用。出《灵枢·经筋》。

目上网（mù shàng wǎng）　**net above the eyes** The net above the eyes，which is formed by the foot *taiyang* conduit，and located at the upper eyelids，serving to manage the openning or closing of the eyelids. See *Ling Shu* chapter 13.

目不瞑　不能闭目入睡。出《灵枢·大惑论》。

目不瞑（mù bù míng）　**inability to close the eyes and sleep** See *Ling Shu* chapter 80.

目风　病名。风邪入侵目系，以目痛目痒，或畏风羞明为主症。出《素问·风论》。

目风（mù fēng）　**eye wind** A disease with eye pain and itching，or anemophobia and photophobia，as the main symptoms. It appears when the wind enters the eye connector. See *Su Wen* chapter 42.

目本　目之本系，即目系，为眼内连于脑的脉络。出《灵枢·寒热病》。

目本（mù běn）　**the base of eyes** The main system of the eyes，in which，the vessel in the eye reaches and connects with the brain. See *Ling Shu* chapter 21.

目运 头目旋晕昏眩。出《灵枢·经脉》。

目运（mù yùn） **eye movements with dizziness** See *Ling Shu* chapter 10.

目系 系，联属之意。为眼球后连于脑的脉络。出《灵枢·大惑论》。

目系（mù xì） **eye connection** "系" means "connection". It is the vessel behind the eyes connecting to the brain. See *Ling Shu* chapter 10.

目转 眩晕貌，视物旋转。出《素问·五常政大论》。

目转（mù zhuàn） **rolling eyes with dizziness** See *Su Wen* chapter 70.

目盲 视觉丧失。出《素问·生气通天论》。

目盲（mù máng） **blindness** See *Su Wen* chapter 3.

目浸 出《灵枢·热病》。（1）泪出不收。见《类经·针刺四十》。（2）目障，俗谓之翳。见《释名·释疾病》。

目浸（mù jìn） **epiphora** See the chapter 23 of *Ling Shu*. (1) Tears that cannot be held back. See the *Lei Jing*（*Classified Classic*）"Needling Chapter 40". (2) Visual

obstruction，commonly known as corneal opacity. See *Shi Ming* "Shi Ji Bing".

目眦 ① 眼角，眼眶。出《灵枢·癫狂病》。② 指目。出《素问·解精微论》。

目眦（mù zì） ① The corners of the eyes, the eye socket. See *Ling Shu* chapter 22. ② Refers to the eyes. See *Su Wen* chapter 81.

目瞏绝系 症状名。指由足少阳经气绝，而致目与目系不相维系的两目直视之症。目瞏，直视如惊貌。绝系，入属于脑的目系已绝，目失灵动。出《素问·诊要经终论》。

目瞏绝系（mù qióng jué xì） **orthophoria** Symptom name. Refers to eyes staring blankly into space. It appears when the qi of the *shaoyang* vessel is finished and the connection between the eyes and the eye connector is severed. *Mù qióng* means the eyes stare as if terrified. *Jué xì* means that the eye connection with the brain has been severed，and thus the eyes fail to move freely. See *Su Wen* chapter 16.

目窠 眼胞。窠（Kē 科），裹之意。出《灵枢·水胀》。

目窠（mù kē） **Eyelids** "窠" means

wrap. See *Ling Shu* chapter 57.

目裏　眼胞。出《素问·平人气象论》。

目裏（mù guǒ）　**Eyelids** See *Su Wen* chapter 18.

目瞑　① 目昏暗不明。出《素问·六元正纪大论》。② 合目而眠。出《灵枢·口问》。

目瞑（mù míng）　① Blurred vision. See *Su Wen* chapter 71. ② Closing eyes to sleep. See *Ling Shu* chapter 28.

目瞳子　指瞳子髎。足少阳胆经之穴，又名太阳、前关。在目外去眦五分。出《素问·气穴论》。

目瞳子（mù tóng zǐ）　Refers to Tong Zi Liao (GB 1), the acupuncture point on the gallbladder meridian of foot *taiyang*, which is also called Tai Yang or Qian Guan. It is located 0.5 *cun* lateral to the outer canthus of the eye. See *Su Wen* chapter 58.

甲子　天干甲与地支子相合之年。干支纪年，以十天干(甲、乙、丙、丁、戊、己、庚、辛、壬、癸)与十二地支(子、丑、寅、卯、辰、巳、午、未、申、酉、戌、亥)依次相配，起于甲子，止于癸亥，其数凡六十，复回甲子轮转，甲子乃六十年之首，故亦简称甲子。出《素问·六微旨大论》。

甲子（jiǎ zǐ）　***jia zi*** The year when the first of the ten Heavenly Stems is combined with the first of the twelve Earthly Branches. The stem-branch combination，a way to mark time，and is the combination of the ten Heavenly Stems（*jia*，*yi*，*bing*，*ding*，*wu*，*ji*，*geng*，*xin*，*ren*，*gui*）and the twelve Earthly Branches（*zi*，*chou*，*yin*，*mao*，*chen*，*si*，*wu*，*wei*，*shen*，*you*，*xu*，*hai*）in sequential order，starting from *Jia zi* and ending with *gui hai* in a sixty-year cycle. *Jia zi* is the first year of the cycle. See *Su Wen* chapter 68.

四支　支，同肢。手足四肢。出《素问·阴阳应象大论》。

四支（sì zhī）　**four limbs** 支 is the same as 肢. See *Su Wen* chapter 5.

四气　① 指春夏秋冬四时之气。出《素问·四气调神大论》。② 运气中六气的四之气，主治大暑至秋分之间。出《素问·至真要大论》。③ 运气中五运的第四步，主治夏至后三十一日至秋分日之间。出《素问·六元正纪大论》。

四气（sì qì）　① Refers to the qi of the four seasons. See *Su Wen* chapter 2. ② The "fourth qi" among the six circuits and qi, which mainly governs the period between the Great Heat (12th solar term) and the Autumn Equinox (16th solar term). See *Su Wen* chapter 74. ③ The fourth phase among the five circuits and qi, which mainly governs the period from the 31st days after the Summer Solstice (10th solar term) to the Autumn Equinox (16th solar term). See *Su Wen* chapter 71.

四气调神大论 《素问》篇名。四气,春夏秋冬四时之气。调,调养。神,精神意志。大论,指内容宏富。此篇主要介绍顺应四时气候特点以调摄精神情志等养生方法。故名。

四气调神大论(sì qì tiáo shén dà lùn) **Major Discussion of Regulation of Spirit According to the Changes of the Four Seasons** Chapter title in *Su Wen*. *Sì qì* refers to the qi of the four seasons. *Tiáo* means to regulate. *Shén* refers to spirit. And *dà lùn* means the content is rich. This chapter mainly introduces health preservation methods such as regulating spirit and emotions according to the changes of the four seasons, thus its name.

四末 ① 泛指四肢。出《灵枢·邪客》。② 四肢远端掌指(趾)处。出《素问·疟论》。

四末(sì mò) ① Refers to the four limbs in general. See *Ling Shu* chapter 71. ② The metacarpal fingers (toes) of the four extremities. See *Su Wen* chapter 35.

四白 唇之四际白肉。出《素问·六节藏象论》。

四白(sì bái) The four white sections in the eyes surrounding the pupils. See *Su Wen* chapter 9.

四关 指两肘、两膝四个关节。出《灵枢·九针十二原》。

四关(sì guān) Refers to the two elbows and two knees, the four joints. See *Su Wen* chapter 1.

四极 四肢。出《素问·汤液醪醴论》。

四极(sì jí) **four extremities** Refers to the four limbs. See *Su Wen* chapter 14.

四时 ① 即春、夏、秋、冬四季,又称四气。出《素问·上古天真论》《素问·八正神明论》。② 指一日之中的四个时间段。出《灵枢·顺气一日分为四时》。

四时(sì shí) ① Namely, the four seasons, also known as the four qi. See *Su Wen* chapter 1 and *Su Wen* chapter 26. ② Refers to the four time periods in a single day. See *Ling Shu* chapter 44.

四时气 《灵枢》篇名。该篇主要论述了四时气候的变化对人体的影响，提出刺灸要根据四时气候的变化，选择相应的穴位及手法。篇中还讨论了温疟、风痹、徒痹、著痹、疠风等病的针刺治疗，以及邪在腑的症状特点、针刺方法等。

四时气(sì shí qì)　**Four Seasonal Qi** Chapter title in *Ling Shu*. This chapter mainly introduces the influence of the climatic changes in the four seasons on the human body, and puts forward a selection of acupuncture points and techniques, in the acupuncture and moxibustion therapy, on which therapy should be based. The acupuncture treatment is specified for diseases such as warm malaria, wind-water-illness, water-illness, fixed arthralgia, and pestilential wind (leprosy). As well, the characteristics and symptoms caused by pathogens in the bowels, and their respective acupuncture treatments, are also discussed.

四时刺逆从论 《素问》篇名。四时，春夏秋冬四季；刺，针刺；逆，违背；从，遵从。此篇从正反两方面论述针刺遵从和违背四时的变化规律对人体脏腑气血的影响。故名。

四时刺逆从论(sì shí cì nì cóng lùn)　**Discussion on Acupuncture Following and Against the Changes of the Four Seasons** Chapter title in *Su Wen*. *Sì shí* refers to the four seasons, *cì* refers to acupuncture, *nì* means opposition and *cóng* refers to compliance. This chapter expounds the positive and negative effects of acupuncture on the organs, qi and blood of the human body when the methods comply or violate the rules of the changing four seasons, thus its name.

四季 ① 一年中春、夏、秋、冬四个季节，又名四时。出《素问·刺要论》。② 指一日之中辰戌丑未四个时辰。出《素问·藏气法时论》。

四季(sì jì)　① The four seasons, i.e. spring, summer, autumn, winter, also called *si shi*. See *Su Wen* chapter 50. ② The four periods in a day, namely *chen* (7-9 a.m.), *xu* (7-9 p.m.), *chou* (1-3 a.m.) and

五画

wei (1 – 3 p.m.). See *Su Wen* chapter 22.

四经 四时正常脉象,即春弦、夏洪、秋浮、冬沉。出《素问·阴阳别论》。

四经(sì jīng) **four normal pulses** Normal pulse conditions in the four seasons,i.e. *xian* (taut) pulse in spring,*hong* (full) pulse in summer,*fu* (floating) pulse in autumn and *chen* (sinking) pulse in winter. See *Su Wen* chapter 7.

四畏 用药时应避畏自然界气候的四种情况,即用热远热、用寒远寒、用凉远凉、用温远温。出《素问·六元正纪大论》。

四畏(sì wèi) **four contraindications** The four climatic conditions which must be abided by when using drugs. That is,if heat dominates the season,one must not offend it by using drugs hot in nature;if cold dominates the season,one must not offend it by using drugs cold in nature;if coolness dominates the season,one must not offend it by using drugs cool in nature; if warmth dominates the season, one must not offend it by using drugs warm in nature. See *Su Wen* chapter 71.

四逆 四肢逆冷。出《素问·阴阳别论》。

四逆(sì nì) **four reversals** Reversal cold of limbs. See *Su Wen* chapter 7.

四海 ① 东、南、西、北四海。出《灵枢·海论》。② 髓海、血海、气海、水谷之海的合称。出《灵枢·海论》。

四海(sì hǎi) ① East Sea,West Sea, South Sea, and North Sea. See *Ling Shu* chapter 33. ② The sea of marrow,the sea of blood, the sea of qi, and the sea of water and grains collectively. See *Ling Shu* chapter 33.

四难 指形气相失、色夭不泽、脉实以坚、脉逆四时四种难治的危重证候。出《素问·玉机真藏论》。

四难(sì nán) **four difficulties** Four kinds of critical symptoms which are difficult to treat, including body constitution and qi fading out; faded lusterless complexion; replete and firm vessels; and pulse going against the four seasons. See *Su Wen* chapter 19.

四淫 痈毒浸淫于四肢。出《灵枢·痈疽》。

四淫(sì yín) **four fold excess** Carbuncles spreading over limbs.

See *Ling Shu* chapter 81.

四维 ① 指东南、东北、西南、西北四隅。出《素问·气交变大论》。② 指辰戌丑未月。出《素问·至真要大论》。③ 指春夏秋冬四季所主的风暑湿寒四种气候。出《素问·生气通天论》。

四维(sì wéi) ① Refers to four corner directions, i.e. southeast, northeast, southwest and northwest. See *Su Wen* chapter 69. ② Refers to the months of *chen*, *xu*, *chou* and *wei* in a year. See *Su Wen* chapter 74. ③ Refers to four climates, i.e. wind, summerheat, dampness and cold, which are dominated by the four seasons (spring, summer, autumn and winter). See *Su Wen* chapter 3.

四厥 四肢厥冷。出《灵枢·五乱》。

四厥(sì jué) **coldness of the four limbs** See *Ling Shu* chapter 34.

四街 头、胸、腹、胫四部气街的合称,是气的径路。出《灵枢·动输》。

四街(sì jiē) **four paths** The four paths of qi in the head, chest, abdomen and leg, and which are shortcuts for the exchanges of qi. See *Ling Shu* chapter 62.

四德 指医生应具备的四种品德素质,内容大致包括结合天地四时阴阳、掌握刺灸砭石毒药的主治作用,了解病人的个体差异及生活环境,精神状态,注意五色与脉象的细微变化,知晓疾病的始末,强调正气等。出《素问·疏五过论》。

四德(sì dé) **four virtues** Refers to the four virtues doctors should possess while giving therapy, including mastering the therapies of acupuncture and moxibustion, stone needling and following indications of toxic drugs according to the rules of heaven and earth, paying attention to the four seasons and the yin and yang; understanding the individual differences in the daily lives and mental states of patients; paying attention to the subtle changes of the five colors and pulse conditions, knowing the whole course of the disease, and valuing healthy qi, etc. See *Su Wen* chapter 77.

生气 ① 阳气。出《素问·生气通天论》。② 生机。出《素问·四气调神大论》。③ 春令生发之气,五行属木,又称木气。出《素问·五常政大论》。

生气(shēng qì) ① Yang qi. See *Su Wen* chapter 3. ② Vitality. See *Su Wen* chapter 2. ③ The qi generated in spring, pertaining to wood in the five elements, and also called wood qi. See *Su Wen* chapter 70.

生气通天论 《素问》篇名。生气,生命之气。包括阴精和阳气。通,通应。天,自然界。生气通天,指人体阴阳之气与自然界阴阳之气互相贯通。此篇的主要内容讨论阳气的重要性,阳气的生理病理以及自然之气的关系;强调阴精与阳气相互协调对人体健康的关系。

生气通天论(shēng qì tōng tiān lùn) **Discussion on the Interrelationship Between Life and Nature** Chapter title in *Su Wen*. *Shēng qì*, namely the qi of life, consists of yin essence and yang qi. *Tōng* means the correspondence. *Tiān* refers to the natural world. *Shēng qì tōng tiān* refers to the mutual correspondence between the yin qi and yang qi of the human body and those of nature. The chapter focuses on the importance and the physiological pathology of yang qi as well as its relationship with the natural qi. In addition, it emphasizes the impact of the relationship between yin essence and yang qi on human health.

生化 万物的产生、发展和变化。出《素问·五运行大论》。

生化(shēng huà) **generation and transformation** The process of emergence, development and transformation of all things. See *Su Wen* chapter 67.

生阳 ① 正月初生之阳气。出《灵枢·阴阳系日月》。② 五脏疾病相传,若按相生次序传变时,是有生机。如疾病为从肝病传心之类。出《素问·阴阳别论》。

生阳(shēng yáng) ① The yang qi generated in the first month. See *Ling Shu* chapter 41. ② Diseases of the five viscera are likely to transmit, and vitality exists if they are transmitted according to the generation order of the five phases, for example, a disease transmitted from the liver to the heart. See *Su Wen* chapter 7.

生阴 七月初生之阴气。出《灵枢·阴阳系日月》。

生阴(shēng yīn) **generating yin** The yin qi generated in the seventh month. See *Ling Shu* chapter 41.

生政 指以生发为特点的物候现象布行。政,施政。出《素问·

五画

五常政大论》。

生政（shēng zhèng） **generating zheng** Refers to the distribution of phenological phenomena characterized by generation and development. *Zheng* refers to governance. See *Su Wen* chapter 70.

生铁洛 又写作生铁落。其气寒而重，能重镇心神，坠热开结，平木火之邪，以此为饮，能治怒狂。是《内经》十三方之一。出《素问·病能论》。

生铁洛（shēng tiě luò） **iron filings** A medicine whose qi is cold and heavy, thus it can be used to tranquilize the mind, clear heat, relieve depression, and free stagnation. Taking it in decoction, anger can be diffused. It is one of the thirteen prescriptions in the *Nei Jing* (*Internal Classic*). See *Su Wen* chapter 46.

生病起于过用 过用，过度劳用。诸如饮食过饱，思虑过度，房室不节，操劳过倦等均属过用之例，这些都是起病的原因。出《素问·经脉别论》。

生病起于过用（shēng bìng qǐ yú guò yòng） **disease emerging from overexertion** *Guò yòng* refers to excessive exertion. Overeating, overthinking, over indulgence and overexertion are some of the causes of disease. See *Su Wen* chapter 21.

生桑灰 即生桑炭。桑木之灰炭火。出《灵枢·经筋》。

生桑灰（shēng sāng huī） **Charcoal of the mulberry tree.** See *Ling Shu* chapter 13.

生桑炭 桑木之炭火。出《灵枢·寿夭刚柔》。

生桑炭（shēng sāng tàn） **Charcoal of the mulberry tree.** See *Ling Shu* chapter 6.

失气 ① 症状名。失同矢，矢通屎。失气即屎气，俗称屁。出《素问·咳论》。② 病机。由针刺不当而致正气败失。出《素问·终始》。

失气（shī qì） ① Symptom name. "失" is the same as "矢" or "屎". *Shī qì* means flatus. See *Su Wen* chapter 38. ② Disease mechanism, in which improper acupuncture techniques impair the healthy qi. See *Ling Shu* chapter 9.

失守 ① 运气术语。一年中，六气各守其位。若出现不迁正、不退位，升降不前时，就是失守其位。出《素问·本病论》。② 脏气不能内守而衰败。出《素问·脉要精微论》。

失守（shī shǒu） ① Terminology of circuits and qi, when in a year，the six qi guard their positions respectively. However，if the six qi didn't maintain their due positions and didn't abdicate，and there are abnormal changes of the intermediate qi at the right and left sides，it is called *Shī Shǒu*（loss of position）. See *Su Wen* chapter 73. ② The qi of five viscera fails to guard and decays. See *Su Wen* chapter 17.

失志　狂言，神志失常。因肾藏精，精舍志，病阴阳交，邪盛精败，志无所舍，故称。出《素问·评热病论》。参"阴阳交"条。

失志（shī zhì）　**mental confusion** Ravings，mental derangement. As the kidney stores essence and the essence houses spirit，when the disease passes on to the yin and yang leading to the domination of evil and defeat of essense，the essence loses its resting place. See *Su Wen* chapter 33. See the term "阴阳交".

失枕　病证名。症状为颈项不能转动伸舒，即今所谓落枕。多因睡卧姿势不当，或局部感受风寒所致。出《素问·骨空论》。

失枕（shī zhěn）　**Neck cannot touch the pillow.** Syndrome name for a stiff neck，or torticollis. It is characterized by difficulty in moving the neck，especially when trying to turn the head side to side. The most common cause of a stiff neck is an awkward sleeping posture or wind-cold. See *Su Wen* chapter 60.

失精　病证名。由于先富后贫，精神忧郁，营养不良，致五脏精气日益亏损的病证。出《素问·疏五过论》。

失精（shī jīng）　**loss of essence** Syndrome name，of when a patient was formerly wealthy and then later became poor，causing depression，malnutrition，and the depletion of the five viscera. See *Su Wen* chapter 77.

乍疏乍数曰死　脉来忽快忽慢，是胃气衰败之象，预后不良。出《素问·平人气象论》。

乍疏乍数曰死（zhà shū zhà shuò yuē sǐ）　**spaced and frequent pulses indicating death** If at times the pulse is spaced，at times frequent，it represents the decline of stomach qi and the prognosis is poor. See *Su Wen* chapter 18.

丘墟　经穴名。足少阳胆经之原穴，在足外踝下微前陷中。出《灵枢·本输》。

丘墟（qiū xū）　**Qiu Xu（GB 40）**

Acupoint name of Qiu Xu (GB 40), which is the source acupoint of the gallbladder meridian of foot *shaoyang*. It is located on the anterolateral aspect of the ankle, in the depression anterior and distal to the lateral malleolus. See *Ling Shu* chapter 2.

代 ① 代脉。脉来缓弱而有规则的间歇,多主脏气衰弱。出《素问·脉要精微论》《灵枢·根结》。② 脉来软弱和缓是脾的正常脉象。出《素问·宣明五气》。

代(dài) ① Intermittent pulse, which is a moderate weak pulse with regular intervals, indicating that the visceral qi has weakened. See *Su Wen* chapter 17 and *Ling Shu* chapter 5. ② The normal pulse of the spleen is weak, moderate and slow. See *Su Wen* chapter 23.

代则气衰 脉有规则的歇止谓之代,是元气虚衰之象。出《素问·脉要精微论》。

代则气衰(dài zé qì shuāi) *Dài* refers to a moderate weak pulse with regular intervals, indicating that the original qi is deficient and weak. See *Su Wen* chapter 17.

白尸鬼 指金疫之邪。出《素问·本病论》。

白尸鬼(bái shī guǐ) **metal pestilence** Refers to the evil of metal pestilence. See *Su Wen* chapter 73.

白气 ① 指肺气。出《素问·调经论》。② 运气术语,即金运之气的代称。出《素问·气交变大论》。③ 当作"雨气"。出《素问·六元正纪大论》。

白气(bái qì) ① Refers to lung qi. See *Su Wen* chapter 62. ② Terminology of circuits and qi, that is the pronoun of the qi of metal movement. See *Su Wen* chapter 69. ③ Qi of rain. See *Su Wen* chapter 71.

白为寒 凡见肤色白或人体病理过程中产生的分泌物呈白色,多为寒象。出《素问·举痛论》。

白为寒(bái wéi hán) **white indicates cold** Any appearance of pale skin, or white secretions produced in the pathological processes of the body, signifies that the patient is usually suffering from retention of cold qi. See *Su Wen* chapter 39.

白肉际 边缘为际。指手足掌指(趾)内(掌)侧与外侧的皮肤交界处。掌侧(阴)面皮肤色泽较白,称白肉;背(阳)侧生毫毛的皮肤色泽较深,称赤肉。故赤白肉交界处，又称赤白肉际。出《灵枢·邪客》。

白肉际（bái ròu jì）　**borderline of the white flesh** Taking the border as the dividing line, it is the skin boundary between the palm or sole（red in color，namely red flesh）and the back of the hand or foot（white in color，namely white flesh），also called the border between the red and white flesh. See *Ling Shu* chapter 71.

白汗　即自汗。出《素问·经脉别论》。

白汗（bái hàn）　**white sweat** Namely, spontaneous sweating. See *Su Wen* chapter 21.

白沙蜜　即白蜜，性味甘平，有补中缓急、润肺止咳的作用，常用作丸药的赋形剂。出《素问·刺法论》。

白沙蜜（bái shā mì）　**white honey** It is mild and sweet in nature and flavor. It has the effects of tonifying the middle，relaxing tensions，and moistening the lung to suppress cough. It is often used in the pill form. See *Su Wen* chapter 72.

白脉　肺脉。白为肺之色，故称。出《素问·五藏生成》。

白脉（bái mài）　**white pulse** The lung pulse. The colour white corresponds to the colour of the lung in the five colors，hence its name. See *Su Wen* chapter 10.

白帝　五天帝之一，主西方。出《灵枢·阴阳二十五人》。

白帝（bái dì）　**white thearch** One of the five lords of heaven ruling the west. See *Ling Shu* chapter 64.

白眼　指眼球的白色部分，即巩膜。肺色白，故与肺相应。出《灵枢·大惑论》。

白眼（bái yǎn）　**white part of the eyes** Refers to the sclera，and corresponds to the lung, as the lung's colour is also white. See *Ling Shu* chapter 80.

白淫　指精浊带下。出《素问·痿论》。

白淫（bái yín）　**white overflow** Refers to turbid vaginal and seminal discharge. See *Su Wen* chapter 44.

卯酉之纪　指纪年地支是卯、酉之年，为阳明燥金司天。纪，纪年。出《素问·六元正纪大论》。

卯酉之纪（mǎo yǒu zhī jì）　**year of *mao* and *you*** Refers to the years in which the Earthly Branches are *mao* and *you* in marking time according to the Stem-

Branch Combination. In these years，*yangming* qi and metal qi dominate the heavens. *Jì* means designating the year. See *Su Wen* chapter 71.

外门 针孔。出《素问·调经论》。

外门（wài mén） **external gate** Needle hole. See *Su Wen* chapter 62.

外内之病 指外内相应之外感内伤病。出《灵枢·寿夭刚柔》。

外内之病（wài nèi zhī bìng） Diseases of the exterior and interior. See *Ling Shu* chapter 6.

外内皆越 身体内外之气泄越耗散。出《素问·举痛论》。

外内皆越（wài nèi jiē yuè） The qi inside the body is leaking and the qi outside the body is dissipating. See *Su Wen* chapter 39.

外关 经穴名。手少阳三焦经之络穴。又是八脉交会穴，通阳维脉，在腕后二寸陷者中。出《灵枢·经脉》。

外关（wài guān） **Wai Guan（TE 5）** Acupoint name for the connecting acupoint of the triple *jiao* meridian and the confluent acupoint of the eight extra meridians，connecting with the *yangwei* meridian. It is located 2 *cun* proximal to the dorsal wrist crease and in the depression between the ulna and radius. See *Ling Shu* chapter 10.

外经 指经脉外行部分，包括四肢、皮肤等，与内行于脏腑部分相对而言。出《灵枢·邪气藏府病形》。

外经（wài jīng） The external conduits of the meridians，including the four limbs，skin，etc，as opposed to the internal conduits of the meridians in the viscera and bowels. See *Ling Shu* chapter 4.

外格 三阳之气盛于外，与三阴之气相格拒，表现为人迎脉大且数，盛于寸口脉四倍的脉象。出《灵枢·终始》。

外格（wài gé） **external blockage** The overflowing qi of the three yang cause blockages of the qi of the three yin，with the manifestation of the *ren ying* pulse being four times greater than that of the *cun kou* pulse. It is large and rapid，indicating a morbid condition known as the blockage of yin qi outside. See *Ling Shu* chapter 9.

外眦 眼眶上边，又指外侧眼角。出《灵枢·癫狂》。

外眦（wài zì） **outer canthus** The superior aspect of the eye socket，also refers to the outer canthus. See *Ling Shu* chapter 22.

外维 足少阳筋直支之分支，结于眼外角者，有维系眼球，左右盼视之用。出《灵枢·经筋》。

外维（wài wéi） **external** *wei* The branch of the gallbladder meridian connecting at the outer canthus as the external defence of the eye. Its function is to maintain eye movement left and right. See *Ling Shu* chapter 13.

外揣 《灵枢》篇名。揣，《说文》曰："量也。"即推测度量之意。外揣，即从体外征象推测内脏之变化。此篇强调人体是一个阴阳内外相应的统一整体，可以通过察外以知内，知内而测外的道理作为分析病情的法则。故名。

外揣（wài chuāi） **Diagnosing the Interior by Examining the Exterior** Chapter title in *Ling Shu*. *Chuāi* means speculation and *wài chuāi* refers to speculating the change of the viscera according to their visible body signs. This chapter stresses the concept of holism. The interior pathological changes of the viscera can be diagnosed by examining the external symptoms and signs of the patient；the exterior syndromes can be diagnosed by studying the interior disorders of the viscera. This is the rule to analyze the disease's condition.

外踝 足踝外侧骨头。出《灵枢·骨度》。

外踝（wài huái） **external malleolus** The bone of the external malleolus. See *Ling Shu* chapter 14.

冬三月 指农历十、十一、十二三月，包括立冬、小雪、大雪、冬至、小寒、大寒六个节气。此时天寒地冻，万物潜藏。出《素问·四气调神大论》。

冬三月（dōng sān yuè） **three months in winter** Refers to the tenth，eleventh and twelfth lunar months，including the six solar terms，namely，the Beginning of Winter，Slight Snow，Great Snow，Winter Solstice，Slight Cold，Great Cold. The three months of winter is the season for storage as the weather is freezing. See *Su Wen* chapter 2.

冬气 ①冬季潜藏之气。与肾相应。出《素问·四气调神大论》《素问·六节藏象论》。②冬季之人体精气，其藏在骨髓中。出《素问·四时刺逆从论》。③冬季中人之病气。出《灵枢·终始》。

冬气（dōng qì） ① The storing

of qi in the human body in winter. See *Su Wen* chapter 2 and *Su Wen* chapter 9. ② The qi of essence stored in the marrow in winter. See *Su Wen* chapter 64. ③ Pathogenetic qi in the human body in winter. See *Ling Shu* chapter 9.

冬分 指骨髓。是冬季人体精气相对集中的部位，与肾相应。出《素问·诊要经终论》。

冬分（dōng fēn） **winter parts** Refers to bone marrow, and also refers to the part of the human body where the qi of essence is concentrated. It corresponds to the kidney. See *Su Wen* chapter 16.

冬脉 沉石之脉。冬季应时之脉，与肾相应。出《素问·玉机真藏论》。

冬脉（dōng mài） **winter pulse** A sunken or deep pulse, which is in accordance with winter, and also corresponds to the kidney. See *Su Wen* chapter 19.

冬脉如营 冬令万物闭藏，人体脉气与之相应，沉而濡滑有力，如营兵内守之状，故营脉为冬季之脉，与肾相应。出《素问·玉机真藏论》。

冬脉如营（dōng mài rú yíng） **winter pulse is encamped** Winter is the period in which all the things in nature go into hiding, and the pulse in winter appears deep, soggy, slippery and forceful, like the ying (camp) guarding internally. Hence, it is "encamped" and is the pulse of winter, which corresponds to the kidney. See *Su Wen* chapter 19.

包络 即心包络。出《灵枢·邪客》。见"心包络"条。

包络（bāo luò） **collateral** That is, the collateral of the pericardium. See *Ling Shu* chapter 71. See "心包络".

主 ① 指心，为君主之官。出《素问·灵兰秘典论》《灵枢·五癃津液别》。② 指先至的脉。出《素问·阴阳类论》。③ 指主气，与客气相对而言。主司一年中的常规气候变化。主气将一年分六步，一步主四个节气，始于厥阴风木，终于太阳寒水，年年不变。出《素问·至真要大论》。④ 指受制约。出《素问·五藏生成》。⑤ 主宰。《灵枢·九针论》。⑥ 主要。出《素问·至真要大论》。⑦ 主治。出《素问·刺热》。

主（zhǔ） ① Refers to the heart, which is the organ similar to a monarch. See *Su Wen* chapter 8 and *Ling Shu* chapter 36.

② Refers to the vessel that arrives first. See *Su Wen* chapter 79. ③ Refers to dominant qi that is opposite to guest qi. Dominant qi controls the regular climate change of a year. It divides one year into six steps with each step ruling four solar terms. Originating from the wind-wood of reverting yin and ending up with the cold-water of *taiyang*, it remains unchanged annually. See *Su Wen* chapter 74. ④ Refers to being limited. See *Su Wen* chapter 10. ⑤ Refers to domination. See *Ling Shu* chapter 78. ⑥ Refers to the main concern. See *Su Wen* chapter 74. ⑦ Refers to indications. See *Su Wen* chapter 32.

主气 运气术语。与客气相对，亦称主时之气。指每年各个季节气候的常规变化，一年分六步，每步主四个节气，起于厥阴风木，终于太阳寒水，年年固定不变。出《素问·六元正纪大论》。

主气（zhǔ qì） **dominant qi** Terminology of circuits and qi, which is opposite to guest qi, and is also called the qi that rules the seasons. It controls the regular climatic changes in a year, and divides one year into six steps with each step ruling four solar terms. Originating from the wind-wood of reverting yin and ending at the cold water of *taiyang*, every year it remains unchanged. See *Su Wen* chapter 71.

主岁 运气术语。五运之气各主一岁。即甲己之年，土运主岁；乙庚之年，金运主岁；丙辛之年，水运主岁；丁壬之年，木运主岁；戊癸之年，火运主岁。出《素问·五运行大论》《素问·六元正纪大论》。

主岁（zhǔ suì） **qi ruling a year** Terminology of circuits and qi, in which each of the five qi rules over one year. *Jia* and *ji* years are governed by earth circuit. *Yi* and *geng* years are governed by metal circuit. *Bing* and *xin* years are governed by water circuit. *Ding* and *ren* years are governed by wood circuit. *Wu* and *gui* years are governed by fire circuit. See *Su Wen* chapter 67 and *Su Wen* chapter 71.

主病 ① 主治病变的要药。出《素问·至真要大论》。② 发病的主要部位。出《灵枢·寒热病》。③ 主要病证。出《素问·至真要大论》。

主病（zhǔ bìng） ① Main drugs in treating the disease. See *Su Wen* chapter 74. ② Main location of the disease. See *Ling Shu* chapter 21. ③ Main disease. See *Su Wen* chapter 74.

玄天之气 古天文学家在张、翼、娄、胃诸宿间看到的黑色之气。其中张、翼二宿位于南方偏东之丙位，娄、胃二宿位于西方偏北之辛位。《内经》以此说明"天干纪运"的方法，即黑属水，故水主治丙辛年。出《素问·五运行大论》。

玄天之气（xuán tiān zhī qì） **qi of dark heaven** The black qi that ancient astronomers observed passing through the stellar divisions of *zhang* and *yi*, and through those of *lou* and *wei*. *Zhang* and *yi* are located in the *bing* position (southern east), whereas *lou* and *wei* are located in the *xin* position (western north). This was used to interpret the way of "calculating the yearly movement according to Heavenly Stems" in *Nei Jing*（ *Internal Classic* ）. For example, water rules the year of *bing* and *xin* as the colour black pertains to water. See *Su Wen* chapter 67.

玄委 九宫之一。西南方之坤宫，主立秋、处暑、白露三个节气。出《灵枢·九宫八风》。

玄委（xuán wěi） *Xuan Wei* One of the nine mansions, which is attributed to the trigram *kun*（坤）that covers the three solar terms of Beginning of Autumn（ *li qiu* ）, Limited Summer Heat（ *chu shu* ）, and White Dew（ *bai lu* ）. See *Ling Shu* chapter 77.

玄府 即汗空。指汗腺。出《素问·六元正纪大论》。

玄府（xuán fǔ） **mysterious mansion** Namely, sweat pores, and refers to the sweat glands. See *Su Wen* chapter 71.

玄珠密语 古医籍名，已佚。内容可能与五运六气有关。出《素问·本病论》。

玄珠密语（xuán zhū mì yǔ） *Xuan Zhu Mi Yu* Name of a classic medical book which has been lost in history. Its contents may be closely related with the theory of the five circuits and six qi. See *Su Wen* chapter 73.

兰 指兰草，即佩兰。气味辛平芳香，能醒脾化湿，清暑辟浊。用以治疗脾瘅（脾热）。出《素问·奇病论》。

兰（lán） **herba eupatorii** Refers

to *lan cao*, that is Pei Lan (*Herba Eupatorii*), which is an aromatic medicine, pungent in taste, moderate in nature, enlivens the spleen and resolves dampness, clears the summer heat and dispels turbidity. The drug can be used to treat spleen-heat syndrome. See *Su Wen* chapter 47.

半刺　五刺法之一。半,形容浅刺之意。浅刺皮肤,很快出针,不伤肌肉,犹如拔毫毛那样,以宣泄浅表部邪气。出《灵枢·官针》。

半刺(bàn cì)　**half needling** One of the five needling methods. *Bàn* means shallow needling. The insertion is superficial, and the needle is withdrawn quickly without harming the flesh. It is a way to purge the superficial evil qi as if plucking out a hair. See *Ling Shu* chapter 7.

半夏　药名。气味辛温,功能燥湿化痰,消痞散结。与秫米制成半夏汤,为《内经》十三方之一,用治不寐症。出《灵枢·邪客》。

半夏(bàn xià)　**Ban Xia** (*Rhizoma Pinelliae*) Name of a medicine. It is pungent in taste, warm in nature, dries dampness to resolve phlegm, and disperses abscesses and nodules. Ban Xia Shu Mi Decoction is one of the thirteen classical formulae in *Nei Jing* (*Internal Classic*) and it can be used to treat sleeping disorders. See *Ling Shu* chapter 71.

半夏汤　《内经》十三方之一,由半夏、秫米组成,又称半夏秫米汤。主治阳不能交阴而致之失寐。出《灵枢·邪客》。

半夏汤(bàn xià tāng)　**Ban Xia Decoction** With Ban Xia (*Rhizoma Pinelliae*) and Shu Mi (husked Chinese sorghum) as the main ingredients, it is also known as Ban Xia Shu Mi Decoction. It is one of the thirteen classical formulas in *Nei Jing* (*Internal Classic*) and can be used to treat insomnia caused by the yang failing to coordinate with the yin. See *Ling Shu* chapter 71.

头半寒痛　偏头冷痛。出《灵枢·厥痛》。

头半寒痛(tóu bàn hán tòng)　**cold and aches of the half head** Half of the head is cold and aches. See *Ling Shu* chapter 24.

头者精明之府　精明,精气神明之谓。府,指聚集之处。头部是精气神明所聚集的地方。出《素问·脉要精微论》。

头者精明之府（tóu zhě jīng míng zhī fǔ）　**The head is the organs where essence，qi and bright spirit gather.** *Jing ming* means essence qi and spirit brilliance，and *fu* refers to the gathering region. The head is the place where essence，qi and bright spirit gather. See *Su Wen* chapter 17.

穴　① 腧穴的简称。是人体脏腑经络气血输注于体表的部位。穴，含有"孔""隙"之意。出《素问·气穴论》。② 针孔。出《灵枢·官能》。

穴（xué）　① Abbreviation for *shu xue*，acupoints. It is the region where the viscera，meridians，qi and blood are infused on the body's surface. Acupoint encompasses the meaning of hole and aperture. See *Su Wen* chapter 58. ② Needling hole. See *Ling Shu* chapter 73.

穴空　穴孔，腧穴。出《素问·气穴论》。

穴空（xué kōng）　**acupoints** See *Su Wen* chapter 58.

穴俞　穴俞，即腧穴，简称穴或俞（腧）。出《素问·生气通天论》。

穴俞（xué shū）　**Acupoints** *Xué shū* is usually abbreviated as *xué* or *shū*. See *Su Wen* chapter 3.

司天　运气术语。谓轮值、主司天令者，为客气之一种。六气分步推移中，司天之气位于正南方（上），当主气的三之气，主管每年上半年的气候、物候变化。司天轮值的推演，以纪年地支为工具，凡逢子、午之年为少阴君火司天。丑、未之年为太阴湿土司天。寅、申之年为少阳相火司天。卯、酉之年为阳明燥金司天。辰、戌之年为太阳寒水司天。巳、亥之年为厥阴风木司天。出《素问·五常政大论》。

司天（sì tiān）　**governing the heaven** Terminology of circuits and qi. Refers to the guest qi controlling the heavens in rotation. In the six qi，the qi dominating the heavens is located in the south（top），and serves as the third qi of the dominant qi，which is in charge of the climatic and phenological changes in the first half of each year. The Earthly Branches is used to speculate the rotation of the qi dominating the heavens. *Shaoyin* and sovereign fire dominate the heavens in the years of *zi* and *wu*. *Taiyin* and damp-earth dominate the heavens in the years of *chou* and *wei*. *Shaoyang* and ministerial fire dominate the heavens in the years of *yin* and *shen*. *Yangming* and dry-metal dominate the heavens in the years of *mao* and *you*. *Taiyang* and cold-water dominate the heavens in the years of *chen* and *xu*. *Jueyin* and wind-wood dominate the heavens in the years of *si* and *hai*. See *Su Wen* chapter 70.

司内揣外 司（sì），探察，《灵枢识》："司，伺通。"揣，推测。言通过探察五脏之病，可以推测其在外的症状。出《灵枢·外揣》。

司内揣外（sì nèi chuǎi wài）
governing interior to infer exterior
Sì refers to inspecting. *Ling Shu Zhi* (*Understanding Ling Shu*) states that "司" is the same as "伺". By inspecting the visceral diseases at the interior, the exterior symptoms can be speculated. See *Ling Shu* chapter 45.

司气 司五运之气。与岁气、主岁义同。出《素问·至真要大论》。

司气（sì qì）　**governing qi** The qi controlling the five movements，which has the same meaning as the heavenly qi and the ruling qi in a year. See *Ling Shu* chapter 74.

司外揣内 司（sì），探察，《灵枢

识》曰："司，伺通。"揣，推测。言通过探察病人外在的表现，可以推测体内五脏的病变。这是中医认识人体生理病理的重要方法。出《灵枢·外揣》。

司外揣内（sì wài chuǎi nèi）
governing exterior to infer interior
Sì refers to inspecting. *Ling Shu Zhi* (*Understanding Ling Shu*) states that "司" is as the same as "伺". *Chuǎi* refers to assessing. One can assess the visceral diseases by examining the condition of the exterior，which is an important method for TCM physicians to understand human physiology and pathology. See *Ling Shu* chapter 45.

司杀府 指阳明燥金司令之秋季，金气肃杀，故云。出《素问·六元正纪大论》。

司杀府（sì shā fǔ）　**palace that controls the killing** Refers to *yangming* and dry-metal qi dominating the heavens in autumn，and the metal qi characterized by clearing and descending. See *Su Wen* chapter 71.

尻 臀部，尾骶部的统称。出《素问·痹论》。

尻（kāo）　**buttock** The general term for buttocks and sacrum. See *Su Wen* chapter 43.

尻尾 指尻骨尾端长强穴处。出《素问·气府论》。

尻尾(kāo wěi) sacrum The end of the sacrum where the acupoint Chang Qiang（GV 1）is located. See *Su Wen* chapter 59.

尻骨 尾骶骨。出《素问·骨空论》。

尻骨（kāo gǔ） sacrum Sacral bone. See *Su Wen* chapter 60.

尻脉 出于尾尻的督脉支络。出《素问·气穴论》。

尻脉（kāo mài） sacrum vessel Branch of the governor vessel exiting from the end of the sacrum. See *Su Wen* chapter 58.

加 ① 加重。出《灵枢·顺气一日分为四时》。② 侵侮。出《素问·六节藏象论》《素问·藏气法时论》。

加（jiā） ① Exacerbation. See *Ling Shu* chapter 44. ② Counter-restriction. See *Su Wen* chapter 9 and chapter 22.

加宫 体质名。阴阳二十五人中土形人之一种。出《灵枢·五音五味》。

加宫（jiā gōng） *jia gong* Name of constitution, one of the earth type constitutions among the twenty-five types of people divided according to yin and yang. See *Ling Shu* chapter 65.

加宫之人 体质名。宫,五音之

一,五行属土。加宫,宫音之一,此代表阴阳二十五人中土形人之一种,其特征是神情喜悦快活。出《灵枢·阴阳二十五人》。参"土形之人"。

加宫之人（jiā gōng zhī rén） *jiagong*-type people Name of constitution. *Gong* is one of five musical notes, and belongs to earth in the five elements. *Jia gong*, one of *gong* notes, refers to one type of earth constitution with a joyous manifestation. See *Ling Shu* chapter 64. See the term "土形之人".

皮毛生肾 五脏相生,肺生肾之意。出《素问·阴阳应象大论》。

皮毛生肾（pí máo shēng shèn） **skin and body hair generates the kidney** Mutual promotion of the five viscera, with the lung generating skin and body hair, and skin and body hair generating the kidney. See *Su Wen* chapter 5.

皮部 十二经脉及其所属络脉在体表皮腠的分部,也是十二经脉之气布散之处。又称十二皮部。出《素问·皮部论》。

皮部（pí bù） **skin sections** Skin sections are divisions of the twelve meridians and their collaterals in the skin and interstices of the body's surface, and are also the places where the qi of the twelve meridians is scattered. They are also known as the twelve cutaneous regions. See *Su Wen* chapter 56.

皮部论　《素问》篇名。皮,皮肤;部,分部。此篇主要论述三阴三阳经在皮肤上的分部,建立了脏腑、经脉、与皮肤相应部位的联系,说明疾病经皮肤由表入里的传变途径,以此强调早期治疗的重要性。

皮部论(pí bù lùn)　**Discussion on Skin Sections** Chapter title in *Su Wen*. *Pí* refers to skin and *bù* refers to section. This chapter mainly discusses the skin sections of the three yin and the three yang meridians, establishes the connections between the viscera, meridians, and the corresponding parts of skin, and explains the transmission path of the disease from the exterior to the interior through the skin, so as to emphasize the importance of early treatment.

皮痹　病证名。五体痹之一。病发于秋季的痹证。因秋主皮毛,故名。出《素问·痹论》。

皮痹(pí bì)　**skin blockage** Syn-

drome name, and one of the five physical skin blockages which happens in autumn. Since the autumn governs skin and hair, it is called the skin blockage. See *Su Wen* chapter 43.

皮𩩲　出《素问·长刺节论》。(1)𩩲为骺之误,指横皮肋骨之端。见《类经·针刺四十七》。(2)脐下五寸之横纹。见《素问》王冰注。(3)一说𩩲同䏶,腹皮肥厚处。见《素问注证发微》。

皮𩩲(pí téng)　See *Su Wen* chapter 55. (1)"𩩲" is "骺" misspelled, and it refers to the end of the ribs. See *Lei Jing* (*Classified Classic*) "Needling Chapter 47". (2) The cross lines, five *cun* below the navel. See *Su Wen* annotated by Wang Bing. (3)"Teng" is equivalent to "䏶", and refers to the thick part of the abdominal skin. See *Su Wen Zhu Zheng Fa Wei* (*Annotation and Elaboration on Su Wen*).

发蒙　刺五节法之一。主要治疗腑病及耳目病。要求在中午时刺听宫穴,使针刺感应达到瞳子及耳中。其效有如去除蒙蔽,故名。出《灵枢·刺节真邪》。

发蒙(fā méng)　**dispersing obstacle** One of the needling in five sections methods，mainly applied for visceral diseases，and ear and eye diseases. Ting Gong （SI 19） acupoint must be needled at noon，in order for the sensation of needling to reach the pupils and ears，and achieve the curative effect of removing the obstacles. See *Ling Shu* chapter 75.

圣人 古代的养生家。他们善于适应自然气候的变化，生活随俗，形劳不倦，思想恬愉自得，精神内守。故可得享天年。出《素问·上古天真论》。

圣人（shèng rén） Expert on health preservation in ancient times. They adapted to changes in the natural climate，accommodated their cravings and desires within the world，did not tax their physical appearance with any affairs or suffer from any pondering，and made every effort to achieve peaceful relaxation. Therefore，they could reach a number of one hundred years. See *Su Wen* chapter 1.

六 画

动脉 能从体表触摸到搏动的经脉,称动脉。古代用以作为诊脉的部位,如三部九候诊法,是诊察全身上、中、下三部有关的动脉。见《素问·三部九候论》。

动脉(dòng mài) **moving vessels** The pulses that can be palpated from the body's surface are called moving vessels. In ancient times, the parts that were used for pulse diagnosis, such as three sections and nine indicators, were used to examine the pulses related to the upper, middle and lower parts of the whole body. See *Su Wen* chapter 20.

动输 《灵枢》篇名。动,指经脉的搏动;输,输注。此篇主要论述手太阴、足阳明、足少阴三条经脉分别在太渊、人迎、太溪穴,搏动不休的原理,以及它们和全身气血输注的关系。故名。

动输(dòng shū) **Throbbing of Channels** Chapter title in *Ling Shu*. *Dòng* refers to the throbbing of the pulse; *Shū* indicates the infusion. This chapter discusses the endless throbbing of the three acupoints of Tai Yuan (LU 9), Ren Ying (ST 9) and Tai Xi (KI 3) in the meridians of hand *taiyin*, foot *yangming* and foot *shaoyin* respectively, and the relationship between these three acupoints and the transmission of blood and vessels. Hence the name.

扞皮开腠理 针法之一种。扞,同揗。在按得分肉的穴位上,用手力以伸展肌肤之纹理,缓缓地垂直进针,浅刺其皮而不伤肉,可开泄腠理,祛邪而不致散乱神气。出《灵枢·邪客》。

扞皮开腠理(dǎ pí kāi còu lǐ) **to pull up the skin and open the skin striae** One kind of needling method, in which 扞 refers to 揗, or pull. On the acupoints of the flesh, hand force is used to stretch the skin, and the needle is inserted slowly and vertically, just until the shallow needling punctures the skin without hurting the flesh. In this way, the interstices can be opened and loosened, in order to remove the evil qi without dissipating or disturbing the spirit. See *Ling Shu* chapter 71.

执法 运气术语。指天符之年，其特点如执法的官吏，故名。出《素问·六微旨大论》。

执法（zhí fǎ） **uphold the law** Terminology of circuits and qi. Refers to the year of *tian fu*（heavenly complement）. It is so named as its characteristics officially uphold the law. See *Su Wen* chapter 68.

地气 指在泉之气。见《素问·六元正纪大论》。

地气（dì qì） **earth qi** Refers to the qi of the earth in the spring. See *Su Wen* chapter 71.

地气通于嗌 饮食五味与人之咽喉相通应。地气，此指饮食五味。出《素问·阴阳应象大论》。

地气通于嗌（dì qì tōng yú yì） **The qi of the earth communicates with the throat.** The five flavors corresponding to the throat of the human body. The qi of the earth refers to the five flavors of food. See *Su Wen* chapter 5.

地化 言临床用药之寒热轻重多少。如气候与证候同属于寒，是谓同清，则治疗须多用感受温热的在泉（地）之气而化生的偏温热之性的药物，故曰地化。

见《素问·六元正纪大论》。

地化（dì huà） **earth transformation** Indicating the usage of cold or hot and heavy or light drugs clinically. For example，if the climate and syndrome belong to cold，which is called *tong qing*，then the treatment should include more warm drugs produced by the qi in the spring（ground）to feel the warm heat，thus it is called earth transformation. See *Su Wen* chapter 71.

地玄 水星位置居天时之称谓。出《素问·刺法论》。

地玄（dì xuán） **Di Xuan** The appellation when Mercury is located in the heavens. See *Su Wen* chapter 72.

地苍 ① 木星位置居地时之称谓。出《素问·刺法论》。② 指苍黑的真脏色。出《素问·脉要精微论》。

地苍（dì cāng） ① Di Cang. The appellation when Jupiter is located on the earth. See *Su Wen* chapter 72. ② Refers to a black complexion indicating deterioration of the visceral essence. See *Su Wen* chapter 17.

地彤 火星位置居天时之称谓。出《素问·刺法论》。

六画

地彤(dì tóng)　**Di Tong** The appellation when Mars is located in the heavens. See *Su Wen* chapter 72.

地阜　土星位置居天时之称谓。出《素问·刺法论》。

地阜(dì fù)　**Di Fu** The appellation when Saturn is located in the heavens. See *Su Wen* chapter 72.

地晶　金星位置居天时之称谓。出《素问·刺法论》。

地晶(dì jīng)　**Di Jing** The appellation when Venus is located in the heavens. See *Su Wen* chapter 72.

地道　①足少阴下部的脉道。出《素问·三部九候论》《素问集注》。②指经水。出《素问·上古天真论》。

地道(dì dào)　① The lower portion of the foot-*shaoyin* meridian. See *Su Wen* chapter 20 and *Su Wen Ji Zhu*（*Collected Annotation of Su Wen*）. ② Refers to the water of the meridian. See *Su Wen* chapter 1.

地数　指在泉之气。见《素问·本病论》。

地数(dì shù)　*di shu* Refers to the qi of the spring（earth）. See *Su Wen* chapter 73.

扬刺　刺法之一。扬，散也。在病变正中刺一针，四周散在刺四针，都用浅刺法，可治寒气稽留邪浅而广的病症。出《灵枢·官针》。

扬刺（yáng cì）　**dissemination piercing** One of the piercing methods meaning dissemination. One needle is inserted into the location of the disease，and four needles are inserted sideways superficially. This method is used to cure massively stagnating cold qi. See *Ling Shu* chapter 7.

耳门　耳屏前的部位。出《灵枢·五色》。

耳门(ěr mén)　Ear gate refers to the opening of the outer ear. See *Ling Shu* chapter 49.

耳中　①耳内。出《素问·缪刺论》《灵枢·经脉》。②穴名。即听宫穴，又名窗笼。出《灵枢·根结》。

耳中(ěr zhōng)　① Center of the ear. See *Su Wen* chapter 63 and *Ling Shu* chapter 10. ② Acupoint name，Ting Gong（SI 19），also called Chuang Long（SI 19）. See *Ling Shu* chapter 5.

耳间青脉　耳朵上的青色络脉。出《灵枢·论疾诊尺》。

耳间青脉(ěr jiān qīng mài)

The greenish vessels above the ears. See *Ling Shu* chapter 74.

耳鸣　耳中鸣响的症状。出《灵枢·口问》。

耳鸣（ěr míng）　**tinnitus** Symptoms of tinnitus. See *Ling Shu* chapter 28.

机　① 部位名。指髋关节部位，相当于环跳穴处。出《素问·骨空论》。② 经气至，得气。出《灵枢·九针十二原》《灵枢·小针解》。③ 事物的枢机、关键。出《灵枢·忧恚无言》《灵枢·刺节真邪》《素问·玉版论》。

机（jī）　① Name of a body part. Refers to the hip joint，and equivalent to the acupoint Huan Tiao（GB 30）. See *Su Wen* chapter 60. ② When the meridian qi arrives. See *Ling Shu* chapter 1 and chapter 3. ③ The pivot and key of things. See *Ling Shu* chapter 69 and chapter 75. See *Su Wen* chapter 15.

机关　指关节。出《素问·痿论》《素问·厥论》。

机关（jī guān）　Refers to the joints. See *Su Wen* chapter 44 and chapter 45.

权衡规矩　权，秤锤；衡，秤杆；规，作圆的工具；矩，作方的工具。权衡规矩，喻四时正常脉象。出《素问·阴阳应象大论》。

权衡规矩（quán héng guī jǔ）　**weight，beam，circle and square** *Quán* indicates the sliding weight of a steelyard；*Héng* indicates the arm of a steelyard；*Guī* indicates a tool for making circles；*Jǔ* indicates a tool for making squares. The weight，beam，circle and square is a metaphor for a normal pulse in the four seasons. See *Su Wen* chapter 5.

臣使之官　① 指膻中，因其接近于心，有为心传递志意、使令的职能，故以此为喻。出《素问·灵兰秘典论》。② 指心包络。见《灵枢·胀论》。

臣使之官（chén shǐ zhī guān）　① minister and envoy-like organ. Refers to Dan Zhong，as it is close to the heart and has the function of transmitting the will and making the order，which is used as a metaphor. See *Su Wen* chapter 8. ② Pericardium. See *Ling Shu* chapter 35.

百病生于气　百病，多种疾病。人以气为本，气和则健康无病，气失调即是疾病，故所谓百病生于气。出《素问·举痛论》。

百病生于气（bǎi bìng shēng yú qì）　**All diseases are generated**

by the qi. *Bǎi bìng* refers to hundreds of diseases. Qi is the root of the human body, and qi harmony is healthy and disease-free. However，qi disorders trigger disease，therefore the hundreds of diseases are generated by qi. See *Su Wen* chapter 39.

百病始生　《灵枢》篇名。百病，泛指多种疾病。此篇主要讨论疾病开始发生的原因、病邪侵犯的部位以及外感病的一般传变规律等，因篇首有"百病始生"句，故名。

百病始生（bǎi bìng shǐ shēng）**Occurrence of Hundreds of Diseases** Chapter title in *Ling Shu*. *Bǎi bìng* refers to various diseases. This chapter mainly discusses the causes of onset of diseases, the locations of disease invasion, and the general laws of transmission of exogenous diseases. The chapter is so named due to its first sentence "generating hundreds of diseases".

有余者折之　治法。折，挫折。言出现有余病症，应当用攻法治疗，挫其病势。出《素问·至真要大论》。

有余者折之（yǒu yú zhě zhé zhī）**What is in surplus，break it.** Therapeutic method. *Zhé* means frustrated. It indicates that if there is a disease of surplus, the purgation method should be used to frustrate it. See *Su Wen* chapter 74.

夺气　正气被劫夺、耗伤。出《素问·脉要精微论》。

夺气（duó qì）**qi deprivation** The deprivation and exhaustion of healthy qi. See *Su Wen* chapter 17.

夺精　① 指精气内伤，不能上营于目导致目盲的病机。出《灵枢·口问》。② 指惊吓而致神散，神散则心之精气被劫夺的病机。出《素问·经脉别论》。

夺精（duó jīng）① Refers to the pathogenesis of blindness caused by the internal damage of essence，which cannot nourish the eyes. See *Ling Shu* chapter 28. ② Refers to a scattered spirit，with consumption of the heart's vital essence，causing the pathogenesis of fright. See *Su Wen* chapter 21.

列缺　经穴名。手太阴经之络穴。又是八脉交会穴之一，通任脉。在桡骨茎突上方，腕横纹上一寸五分。出《灵枢·经脉》。

列缺（liè quē）**Lie Que（LU 7）** Acupoint name. The collateral

六画

acupoint on the hand *taiyin* meridian. Also one of the crossing acupoints of the eight meridians, connecting with the conception vessel. Above the styloid process of the radius, one and a half *cun* above the transverse line of the wrist. See *Ling Shu* chapter 10.

死心脉 即心之真脏脉。其脉来洪大而不滑利,全无冲和之象,是胃气大败,心之藏真之气暴露的危候。出《素问·平人气象论》。

死心脉(sǐ xīn mài) **dying heart pulse** That is the genuine *zang* pulse of the heart. The pulse is full, large and unsmooth when it comes, without a complete harmonious flow. This critical symptom reflects the failure of stomach qi and explosion of genuine heart zang qi. See *Su Wen* chapter 18.

死阴 病邪在五脏的传变,按五行相克次序而传,如心病传肺等,因预后较差,与"生阳"相对而言,故称死阴。出《素问·阴阳别论》。

死阴(sǐ yīn) **dying yin** The transmission of pathogenic factors in the five viscera, according to the restraining order of the five elements, such as diseases of the heart transmitted into the lung. As it is the opposite of generating yang, it is thus called dying yin. See *Su Wen* chapter 7.

死肝脉 指肝之真脏脉。脉来弦急强劲,毫无和缓从容之意,是无胃气之危候。出《素问·平人气象论》。

死肝脉(sǐ gān mài) **dying liver pulse** Refers to the genuine zang pulse of the liver. The pulse appears wiry, rapid and tense when it comes, without complete harmonious flow. It is a critical sign of the failure of stomach qi. See *Su Wen* chapter 18.

死肾脉 指肾之真脏脉,是病人垂危时出现的一种脉象。其脉来坚劲,如按在两人争夺的绳索上一样,或脉来坚实,如指弹石上辟辟然,毫无胃气之象,故死。出《素问·平人气象论》。

死肾脉(sǐ shèn mài) **dying kidney pulse** Refers to the genuine zang pulse of the kidney. The pulse appears hard and powerful when it comes, as if a rope was being pulled away, or the pulse appears hard and solid when it comes, as a hand knocking on a stone. It is a sign of the failure of stomach qi, and the patient will die. See *Su Wen* chapter 18.

死肺脉　指肺之真脏脉,其脉虚浮无根,散乱无绪,绝少从容和缓之象,是无胃气之危候。出《素问·平人气象论》。

死肺脉(sǐ fèi mài)　**dying lung pulse** Refers to the genuine zang pulse of the lung. The pulse appears weak, a floating pulse without a root, irregular and inharmonious. It is a sign of the failure of stomach qi. See *Su Wen* chapter 18.

死脾脉　指脾的真脏脉,其脉或如禽鸟之喙、距那样坚锐而不柔;或如屋漏之水,点滴无伦而无规则;或如水之流,去而不复来,皆是脾气败绝无胃之危候。出《素问·平人气象论》。

死脾脉(sǐ pǐ mài)　**dying spleen pulse** Refers to the genuine zang pulse of the spleen. The pulse is pointed and firm, as if a crow's beak, or as if a bird's spur; or like water dripping into a house irregularly; or like the flow of running water never return. All of these are signs of the failure of stomach qi. See *Su Wen* chapter 18.

成骨　《素问·刺腰痛》。(1)骭骨上端突起部。见《素问识》《类经·针刺四十九》。(2)胫骨,即骭骨。见《医宗金鉴》。

成骨(chéng gǔ)　**support bone** See *Su Wen* chapter 41. (1) Protuberance of upper part of the sphenoid bone. See *Su Wen Zhi* (*Understanding Su Wen*) and *Lei Jing* (*Classified Classic*) "Needling Chapter 49". (2) Tibia, that is, trochanteric bone. See *Yi Zong Jin Jian* (*Golden Mirror of the Medical Ancestors*).

夷则　阳六律之一,为徵音,即火音。出《素问·本病论》。

夷则(yí zé)　One of the six yang tones, that is the fire tone. See *Su Wen* chapter 73.

邪　① 即邪气,泛指各种致病因素。出《素问·调经论》。② 邪恶,不正当。出《灵枢·本藏》。③ 通"斜"。出《灵枢·经脉》。④ 同"耶",相当于"吗"的意思。出《素问·上古天真论》。

邪(xié)　① Evil qi. Generally refers to different kinds of pathogenic factors. See *Su Wen* chapter 62. ② Evil, bad or harmful. See *Ling Shu* chapter 47. ③ An alternative word for "斜". See *Ling Shu*

六画

chapter 10. ④ Same as "耶", meaning "What?" See *Su Wen* chapter 1.

邪气　泛指各种致病因素,与正气相对而言。出《灵枢·刺节真邪》《灵枢·小针解》。

邪气(xié qì)　**evil qi** Generally refers to various pathogenic factors, and is the opposite to the healthy qi. See *Ling Shu* chapter 75 and chapter 3.

邪气藏府病形　《灵枢》篇名。邪气,指致病因素;病形,即发病的形态,此篇主要论述邪气侵犯人体不同部位的机制,疾病发生的一般规律,以及脏腑受邪所表现的症状和诊断、治疗方法。

邪气藏府病形(xié qì zàng fǔ bìng xíng)　**Symptoms of Viscera and Bowels Due to Attack of Pathogenic Factors** Chapter title in *Ling Shu*. *Xié qì* refers to the pathogenic factors; *Bìng xíng* refers to the symptoms of the disease. This chapter mainly discusses the mechanism of evil qi invading different parts of the human body, the general law of disease occurrence, and the symptoms, diagnosis and therapeutic methods of diseases of the viscera and bowels due

to the attack of pathogenic factors.

邪风　① 泛指四时不正之气。出《素问·阴阳应象大论》。② 指风邪。出《灵枢·九宫八风》。

邪风(xié fēng)　① Generally refers to the abnormal qi of the four seasons. See *Su Wen* chapter 5. ② Refers to wind evil. See *Ling Shu* chapter 77.

邪客　《灵枢》篇名。客,侵犯。邪客,指邪气侵犯人体。该篇以邪气侵人后产生的不眠证,来说明宗气、营气、卫气的循行与作用。

邪客(xié kè)　**Invasion of Pathogenic Factors** Chapter title in *Ling Shu*. *Kè* means attack. *Xié kè* refers to the pathogenic factors attacking the human body. This chapter explains the circulation and function of thoracic qi, nutrient qi and defensive for insomnia after the invasion of evil qi.

邪僻　同义复词。僻(pì 辟),不正的意思,即邪。出《素问·六节藏象论》。

邪僻(xié pì)　**evils** *Xié* and *pì* are synonymous words. *Pì* means evil. See *Su Wen* chapter 9.

至人　理想中中古时代的养生家。他们具有淳厚的道德品质,深谙养生之道,令身体与天地阴阳、四时气候相适应,达到强身益寿的境界。其养生成就仅次于"真人"。出《素问·上古天真论》。

至人(zhì rén) **accomplished people** An ideal health preserving expert at the time of middle antiquity of honest moral character, and who are familiar with the ways of health preservation. They adapt their bodies to the yin and yang, heaven and earth, four seasons and climate, so that they can reach the realm of strengthening the body, and longevity. Their health preservation achievements are second only to "true people". See *Su Wen* chapter 1.

至而不至 言时令已到而气候尚未到来,为应至之气不足的表现。出《素问·六微旨大论》。

至而不至(zhì ér bù zhì) **[Time] has arrived but [the climate] has not arrived.** This indicates that the time has arrived, but the climate has not arrived, thus the seasonal qi is insufficient. See *Su Wen* chapter 68.

至而不至者病 出《素问·至真要大论》。

至而不至者病(zhì ér bù zhì zhě

bìng) **When [the time] arrives but [the climate] does not arrive, there is a disease.** See *Su Wen* chapter 74.

至而太过 谓时令方至而气候已太过,属来气有余的表现。出《素问·六微旨大论》。

至而太过(zhì ér tài guò) **[Time] has arrived and [the qi of] the climate is greatly excessive.** This indicates that when [its time] has arrived and [the qi of] the climate is excessive, there is a surplus of incoming qi. See *Su Wen* chapter 68.

至而反者病 出《素问·至真要大论》。

至而反者病(zhì ér fǎn zhě bìng) **When [the time] that arrives is contrary [to the climate], then there is disease.** See *Su Wen* chapter 74.

至而至 言气候应时而来。凡六气按时令如期而到者,为和平之年。出《素问·六微旨大论》。

至而至(zhì ér zhì) **[Time] has arrived and [the qi of] the climate has also arrived.** This indicates that the time, as well as the six qi, have both arrived, and it is a harmonious year. See *Su Wen* chapter 68.

至而甚则病 出《素问·至真要

大论》。

至而甚则病(zhì ér shèn zé bìng)
**When〔the qi〕that arrives is
extreme，then there is disease.**
See *Su Wen* chapter 74.

至阳 ① 指天。出《素问·方盛
衰论》。② 至，极也，谓阳气极
盛。出《素问·著至教论》。

至阳（zhì yáng） ① Refers to
heaven. See *Su Wen* chapter
80. ② *Zhì* means extreme，
which is extreme yang qi. See
Su Wen chapter 75.

至阴 ① 指土气。土位乎下，为
至阴，能生长万物，出《素问·
五常政大论》。② 指肾，肾精。
出《素问·水热穴论》《素问·
解精微论》。③ 指太阴脾。出
《素问·金匮真言论》《素问·
评热病论》。④ 指至阴穴，属足
太阳膀胱经，在小趾外侧甲角
旁。出《灵枢·本输》。⑤ 指长
夏季节。至，达也。脾外应长
夏，居夏秋之交。由阳入阴故谓
至阴。出《素问·咳论》。⑥ 指
地气。出《素问·方盛衰论》。

至阴（zhì yīn） ① Refers to
earth qi，located in the lower
areas，and is the extreme yin，
which grows in all the living
things. See *Su Wen* chapter 70.
② Refers to the kidney，or
kidney essence. See *Su Wen*

chapter 61 and chapter 81. ③ Refers to *taiyin*-spleen. Seen *Su
Wen* chapter 4 and chapter 33.
④ Refers to *zhi yin* acupoint，
which belongs to the bladder
meridian of foot *taiyang*. It is
located next to the lateral nail
of the little toe. See *Ling Shu*
chapter 2. ⑤ Refers to the late
summer season. *Zhì* means arrive. The spleen corresponds to
the late summer outside，which
is in between summer and autumn. When the yang enters
into the yin，it is called extreme
yin. See *Su Wen* chapter 38.
⑥ Refers to earth qi. See *Su
Wen* chapter 80.

至治 最好的治疗原则。出《素
问·六元正纪大论》。

至治（zhì zhì） **perfect treatment**
The best therapeutic principle.
See *Su Wen* chapter 71.

至真要大论 《素问》篇名。至，
最也；真，真实，正确；要，重要；
大论，内容宏富之论。此篇是
对前六篇大论的总结，并在此
基础上从五运六气推演中医辨
证论治的理论体系及临床运用
的规律，尤其是"病机十九条"，
更被历代医家推崇。为强调该篇
内容极其重要，故名"至真要"。

至真要大论(zhì zhēn yào dà lùn)

Comprehensive Discourse on the Essentials of the Most Reliable Chapter title in *Su Wen*. *Zhì* refers to comprehensive; *Zhēn* refers to reliable, or truth; *Yào* refers to essential; *Dà lùn* refers to discourse, or rich contents. This chapter is a summary of the first six chapters. On this basis, it deduces the theoretical system of TCM syndrome differentiation and treatment, and the principle of clinical application with the five circuits and six qi, especially the "nineteen pathogenesis", which is highly praised by doctors of all ages. In order to emphasize the importance of the content of this article, thus it is called "Zhi Zhen Yao".

师传　《灵枢》篇名。师传,言所述内容系先师传授,以示重要,故名。此篇主要论述问诊的重要性和方法,以及相应的治疗原则;望形体大小以测知内脏盛衰常变的一般规律。

师传(shī chuán)　**Transmissions from the Teachers** Chapter title in *Ling Shu*. "Transmissions from the teachers" elaborates that the content is taught by teachers to show its importance, hence

the name. This chapter mainly discusses the importance and methods of consultation, as well as the corresponding treatment principles, such as to determine the general law of the rise and fall of the internal organs by inspecting the size of the body.

光明　经穴名。足少阳胆经的络穴。在足外踝上五寸,当腓骨前缘处。出《灵枢·经脉》。

光明(guāng míng)　**Guang Ming (GB 37)** Acupoint name. It is the collateral acupoint on the gallbladder meridian of foot *shaoyang*, located five *cun* above the lateral aspect of the ankle, at the anterior border of the fibula. See *Ling Shu* chapter 10.

当位　运气术语。出《素问·六微旨大论》。

当位(dāng wèi)　**to occupy the proper position** Terminology of circuits and qi. See *Su Wen* chapter 68.

虫瘕　虫,指肠内寄生虫。瘕,集结成块,聚散无常。出《灵枢·厥病》。

虫瘕(chóng jiǎ)　**worm mass** *Chóng* refers to intestinal parasite. *Jiǎ* refers to the mass of parasites have gathered or are

六画

六画

moving irregularly in the intestines. See *Ling Shu* chapter 24.

曲牙 ① 经穴名。即颊车穴。出《素问·气穴论》。② 部位名。指下颌角的上方处。出《灵枢·经筋》。

曲牙（qǔ yá） ① Acupoint name, that is Jia Che (ST 6). See *Su Wen* chapter 58. ② Location name. The upper part of the mandibular angle. See *Ling Shu* chapter 13.

曲池 经穴名。为手阳明大肠经合穴，在肘窝横纹桡侧端与肱骨外上髁之中点，屈肘取之。出《灵枢·本输》。

曲池（qǔ chí） **Qu Chi（LI 11）** Acupoint name, which is the *He*-sea acupoint of the large intestine meridian of hand *yangming*. It lies in the middle point between the radial end of the transverse stria of the cubital fossa and the lateral epicondyle of the humerus. It is located by bending the arm. See *Ling Shu* chapter 2.

曲周动脉 指颊车穴。出《灵枢·杂病》。

曲周动脉（qǔ zhōu dòng mài） **circularly wandering moving vessel** Refers to Jia Che (ST 6). See *Ling Shu* chapter 26.

曲泽 经穴名。手厥阴心包经之合穴，在肘横纹中，略偏尺侧凹陷处，屈肘可得。出《灵枢·本输》。

曲泽（qǔ zé） **Qu Ze（PC 3）** Acupoint name, which is the *he*-sea acupoint of the large intestine meridian of hand *yangming*. It lies in the transverse lines of the elbow, slightly deviating from the depression on the ulnar side. It is located by bending the arm. See *Ling Shu* chapter 2.

曲泉 经穴名。足厥阴肝经之合穴。在膝内侧辅骨下，大筋上，小筋下陷中，屈膝得之。出《灵枢·本输》。

曲泉（qǔ quán） **Qu Quan（LR 8）** Acupoint name, which is the *he*-sea acupoint of the liver meridian of foot *jueyin*. It is found below the supporting bone, and above the big sinew. It is located by bending the knee. See *Ling Shu* chapter 2.

曲颊 在颊曲骨端。出《灵枢·本输》。

曲颊（qǔ jiá） *qu jia* Located exactly at the bone of the cheek curve. See *Ling Shu* chapter 2.

同天化 运气术语。天，指司天之气。言中运与司天之气的五运属性相同，即天符之年。如戊午年，天干戊年中运为火，地支午年，司天为少阴君火，中运与司天同为火化，即为同天化。甲子一周六十年中，属岁运太过而同天化者有三组：戊子、戊午；戊寅、戊申；丙辰、丙戌。属岁运不及而同天化者亦有三组：丁巳、丁亥；乙卯、乙酉；己丑、己未。出《素问·六元正纪大论》。

同天化（tóng tiān huà）　*heaven complement* Terminology of circuits and qi. *Tian* means the qi governing the heaven. It is said that the five circuits of qi governing the heaven, and the middle circuits are the same, that is, the year of *tian fu* （heavenly complement）. For example, in the year of *wu wu*. Heavenly Stem and *wu* Earthly Branch, the middle movement corresponds with fire and also governs the heaven, thus the middle movement and governor heaven are all fire, that is the heavenly complement. There are three groups, which are all named heavenly complements caused by the excess of yearly movement in sixty years：*wu zi* and *wu wu*；*Wuyin* and *wu shen*；*bing chen* and *bing xu*. Furthermore, there are three groups, which are all named heavenly complements caused by deficiency of yearly movement in sixty years：*Ding ji* and *Ding hai*；*yi mao* and *yi you*；*ji chou* and *ji wei*. See *Su Wen* chapter 71.

同气　《素问·标本病传论》。（1）作固气。指体内固有之邪气。见《黄帝内经素问译释》。（2）指主气。见《类经·标本四》。（3）指病气。见《素问注证发微》。（4）指人身三阴三阳与自然界风热湿火燥寒之气的相应联系。见《素问直解》。（5）与天之六气相应的人体内生六气。见《素问集注》。

同气（tóng qì）　**identical qi** See *Su Wen* chapter 65. (1) Innate qi. Refers to the innate evil qi in the human body. See *Huang Di Nei Jing Su Wen Yi Shi*（*Interpretation and Explanation on Huang Di Nei Jing*）. (2) Main qi. See *Lei Jing*（*Classified Classic*）"Branch and Root Chapter 4". (3) Pathogenic qi. See *Su Wen Zhu Zheng Fa Wei*（*Annotation and Elaboration on Su Wen*）. (4) Refers to the corresponding relationship be-

六画

tween the qi of three yin and three yang of the human body and qi of wind, heat, dampness, fire, dryness, cold, in nature. See *Su Wen Zhi Jie* (*Direct Interpretation on Su Wen*). (5) Six qi generated by the human body corresponding to the six qi in nature. See *Su Wen Ji Zhu* (*Collected Annotation of Su Wen*).

同化 运气术语。五运六气之化，其化相同。即气候变化在时令、性质或作用上相同，可以归属一类的事物或现象，无论胜气与复气，皆有同化现象。出《素问·六元正纪大论》。

同化(tóng huà) **transformation** Terminology of circuits and qi. The transformation of the five circuits and six qi are the same. That is to say, the climatic changes are the same in season, nature or function, and belong to one kind of thing or phenomena. No matter whether winning qi or regaining qi, there is transformation. See *Su Wen* chapter 71.

同地化 运气术语。地，指在泉之气。言中运与在泉之气的五行属性相同。如甲辰年，天干甲年中运为土，地支辰年，在泉之气为太阴湿土，中运与在泉同为土化，即为同地化。甲子一周六十年中，属于岁运太过，而同时又为同地化的年份有三组：甲辰、甲戌；壬寅、壬申；庚子、庚午年。属于岁运不及，同时又为同地化的年份也有三组：癸巳、癸亥；辛丑、辛未；癸卯、癸酉年，此六年又属同岁会。出《素问·六元正纪大论》。

同地化(tóng dì huà) **earth complement** Terminology of circuits and qi. *Dì* means the qi governing the earth. It is said that the five circuits of qi governing the earth and middle circuit are the same. For example, in the year of *jia* heavenly stem and *chen* earthly branch, the middle movement corresponds with damp earth and it also governs the earth, thus the middle movement and governor are all earth, that is the earth complement. There are three groups, which are all named earth complements caused by the excess of yearly movement in sixty years: *jia chen* and *jia xu*; *Ren yin* and *ren shen*; *geng zi* and *geng wu*. Furthermore, there are three groups, which are all named earth complements caused by the deficiency of yearly movement in sixty years: *gui si* and *gui hai*; *xin chou* and *xin wei*; *gui mao* and *gui you*. See *Su Wen* chapter 71.

同病异治　① 同一病证因病机不同,治法不同。出《素问·病能论》。② 因患者所处地理位置不同,虽发病相同,但治法不同。出《素问·五常政大论》。

同病异治(tóng bìng yì zhì)
① Different therapeutic methods should be used to treat same diseases with different pathogenesis. See *Su Wen* chapter 46. ② Although the onset of a disease is the same, due to the different geographical locations, the treatment is different. See *Su Wen* chapter 70.

因时之序　人顺应春夏秋冬四时气候变化之序。因,顺应。时,四时。出《素问·生气通天论》。

因时之序(yīn shí zhī xù)　**to follow the sequence of the seasons** People should follow the order of climatic changes in spring, summer, autumn and winter. *Yīn* refers to conform. *Shí* refers to the four seasons. See *Su Wen* chapter 3.

因其轻而扬之　治法。病轻浅时,可用发散宣扬的方法进行治疗。出《素问·阴阳应象大论》。

因其轻而扬之(yīn qí qīng ér yáng zhī)　**dispersing method for the treatment of mild disease** Therapeutic method. When the disease is mild, it can be treated by the dispersing method. See *Su Wen* chapter 5.

因其重而减之　治法。病势严重的,治疗时宜于逐步使其轻减。出《素问·阴阳应象大论》。

因其重而减之(yīn qí zhòng ér jiǎn zhī)　**eliminating method for the treatment of severe disease** Therapeutic method. When the disease is severe, it can be treated by the eliminating method. See *Su Wen* chapter 5.

因其衰而彰之　治法。气血虚衰者,用补益方法治疗使之恢复正常。出《素问·阴阳应象大论》。

因其衰而彰之(yīn qí shuāi ér zhāng zhī)　**supplementing method for the treatment of weak disease** Therapeutic method. When a disease manifests with deficiency of blood and qi, it can be treated by the supplementing method. See *Su Wen* chapter 5.

岁　① 年。出《灵枢·邪客》。② 年龄。出《素问·上古天真

六画

论》。③ 运气学说中的岁运、岁气。出《素问·至真要大论》。

岁（suì）　① Year. See *Ling Shu* chapter 71. ② Age. See *Su Wen* chapter 1. ③ Annual period. See *Su Wen* chapter 74.

岁土　土，五行之一。岁，年。即土运主岁之年。出《素问·气交变大论》。

岁土（suì tǔ）　**earth year** Earth, one of the five elements, indicates the year dominated by earth. See *Su Wen* chapter 69.

岁土不及　运气术语。凡天干逢"己"之年，为岁土不及，又名卑监之纪。一甲子六十年中凡六见。土运不及之年，木运乘之，气候多风。临床多见脾虚肝乘的病证。出《素问·气交变大论》。

岁土不及（suì tǔ bù jí）　**deficiency of earth circuit in a year** Terminology of circuits and qi. When the Heaven Stem meets the year of *ji*, there is deficiency of earth circuit that year, and it is also named the year of *bei jian*. It occurs six times in sixty years, and it is a year when the earth is over-restrained by wood, and the climate is windy. A common clinical syndrome is spleen deficiency over-restrained by liver.

See *Su Wen* chapter 69.

岁土太过　岁，岁运。凡天干逢"甲"之年，均属岁土太过，是年湿气偏胜，雨湿流行。多见暴雨、久雨的气候。土运太过，乘水侮木，可出现木气来复，而有大风出现。对动植物生长有一定影响，临床多见脾运失司，脾病侮肝等肝脾病症，还可出现肾病。出《素问·气交变大论》。

岁土太过（suì tǔ tài guò）　**excessive earth circuit in a year** *Suì* means the yearly circuit. When the Heaven Stem encounters the year of *jia*, there is excessive earth circuit in that year, and rain and dampness prevail everywhere. The heavenly storms or prolonged rainy days are commonly seen in this year. Excessive earth over-restricts water and the reverse restricts the wood, followed by the arrival of wood qi and strong winds, which influences the growth of animals and plants. Clinically, liver and spleen diseases are common, as well as kidney diseases. For example, the dysfunction of the spleen, and disease of the spleen reversely restraining the liver. See *Su Wen* chapter 69.

岁木　木,五行之一。岁,年。即木运主岁之年。出《素问·气交变大论》。

岁木(suì mù)　**wood year** Wood, one of the five elements. *Suì* refers to year. That is the year dominated by wood movement. See *Su Wen* chapter 69.

岁木不及　运气术语。凡天干逢"丁"之年,为岁木不及,又名委和之纪。一甲子六十年中凡六见。木运不及之年,金运乘之,出现春行秋令,应温反凉,燥气流行的气候。临床多见肝病及肺病。出《素问·气交变大论》。

岁木不及(suì mù bù jí) **deficiency of wood circuit in a year** Terminology for circuits and qi, and according to the twelve Heavenly Stem, the year with *ding* will be called the year of insufficient wood circuit, also known as the year with loss of harmony. In a period of sixty years, there will be 6 years with insufficient wood circuit. In a year of insufficient wood circuit, there is excessive metal circuit, which manifests as abnormal climate, where instead of being warm, in fact the climate is cold with prevalence of dry qi. Liver and lung diseases are commonly seen clinically. See *Su Wen* chapter 69.

岁木太过　岁,岁运。凡天干逢"壬"之年,均属岁木太过,是年风气偏胜,温暖太过。木气过盛,乘土侮金,可致金气来复,而有暴凉的反常气候,对动植物生长有一定影响。临床多见肝气偏盛、肝脾同病、肺病等疾患。出《素问·气交变大论》。

岁木太过(suì mù tài guò) **excessive wood circuit in a year** *Suì* means the yearly movement. When the Heavenly Stem encounters the year of *ren*, there is excessive wood circuit in that year, and wind qi will prevail and it is warm everywhere. Excessive wood qi over-restricts earth and reversely metal is restricted, causing metal qi to appear with uncommon and suddenly cold climate. The growth of the animals and plants is also affected. Clinically, there is a predominance of liver qi, with simultaneous liver and spleen syndromes, and lung diseases etc. See *Su Wen* chapter 69.

岁水　水,五行之一。岁,年。即水运主岁之年。出《素问·气交变大论》。

岁水（suì shuǐ）　**water year** Water, one of the five elements. *Suì* refers to year, that is a year dominated by water. See *Su Wen* chapter 69.

岁水不及　运气术语。天干逢"辛"之年，为岁水不及，又名涸流之纪。一甲子六十年中凡六见。出《素问·气交变大论》。

岁水不及（suì shuǐ bù jí）　**deficiency of water circuit in a year** Terminology of circuits and qi. When the Heavenly Stem meets the year of *xin*, there is deficiency of water circuit in that year, and it is also named the year of *he liu* which occurs six times in sixty years. See *Su Wen* chapter 69.

岁水太过　运气术语。凡天干逢"丙"之年。为岁水太过，又名流衍之纪。一甲子六十年中凡六见。水运太过之年，气候寒冷，寒气太盛，则乘火侮土，土郁之气来复，又可出现大雨。临床多见心肾病证。出《素问·气交变大论》。

岁水太过（suì shuǐ tài guò）　**excessive water circuit in a year** Terminology of circuits and qi. When the Heavenly Stem belongs to the year of *bing*, there is excessive water circuit in that year, and it is also named the year of *liu yan* which occurs six times in sixty years. In a year of excessive water circuit, the climate is cold. Excessive cold qi restricts fire and the reverse restricts earth. Earth qi becomes stagnant and there is heaven rain, causing heart and kidney syndromes to manifest clinically. See *Su Wen* chapter 69.

岁火　火，五行之一。岁，年。即火运主岁之年。出《素问·气交变大论》。

岁火（suì huǒ）　**fire year** Fire, one of the five elements. *Suì* refers to year. That is indicating a year dominated by fire. See *Su Wen* chapter 69.

岁火不及　运气术语。凡天干逢"癸"之年，为岁火不及，又名伏明之纪。一甲子六十年中凡六见。火运不及之年，水运乘之，出现南风偏少，寒雨偏多，应热不热的气候。临床多见心肾病证。出《素问·气交变大论》。

岁火不及（suì huǒ bù jí）　**deficiency of fire movement in a year** Terminology of circuits and qi. When the Heavenly Stem meets the year of *gui*, there is deficiency of fire movement in that year. It is also named the year of *fu ming*, which occurs six times in sixty years. It is a year of fire deficiency，which is over-restrained by water，thus there is less wind from the south，and more cold rain. As the climate should be hot，however it is not，heart and kidney syndromes abound clinically. See *Su Wen* chapter 69.

岁火太过　运气术语。天干逢"戊"之年，为岁火太过，又名赫曦之纪。一甲子六十年中凡六见。出《素问·气交变大论》。

岁火太过（suì huǒ tài guò）　**excessive fire movement in a year** Terminology of circuits and qi. *Suì* means yearly circuit. When the Heavenly Stem belongs to the year of *wu*，there is excessive fire circuit in a year. It is also named the year of *he xi* which occurs six times in sixty years. See *Su Wen* chapter 69.

岁正　当位之岁。即值年气候应时而至。出《素问·本病论》。

岁正（suì zhèng）　**proper year** Yearly circuit corresponding to the position of the five elements. That is to say, the cli-

mate of the year corresponding to the season. See *Su Wen* chapter 73.

岁主　风寒暑湿燥火，六气所主之年岁。出《素问·至真要大论》。

岁主（suì zhǔ）　**year governance** The year dominated by the six qi：wind，cold，summer-heat，dampness，dryness and fire. See *Su Wen* chapter 74.

岁立　运气术语。岁气确立之谓。干支纪年法，以阳干配阳支，阴干配阴支，干支相合以立六十年之岁气。出《素问·六微旨大论》。

岁立（suì lì）　**year establishment** Terminology of circuits and qi. The yearly qi is established. According to the chronology of the branches，the yang stem is matched with the yang branch，and the yin stem is matched with the yin branch. The combination of the stems and the branches is to establish the yearly qi of sixty years. See *Su Wen* chapter 68.

岁会　运气术语。凡是值年中运与年支的五行属性相同，称为岁会，属平气之年。六十年中，有八年为岁会。即丁卯、戊午、甲辰、甲戌、己丑、己未、乙酉、丙子。属平气之年。出《素问·

六微旨大论》。

岁会（suì huì）　**yearly meeting** Terminology of circuits and qi. When the circuit of the year is the same as the property of the five elements of the year, it is named yearly meeting. This is a year with balanced qi, which occurs every eight out of sixty years. Namely, *ding mao*, *wu wu*, *jia chen*, *jia xu*, *ji chou*, *ji wei*, *yi you*, and *bing zi*, which are all years with balanced qi. See *Su Wen* chapter 68.

岁纪　指全年的气候变化规律。纪，规律。出《素问·六元正纪大论》。

岁纪（suì jì）　**yearly rule** Refers to the law of climatic change throughout the year. *Jì* refers to the rule. See *Su Wen* chapter 71.

岁运　统主全年的五运之气，又称中运、大运。出《素问·气交变大论》。

岁运（suì yùn）　**yearly circuit** Yearly circuit governs the qi of the five circuits in a whole year, and it is also named middle motion, or large motion. See *Su Wen* chapter 69.

岁位　即岁会。出《素问·六微旨大论》。

岁位（suì wèi）　**yearly location**

That is, yearly meeting. See *Su Wen* chapter 68.

岁直　运气术语。即岁会。直，会之意。出《素问·天元纪大论》。

岁直（suì zhí）　**year straight** Terminology of circuits and qi, and means yearly meeting, *Suì* refers to meeting. See *Su Wen* chapter 66.

岁金　金，五行之一。岁，年。即金运主岁之年。出《素问·气交变大论》。

岁金（suì jīn）　**metal year** Metal, one of the five elements. *Suì* refers to year, that is a year dominated by metal. See *Su Wen* chapter 69.

岁金不及　运气术语。凡天干逢"乙"之年，为岁金不及，又名从革之纪。一甲子六十年中凡六见。岁金不及之年，火运乘之，故夏季气候特别炎热。临床多见肺、心为病。出《素问·气交变大论》。

岁金不及（suì jīn bù jí）　**deficiency of metal circuit in a year** Terminology of circuits and qi. When the Heavenly Stem meets the year of *yi*, there is deficiency of metal circuit in that year, and it is also named the year of *cong ge*, which occurs six times in sixty years. It is a year of metal deficiency over-restrained by fire, thus it is very hot in the summer. The lung and heart diseases are commonly seen clinically. See *Su Wen* chapter 69.

岁金太过　运气术语。凡天干逢"庚"之年，为岁金太过，又名坚成之纪。一甲子六十年中凡六见。金运太过之年，气候偏凉而干燥。临床多见肺病。出《素问·气交变大论》。

岁金太过（suì jīn tài guò）**excessive metal circuit in a year** Terminology of circuits and qi. When the Heavenly Stem belongs to the year of *geng*, there is excessive metal movement in that year, and it is also named the year of *jian cheng*, which occurs six times in sixty years. In a year of excessive metal circuit, the climate is cool and dry, and lung diseases are common clinically. See *Su Wen* chapter 69.

岁星　木星，为五大行星之一，与五行中的木、五脏中的肝相通应。出《素问·金匮真言论》。

岁星（suì xīng）**sui star** Jupiter, one of the five stars, corresponds to wood in the five elements and to the liver in the five viscera. See *Su Wen* chapter 4.

岁候　全年的气候情况。出《素问·六微旨大论》。

岁候（suì hòu）**yearly climate** The climate in a whole year. See *Su Wen* chapter 68.

岁露论　《灵枢》篇名。岁，年也；露，败也。岁露，指一年中非时之风雨，此篇主要论述一年四季不正常的风雨侵害人体的发病规律，以及预测一年气候变化的方法。故名。

岁露论（suì lù lùn）**Discussion on Abnormal Wind and Rain in a Year** Chapter title in *Ling Shu*. *Suì* refers to year, and *lù* refers to defeat. *Suì lù* refers to the abnormal wind and rain in a year. This chapter mainly discusses the incidence of abnormal wind and rain in the four seasons and the methods of predicting the climatic changes in one year. Hence the name.

回肠　大肠。出《灵枢·肠胃》《灵枢·平人绝谷》。

回肠（huí cháng）**curved intestine** Refers to the large intestine. See *Ling Shu* chapter 31 and chapter 32.

刚风　八风之一。指由西方刮来的风。出《灵枢·九宫八风》。

刚风（gāng fēng） **gang** wind One of the eight winds coming from the west. See *Ling Shu* chapter 77.

肉人 体质名。指形体宽大充实，皮肉不相离者。出《灵枢·卫气失常》。该篇根据人体的肥瘦分为肉、膏、脂三种体质，肉人的生理特点为血多，寒热平和。

肉人（ròu rén） **fleshy people** Name of constitution. Refers to people who are full in shape and inseparable in flesh and skin. See *Ling Shu* chapter 59. According to fatness and thinness of the human body, people can be divided into three kinds of constitutions: fleshy, greasy and fat. The physiological characteristics of fleshy people are people with more blood, as well as balanced between cold and hot.

肉分 肌肉间的纹理。出《素问·气穴论》。

肉分（ròu fēn） **muscle texture** It refers to partings of the flesh. See *Su Wen* chapter 58.

肉里之脉 （1）少阳所生之脉。见《素问·刺腰痛》。（2）指阳辅穴。见《类经·针刺四十九》。

肉里之脉（ròu lǐ zhī mài） **vessel** of the fleshy structures (1) The vessel generated by *shaoyang*. See *Su Wen* chapter 41.（2）Refers to Yang Fu（GB 38）. See *Lei Jing*（*Classified Classic*）"Needling Chapter 49".

肉肓 肌肉会合的空隙处。出《灵枢·胀论》。

肉肓（ròu huāng） **flesh and the** *huang* **space** The space where the muscles meet. See *Ling Shu* chapter 35.

肉苛 症状名。苛，沉重。肉苛，指肌肉虽外形如常，而顽木沉重不用。由营卫俱虚，气血俱病所致。出《素问·逆调论》。

肉苛（ròu kē） **flesh numbness** A symptom. *Kē* here refers to heaviness. It means that although the flesh looks normal, it feels too heavy to function. It is caused by deficiency of nutrient qi, defensive qi, qi and blood. See *Su Wen* chapter34.

肉度 度，度数。肌肉的大小长短度数。出《素问·方盛衰论》。

肉度（ròu dù） **flesh measurement** *Dù* refers to the measurement of both the size and length of the muscles. See *Su Wen* chapter 80.

肉烁 症状名。烁通铄，消之意。肉烁指肌肉消瘦，由于阳盛阴虚所致。出《素问·逆调论》。

肉烁（ròu shuò）　**emaciated flesh** Symptom name. "烁" is the same as "铄"，means emaciation. Emaciated flesh refers to muscle emaciation caused by yang excess and yin deficiency. See *Su Wen* chapter 34.

肉疽　病名，即肉瘤。由于邪气结聚于肌肉，卫气归之，日久互结而成。出《灵枢·刺节真邪》。

肉疽（ròu jū）　**flesh impediment** Disease name. Refers to sarcoid. Together combined with each other over a long period. See *Ling Shu* chapter 75.

肉理　理，腠理，义同肉腠。出《素问·生气通天论》。

肉理（ròu lǐ）　**muscular interstices** *Lǐ* means interstices and refers to the muscular interstices. See *Su Wen* chapter 3.

肉清　清，通凊。肉清为肌肉清冷。出《灵枢·癫狂》。

肉清（ròu qīng）　**cool muscle** "清" is the same as "凊". Refers to the muscles being cool. See *Ling Shu* chapter 22.

肉腠　肌肉腠理。出《素问·生气通天论》。

肉腠（ròu còu）　**muscular interstices** Refers to the muscular interstices. See *Su Wen* chapter 3.

肉痹　又称肌痹。病邪痹阻于肌肉，出现麻木不仁的一类病证。出《素问·四时刺逆从论》。

肉痹（ròu bì）　**flesh numbness** Also named muscular numbness. A disease，in which the pathogenic factors are trapped inside the muscles causing numbness. See *Su Wen* chapter 64.

肉痿　病证名。脾为水湿或郁热所伤，出现肌肉不仁的病证。出《素问·痿论》。

肉痿（ròu wěi）　**flesh limpness** Disease name. The spleen is attacked by dampness or stagnated heat，which causes the disease of flesh limpness. See *Su Wen* chapter 44.

年忌　即有所禁忌的年龄。古人认为从七岁始，每隔九年的年龄都是人之大忌，即七岁、十六岁、二十五岁、三十四岁、四十三岁、五十二岁、六十一岁。出《灵枢·阴阳二十五人》。

年忌（nián jì）　**prohibition age** Refers to all the ages with prohibition. It begins at the age of seven and occurs once every nine years in one's life, usually including the years when one is seven，sixteen，twenty-five，thirty-four，forty-three，fifty-two and sixty-one. See *Ling*

Shu chapter 64.

先天 当运气太过之年,气候先于时令。出《素问・气交变大论》。

先天(xiān tiān) **precede heaven** When there is an excess of the circuits and qi, the climate comes earlier. See *Su Wen* chapter 69.

先师 即僦贷季。传说中远古时代的医学家,岐伯之师,善色脉诊法。出《素问・六节藏象论》。

先师(xiān shī) **former teacher** Refers to Jiu Daiji, the ancient physician, and the teacher of Qi Bo, who was good at the inspection of complexion color, and pulse diagnosis. See *Su Wen* chapter 9.

先巫 上古时代掌握医学道理,善用祝由法治疗疾病的一类医生。出《灵枢・贼风》。

先巫(xiān wū) **ancient sorcerers** In ancient times, doctors who mastered medical principles and made good use of *zhu you* therapy (partly related to sorcery) to treat diseases. See *Ling Shu* chapter 58.

牝藏 牝(pìn 聘),雌性鸟兽,引申为阴性。肺、脾、肾三脏属阴,均为牝脏。出《灵枢・顺气一日分为四时》。

牝藏(pìn zàng) **female viscera** *Pìn* refers to female animals, extended in meaning to yin characteristic. The lung, spleen and kidney are three female viscera which belong to yin. See *Ling Shu* chapter 44.

廷孔 出《素问・骨空论》。(1) 女子之溺孔。见《类经・经络二十七》。(2) 阴户。见《素问集注》《素问识》。

廷孔(tíng kǒng) See *Su Wen* chapter 60. (1) External orifice of urethra. See *Lei Jing* (*Classified Classic*) "Meridians and Collaterals Chapter 27". (2) Vulva. See *Su Wen Ji Zhu* (*Collected Annotation of Su Wen*) and *Su Wen Zhi* (*Understanding Su Wen*).

舌本 即舌根。诸多经脉如足太阴、足少阴、足厥阴、手少阴等皆络于此,故与经络脏腑关系十分密切。出《灵枢・经脉》。② 穴名。风府穴的别称。出《灵枢・寒热病》。

舌本(shé běn) **base of the tongue** It refers to the base of the tongue. Many meridians such as foot *taiyin*, foot *shaoyin*, foot *jueyin* and hand *shaoyin* all connect at the base of the tongue, thus it is closely related to the meridians and viscera. See

六画

Ling Shu chapter 10. ② Acupoint name，and another name for Feng Fu（DU 16）acupoint. See *Ling Shu* chapter 21.

舌卷　舌体卷曲。出《素问·脉要精微论》《灵枢·五阅五使》。

舌卷（shé juǎn）　**curled tongue** A curled tongue. See *Su Wen* chapter 17 and *Ling Shu* chapter 37.

舌柱　指舌下系带。出《灵枢·终始》。

舌柱（shé zhù）　**tongue support** Refers to the sublingual frenum. See *Ling Shu* chapter 9.

舌萎　舌体萎软。出《灵枢·经脉》。

舌萎（shé wěi）　**withered tongue** Refers to a tongue that withers. See *Ling Shu* chapter 10.

迁正　运气术语。指旧年司天左间气，迁为新年司天之正位；旧年在泉左间气，迁为新年在泉之正位。此为客气司天、在泉、四间气转移变化的规律。出《素问·本病论》。

迁正（qiān zhèng）　**to move to the due position** Terminology of the circuits and qi, meaning that the left intermediate qi that dominates the heavens in the old year moves to the due position that dominates the heavens in the coming year；and the left intermediate qi

that is in the spring in the old year moves to the due position that is in spring in the coming year. This is the regular pattern in which the guest qi dominates the heavens or is in spring，and the four intermediate qi transforms and changes. See *Su Wen* chapter 73.

乔摩　乔，通"跷"。出《灵枢·病传》。

乔摩（qiáo mó）　**massage** "乔" is the same as "跷". See *Ling Shu* chapter 42.

传化　① 传导消化。指六腑的生理功能。出《素问·五藏别论》。② 发病部位的转移和性质的变化。出《素问·生气通天论》。

传化（chuán huà）　**transmission and transformation** ① Transformation and digestion. It refers to the physiological functions of the six bowels. See *Su Wen* chapter 11. ② Changes in the location or nature of diseases. See *Su Wen* chapter 3.

传化之府　六腑中胃、大肠、小肠、三焦、膀胱五个脏器功能的总称，它们共同完成水谷食物的消化、传送和排泄。出《素问·五藏别论》。

传化之府（chuán huà zhī fǔ）　**or-**

gans of transmission and transformation A general term for the functions of the stomach, large intestine, small intestine, triple *jiao* and bladder in the six bowels, which function to digest, transmit and excrete water and grains together. See *Su Wen* chapter 11.

传道之府 指大肠，其功能主传送糟粕。出《灵枢·本输》。

传道之府（chuán dào zhī fǔ） **transmission organ** Refers to the large intestine, whose function is to transport and transform waster matters. See *Ling Shu* chapter 2.

传道之官 指大肠。出《素问·灵兰秘典论》。

传道之官（chuán dào zhī guān） **transmission governor** Refers to the large intestine. See *Su Wen* chapter 8.

伏冲之脉 指冲脉伏行于脊内者。出《灵枢·岁露论》。

伏冲之脉（fú chōng zhī mài） **hidden thoroughfare vessel** Refers to the thoroughfare vessel that runs deep inside the spine. See *Ling Shu* chapter 79.

伏阳 阳热内伏之病证。症见内热而烦，心神不宁，惊悸，往来寒热。出《素问·本病论》。

伏阳（fú yáng） **stagnant yang** Refers to the disease of yang heat stagnating inside the body, with symptoms of internal heat and vexation, restlessness, palpitation, and chills and feverishness. See *Su Wen* chapter 73.

伏兔 ① 部位名。大腿前方偏外侧的肌肉突起，相当于股直肌隆起部，其状如伏兔，故名。《素问·气府论》作"伏菟"。出《灵枢·经筋》。② 穴位名。属足阳明胃经，别名外勾。在大腿前外侧，髂前上棘与髌骨外侧连线上，膝膑上六寸处。出《灵枢·经脉》。

伏兔（fú tù） ① Name of a body part, that is the muscle protruding out the front and side of the thigh, the rectus femoris, which appears like a crouching rabbit. It is written as "伏菟" in *Su Wen* chapter 59. See *Ling Shu* chapter 13. ② Acupoint name. The acupoint is located on the stomach meridian of foot *yangming*, also named Wai Gou (ST 32), at the anterolateral thigh, on the line between the anterolateral superior iliac spine and the lateral patella, six *cun* above the patella. See *Ling Shu* chapter 10.

伏菟　同伏兔。出《素问·气府论》。

伏菟(fú tù)　**crouching rabbit** See *Su Wen* chapter 59.

伏梁　病名。伏,藏伏。梁,强梁坚硬。① 心之积证,可见心下痞块、唾血等症。见《灵枢·邪气藏府病形》《灵枢·经筋》。② 腹中之积证。见《素问·腹中论》。③ 体肿腹痛之病。见《素问·奇病论》。

伏梁(fú liáng)　*fu liang* Disease name. *Fu* means hidden, and *Liang* means hard beams. ① Stagnation symptom of the heart, which is characterized by a mass below the heart, and blood spitting. See *Ling Shu* chapter 4 and chapter 13. ② Stagnation symptom in the abdomen. See *Su Wen* chapter 40. ③ Disease with the symptoms of a swollen body and abdominal pain. See *Su Wen* chapter 47.

伏膂之脉　出《素问·疟论》。(1) 即太冲脉、伏冲脉。是冲脉循脊膂而伏行者。膂,即吕,谓脊骨。见《类经·疾病四十八》《新校正》《素问识》。(2) 肾脉之伏行者。

伏膂之脉(fú lǚ zhī mài)　**hidden spine meridian** See *Su Wen* chapter 35. (1) Refers to the *tai chong* and *fu chong* meridians, which are hidden thoroughfare vessels that run deep inside the spine. "膂" means spine. See the *Lei Jing* (*Classified Classic*) "On Diseases Chapter 48", *Xin Jiao Zheng* (*New Revisions of Su Wen*) and *Su Wen Zhi* (*Understanding Su Wen*). (2) Hidden kidney meridian.

伛偻　腰弯背曲。出《灵枢·厥病》。

伛偻(yǔ lǚ)　**Hunchback** It means that the back is bent. See *Ling Shu* chapter 24.

仲冬痹　仲冬,冬季三月之中月,为手太阴经所主之月。仲冬痹,即手太阴经筋在仲冬所发之痹证,可见下肢转筋疼痛,吐血等症。出《灵枢·经筋》。

仲冬痹(zhòng dōng bì)　**winter bi syndrome** *Zhòng dōng* means the second month of winter, which is governed by the hand *taiyin* meridian. Winter Bi-syndrome refers to the blockage illness of the hand *taiyin* meridian onset in the second month of winter. Symptoms include pain in the lower extremities and vomiting of blood, etc. See *Ling Shu* chapter 13.

仲春痹　仲春,春季三月之中月,

为足太阳经所主之月。仲春痹,即足太阳经筋在仲春所发之痹证。可见足跟肿痛等症。出《灵枢·经筋》。

仲春痹(zhòng chūn bì) **spring bi syndrome** *Zhòng chūn* means the second month of spring, which is governed by the foot *taiyang* meridian. Spring Bi-syndrome refers to the blockage illness of the foot *taiyang* meridian onset in the second month of spring. Symptoms include swollen and painful heels. See *Ling Shu* chapter 13.

仲秋痹　仲秋,秋季三月之中月,为足太阴经所主之月。仲秋痹,即足太阴经筋在仲秋所发之痹证。可见转筋、疼痛等症。出《灵枢·经筋》。

仲秋痹(zhòng qiū bì) **autumn bi syndrome** *Zhòng qiū* means the second month of autumn, which is governed by the foot *taiyin* meridian. Autumn Bi-syndrome refers to the blockage illness of the foot *taiyin* meridian onset in the second month of autumn. Symptoms include spasms and pain. See *Ling Shu* chapter 13.

仲夏痹　仲夏,夏季三月之中月,为手太阳经所主之月。仲夏痹,即手太阳经筋在仲夏所发之痹证。可见转筋、小指痛、耳鸣等症。出《灵枢·经筋》。

仲夏痹(zhòng xià bì) **summer bi syndrome** *Zhòng xià* means the second month of summer, which is governed by the hand *taiyang* meridian. Summer Bi-syndrome refers to the blockage illness of the hand *taiyang* meridian onset in the second month of summer. Symptoms include spasms, pain in the little finger, and tinnitus. See *Ling Shu* chapter 13.

任脉　奇经八脉之一。起于中极之下的胞中,下出会阴,上毛际,沿腹部及胸部正中线上行,经关元,至咽喉,上行至下颌部,绕口唇,沿面颊,分行至目眶下。分支从胞中出,向后与冲脉偕行于脊内。总任一身阴经之脉气,调节阴经之气血,为“阴脉之海”。与女子生殖生育有关。出《素问·骨空论》。

任脉(rèn mài) **conception vessel** One of the eight extraordinary meridians. It starts from the uterus below the Zhong Ji (CV 3), goes out of the perineum and the hairline, goes up along the midline of the abdomen and chest, passes through Guan

Yuan (CV 4), goes to the throat, goes up to the chin, wraps around the lips, goes along the cheek, and branches under the eye orbit. The branches come out of the uterus and go back in the ridge together with the thoroughfare vessel. It belongs to the sea of yin vessels, and governs the vessel qi of the yin vessels of the whole body, and regulates the qi and blood of the yin vessels. Related to female reproduction. See *Su Wen* chapter 60.

任脉之别　为十五别络之一,穴名尾翳(鸠尾)。其络从鸠尾向下,散布于腹部。出《灵枢·经脉》。

任脉之别(rèn mài zhī bié)　**divergent of the conception vessel** One of the fifteen divergent collaterals, which is called Wei Yi (Jiu Wei, CV 15). The divergent collateral descends from Jiu Wei (CV 15) and disseminates in the abdomen. See *Ling Shu* chapter 10.

伤寒　出《素问·热论》。(1)病因。泛指伤于一切外邪。见《素问集注》。(2)病因,指伤于寒邪。见《太素·热病决》。(3)病名。泛指一切以发热为主症的外感疾病。见《难经·五十八难》《素问直解》。

伤寒(shāng hán)　**cold damage** See *Su Wen* chapter 31. (1) Cause of diseases, refers to the all the external evils generally. See *Su Wen Ji Zhu* (*Collected Annotation of Su Wen*). (2) Cause of diseases, refers to diseases caused by cold evil. See *Tai Su* (*Grand Plain*) "Warm Diseases". (3) Disease name. Generally refers to all exogenous diseases with fever as the main symptom. See *Nan Jing* (Classic of Difficult Issues) The 58th Difficult *Issues* and *Su Wen Zhi Jie* (*Direct Interpretation on Su Wen*).

血　运行于脉中的红色液体,循脉流注全身,具有很强的营养和滋润作用,是构成人体和维持人体生命活动的基本物质之一。其由中焦脾胃消化、吸收水谷中的精微物质化生而成。出《灵枢·决气》《灵枢·营卫生会》。

血(xuè)　**blood** The red liquid running in the vessels and flowing through the whole body. It has a strong nutrition and moistening effect. It is one of the basic substances that constitutes the human body and maintains human life activities. It is formed by the digestion and absorption of fine substances, from the water and grain, by the spleen and stomach in the middle *jiao*. See *Ling Shu* chapter 30 and chapter 18.

血之精为络 心主血脉,血之精乃血脉之精,即心之精,络,指目眦内之血络。故眦络能反映心之生理病理状态。出《灵枢·大惑论》。

血之精为络(xuè zhī jīng wéi luò) **essence of the blood as collaterals** The heart governs the blood, and the essence of the blood is the essence of the vessels, that is, the essence of the heart. Collaterals refer to the blood collaterals within the canthus. Therefore, the canthus can reflect the physiological and pathological state of the heart. See *Ling Shu* chapter 80.

血气形志 《素问》篇名。血,指流贯六经之血;气,指六经之气;形,形体;志,情志。此篇主要论述六经气血多少;各种形志苦乐可产生不同的病证,治疗时要采用不同的方法。故名。

血气形志(xuè qì xíng zhì) **Blood, Qi, Physique and Emotion** Chapter title in *Su Wen*. Blood refers to the blood flowing through the six meridians; qi refers to the qi of the six meridians; physique refers to body and appearance; emotion refers to moods and the mind. This chapter mainly discusses the amount of qi and blood in the six meridians. Different kinds of physiques and mindsets, along with sadness and joy, can generate different diseases and syndromes. Different therapeutic methods should be adopted for the treatment of different diseases. Hence its name.

血有余则怒,不足则恐 肝藏血,血有余,不足,实指肝的有余不足。出《灵枢·本神》《素问·调经论》。

血有余则怒,不足则恐(xuè yǒu yú zé nù, bù zú zé kǒng) **When there is a surplus in blood, anger proceeds; when blood is insufficient, fear arises.** Liver stores blood, and the exuberance or insufficiency of blood reflects the exuberance or insufficiency of the liver. See *Ling Shu* chapter 8 and *Su Wen* chapter 62.

血并 并,偏盛。气血阴阳常相对平衡,血偏盛则气虚。出《素问·调经论》。

血并（xuè bìng）　**blood excess**
Bìng refers to excess. The yin and yang of the qi and blood are always in relative balance，although excess of blood leads to qi deficiency. See *Su Wen* chapter 62.

血泣　泣，古通涩。血泣，指血行涩滞不通。出《素问·五藏生成篇》。

血泣（xuè qì）　**blood stagnation**
"泣" is the same as "涩" in ancient Chinese，which means stagnation of blood. Blood stagnation refers to the retarded flow or blockage of blood. See *Su Wen* chapter10.

血实　① 血气充盛。出《素问·刺志论》。② 瘀血壅滞。出《素问·阴阳应象大论》。

血实（xuè shí）　① The blood is replete. See *Su Wen* chapter 53. ② Blood stasis. See *Su Wen* chapter 5.

血实宜决之　治法。决之，指逐瘀、放血法之类。血气壅实之证，宜用泻血法治疗。出《素问·阴阳应象大论》。

血实宜决之（xuè shí yí jué zhī）
Blood excess should be treated by the eliminating method. Therapeutic method. The eliminating method refers to removing blood stasis，or bloodletting methods etc. Syndromes of blood stagnation and qi should be treated with the bloodletting method. See *Su Wen* chapter 5.

血枯　血液枯涸之病证。由年少脱血，房室过度，而见胸胁支满、纳差、唾血、便血等症。出《素问·腹中论》。

血枯（xuè kū）　**blood depletion**
The disease of blood desiccation，with symptoms of fullness in the chest and hypochondriac branches，poor appetite，blood spitting and passing bloody stools，etc. These are seen in young patients after massive blood loss or excessive sexual activity. See *Su Wen* chapter 40.

血食之君　指生活富裕有权势的人。出《灵枢·根结》。

血食之君（xuè shí zhī jūn）　**Man that consumes blood.** Refers to a man of wealth and power. See *Ling Shu* chapter 5.

血络　即络脉。血脉的分支为血络。出《灵枢·血络论》《灵枢·脉度》《素问·调经论》。

血络（xuè luò）　**blood collaterals**
Refers to the collaterals. The branches of blood vessels are blood collaterals. See *Ling Shu* chapter 39 and chapter 17，and *Su Wen* chapter 62.

血络论　《灵枢》篇名。血络，即络脉。此篇主要讨论奇邪客于血络，刺络泻血的方法；刺血络后的不良反应及机制等。故名。

血络论（xuè luò lùn）　**Discussion on Blood Collaterals** Chapter title in *Ling Shu*. Blood collaterals refer to collaterals. This chapter mainly discusses uncommon pathogenic factors attacking the blood collaterals being treated by pricking collaterals and bloodletting methods, and the adverse reactions and its mechanism after pricking the blood collaterals. Hence the name.

血㕄　㕄（pēi 胚），又名"㕄血"，瘀败凝结之血块。出《素问·五藏生成》《灵枢·五禁》。

血㕄（xuè pēi）　**stagnated blood** 㕄, also named "blood stagnation", refers to blood stasis caused by stagnation. See *Su Wen* chapter 10 and *Ling Shu* chapter 61.

血海　指冲脉。又称十二经之海。其脉既与先天之本肾经相并相注，又与后天之本胃经相合，而肾与胃是精血所生所藏之脏，故冲脉藏血最盛，分布最广，其能渗灌脏腑诸经，故名。海，百川汇聚之处。出《灵枢·海论》。

血海（xuè hǎi）　**blood sea** Refers to the thoroughfare vessel, also known as the sea of the twelve meridians. Its meridian is not only in combination with the innate kidney meridian, but also in combination with the acquired stomach meridian. The kidney and stomach are the viscera of the blood and essence. Therefore, blood of the thoroughfare vessel is the most abundant and is widely distributed, and it can permeate the viscera channels, hence its name. Sea, where all rivers or streams converge. See *Ling Shu* chapter 33.

血虚　血不足。出《素问·刺志论》。

血虚（xuè xū）　**blood deficiency** Deficient blood. See *Su Wen* chapter 53.

血崩　病证名，妇女下血，量多如崩的病证。出《素问·六元正纪大论》。

血崩（xuè bēng）　**hemorrhage** Disease name, manifested as loss of blood or sudden metrorrhagia in women. See *Su Wen* chapter 71.

血脱　即突然大量失血。出《灵枢·决气》。

血脱（xuè tuō）　**blood depletion**

Refers to a sudden excessive loss of blood. See *Ling Shu* chapter 30.

血痹　病名。指邪入血分，气血闭阻不通，出现身体麻木不仁为主症的病证。出《灵枢·九针论》《素问·五藏生成》。

血痹（xuè bì）　**blood blockage syndrome** Disease name. Refers to a disease with the main symptom of body numbness caused by attacks of evil pathogens entering the blood and triggering blockages of qi and blood. See *Ling Shu* chapter 78 and *Su Wen* chapter 10.

血瘕　病证名。属血瘀积聚之病。出《素问·阴阳类论》。

血瘕（xuè jiā）　**blood mass** Disease name, caused by blood stasis and abdominal mass. See *Su Wen* chapter 79.

囟会　经穴名。属督脉经。在头部正中线，入前发际二寸，即百会前三寸处，别名顶门。出《灵枢·热病》。

囟会（xìn huì）　**Xin Hui（GV 22）** Acupoint name，belonging to the governor vessel, and located in the middle line of the head, two *cun* into the front hairline, that is，three *cun* before Bai Hui（GV 20），also known as

Ding Men acupoint. See *Ling Shu* chapter 23.

囟顶　头顶部。囟（xìn 信），谓婴儿期左右顶骨等接合不紧而出现的骨缝。闭合后即为顶骨。出《素问·气交变大论》。

囟顶（xìn dǐng）　**fontanel** Apex of the head. *Xìn* refers to the spaces between the uncompleted angles of the right and left parietal bones of infants. It is called parietal bone after the space closes. See *Su Wen* chapter 69.

后天　当运气不及之年，气候晚于时令。出《素问·气交变大论》。

后天（hòu tiān）　**behind heaven** When the five circuits and six qi in a year is inadequate，the climate is later than the season. See *Su Wen* chapter 69.

后血　即大小便下血。出《灵枢·百病始生》。

后血（hòu xuè）　**discharge blood** Refers to blood in the stools or urine. See *Ling Shu* chapter 66.

后泄　大便泄泻。出《素问·平人气象论》。

后泄（hòu xiè）　**outflow behind** Refers to diarrhea. See *Su Wen* chapter 18.

后廉　指肢体的后缘。出《灵枢·经筋》。

后廉（hòu lián）　**posterior edge** Refers to the posterior edge of the limbs. See *Ling Shu* chapter 13.

后溪　经穴名。手太阳小肠经之输穴。在手小指外侧本节后陷者中。出《灵枢·本输》。

后溪（hòu xī）　**Hou Xi（SI 3）** Acupoint name，which belongs to the small intestine meridian of hand *taiyang*，and is located at the lateral side of the little finger. See *Ling Shu* chapter 2.

行水　① 指药液。出《素问·五常政大论》。② 水，指肾。行水。即调治肾。出《灵枢·经筋》。

行水（xíng shuǐ）　① Refers to medicinal liquids. See *Su Wen* chapter 70. ② Water，refers to the kidney. Running water refers to regulating the kidney. See *Ling Shu* chapter 13.

行令　运气术语。指岁会之气，如同施行政令。出《素问·六微旨大论》。

行令（xíng lìng）　**carrying out orders** Terminology of the five circuits and six qi. Refers to the qi of the yearly meetings，as if the official is carrying out orders. See *Su Wen* chapter 68.

行针　①《灵枢》篇名。行，施行。此篇主要论述施行针刺治疗的情况，故名。篇中指出由于体质的差异对针刺的反应也不同，针刺操作的正确与否与疗效有密切关系。② 指施行和运用针刺疗法。出《灵枢·官能》。

行针（xíng zhēn）　① Chapter title in *Ling Shu*. *Xíng* refers to manipulation. This chapter mainly discusses the application of acupuncture treatment，hence the name. It points out that the correct manipulation of acupuncture is closely related to its curative effect because of the different physical constitutions having different responses to acupuncture. ② Refers to the implementation and application of acupuncture therapy. See *Ling Shu* chapter 73.

行间　经穴名。足厥阴肝经之荥穴。在足大趾，次趾。出《灵枢·本输》。

行间（xíng jiān）　**Xing Jian（LR 2）** Acupoint name. The spring acupoint of the liver meridian of foot *jueyin*. It is located between the big toe and the second toe. See *Ling Shu* chapter 2.

行痹　病证名。行，游走之意。为疼痛游走之痹证。因风寒湿三邪之中，风邪较胜，风性多动，故呈游走状。出《素问·痹论》。

六画

行痹(xíng bì)　**migratory blockage** Disease name. *Xíng* means migratory. It is a disease characterized by a wandering blockage caused by the three evils, including wind, cold and dampness. The wind is stronger and more active, therefore similar to wandering. See *Su Wen* chapter 43.

会厌　位于喉咽交会处之软骨组织,覆于喉管之上,能张能收,呼吸发声则张,为声音之门户。吞咽则阖,以防异物进入气道。出《灵枢·忧恚无言》。

会厌(huì yàn)　**epiglottis** The cartilage tissue is located at the intersection of the laryngopharynx and the larynx, covering the larynx, and can be opened and closed. It is open while breathing and speaking. As the door of the voice, it is closed while swallowing to prevent substances from entering the airway. See *Ling Shu* chapter 69.

会阴　在前阴和肛门之间的部位。出《素问·刺腰痛》。

会阴(huì yīn)　**yin meeting vessel** The area between the vagina or scrotum and the anus. See *Su Wen* chapter 41.

会阴之脉　指任、冲、督等聚于前后二阴间会阴部的脉。出《素问·刺腰痛》。

会阴之脉(huì yīn zhī mài)　**vessels of yin meeting** Refers to the area between external genitalia and anus, where the three-yin vessels, the thoroughfare vessel, conception vessel and governor vessel, all gather. See *Su Wen* chapter 41.

合　① 合穴。五腧穴之一,位于肘膝附近,多用于治疗脏腑疾患。十二经各有一个合穴,即尺泽(肺经)、曲泽(心包经)、阴陵泉(脾经)、曲泉(肝经)、阴谷(肾经)、曲池(大肠经)、天井(三焦经)、小海(小肠经)、足三里(胃经)、阳陵泉(胆经)、委中(膀胱经)。出《灵枢·九针十二原》《灵枢·邪气藏府病形》。② 配合。如脏腑之表里相合。出《灵枢·本输》。③ 闭合。出《灵枢·经筋》。④ 交合。出《素问·六节藏象论》。⑤ 混合。出《素问·痹论》。⑥ 容量单位,市制十合为一升。合(读 gě),出《灵枢·平人绝谷》。⑦ 参合。出《素问·五藏生成篇》。⑧ 合计。出《素问·六节藏象论》。

合(hé)　① *He*-sea acupoints. One of the five kinds of transport acupoints that are close to

六画

the elbows and knees, and are generally used to treat diseases of the viscera and bowels. Each of the twelve channels has a sea acupoint, that is, Chi Ze (LU 5, the lung meridian), Qu Ze (PC 3, the pericardium meridian), Yin Ling Quan (SP 9, the spleen meridian), Qu Quan (LR 8, the liver meridian), Yin Gu (KI 10, the kidney meridian), Qu Chi (LI 11, the large intestine meridian), Tian Jing (SJ 10, the triple *jiao* meridian), Xiao Hai (SI 8, the small intestine meridian), Zu San Li (ST 36, the stomach meridian), Yang Ling Quan (GB 34, the gallbladder meridian) and Wei Zhong (BL 40, the bladder meridian). See *Ling Shu* chapter 1 and chapter 4. ② Unity. For instance, unity of the viscera at the interior and of the bowels at the exterior. See *Ling Shu* chapter 2. ③ To close. See *Ling Shu* chapter 13. ④ To communicate. See *Su Wen* chapter 9. ⑤ To merge. See *Su Wen* chapter 43. ⑥ *Ge*, a unit of capacity in the Chinese system of weights and measures. Ten *ge* equals a liter. See *Ling Shu* chapter 32. ⑦ To match. See *Su Wen* chapter 10. ⑧ To add up. See *Su Wen* chapter 9.

合阴　谓营卫之气于夜半子时而会合于内脏。出《灵枢·营卫生会》。

合阴（hé yīn）　**to link up the yin** It means that the nutrient qi and the defensive qi meet in the viscera at midnight. See *Ling Shu* chapter 18.

合谷　经穴名。手阳明大肠经之原穴。在手大指次指歧骨间（即第一，二掌骨间）。出《灵枢·本输》。

合谷（hé gǔ）　**He Gu (LI 4)** Acupoint name, which is the source acupoint of the large intestine meridian of hand *yangming*. It is located between the first and the second metacarpal bones. See *Ling Shu* chapter 2.

合谷刺　刺法之一。在肌肉比较丰厚处，将针刺入一定深度，直达分肉之间，再退至皮下，依次将针尖向两侧各斜刺一针，形为鸡爪的分叉，此手法，适用于肌肉的痹症。因脾主肌肉，所以这是和脾相应的刺法。并非指针刺合谷穴。出《灵枢·官针》。

合谷刺（hé gǔ cì）　**united valley piercing** One of the needling methods. In this method，the needle is inserted to a certain depth in the thick muscles，reaches the muscular interstices and then is withdrawn to under the skin. The needle point is inserted obliquely at both sides in turn to shape like the fork of a chicken's paw. This manipulation applies to impediments in the muscles. The spleen dominates the muscles，so this needling method is in correspondence to the spleen. It does not mean needling the He Gu（LI 4）acupoint. See *Ling Shu* chapter 7.

众之为人　体质名。众，常也，即众羽，为羽音之一，此代表阴阳二十五人中水形人之一种，其特征是文静如水。出《灵枢·阴阳二十五人》。

众之为人（zhòng zhī wéi rén）**people of the general *yu* tone** Name of constitution. General *yu* is one of the *yu* tones. It belongs to water-type people among the twenty-five types of people divided according to yin and yang. People with this constitution are quiet as water. See *Ling Shu* chapter 64.

众羽　体质名。阴阳二十五人中水形人之一种。出《灵枢·五音五味》。

众羽（zhòng yǔ）**general *yu*** Name of constitution，which belongs to water-type people among the twenty-five types of people divided according to yin and yang. See *Ling Shu* chapter 65.

众痹　病证名。为痛处固定，呈左右对称，发作与停止无规律的痹证。其邪在分肉之间。出《灵枢·周痹》。

众痹（zhòng bì）**general blockage-illnesses** A syndrome characterized by fixed pain that is symmetrical and occurs and stops without irregularly. The pathogen is located in the muscular interstices. See *Ling Shu* chapter 27.

肌肉之精为约束　脾主肌肉，肌肉之精即脾之精。约束，即眼胞，能反映脾之生理病理状态。出《灵枢·大惑论》。

肌肉之精为约束（jī ròu zhī jīng wéi yuē shù）**essence of the flesh collects in the eyelids** The spleen dominates the flesh，and essence of the flesh is essence of the spleen. Thus，the eyelids can reflect the physiological and pathological conditions of the spleen. See *Ling*

六画

Shu chapter 80.

肌痹 病证名。五体痹之一。病发于长夏的痹证。因长夏主肌肉,故名。出《素问·痹论》。

肌痹（jī bì） **muscle blockage** Syndrome name of one kind of blockage among the five body constituents. It occurs in the late summer, and it is so named as the late summer dominates the muscles. See *Su Wen* chapter 43.

杂病 《灵枢》篇名。该篇主要讨论了厥气上逆、喉痹、疟、齿痛、聋、衄、腰痛、腹满、心痛、痿厥、呃逆等杂病的症状和治疗方法,故名。

杂病（zá bìng） **Miscellaneous Diseases** Chapter title in *Ling Shu*. In this chapter, the symptoms and treatment methods of miscellaneous diseases including the upward flow of *jue* qi (adverse-qi), throat impediment, malaria, toothache, deafness, spontaneous external bleeding, lumbago, abdominal distension, heart pain, *wei jue* (weakness of the limbs) and hiccups etc., are discussed. Hence the name.

壮 ① 指年龄在二十岁以上,五十岁以下者,出《灵枢·卫气失常》。② 艾炷灸的计数单位,每灸一艾炷称为一壮。出《灵枢·癫狂病》。③ 健壮。出《素问·上古天真论》。

壮（zhuàng） ① Refers to a person over the age of 20 and under the age of 50. See *Ling Shu* chapter 59. ② Moxa-cone, the counting unit of moxa sticks, each moxa stick is called one *Zhuang*. See *Ling Shu* chapter 22. ③ Strong. See *Su Wen* chapter 1.

壮火 出《素问·阴阳应象大论》。（1）药食气味纯阳者为壮火。见《素问注证发微》。（2）亢盛的阳气为壮火,属病理之火。见《类经·阴阳一》。

壮火（zhuàng huǒ） **strong fire** See *Su Wen* chapter 5.（1）Strong fire is when the property and taste of the medicine and food is pure yang. See *Su Wen Zhu Zheng Fa Wei*（*Annotation and Elaboration on Su Wen*）.（2）Hyperactivity of yang qi is strong fire, which belongs to pathogenic fire. See *Lei Jing*（*Classified Classic*）"Yin and Yang Chapter 1".

冲头痛 病证名。① 由邪气上冲而见脑后、眉间疼痛。出《素问·至真要大论》。② 为足太阳膀胱经"是动病"症状之一。出《灵枢·经脉》。

冲头痛（chōng tóu tòng） **rushing upwards headache** Disease name. ① Pain at the back of the head and between the eyebrows is caused by the evil qi rushing upwards. See *Su Wen* chapter 74. ② One of the symptoms of a "disease transmitted by meridians" such as the bladder meridian of foot *taiyang*. See *Ling Shu* chapter 10.

冲阳　经穴名。别名会原、跗阳。足阳明胃经之原穴。在足跗上五寸，骨间动脉上，当摇足取之。出《灵枢·本输》。

冲阳（chōng yáng）　**Chong Yang (ST 42)** Acupoint name, also called Hui Yuan or Fu Yang, or the source acupoint of the stomach meridian of foot *yangming*. This acupoint is at five *cun* above the tarsal bone and interosseous artery, and can be located by shaking the foot. See *Ling Shu* chapter 2.

冲疝　病证名。疝之一种，后世称之奔豚疝。症见气从少腹上冲心而疼痛。出《素问·骨空论》。

冲疝（chōng shàn）　**rushing upwards hernia** Disease name. One kind of hernia, also called running piglet hernia by later generations. It is manifested by pain caused by qi rushing from the lower abdomen upwards to the heart. See *Su Wen* chapter 60.

冲脉　奇经八脉之一。其循行路线,起于小腹中(胞中),从气街部(腹股沟动脉处)与足少阴经交会,沿腹部两侧上行,散布于胸中。上达咽喉,环绕唇口,抵于眶下。下行之脉,输注于足少阴之大络,行股内侧,腘内,伏行于胫骨内侧,下至内踝后,渗灌足三阴,前出于足背及大趾间;其内行支,从胞中出,贯脊,上循脊里,与督脉相通。冲脉为十二经脉之海,五脏六腑之海,有促进生殖的功能,同妇女的月经有着密切的联系。出《灵枢·逆顺肥瘦》《素问·骨空论》《灵枢·动输》。

冲脉（chōng mài）　**thoroughfare vessel** It is one of the eight extraodinary meridians. Its upper part starts from lower abdomen (bladder), intersects with foot *shaoyin* meridian in *qi jie* (the part of the artery in groin), then runs up along both sides of the abdomen, disperses in the chest, then moves upward to the throat, runs around the lips and ends at the region below the eye socket. Its lower part infuses into the great collateral vessel of foot *shaoyin* meridian，then reaches to the back of the malleolus medialis，infuses into the three yin meridians of the foot and ends at the dorsal aspect of the foot and the part between the hallux and the second toe. Its inner branch alsō starts from the lower abdomen（bladder），penetrates the spine，runs along the interior of the back and connects with the governor vessel. The thoroughfare vessel is the sea of the twelve meridians and the five viscera and six bowels. It has the function of promoting reproduction and is closely related to women's menstruation. See *Ling Shu* chapter 38，*Su Wen* chapter 60，and *Ling Shu* chapter 62.

齐刺 刺法之一。又称三刺。先刺一针，并于两旁各刺一针，三针齐用，故名。治疗病变小而深的痹痛等症。出《灵枢·官针》。

齐刺（qí cì） **even piercing** One of the needling methods. It is also named triple piercing. In this method，one needle is inserted first，and two needles are inserted sideways. Totally three needles are inserted，hence named even or triple piercing. It is used to treat diseases like impediment pain with small and deep lesions. See *Ling Shu* chapter 7.

决气 《灵枢》篇名。决，区别、分开；气，指精、气、津、液、血、脉六气。此篇主要讨论了六气的概念以及六气虚证的临床特征，指出六气总由水谷一气所化，一气而分为六气。故名。

决气（jué qì） **Differentiation of Qi** Chapter title in *Ling Shu*. *Jué* means to distingush，differentiate. *Qì* refers to the six qi：essence，qi，liquids，body fluids，blood and meridians. This chapter mainly discusses the concept of the six qi and their clinical characteristics of deficiency syndrome. It explains that the six kinds of qi are transformed from water and grain. One qi can be divided into six types of qi. Hence the name.

决渎之官 指三焦。见"三焦者，决渎之官，水道出焉"条。出《素问·灵兰秘典论》。

决渎之官（jué dú zhī guān） **organ in charge of water drainage** Refers to the triple *jiao*. See the term "triple *jiao* is the organ in charge of water drainage. The body liquids are stored in it". See *Su Wen* chapter 8.

妄言 ① 指病人因神明受扰而出现的谵语。出《灵枢·刺节真邪》。② 谓医者谈病不合实际。出《素问·徵四失论》。

妄言（wàng yán）　① Delirium, a mental state where the patient becomes delirious because of illness. See *Ling Shu* chapter 75. ② It means that the doctor makes absurd statements in talking about illness. See *Su Wen* chapter 78.

闭药　指通闭的药物，即利水药。出《灵枢·四时气》。

闭药（bì yào）　**medicinals that relieve obstruction** Refers to the drugs which have the function of dredging stagnation, hence the water-disinhibiting medicinals. See *Ling Shu* chapter 19.

关　① 部位名。见《素问·骨空论》。（1）膝弯上骨节活动处，即骸关。见《类经·经络十九》。（2）指承扶穴部位。见《素问注证发微》。② 出入要道，要冲。见《素问·水热穴论》《灵枢·忧恚无言》。③ 病理名称。指阴气太盛，阻遏阳气运行的一种病理现象。见《灵枢·脉度》。④ 关系、关连。见《素问·咳论》。⑤ 指四肢形体。见《灵枢·小针解》。⑥ 指固密和卫外的功能。见《灵枢·根结》《素问·皮部论》。

关（guān）　① Body part name. See *Su Wen* chapter 60. (1) The knee joint is where the curve above the knee moves. See *Lei Jing*（*Classified Classic*）"Meridians and Collaterals Chapter 19". (2) Refers to Cheng Fu（BL 36）. See *Su Wen Zhu Zheng Fa Wei*（*Annotation and Elaboration on Su Wen*）. ② Important access, important gate. See *Su Wen* chapter 61 and *Ling Shu* chapter 69. ③ Pathological name. It refers to the pathological phenomenon in which the yin qi is too excessive and obstructs yang qi. See *Ling Shu* chapter 17. ④ Relationship, connection. See *Su Wen* chapter 38. ⑤ Refers to the physique of the four limbs. See *Ling Shu* chapter 3. ⑥ Refers to the functions of securing and guarding. See *Ling Shu* chapter 5 and *Su Wen* chapter 56.

关元　经穴名。属任脉，为小肠之募穴，足三阴任脉之会。在脐正中线当脐下三寸处。出《灵枢·寒热病》。

关元（guān yuán） **Guan Yuan (CV 4)** Acupoint name，belonging to the conception vessel and located three *cun* below the navel. It is the front-mu acupoint of the small intestine meridian，and the convergence point of the conception vessel of the three foot-yin meridians. See *Ling Shu* chapter 21.

关冲 经穴名。手少阳三焦经井穴，在环指尺侧，支指甲角一寸。出《灵枢·本输》。

关冲（guān chōng） **Guan Chong (TE 1)** Acupoint name，and the well acupoint of the triple *jiao* meridian of hand *shaoyang*，which is located on the ulnar aspect of the ring finger，one *cun* from the nail angle. See *Ling Shu* chapter 2.

关阴 关，关闭，隔绝。关阴，指气血盛于阴，与三阳隔绝，阴阳不相交通。又称"溢阴""内关"。出《素问·六节藏象论》《灵枢·终始》。

关阴（guān yīn） *guan yin Guān* refers to close，or isolated. *Guān yīn* refers to qi and blood that are abundant in yin，and isolated from the three yang，as yin and yang do not communicate with each other.

Also called *yi yin*，or *nei guan*. See *Su Wen* chapter 9 and *Ling Shu* chapter 9.

关枢 太阳经之皮部。六经皮部之一。关枢，是关键，转枢的意思。三阳经主表证，以太阳当关，故名。出《素问·皮部论》。

关枢（guān shū） *guan shu* The skin section of the *taiyang* meridian，and one of the skin sections of the six meridians. It refers to the key pivot. The three yang meridians dominate the exterior syndromes，and *taiyang* is the key pivot. Hence the name. See *Su Wen* chapter 56.

关刺 五刺法之一。关，即关节。其法直刺四肢关节部分，筋的尽端处。可治筋痹之证，刺时当注意勿伤脉出血。肝主筋，本法与肝相应。又名"渊刺""岂刺"。见《灵枢·官针》。

关刺（guān cì） **joint piercing** One of the five needling methods. *Guān*，namely the joints. This method is to insert the needles perpendicularly into the joints of the limbs，and at the end of tendons. It can be used to treat syndromes of sinew blockage-illnesses. However heed must be taken not to hurt the blood vessels when needling. The liver dominates the tendons，and this method corresponds to liver. It is also known as "abyss piercing" or "triumphant piercing". See *Ling Shu* chapter 7.

关格　病证名。指阴阳俱盛，不相协调的病证，其脉象表现为人迎与寸口俱盛。出《素问·脉要精微论》《灵枢·脉度》《素问·六节藏象论》。

关格（guān gé）　**obstruction and rejection** Disease name，refers to the syndrome of excess and imbalance of both yin and yang. The condition of the pulse shows an overabundance of both *ren ying* and *cun kou* pulses. See *Su Wen* chapter 17，*Ling Shu* chapter 17 and *Su Wen* chapter 9.

关蛰　六经皮部之一，指手足太阴经所属的体表部位。关蛰，是关键和潜藏的意思，三阴经主里证，太阴为关，故名。出《素问·皮部论》。

关蛰（guān zhé）　*guan zhe* One of the skin sections of the six meridians. It refers to the body surface of the hand and foot *taiyin* meridians. *Guān zhé* means crucial and hidden. The three yin meridians dominate

the internal syndromes，and the *taiyin* meridian is the most crucial. Hence the name. See *Su Wen* chapter 56.

米疽　病名。为发于腋下，形小而深赤色坚硬的疽。后世又称腋疽。出《灵枢·痈疽》。

米疽（mǐ jū）　**subaxillary carbuncle** Disease name，of one that breaks out in the armpit，and is small，dark red and hard. It was also known as axillary carbuncle in later generations. See *Ling Shu* chapter 81.

州都之官　指膀胱。出《素问·灵兰秘典论》。

州都之官（zhōu dū zhī guān）　**governor of regional reservoir** Refers to the bladder. See *Su Wen* chapter 8.

汗者不以奇　谓发汗解表的方剂，宜用药味组合相对较多，药力较足的偶方，而不用药味相对较少的奇方。出《素问·至真要大论》。

汗者不以奇（hàn zhě bù yǐ qí）　**to promote sweating，odd-numbered prescriptions should be avoided** Refers to even-numbered formulas，with more medicinal ingredients and stronger effects，should be used to promote sweating and relieve the exterior，

六画

instead of the odd-numbered prescriptions with relatively fewer ingredients. See *Su Wen* chapter 74.

汤液醪醴论 《素问》篇名。汤液，用五谷煮成的清汤。醪（láo 劳）醴（lǐ 礼），用五谷制成的酒类，醪为浊酒，醴为甜酒。此篇因首论汤液醪醴的制作方法及治疗作用，故名。内容主要讨论五脏损伤的病因及水肿病的治疗等。

汤液醪醴论（tāng yè láo lǐ lùn） **Discourse on Decoctions and Wines** Chapter title in *Su Wen*. *Tāng yè* refers to a clear soup made of five grains. *Láo lǐ* refers to wine, which is made from five grains. *Láo* is turbid wine and *lǐ* is sweet wine. This chapter is named for the first discussion on the production methods and therapeutic effects of decoctions and wines. It mainly discusses the causes of injury of the five viscera, and the treatment of edema.

汤熨 汤，用热汤洗浴。熨，用药热敷。皆是以热驱寒的一类疗法。出《素问·玉机真藏论》。

汤熨（tāng yùn） **bath and compress** *Tāng* refers to taking a bath in hot water. *Yùn* refers

to hot compresses. Both of them are therapeutic methods for expelling the cold with hot medicine. See *Su Wen* chapter 19.

论勇 《灵枢》篇名。勇，勇敢。在此指一种体质的特征。此篇提出人的体质分为勇、怯两种，并论述了其外部形态，组织结构，性格表现方面的特征和对发病，辨证及预后的临床意义，故名。

论勇（lùn yǒng） **Discussion on Bravery** Chapter title in *Ling Shu*. *Yǒng* refers to brave, and here refers to a physical characteristic. This chapter points out that human constitutions can be divided into courage and timidity, and discusses the characteristics of its external features, tissue structure, and personality performance, as well as its clinical significance for diseases, syndrome differentiation and prognosis. Hence the name.

论疾诊尺 《灵枢》篇名。尺，尺肤，指前臂内侧面。此篇主要讨论通过诊察尺肤的缓、急、大、小、滑、涩以判断疾病，同时强调诊尺肤必须和望诊、切诊以及四时季节的变化相参。故名。

论疾诊尺（lùn jí zhěn chǐ） **Dis-**

cussion on Diagnosis of Diseases through Examination of the Skin from Elbow to Wrist Chapter title in *Ling Shu*. *Chǐ* and *chǐ fū* refer to the inner side of the forearm. This chapter mainly discusses how to judge a disease by examining the slowness, urgency, largeness, smallness, slipperiness and astringency of the skin from the elbow to the wrist, and emphasizes that the examination must be related to inspection, palpation and pulse taking, and changes of the four seasons. Hence the name.

论痛　《灵枢》篇名。痛，疼痛。此篇主要论述不同的体质，对针灸所致疼痛的耐受性亦不同，故名。

论痛（lùn tòng）　**Discussion On Pain** Chapter title in *Ling Shu*. *Tòng* refers to pain. This chapter mainly discusses different body type constitutions and their tolerance to pain caused by acupuncture, hence the name.

导气　针刺导引经气之法。出《灵枢·邪客》。

导气（dǎo qì）　**inducing qi** An acupuncture method to induce qi. See *Ling Shu* chapter 71.

导引　是古代一种健身方法。以调节呼吸、运动肢体和自我按摩等方法为特点，以达到行气活血、强筋健骨、祛病延年的目的。目前所称气功、按摩、健身操均属其范围。出《素问·异法方宜论》。

导引（dǎo yǐn）　*dao yin* A kind of physical exercise in ancient times characterized by regulating the breath, moving the limbs, and self massage, so as to achieve the purpose of promoting the flow of qi and blood circulation, strengthening muscles and bones, eliminating diseases and prolonging life. At present, *qi gong*, massage and exercise belong to its scope. See *Su Wen* chapter 12.

导而下之　凡是上部病气有余的，应采取上病下取的方法，针刺下部穴位以引导病气下行。出《灵枢·阴阳二十五人》。

导而下之（dǎo ér xià zhī）　**to induce the qi to descend** If the upper part of the disease has excess qi, it is necessary to use the method of needling the lower part to treat upper, or needling the acupoints in the lower parts to induce the evil qi to descend. See *Ling Shu* chapter 64.

导而行之　如果有寒热交争的现

六画

象,根据其阴阳偏胜的不同情况,引导其气血运行而达到阴阳平衡。出《灵枢·阴阳二十五人》。

导而行之(dǎo ér xíng zhī) **to induce the qi to move** If there is conflict between hot and cold, according to the different conditions of the predominance of yin and yang, the movement of qi and blood should be guided to achieve a balance of yin and yang. See *Ling Shu* chapter 64.

异法方宜论 《素问》篇名。异法,指不同的治疗方法。方宜,指地域环境各有所宜。此篇主要论述由地域不同,人们的生活特点、所患疾病也不同。因之治病的方法亦不同,强调医生必须综合掌握这些情况和治法,始能达到各得其宜。故名。

异法方宜论(yì fǎ fāng yí lùn) **Discussion on Different Therapeutic Methods for Different Diseases** Chapter title in *Su Wen*. *Yì fǎ* refers to the different therapeutic methods. *Fāng yí* refers to different regions having different environments. This chapter mainly discusses that people from different regions have different characteristics, and different diseases, therefore they should be treated with different methods. It emphasizes that doctors should consider these factors and therapeutic methods comprehensively, in order to achieve satisfying therapeutic effects. Hence the name.

孙脉 细小的络脉,又称孙络。孙脉与络脉都通向经脉。见《素问·调经论》。

孙脉(sūn mài) **tertiary vessel** Refers to the tiny collaterals, also called tertiary collaterals. All tertiary vessels and collaterals lead to the meridians. See *Su Wen* chapter 62.

孙络 最细小的络脉,又称孙脉。见《素问·气穴论》《类经·经络八》《灵枢·脉度》。

孙络(sūn luò) **tertiary collateral** The thinnest collateral, also called the tertiary vessel. See *Su Wen* chapter 58, *Lei Jing* (*Classified Classic*) "Meridians and Collaterals Chapter 8" and *Ling Shu* chapter 17.

阳 ① 古代哲学概念。与阴相对,凡向上、炎热、运动、光明、亢盛等特性的事物或现象均属阳。出《素问·阴阳应象大论》。② 代表人体组织结构中阳经(如手足三阳经)、阳脏(如心、肝)、六腑,以及表浅的、外侧的、上部的部位等。出《素问·热论》《灵枢·寿夭刚柔》《素问·六节藏象论》《素问·金匮真言论》。③ 代表生命过程中具有推动、温煦、兴奋等作用或表现的物质及功能。出《素问·生气通天论》。④ 代表致病因素中的外邪、外邪中的风邪、热邪、火邪、暑邪以及亢盛的邪气等。出《素问·阴阳应象大论》《素问·太阴阳明论》。⑤ 代表阳有余的病证脉象。出《素问·阴阳别论》《素问·阴阳应象大论》。⑥ 代表药物的性味功能,辛、甘、淡者为阳。出《素问·至真要大论》。

阳(yáng)　① A philosophical concept in ancient times, in contrast to yin. Things or phenomena characterized by upwardness, heat, movement, brightness and hyperactivity all belong to yang. See *Su Wen* chapter 5. ② It represents the yang meridians (three yang meridians of hand and foot), yang viscera (heart, liver), six bowels, and superficial, lateral and upper parts of the human tissue structure. See *Su Wen* chapter 31, *Ling Shu* chapter 6, and *Su Wen* chapter 9 and chapter 4. ③ It represents that which has the function of promoting, warming, and stimulating in the processes of life. See *Su Wen* chapter 3. ④ It represents the pathogenic factors, such as external evil, wind evil, heat evil, fire evil, summer-heat evil and hyperactivity of evil qi. See *Su Wen* chapter 5 and chapter 29. ⑤ It represents the syndrome or pulse condition with excess yang. See *Su Wen* chapter 7 and *Su Wen* chapter 5. ⑥ It represents the property, flavor and function of medicinals, and those pungent, sweet and tasteless belong to yang. See *Su Wen* chapter 74.

阳人　指偏于阳性体质的人。出《灵枢·通天》。阳人包括多阳无阴的太阳之人,多阳少阴的少阳之人,他们在生理、性格心理,外形、病理反应各方面有差异。参"太阳之人""少阳之人"。

阳人(yáng rén)　**yang people** Refers to those with a yang body constitution. See *Ling Shu* chapter 72. It includes the people of *taiyang* constitution with more yang and without yin, and the people of *shaoyang* constitution with more yang and less yin，and they all possess differences in physiology，personality，psychology，physique and pathological reactions. See "太阳之人" and "少阳之人"。

阳中之太阳　① 指心。位居膈上，属阳，又为阳脏，故称。出《灵枢·九针十二原》《类经·经络十五》。② 指手之阳侧。手在上，属阳，手的阳面外侧，阳气隆盛，故称。出《灵枢·阴阳系日月》。

阳中之太阳（yáng zhōng zhī tài yang）　① *Taiyang* in the yang. Refers to the heart，which is located above the diaphragm，and belonging to yang. It is also called the yang viscera. See *Ling Shu* chapter 1 and *Lei Jing*（*Classified Classic*）"Meridians and Collaterals Chapter 15". ② Refers to the yang side of the hand. The upper part of the hand belongs to yang，and at the outside of the yang side of the hand，the yang qi is prosperous. Hence the name. See *Ling Shu* chapter 41.

阳中之太阴　指肺。出《素问·六节藏象论》《灵枢·九针十二原》《灵枢·阴阳系日月》。

阳中之太阴（yáng zhōng zhī tài yīn）　*taiyin* in the yang Refers to the lung. See *Su Wen* chapter 9，*Ling Shu* chapter 1，and *Ling Shu* chapter 41.

阳中之少阳　指肝。出《素问·六节藏象论》。

阳中之少阳（yáng zhōng zhī shào yáng）　*shaoyang* in the yang Refers to the liver. See *Su Wen* chapter 9.

阳中之少阴　阴阳之中又有阴阳之分。然阳中之阴阳，其阴无多，故曰少阴。① 指肺。位居膈上，属阳位，但为阴脏，故称。出《灵枢·九针十二原》。② 指手之阴侧。手在上，属阳，其阴面里侧，阴气较弱，为阳中的少阴。出《灵枢·阴阳系日月》。

阳中之少阴（yáng zhōng zhī shào yīn）　*shaoyin* in the yang Yin and yang can be subdivided into yin and yang. However，when there are yin and yang in the yang，it has less yin，thus it is called *shaoyin*. ① Refers to the lung. Located above the diaphragm，which is in the yang position，but is a yin organ，hence the name. See *Ling Shu* chapter 1. ② Refers to the yin side of the hand. The upper side of the hand belongs to yang, and the yin qi is weak on the inner side of the yin side, therefore it is called the *shaoyin* in yang. See *Ling Shu* chapter 41.

阳中之阳　① 指日出至中午一段时间。白昼为阳,其阳气最为隆盛,故称。出《素问·金匮真言论》。② 指心。其为阳藏,又居于上焦阳位故称。出《素问·金匮真言论》。

阳中之阳(yáng zhōng zhī yáng) ① Yang in the yang. Refers to the period from dawn to noon. The daytime is yang, and the yang qi is prosperous at daytime, thus the name. See *Su Wen* chapter 4. ② Refers to the heart. The heart is the yang organ located at the upper *jiao*, hence the name. See *Su Wen* chapter 4.

阳中之阴　① 指中午至日落一段时间。其时阳气渐衰,阴气渐盛,故称。出《素问·金匮真言论》。② 指肺。其居上焦阳位,而为阴脏,故称。出《素问·金匮真言论》。

阳中之阴(yáng zhōng zhī yīn) ① Yin in the yang. Refers to the period from noon to dusk. At that time, the yang qi is gradually declining, and the yin qi is gradually flourishing,

thus the name yin in the yang. See *Su Wen* chapter 4. ② Refers to the lung, which is located in the upper *jiao*. It is a yin viscera, hence the name. See *Su Wen* chapter 4.

阳气　① 与人体阴气相对,有温养、气化等功能。出《素问·生气通天论》《素问·阴阳应象大论》。② 指天气。出《素问·四气调神大论》。③ 指阳邪。出《素问·疟论》。④ 指自然界具有生发作用的温热之气。出《素问·脉要精微论》。

阳气(yáng qì) ① Yang qi. Opposite to the yin qi in the human body, with the functions of warming, and qi transforming, etc. See *Su Wen* chapter 3 and *Su Wen* chapter 5. ② Refers to the climate. See *Su Wen* chapter 2. ③ Refers to the yang evil. See *Su Wen* chapter 35. ④ Refers to the warm qi whose function is to help grow and develop in nature. See *Su Wen* chapter 17.

阳加于阴谓之汗　出《素问·阴阳别论》。(1) 指阳气加于阴液而汗出。见《素问集注》。(2) 阳脉出现于阴位,主汗出。见《类经·脉色二十九》。

阳加于阴谓之汗(yáng jiā yú yīn

六画

wèi zhī hàn）　See *Su Wen* chapter 7.（1）When yang qi is added to yin fluids，sweat results. See *Su Wen Ji Zhu*（*Collected Annotation of Su Wen*）.（2）When the yang pulse appears in the yin position，sweating results. See *Lei Jing*（*Classified Classic*）"Pulse and Color Chapter 29".

阳邪　侵犯阳分或阳经的邪气。出《灵枢·官针》。

阳邪（yáng xié）　**yang evil** The evil qi which attacks the yang or the yang meridians. See *Ling Shu* chapter 7.

阳杀　杀，消亡。阳杀，阳气消亡不生。出《素问·阴阳类论》。《素问·阴阳应象大论》有"阳生阴长，阳杀阴藏"，见该条。

阳杀（yáng shā）　**killed yang** *Shā* refers to kill, or eliminate. Killed yang refers to that the yang qi is eliminated and cannot be generated. See *Su Wen* chapter 79. See "阳生阴长，阳杀阴藏" in *Su Wen* chapter 5.

阳池　经穴名。手少阳三焦经之原穴。在手腕上陷者中。出《灵枢·本输》。

阳池（yáng chí）　**Yang Chi（SJ 4）**Acupoint name，and source acupoint of the triple *jiao* me-

ridian of hand *shaoyang*. Located in the depression of the wrist. See *Ling Shu* chapter 2.

阳谷　经穴名。手太阳小肠经之经穴。在手外侧腕中锐骨下方凹陷中。出《灵枢·本输》。

阳谷（yáng gǔ）　**Yang Gu（SI 5）**Acupoint name on the small intestine meridian of hand *taiyang*. Located in the depression below the protuberant bone in the lateral aspect of the wrist. See *Ling Shu* chapter 2.

阳明　① 二阳。出《素问·阴阳类论》。② 指两阳合明。出《素问·至真要大论》。③ 指两火并合。《灵枢·阴阳系日月》："两火并合，故为阳明。"见该条。④ 单指或统指手、足阳明大肠、胃及其经脉。出《素问·诊要经终论》《素问·五常政大论》《素问·六元正纪大论》。

阳明（yáng míng）　① *Yangming*. Refers to the second yang. See *Su Wen* chapter 79. ② Refers to the combination of two yang. See *Su Wen* chapter 74. ③ Refers to the combination of two fires. See "两火并合，故为阳明" in *Ling Shu* chapter 41. ④ Refers to the large intestine meridian or stomach meridian of hand or foot *yangming* individually or unified. See *Su Wen* chapter 16，chapter 70 and chapter 71.

阳明之政　即阳明司天之政。出《素问·六元正纪大论》。

阳明之政（yáng míng zhī zhèng）**policy of** *yangming* Namely，the policy of *yangming* which dominates the heaven. See *Su Wen* chapter 71.

阳明之复　运气术语。复，即六气偏胜情况下，而产生的复气。此指厥阴风木之气偏胜至一定程度，阳明燥金凉气来复，气候由温转凉，人体多见燥气伤肺损肝之病。出《素问·至真要大论》。

阳明之复（yáng míng zhī fù）**retaliation of** *yangming* Terminology of the circuits and qi. *Fù* refers to the reversal qi caused by the predominate six qi. It means that the qi of *jueyin* wind-wood is so exuberant that the cool dry metal qi of *yangming* returns, and the climate changes from warm to cool. Damage to the lung and the liver by dry qi is common in the human body. See *Su Wen* chapter 74.

阳明之胜　运气术语。指阳明燥金偏胜之气，如阳明司天在泉之时燥气偏盛，气候清凉而干燥，人体多见凉燥之气偏胜的肺病。出《素问·至真要大论》。

阳明之胜（yáng míng zhī shèng）**predominance of** *yangming* Terminology of the five circuits and six qi. Refers to the predominant dry-metal qi of *yangming*. For example，when *yangming* governs the heavens in the spring，dry qi is predominant，and with a cool and dry climate，people may suffer from lung diseases. See *Su Wen* chapter 69.

阳明之厥　六经厥之一。其病机为阳明经气逆乱，神明受扰。症见癫狂走呼，面赤身热，腹满，谵言、幻视等。出《素问·厥论》。

阳明之厥（yáng míng zhī jué）**recession in** *yangming* One of the six-meridian *jue* qi. The pathogenesis of the disease is the disorder of the *yangming* meridian qi and of the disturbance of spirit brilliance. Symptoms include mania，red complexions，fever，abdominal fullness，delirium，and hallucination，etc. See *Su Wen* chapter 45.

阳明为阖　出《灵枢·根结》。见"三阳之离合也……少阳为枢"条。

阳明为阖（yáng míng wéi hé）

Yangming is the gate. See *Ling Shu* chapter 5. See "三阳之离合也……少阳为枢".

阳明主肉 足阳明胃之经脉与脾相表里,脾主肌肉,故阳明所主亦为肉。见《素问·热论》参"脾主肉"条。

阳明主肉（yáng míng zhǔ ròu）

Flesh is dominated by *yangming*. The stomach meridian of foot *yangming* corresponds to the spleen meridian. As the spleen governs the muscles, therefore *yangming* also dominates the muscles. See *Su Wen* chapter 31. See "脾主肉".

阳明司天 运气术语。指上半年由阳明燥金之气主事时的气候病候等情况。凡纪年地支逢卯、酉之年,均属阳明燥金司天。该年上半年气候偏凉干燥。金能制木,临床多见肝病。出《素问·五常政大论》。

阳明司天（yáng míng sī tiān）

Yangming governs the heaven. Terminology for the five circuits and six qi. Refers to the climatic conditions and disease patterns in the first half of the year when dry-metal qi of *yangming* governs the heavens. *Yangming* dry-metal governing the heavens includes all the year of *mao* and *you* according to the Earthly Branches. In this half year, the climate is a little cool and dry. As metal restricts wood, liver diseases are commonly seen clinically. See *Su Wen* chapter 70.

阳明司天之政 指阳明燥金司天的气候、物候及疾病流行情况。凡逢纪年地支是卯、酉的年份为阳明燥金司天,其特点是:阳明主凉,主燥。该年上半年气候偏凉,干燥。物候以稻、麦类谷物生长良好,介虫、羽虫生育良好,毛虫生育不利。临床多见肝经失调,肺肝同病的疾病。政,主事,施政之意。出《素问·六元正纪大论》。

阳明司天之政（yáng míng sī tiān zhī zhèng） **policy of *yangming* governing the heaven** Refers to the climate, phenology and disease prevalence when *yangming* dry-metal governs the heavens. In the year of *mao* and *you*, according to the Earthly Branches, *yangming* dry-metal governs the heavens, and it is characterized by controlling coolness and dryness. Thus, the climate in the first half of the year will be cool and dry. In phenology, rice and wheat grains grow very well, creatures with shells and those with feathers also grow well, however caterpillars do not. Disorders of the liver meridian, and disorders of both the lung and liver are commonly seen clinically. *Zhèng* means management and policy. See *Su Wen* chapter 71.

阳明在泉 运气术语。指下半年由阳明燥金之气主事时的气候物候等情况。凡纪年地支逢子、午之年,均属阳明燥金在泉。该年下半年气候偏凉,偏燥。其所生成的药物或食物,在气味上也偏于凉燥,而具有滋润作用的药食物则生长不良。出《素问·五常政大论》。

阳明在泉(yáng míng zài quán) *yangming* in spring Terminology of the circuits and qi. Refers to the climate and phenology in the second half of the year when dry-metal qi of *yangming* supervises. In the year of *zi* and *wu*, according to the Earthly Branches, *yangming* dry-metal governs in spring. The climate in the second half of the year is a little bit cool and dry. Herbs and food grown are cool and dry in flavor, while herbs and food for nourishment do not grow very well. See *Su Wen* chapter 71.

阳明脉 指十二经脉中手阳明和足阳明经脉。出《素问·上古天真论》。

阳明脉(yáng míng mài) *yangming* meridian Refers to the hand *yangming* meridian and foot *yangming* meridian of the twelve regular meridians. See *Su Wen* chapter 1.

阳明脉解 《素问》篇名。阳明脉,指足阳明胃经。此篇主要解释阳明经有关情志病变的问题,故名。

阳明脉解(yáng míng mài jiě) **Explanation of the Yangming Meridian** Chapter title in *Su Wen*. The *yangming* meridian refers to the stomach meridian of foot *yangming*. This chapter mainly explains the problem of emotional diseases related with the *yangming* meridian, hence the name.

阳明厥逆 十二经厥之一,为足阳明经气厥逆之证。症见喘咳身热,容易发惊,衄血、呕血。出《素问·厥论》。

阳明厥逆(yáng míng jué nì) *jue*

ni of yangming One of the twelve meridians with symptoms of the reverse flow of foot *yangming*, such as panting and coughing, feverishness, tendency to be frightened, nosebleeds and vomitting blood. See *Su Wen* chapter 45.

阳明藏　指阳明经脉。藏，指脏腑。脏腑与经脉相连属，言阳明经脉，必赅括其所属脏腑。出《素问・经脉别论》。

阳明藏（yáng míng zàng）*yangming* **viscera** Refers to the *yangming* meridian. *Zàng* refers to the viscera and bowels, which are connected to the meridians. If the *yangming* meridians are mentioned, the viscera and bowels belonging to them are included as well. See *Su Wen* chapter 21.

阳明燥化　运气术语。化，制化，制则生化之意。根据五行原理，阳明凉燥之金气，可以制约风温之木气，不使过于偏胜，从而维持自然气候的正常，有利于万物的生长化成。出《素问・六元正纪大论》。

阳明燥化（yáng míng zào huà）**dryness transformation of** *yangming* Terminology for the five circuits and six qi. *Huà* means trans-formation. According to the principles of the five elements, the cool and dry metal qi of *yangming* restricts wind-warm wood qi in order to avoid its predominance, thus maintaining a normal natural climate and promoting the growth and transformation of all things on earth. See *Su Wen* chapter 71.

阳经　属阳的经脉。如太阳、少阳、阳明经者均是。出《素问・调经论》。

阳经（yáng jīng）**yang meridian** Meridians belonging to yang, such as *taiyang*, *shaoyang* and *yangming*. See *Su Wen* chapter 62.

阳脉　① 十二经脉中的手足三阳经脉，分属于六腑。出《灵枢・脉度》。② 盛阳之经脉，又称盛经。出《素问・水热穴论》《素问・腹中论》。③ 上部之脉。出《素问・脉解》。

阳脉（yáng mài）　① Three yang meridians of hand and foot, which belong to the six bowels. See *Ling Shu* chapter 17. ② Excessive yang meridian, also named excessive meridian. See *Su Wen* chapter 61 and chapter 40. ③ Upper meridian. See *Su*

六画

Wen chapter 49.

阳络 ①与阴络相对言,指在上、在表的络脉。出《灵枢·百病始生》。②阳明经之络。出《素问·调经论》。

阳络(yáng luò) ① Yang collaterals. Opposite to the yin collaterals, and refers to the upper or superficial collaterals. See *Ling Shu* chapter 66. ② Collaterals of the *yangming* meridian. See *Su Wen* chapter 62.

阳病 属阳分的病变,如气病,阳经、六腑、阳脏或病位表浅的病,均可称阳病。出《素问·阴阳应象大论》《素问·太阴阳明论》。

阳病(yáng bìng) **yang diseases** Diseases belonging to yang, such as diseases related to the qi, yang meridians, six bowels, yang viscera or diseases located superficially, all of them can be called yang diseases. See *Su Wen* chapter 5 and chapter 29.

阳陵泉 经穴名。出《灵枢·邪气藏府病形》。

阳陵泉(yáng líng quán) **Yang Ling Quan（GB 34）** Acupoint name. See *Ling Shu* chapter 4.

阳盛生外热 指外邪入侵所致的热证。其机制是:外盛寒邪,上焦不通,腠理闭塞,卫气郁遏而致肌表发热。出《素问·调经论》。

阳盛生外热(yáng shèng shēng wài rè) **Yang exuberance generates external heat.** Refers to the heat patterns caused by the external evils. Its mechanism is: exuberant cold evil outside obstructing the upper *jiao*. The interstices and sweat pores are obstructed, causing the skin to be hot because of the stagnation of defensive qi. See *Su Wen* chapter 62.

阳盛则热 出《素问·疟论》。义同"阳胜则热"。见"阳胜则热,阴胜则寒"条。

阳盛则热(yáng shèng zé rè) **When the yang is exuberant, there is heat.** See *Su Wen* chapter 35. The meaning is the same as "阳胜则热". See "阳胜则热,阴胜则寒".

阳辅 经穴名。属足少阳胆经。在足外踝上四寸,辅骨前,绝骨端,为经穴。出《灵枢·本输》。

阳辅(yáng fǔ) **Yang Fu（GB 38）** Acupoint name belonging to the gallbladder meridian of foot *shaoyang*. It is located 4 *cun* above the exterior malleolus, in front of the supporting bone, at the tip of the calf bone, also a stream acupoint. See *Ling Shu* chapter 2.

阳虚　阳气虚弱不足。表现畏寒、肢冷、疼痛等症状。出《素问·调经论》。

阳虚（yáng xū）　**yin deficiency** Deficiency of yang qi, which is characterized by the symptoms of aversion to cold, cold limbs, and pain. See *Su Wen* chapter 62.

阳脱　阳气亡脱。出《灵枢·终始》。

阳脱（yáng tuō）　**yang depletion** Depletion of yang qi. See *Ling Shu* chapter 9.

阳维之脉　奇经八脉之一，维络全身诸阳经并与阴维脉相互维系之脉，有调节气血盛衰的作用。出《素问·刺腰痛》。

阳维之脉（yáng wéi zhī mài）　*yangwei* **meridian** One of the eight extraordinary meridians, connecting with all the yang meridians and *yinwei* meridian, with the function of regulating qi and blood. See *Su Wen* chapter 41.

阳厥　①病证名。指怒狂之神志异常疾患。因情志猝受刺激，致阳气厥逆化火，扰乱神明，故名。出《素问·病能论》。②足少阳经脉之气厥逆的病候。出《灵枢·经脉》。

阳厥（yáng jué）　① Disease name, refers to diseases characterized by abnormal mental

disorders caused by anger and mania. Due to the sudden emotional stimulus, yang qi reversely turns into fire and disturbs the spirit brilliance, hence the name. See *Su Wen* chapter 46. ② Diseases or symptoms caused by the reverse flow of qi of the foot *shaoyang* meridian. See *Ling Shu* chapter 10.

阳跷　即阳跷脉。奇经八脉之一，其循行路线，从足太阳经分出，起于足跟外侧，从外踝后上行，经腹部，沿胸部后外侧，经肩部，颈外侧，上挟口角，到目内眦，与手足太阳经、阴跷脉会合，上行入风池，在项中的两筋间入脑。出《素问·缪刺论》。

阳跷（yáng qiáo）　*yangqiao* **meridian** One of the eight extraordinary meridians, which runs divergent from the *taiyang* meridian of the foot and starts from the lateral aspect of the heel. It ascends behind the external malleolus, passes the abdomen and converges with the *taiyang* meridian of the foot and hand as well as the *yinqiao* meridian at inner canthus along the posterolateral aspect of the chest, shoulder, lateral neck and angulus oris successively. Then it ascends to Feng Chi (GB 20) acupoint and enters the brain through the two sinews in the neck. See *Su Wen* chapter 63.

阳溪　经穴名。手阳明大肠经之经穴。在手腕上侧横纹前，两筋间凹陷中。出《灵枢·本输》。

阳溪（yáng xī）　**Yang Xi (LI 5)** Acupoint name on the large intestine meridian of hand *yangming*，and located in front of the striation on the upper side of the wrist，in the indentation between the two sinews. See *Ling Shu* chapter 2.

阳精　谓东南方的阳气。出《素问·五常政大论》。

阳精（yáng jīng）　**yang essence** It refers to the yang qi from the southeast. See *Su Wen* chapter 70.

阴　① 古代哲学概念。与阳相对，凡具向下、寒冷、安静、晦暗、低下等特性的事物或现象均属阴。出《素问·阴阳应象大论》。② 代表人体组织结构中阴经（如手足三阴经）、阴脏（如脾、肾）、五脏，以及在里的、内侧的、下部的部位等。出《灵枢·寿夭刚柔》《素问·六节藏象论》。③ 代表生命过程中具有凝聚、滋润、抑制等作用或表现的物质及功能，统属于阴。出《素问·生气通天论》《素问·阴阳应象大论》。④ 代表阴有余的病证脉象。出《素问·阴阳别论》。⑤ 代表药物的性味功能，酸苦属阴。出《素问·阴阳应象大论》。

阴（yīn）　① Yin. A concept in ancient philosophy. In contrast to yang, all things or phenomena with characteristics of downward，cold，quiet，dark，low，etc. all belong to yin. See *Su Wen* chapter 5. ② It represents the yin meridians (such as the three yin meridians of hands and feet)，yin viscera (such as spleen and kidney)，five viscera，and the inner，inside or lower parts of the human body. See *Ling Shu* chapter 6 and *Su Wen* chapter 9. ③ It represents the substances and functions in the processes of life，such as condensation，moistening and inhibition，all belong to yin. See *Su Wen* chapter 3 and chapter 5. ④ It represents the pulse of the disease with excess yin. See *Su Wen* chapter 7. ⑤ It represents the nature，taste and function of materia medica. Sour and bitter flavors belong to yin. See *Su Wen* chapter 5.

阴人　指偏于阴性体质的人。阴人包括多阴无阳的太阴之人，多阴少阳的少阴之人，他们在生理、性格心理、外形、病理反应各方面有差异。参"太阴之人""少阴之人"。出《灵枢·通天》。

阴人（yīn rén）　**yin person** Refers to a person with a yin constitution. Yin people include *taiyin* people with the superabundance of yin and the absence of yang, and the *shaoyin* people with superabundant yin and less yang. There are differences in physiology, personality, psychology, appearance, and pathological reactions among them. See "太阴之人" and "少阴之人". See *Ling Shu* chapter 72.

阴中之太阴　阴阳之中有阴阳之分。阴中之阴阳，其阴尤盛，故谓太阴。① 指肾，位居于下，属阴位，故称。出《灵枢·九针十二原》。② 指足之阴侧。足在下。阴气尤盛，为阴中之太阴。出《灵枢·阴阳系日月》。

阴中之太阴（yīn zhōng zhī tài yīn）　*taiyin* in the yin Yin and yang can be subdivided into yin and yang. Yin and yang in yin, or with excessive yin, is called *taiyin* . ① Refers to the kidney, which is located in the lower position, or yin position. See *Ling Shu* chapter 1. ② Refers to the yin side of the foot. The foot is at the lower part of the body where yin qi is excessive, thus it is the *taiyin* in yin. See *Ling Shu* chapter 41.

阴中之少阳　① 指肝。位居膈下属阴，但为阳脏，故称。出《灵枢·九针十二原》。② 指足之阳侧。足在下，属阴，其外侧阳面，阳气相对偏弱，故称。出《灵枢·阴阳系日月》。

阴中之少阳（yīn zhōng zhī shào yáng）　① *Shaoyang* in the yin. Refers to the liver. It is located under the diaphragm and belongs to yin, but it is a yang viscera. See *Ling Shu* chapter 1. ② Refers to the yang side of the foot. The foot at the lower part of the body belongs to yin, and the outside of it is yang, however the yang qi is relatively weak and hence the name. See *Ling Shu* chapter 41.

阴中之少阴　① 指足少阴肾之经脉。肾本阴脏，其脉起于足心之涌泉穴是居于阴分，故称。出《素问·阴阳离合论》。② 指肺。为"阳中之少阴"之误。出

六画

《灵枢·阴阳系日月》。

阴中之少阴（yīn zhōng zhī shào yīn）　① *Shaoyin* in the yin. Refers to the kidney meridian of foot *shaoyin*. The kidney is a yin viscera，whose meridian starts at Yong Quan（KI 1）acupoint at the sole of the foot located in the yin phase. See *Su Wen* chapter 6. ② Refers to the lung. It is the mistaken "*shaoyin* in yang". See *Ling Shu* chapter 41.

阴中之至阴　指脾。脾居中焦，为阴脏，位于心肺与肝肾之间；外应长夏，处于春夏与秋冬之交，由阳入阴，故为阴中之至阴。至，有达之义。出《素问·金匮真言论》。

阴中之至阴（yīn zhōng zhī zhì yīn）　*zhiyin* in the yin Refers to the spleen. The spleen is located in the middle *jiao*，and is the yin organ between the heart，lung，liver and kidney. It corresponds with the late summer，at the turn of spring-summer and autumn-winter. As the yang proceeds to yin，thus it is so called. Zhi means extreme. See *Su Wen* chapter 4.

阴中之阳　① 指半夜至凌晨一段时间。夜为阴，自夜半鸡鸣至平旦日出之时，阴气渐衰，阳气渐生，故为阴中之阳。鸡鸣，夜半；平旦，凌晨日出之时。出《素问·金匮真言论》。② 指肝。其为阳脏，而居于腹中阴位，故称。出《素问·金匮真言论》。③ 指植物初冒出土。地为阴，万物初生，长出地面，为阴中之阳。出《素问·阴阳离合论》。④ 指足太阳膀胱经脉。足太阳膀胱经与足少阴肾经相表里，阴阳相离又相合，故称。出《素问·阴阳离合论》。⑤ 指足阳明胃之经脉。足阳明胃经与足太阴经相表里，阴阳相离又相合，故称。出《素问·阴阳离合论》。

阴中之阳（yīn zhōng zhī yang）　① Yang in the yin. Refers to the period from midnight to early morning. Night is yin. From the crowing of the cocks to dawn，yin qi gradually declines and yang qi augments，thus it is the yang in yin. The crowing of the cocks refers to midnight；*Píng dàn* refers to dawn or sunrise. See *Su Wen* chapter 4. ② Refers to the liver. It is the yang organ，which is located in the yin position of the abdomen，hence the name. See *Su Wen* chapter

六画

4. ③ Refers to newly unearthed plants. The earth is yin, all things are born and grow out of the ground. It is the yang in yin. See *Su Wen* chapter 6. ④ Refers to the bladder meridian of foot *taiyang*. The bladder meridian of foot *taiyang* and the kidney meridian of foot *shaoyin* are interiorly and exteriorly related to each other. Yin and yang are opposed to and depend on each other. Hence its name. See *Su Wen* chapter 6. ⑤ Refers to the stomach meridian of foot *yangming*. The stomach meridian of foot *yangming* and foot *taiyin* are interiorly and exteriorly related to each other. Yin and yang are opposed to and depend on each other, hence the name. See *Su Wen* chapter 6.

阴中之阴 ① 指一日之中日落至半夜一段时间,阴气最盛,故为阴中之阴。夜为阴,黄昏合夜至半夜鸡鸣之时。出《素问·金匮真言论》。② 指肾。其为阴脏,又处于下焦阴位,故称。出《素问·金匮真言论》。③ 指阴处。天地之间,万物初生,未长出地面时,叫阴处,又称为阴中之阴。出《素问·阴阳离合论》。④ 指足太阴脾之经脉。脾居腹中为阴,其脉起于足大趾端之隐白穴,下者为阴,是居于阴分,故为阴中之阴。出《素问·阴阳离合论》。

阴中之阴 (yīn zhōng zhī yīn)

① Yin in the yin. Refers to the period from sunset to midnight in a day, when yin qi is the most abundant, thus it is the yin within yin. The night pertains to yin, this phrase refers to the period from dusk to the midnight. See *Su Wen* chapter 4. ② Refers to the kidney, which is the yin organ located in the yin position of the lower *jiao*, hence the name. See *Su Wen* chapter 4. ③ Refers to the location of yin between heaven and earth, when all things are born yet do not grow out of the ground, and it is called the location of yin, or yin in the yin. See *Su Wen* chapter 6. ④ Refers to the spleen meridian of foot *taiyin*. The spleen is the yin organ which is located in the abdomen. The spleen meridian starts at Yin Bai (SP 1) at the end of the big toe. The lower part of the body is Yin, and thus the yin position gives it its name of yin in the yin. See *Su Wen* chapter 6.

阴气　① 与人体阳气相对,有制约阳气,达到阴阳平衡的作用。出《素问·生气通天论》。② 指阴精。出《素问·阴阳应象大论》。③ 指五神脏。出《素问·痹论》。④ 指自然界具有收藏作用的寒凉之气。出《素问·脉要精微论》。⑤ 指水邪。出《素问·脉解》。

阴气(yīn qì)　① Yin qi. Opposite to yang qi in the human body, and whose function is to restrain yang qi to achieve balance between yin and yang. See *Su Wen* chapter 3. ② Refers to yin essence. See *Su Wen* chapter 5. ③ Refers to the five spirit viscera. See *Su Wen* chapter 43. ④ Refers to the cold qi with the function of storing in nature. See *Su Wen* chapter 17. ⑤ Refers to water evil. See *Su Wen* chapter 49.

阴尺动脉　指手太阴尺泽穴上三寸动脉处。是阴气所在之处,古人认为应禁针。出《灵枢·本输》。

阴尺动脉(yīn chǐ dòng mài) *yin chi* **pulsating point** Refers to the location of the pulsating point three *cun* above Chi Ze (LU 5) acupoint on the hand *taiyin* meridian. It is the location of yin qi, which was forbidden to be pierced in ancient times. See *Ling Shu* chapter 2.

阴邪　① 侵犯阴分的邪气。出《素问·疟论》。② 部位较深的邪气。出《灵枢·官针》。③ 指湿邪。出《素问·水热穴论》。

阴邪(yīn xié)　① The evil attacks the yin aspect. See *Su Wen* chapter 35. ② The evil qi is deeply located. See *Ling Shu* chapter 7. ③ Refers to wet evil. See *Su Wen* chapter 61.

阴阳　① 古代哲学概念。代表相关事物的相对属性,或一个事物内部相互对应的两个方面,以此说明自然界万物发生、发展、变化的规律。出《素问·阴阳应象大论》《灵枢·阴阳系日月》。② 代表人体的组织结构。出《素问·宝命全形论》《素问·金匮真言论》《灵枢·寿夭刚柔》《灵枢·九针论》。③ 代表营卫气血等物质。出《灵枢·营卫生会》《素问·阴阳应象大论》。④ 概括人的生理病理。出《素问·生气通天论》《素问·阴阳应象大论》。⑤ 代表证候与脉象。出《素问·阴阳应象大论》《灵枢·终始》。⑥ 代表药物性味。出《素问·至真要大论》。⑦ 表示体质类型。出《灵枢·通天》。⑧ 古医籍名。已佚。出《素问·病能论》。⑨ 病因。指房事。出《素问·调经论》。

阴阳(yīn yáng) ① Yin yang. A concept in ancient philosophy, which represented the relative property of related things or the two corresponding aspects of one thing, so as to explain the law of occurrence, development and change of all things in nature. See *Su Wen* chapter 5 and *Ling Shu* chapter 41. ② Refers to the tissue structure of the human body. See *Su Wen* chapter 25 and chapter 4, *Ling Shu* chapter 6 and chapter 78. ③ Refers to the nutrient qi, defensive qi, and qi and blood. See *Ling Shu* chapter 18 and *Su Wen* chapter 5. ④ Summarizes the physiology and pathology of the human body. See *Su Wen* chapter 3 and chapter 5. ⑤ Refers to symptoms and pulse conditions. See *Su Wen* chapter 5 and *Ling Shu* chapter 9. ⑥ Refers to the property and flavor of medicinal plants. See *Su Wen* chapter 74. ⑦ Refers to the constitutional patterns. See *Ling Shu* chapter 72. ⑧ Name of ancient medical book that has been lost in history. See *Su Wen* chapter 46. ⑨ Cause of disease. Refers to sexual activity. See *Su Wen* chapter 62.

阴阳二十五人 ① 指二十五种体质类型。古人运用阴阳五行学说,结合人体肤色、体形、禀性及对自然变化的适应能力等方面的特征,总结了木、火、土、金、水五种体质类型,然后又根据五音太少、阴阳属性以及手足之阳经的左右上下、气血多少之差异,将上述每一类型再推演为五类,即五五二十五种体质类型。出《灵枢·阴阳二十五人》。②《灵枢》篇名。此篇主要讨论二十五种人的体质特性,并提出不同的治疗原则。

阴阳二十五人(yīn yáng ér shí wǔ rén) ① Twenty-five types of people divided according to yin and yang. Combined with the characteristics of skin color, body shape, nature, and adaptability to natural changes in human body, the ancients concluded that there were five types of body constitutions, namely wood, fire, earth, metal and water based on the yin-yang theory. Then，according to the five tones，nature of yin and yang, as well as the difference between the left and right sides of the yang meridians of hand and foot，and the amount of qi and blood，each of the above types was further divided into five categories，thus five times five was twenty-five, and the name came about. See *Ling Shu* chapter 64. ② Chapter title in *Ling Shu*. This chapter mainly discusses the physical characteristics of the twenty-five types of people，and puts forward the different treatment principles for each physical constitution.

阴阳十二官相使　古医籍名,已佚。从本篇所述推测,它可能是一本关于脏腑病证及治疗的医著。出《素问·奇病论》。

阴阳十二官相使（yīn yáng shí èr guān xiāng shǐ）*Mutual Engagement Among the Twelve Officials of Yin and Yang* Name of an ancient chinese medical book，which has been lost in history. It can be speculated from this chapter that it may be a medical book on the syndrome and treatment of diseases in the viscera and bowels. See *Su Wen* chapter 47.

阴阳之人　即阴阳二十五人。详见该条。出《灵枢·阴阳二十五人》。

阴阳之人（yīn yáng zhī rén）**yin-yang type people** Refers to the twenty-five types of people divided according to yin and yang. See "阴阳二十五人". See *Ling Shu* chapter 64.

阴阳之政　政,主事、施政的意思。阴阳,指三阴三阳。即少阴、太阴、厥阴、太阳、阳明、少阳值年的气候、物候及疾病流行的特点。《素问·六元正纪大论》。参"厥阴之政""少阴之政""太阴之政""少阳之政""阳明之政""太阳之政"诸条。

阴阳之政（yīn yáng zhī zhèng）**policies of yin and yang** *Zhèng* means policy. *Yīn yáng* refers to the three yin and the three yang. Namely，the characteristics of the climate，phenology and epidemic diseases of the *shaoyin*，*taiyin*，*jueyin*，*taiyang*，*yangming* and *shaoyang* years. See *Su Wen* chapter 71. See "厥阴之政""少阴之政""太阴之政""少阳之政""阳明之政" and "太阳之政".

阴阳不奇　奇（yǐ 倚）,倚,偏于一

六画

边。阴阳不倚,即阴阳协调不偏。出《灵枢·官能》。

阴阳不奇(yīn yáng bù yǐ) **unbiased yin and yang** "奇" is the same as "倚", and refers to unbiased. Unbiased yin and yang means neither yin nor yang dominate unilaterally. See *Ling Shu* chapter 73.

阴阳不通 指阴阳气血阻滞不畅。见《灵枢·玉版》。

阴阳不通(yīn yáng bù tōng) **obstruction of yin and yang** Refers to the obstruction of yin, yang, qì and the blood. See *Ling Shu* chapter 60.

阴阳内夺 夺,失去、耗损。阴阳内夺,即体内的阴阳之气均耗损。见《素问·脉解篇》。

阴阳内夺(yīn yáng nèi duó) **inner depletion of yin and yang** *Duó* means lost, or depletion. The inner depletion of yin and yang refers to the depletion of the qi of yin and yang in the body. See *Su Wen* chapter 49.

阴阳反他 阴阳不协调之意。"他" 是"作"之形误。出《素问·玉版论要》。

阴阳反他(yīn yáng fǎn tā) **Yin and yang oppose each other.** Refers to disharmony between yin and yang. 他 is the form error

of 作. See *Su Wen* chapter 15.

阴阳匀平 指阴阳均匀平衡、相互协调、无太过、无不及之象。出《素问·调经论》。

阴阳匀平(yīn yáng yún píng) **Yin and yang are evenly balanced.** Refers to the balance and harmony between yin and yang, without any manifestations of excess or deficiency. See *Su Wen* chapter 62.

阴阳平复 平,平衡;复,恢复。病有余用泻法,病不足用补法,其根本目的是使阴阳恢复平衡协调。出《灵枢·刺节真邪》。

阴阳平复(yīn yáng píng fù) **Yin and yang are to rebalanced.** The dredging method is used where there is a surplus, and the supplementing method is used where there is an insufficiency. The ultimate goal is to restore the balance of yin and yang. See *Ling Shu* chapter 75.

阴阳四溢 溢,盈满流失。阴阳四溢,原意是指因针刺不懂得逆顺补泻,致使阴阳气血溢失。出《灵枢·根结》。

阴阳四溢(yīn yáng sì yì) **Yin and yang spill over at all four ends.** "溢" refers to spill over. The original meaning of "yin and yang spill over at all four ends" is that the acupuncturist does not know the proper reinforcing and reducing manipulations, resulting in the loss of yin, yang, qi and blood. See *Ling Shu* chapter 5.

阴阳传　古籍名。已佚，据书名推测，是一部阐释阴阳学说的专著。出《素问·著至教论》。

阴阳传（yīn yáng zhuàn）　***Discussions on Yin and Yang*** Name of an ancient book which was lost in history. According to the title of the book, it was a monograph expounding the yin and yang theory. See *Su Wen* chapter 75.

阴阳交　① 病名。为热病中阳邪交入阴分而不解，邪盛精败的危重证候，多出现于热病后期，症见汗出而热不能退，脉仍躁动疾数，不能进食，神情躁狂。其病机为邪热炽盛，阴液枯涸，胃气败绝，神明受扰。出《素问·评热病论》《素问·阴阳类论》。② 指脉。阴即右脉，阳即左脉，交为交叉之义。出《素问·五运行大论》。

阴阳交（yīn yáng jiāo）　① **Yin and yang interaction**. A disease in which the critical syndrome of exuberant *xie* (Evil) and corrupted essence causes the invasion of yang *xie* (Evil) into the yin aspect. It occurs mostly in the later stages of febrile diseases and manifests with sweating and lingering fever, a rapid and agitated pulse, the inability to eat and mania. The pathogenesis is exuberant pathogenic heat, exhausted yin fluid, vanquished stomach qi and disturbed spirit brilliance. See *Su Wen* chapter 33 and chapter 79. ② Refers to the pulse. Yin is the right pulse and yang is the left pulse, and yin yang cross each other. See *Su Wen* chapter 67.

阴阳异位　出《素问·太阴阳明论》。（1）阴阳所主之位不同。如春夏从阳，秋冬从阴；阴主内、阳主外；阴在下、阳在上；营阴在脉中、卫阳在脉外；阴脉上行、阳脉下行；太阴在内、阳明主外等。（2）阴阳反常之位。如阴在下而反上，阳在上而反下。

阴阳异位（yīn yáng yì wèi）　**Yin and yang occupy different positions**. See *Su Wen* chapter 29. （1）Yin and yang dominate different positions. For instance, spring and summer pertains to yang, while autumn and winter pertains to yin. Yin dominates the interior and yang dominates the exterior. Yin is at the lower places，while yang is at the upper places. Nutrient yin is inside the vessels and defensive yang is outside the vessels. *Yin meridians run upwards and yang meridians go downwards. Taiyin is in the interior and yangming dominates the exterior.* (2) Abnormal positions of yin and yang. For instance，yin is at the upper places and yang is at the lower places.

阴阳如一 出《灵枢·邪客》。(1)指阴阳表里气血俱败伤。(2)指人迎、气口脉若一。

阴阳如一（yīn yáng rú yī） **Yin and yang are like one.** See *Ling Shu* chapter 71. (1) Indicates the damage to yin and yang, interior and exterior，qi and blood. (2) It means that the *ren ying* pulse and the *qi kou* pulse are like one.

阴阳更胜 更，更迭。阴阳更胜，即阴阳更迭，消长盛衰的变化。出《素问·疟论》。或言人体及自然界阴阳之气更胜。出《素问·五常政大论》。

阴阳更胜（yīn yáng gēng shèng） **alternating domination of yin and yang** Indicates the changes of waning and waxing of yin and yang. See *Su Wen* chapter 35. Or，it means the alternating domination of yin qi and yang qi in the human body and in nature. See *Su Wen* chapter 70.

阴阳别论 《素问》篇名。别，区别。此篇主要论述阴阳，辨别真脏脉、病脉的方法，故名。

阴阳别论（yīn yáng bié lùn） **Separate Discussion on Yin and Yang** Chapter title in *Su Wen*. In this chapter，yin and yang，and methods to identify visceral exhaustion pulses and abnormal pulses are discussed. Hence the name.

阴阳系日月 《灵枢》篇名。系，联系。阴阳系日月，即通过联系日月运转的情况来说明阴阳的盛衰消长。此篇以天人相应的观点，把自然界天地阴阳日月运转的情况与人体手足阴阳经脉联系起来，并据此提出针刺方面的注意事项。故名。

阴阳系日月（yīn yáng xì rì yuè） **Correspondence Between Yin and Yang and the Sun and the Moon** Chapter name in *Ling Shu*. The correspondence between yin and yang and the sun and the moon is used to indicate exuberance and debilitation,

六画

and the rising and falling of yin and yang in consideration to the movement of the sun and the moon. In this chapter, from the viewpoint of correspondence between nature and humans, the movement of heaven and earth, yin and yang, sun and moon, is connected with the yin and yang channels of the hands and feet of the body, and needling precautions are outlined. Hence its name.

阴阳应象大论　《素问》篇名。阴阳,是中国古代哲学的一对范畴。应,应验。象,征象、现象。此篇主要论述阴阳的基本概念、相互关系以及在医学中的具体应用,其内容十分丰富,故名为"大论"。

阴阳应象大论（yīn yáng yìng xiàng dà lùn）　**Major Discussion on the Theory of Yin and Yang and the Corresponding Relationships Among all the Things in Nature** Chapter title in *Su Wen*. Yin and yang are a pair of concepts in ancient Chinese philosophy. *Yìng* refers to corresponding. *Xiàng* refers to manifestation or sign. In this chapter, the basic concepts of yin and yang, their relationship

and specific applications in medicine are discussed in detail. The content is very rich, so it is called "Major Discussion".

阴阳易　易,变易,言脉象之阴阳与时令、天气之阴阳不相应。如阴位见阳脉,阳位见阴脉,此为阴阳之乱,属危候。出《素问・至真要大论》。

阴阳易（yīn yáng yì）　**changes of yin and yang** *Yì* refers to changes, which means that the yin and yang of pulse manifestations are not corresponding to the seasons or the yin and yang of the celestial qi. For instance, a yang pulse is seen in the yin position and vice versa. This is a yin and yang disorder and indicates a critical disease. See *Su Wen* chapter 74.

阴阳易居　易,变易。阴阳易居,因邪入经脉而使阴阳气血的运行变易逆乱。出《灵枢・终始》。

阴阳易居（yīn yáng yì jū）　**yin and yang exchanging places** *Yì* means exchange. It refers to that pathogenic qi enters the channels and leads to disordered movement of yin and yang, and qi and blood. See *Ling Shu* chapter 9.

阴阳和　出《素问・上古天真论》。

六画

（1）男女两性交合。（2）阴阳气血调和。

阴阳和（yīn yáng hé） **harmony of yin and yang** See *Su Wen* chapter 1. (1) Intercourse between men and women. (2) Harmony between yin and yang, and qi and blood.

阴阳和平之人 体质名,属五志之人中阴阳气和者。其人血脉调和,心安不惧,志闲少欲,位尊而自谦,顺从四时的变化,无为而治。外表和蔼可亲,言行得体。故治疗必须仔细诊其阴阳虚实,采用相应的治疗原则。出《灵枢·通天》。

阴阳和平之人（yīn yáng hé píng zhī rén） **people with a harmonious balance of yin and yang** Name of constitution. Refers to people among the five-emotion types with harmony in yin and yang. These people have harmonious blood vessels and live in peace and contentment without any fear, they are modest in a high position and obedient to the changes of the four seasons, and do not go against nature. They look amiable and behave properly. So in treatment, yin and yang, deficiency and excess should be differentiated carefully to determine the corresponding treatment principles. See *Ling Shu* chapter 72.

阴阳相过曰溜 长夏之时,阴阳之气微上微下而相过,其脉滑利。溜,古通流,流利之意。出《素问·阴阳别论》。

阴阳相过曰溜（yīn yáng xiāng guò yuē liū） **stream-like when yin and yang surpass each other** In the late summer, yin qi and yang qi ascend and descend slightly and surpass each other, and the pulse is slippery. "溜" is the same as "流", which refers the slippery. See *Su Wen* chapter 7.

阴阳相倾 阴阳失调,偏倾于一方,造成阴阳的偏胜与偏衰。出《素问·调经论》。

阴阳相倾（yīn yáng xiāng qīng） **Yin and yang lose their balance.** Imbalance of yin and yang leads to abnormal exuberance or debilitation of yin or yang. See *Su Wen* chapter 62.

阴阳相移 阴阳交争,虚实更移,或阳虚阴实,或阳实阴虚,此指疟疾发作的机理。出《素问·疟论》。

阴阳相移（yīn yáng xiāng yí） **Yin and yang moves into each other's section.** Yin qi and yang qi rise and descend, and interact in struggle，leading to yang deficiency and yin excess，or yang exccss and yin deficiency，which is the pathogenesis of malaria. See *Su Wen* chapter 35.

阴阳相错　① 阴阳错乱。出《素问·八正神明论》。② 阴阳交错。天地阴阳之气相互作用，变生万物。出《素问·天元纪大论》。

阴阳相错（yīn yáng xiāng cuò）

① Disorder of yin and yang. See *Su Wen* chapter 26. ② Intersection of yin and yang. Yin qi and yang qi in heaven and earth intersect with each other and all things come into being. See *Su Wen* chapter 66.

阴阳相薄　薄（bó 搏），通"搏"，抗争的意思，阴阳相薄，即阴阳相争。出《素问·脉解》。

阴阳相薄（yīn yáng xiāng bó）

Yin qi and yang qi strike at each other. "薄" is the same as "搏". Means the struggle between yin and yang. See *Su Wen* chapter 49.

阴阳类论　《素问》篇名。阴阳，指三阴三阳经脉；类，类聚。此篇主要讨论三阴三阳经脉名称的含义，及三阴三阳的变化而产生的疾病和脉象，并论述了疾病的预后与四时阴阳关系。这些内容都是以阴阳类聚加以

阐述的，故名。

阴阳类论（yīn yáng lèi lùn）　**Discussion on the Categorization of Yin and Yang** Chapter title in *Su Wen*. Yin and yang refer to the three yin and three yang channels. In this chapter, consideration to the categorization of yin and yang, the meaning of the names of the channels, changes in the channels and the diseases ensued, and pulse manifestations is prioritized, and the relationship between disease prognosis and the yin and yang in the four seasons is expounded.

阴阳结斜　出《素问·阴阳别论》。（1）斜，同邪。邪气郁结于阴经、阳经。（2）斜，指偏。阴阳偏于一方，或寒，或热。

阴阳结斜（yīn yáng jié xié）

Pathogenic factors stagnates in both yin and yang meridians. See *Su Wen* chapter 7. (1) "斜" is the same as "邪". Pathogenic qi stagnating in both yin and yang meridians. (2) Xié refers to move to one side. Yin and yang are one-sided，tending towards hot or cold.

阴阳俱感　① 阴、阳经脉均感受邪气。出《素问·缪刺论》。② 内

六画

外皆伤。出《灵枢·邪气藏府病形》。

阴阳俱感（yīn yáng jù gǎn）
① Both yin and yang channels are attacked by pathogenic qi. See *Su Wen* chapter 63. ② Damage to both the interior and exterior. See *Ling Shu* chapter 4.

阴阳俱溢　溢，满溢、极盛的意思，人迎脉盛，且大且数，名溢阳；寸口脉盛，且大且数，名溢阴；人迎与寸口脉比平时大三倍以上，此为阴阳极盛的表现，称为阴阳俱溢。出《灵枢·终始》。

阴阳俱溢（yīn yáng jù yì）　**Both yin qi and yang qi spill over.** Spilling over means extreme exuberance. Yang qi spills over when the qi is abundant at the *ren ying* opening with a large and rapid pulse，and yin qi spills over when the qi is abundant at the *cun kou* with a large and rapid pulse. Both yin qi and yang qi spill over when the qi is three times or more abundant than normal，both at the *ren ying* and *cun kou*，indicating extreme exuberance of yin qi and yang qi. See *Ling Shu* chapter 9.

阴阳离合论　《素问》篇名。

阴阳离合论（yīn yáng lí hé lùn）　Separation and Combination of Yin and Yang Chapter title in *Su Wen*.

阴阳清浊　《灵枢》篇名。清，清气；浊，浊气。此篇主要论述人体清气、浊气的输注过程，并根据阴阳规律，说明清中有浊，浊中有清的道理，以指导针刺治疗，故名。

阴阳清浊（yīn yáng qīng zhuó）　**Yin and Yang, Clear and Turbid** Chapter title in *Ling Shu*. *Qīng* refers to the clear qi，and *zhuó* refers to the turbid qi. In this chapter，infusion of the clear and turbid qi of the human body is discussed，and in accordance with the law of yin and yang，the truth of turbid qi in clear qi and vice versa is explained to guide the acupuncture treatment. Hence its name.

阴阳喜怒　见《素问·调经论》。（1）七情随人体气质之不同而有所偏，如喜之属阳，怒之属阴。（2）言房事与情志。阴阳指房事、喜怒概括七情。

阴阳喜怒（yīn yáng xǐ nù）　**sexual union of yin and yang and emotions such as joy or anger** See *Su Wen* chapter 62.（1）The seven emotions are biased depen-

六画

ding on human temperament, for example, joy pertains to yang and anger yin. (2) Sexual intercourse and emotions. Yin and yang are used to talk about sexual intercourse, and joy and anger refer to the seven emotions in general.

阴阳跷　阴跷脉和阳跷脉的合称。出《素问·气府论》。

阴阳跷（yīn yáng qiáo）　*yinqiao and yangqiao* meridians Combined term for the *yinqiao* and *yangqiao* meridians. See *Su Wen* chapter 59.

阴谷　经穴名。足少阴肾经之合穴。在辅骨后，大筋下，小筋上，按之应手，屈膝得之。出《灵枢·本输》。

阴谷（yīn gǔ）　**Yin Gu（KI 10）** Acupoint name of the *he*-sea acupoint of the kidney meridian of foot *shaoyin*. It is located behind the auxiliary bone, below the big sinew, and above the small sinew. If one presses the Yin Gu acupoint, the hand will feel a response. It can be located by bending the knee. See *Ling Shu* chapter 2.

阴卵　睾丸。出《素问·骨空论》。

阴卵（yīn luǎn）　**testicles** See *Su Wen* chapter 60.

阴刺　① 刺法之一。指左右配穴针刺法，如下肢寒厥的病症，可同时针左右两侧的足少阴经穴。出《灵枢·官针》。② 阳刺或扬刺之误。出《素问·长刺节论》。

阴刺（yīn cì）　① Yin needling. One of the needling techniques. Refers to the needling with a combination of right and left acupoints. For example, to treat cold reversal in legs, foot *shaoyin* meridians should be pierced bilaterally. See *Ling Shu* chapter 7. ② Mistaken *yang* needling or dissemination needling. See *Su Wen* chapter 55.

阴股　大腿内侧。出《素问·刺禁论》。

阴股（yīn gǔ）　**yin thigh** Refers to the inner side of the thighs. See *Su Wen* chapter 52.

阴经　指手足三阴经脉，包括太阴、少阴、厥阴经。出《灵枢·邪气藏府病形》。

阴经（yīn jīng）　**yin meridian** Refers to the three yin meridians of the hands and feet, including the *taiyin* meridian, *shaoyin* meridian, and *jueyin* meridian. See *Ling Shu* chapter 4.

阴脉　① 足三阴经脉。出《素问·厥论》，见《素问集注》。② 属

六画

阴的脉象,如细脉、沉脉。出《灵枢·动输》。

阴脉(yīn mài)　① Yin meridian. Refers to the three yin meridians of the feet. See *Su Wen* chapter 45. See *Su Wen Ji Zhu* (*Collected Annotation of Su Wen*). ② The pulse condition pertaining to yin,such as a thin deep pulse. See *Ling Shu* chapter 62.

阴洛　九宫之一,即巽宫,居于东南方位。出《灵枢·九宫八风》。

阴洛(yīn luò)　*yin luo* One the of nine mansions,namely the *xun* mansion,located in the Southeast direction. See *Ling Shu* chapter 77.

阴病　属阴分的病变,如血病,阴经、阴脏或病位较深的病,均可称阴病。出《素问·阴阳应象大论》《素问·太阴阳明论》。

阴病(yīn bìng)　**yin diseases** Diseases pertaining to the yin aspect,such as blood diseases, or diseases related to the yin meridians,yin viscera,or located in deep parts,are all called yin diseases. See *Su Wen* chapter 5 and chapter 29.

阴陵泉　经穴名。足太阴脾经之合穴,在小腿内侧,胫骨内侧踝下缘凹陷中。出《灵枢·四时气》。

阴陵泉(yīn líng quán)　**Yin Ling Quan**(**SP 9**) Acupoint name. The *he*-sea acupoint of the spleen meridian of foot *taiyin*. It is located on the medial side of the leg,in the depression of the medial tibia and the lower edge of the ankle. See *Ling Shu* chapter 19.

阴盛生内寒　阴寒之气积于胸中,损伤阳气而出现内寒证。《素问·调经论》。

阴盛生内寒(yīn shèng shēng nèi hán)　**Yin abundance generates internal cold.** Yin cold qi accumulates in the chest and damages yang qi,resulting in an internal cold syndrome. See *Su Wen* chapter 62.

阴盛则内寒　出《素问·调经论》。见"阴盛生内寒"条。

阴盛则内寒(yīn shèng zé nèi hán)　**When yin is exuberant, there is internal cold.** See *Su Wen* chapter 62. See the term "阴盛生内寒".

阴虚　① 阴精虚弱不足。出《灵枢·本神》。② 脾气虚弱不足。出《素问·调经论》。

阴虚(yīn xū)　① The deficiency or weakness of yin essence. See *Ling Shu* chapter 8. ② The deficiency or weakness of spleen qi. See *Su Wen* chapter 62.

阴虚生内热　指脾虚发热。脾属阴,故称阴虚。其机制是：因劳倦太过,损伤脾气,清阳不升,浊阴不降,谷气留而不行,郁而化热。出《素问·调经论》。

阴虚生内热(yīn xū shēng nèi rè) **Yin deficiency generates internal heat.** Refers to heat caused by spleen deficiency. The spleen belongs to yin, thus it is called yin deficiency. Its mechanism is: the spleen qi is damaged by overstrain, followed by the clear yang failing to ascend and the turbid yin failing to descend. Also, the grain qi fails to transform, thus the depression transforms into fire. See *Su Wen* chapter 62.

阴虚则内热　出《素问·疟论》《素问·调经论》。

阴虚则内热(yīn xū zé nèi rè) **When yin is deficient, there is internal heat.** See *Su Wen* chapter 35 and chapter 62.

阴虚阳搏谓之崩　出《素问·阴阳别论》。(1)阴,指阴脉。阳,指阳脉。(2)阴,指诊脉沉取。阳,指诊脉浮取。(3)阴,指尺脉。阳,指寸脉。搏,形容脉来盛大搏指。崩,大出血,包括吐血、便血、溲血、妇女血崩等。因阴虚阳盛,迫血离经,故为崩。

阴虚阳搏谓之崩(yīn xū yáng bó wèi zhī bēng) **When the yin is deficient and the yang wins, it is called collapse.** See *Su Wen* chapter 7. (1) Yin refers to the yin meridian. Yang refers to the yang meridian. (2) Yin refers to the heavy taking of pulse. Yang refers to the light taking of pulse. (3) Yin refers to the *chi* pulse. Yang refers to the *cun* pulse. Bó describes a pulse that is large and forceful and can be felt easily by pulse taking. Bēng refers to massive hemorrhaging, including hematemesis, bloody stools, bloody urine, metrorrhagia, etc. Because of yin deficiency and yang excess, the blood is forced to depart the meridians, thus it collapses.

阴脱　阴,指五脏精血。脱,虚脱。由于刺络血出过多,致阴经血虚,进而导致相应的五脏精血虚脱。出《灵枢·血络论》。

阴脱(yīn tuō) **yin collapse** Yin refers to the essence and blood of the five viscera. Collapse refers to depletion. Due to the excessive blood letting out of the collaterals, blood in the yin

六画

meridians is deficient. Afterwards, both essence and blood in the five viscera are relatively deficient. See *Ling Shu* chapter 39.

阴维 即阴维脉，奇经八脉之一。其循行路线，从足少阴肾经的筑宾穴开始，沿下肢内侧向上，进入小腹，通过胁肋，胸腔，上至咽部。见《素问·刺腰痛》。

阴维(yīn wéi) *yinwei* Refers to the *yinwei* meridian, one of the eight extraordinary meridians. Its route starts from Zhu Bin（KI 9）on the kidney meridian of foot *shaoyin*, goes up along the inner side of the lower limbs, enters the lower abdomen, passes through the ribs and chest, and goes up to the pharynx. See *Su Wen* chapter 41.

阴厥 寒气厥逆。出《素问·气交变大论》。

阴厥(yīn jué) **yin *jue*** Reverse flow of cold qi. See *Su Wen* chapter 69.

阴跷 即阴跷脉。奇经八脉之一。其循行路线，从足少阴经分出，起于然谷之后，沿内踝后直上下肢内侧，经前阴，沿腹胸进入缺盆，出行于人迎穴之前，经鼻旁，到目内眦，与手足太阳经，阳跷脉会合。见《灵枢·寒

热病》。《灵枢·脉度》，此跷脉实指阴跷脉。

阴跷(yīn qiào) *yinqiao* **meridian** One of the eight extraordinary meridians which diverges from the foot *shaoyin* meridian, starts from the posterior aspect of Ran Gu（KI 2）acupoint, proceeds straight up to the medial aspect of the lower extremities along the regiones retromalleolaris medialis. Passing through the external genitalia, it enters the supraclavicular fossa along the abdomen and chest. Before arriving to Ren Ying（ST 9）acupoint, it passes through the region near the nose, then the inner canthus and converges with *taiyang* meridians of the hand and foot, as well as the *yangqiao* meridian. See *Ling Shu* chapter 21. In *Ling Shu* chapter 17, the *qiao* meridian mentioned refers to *yinqiao* meridian.

阴痹 病证名。① 局部疼痛不温之寒痹。出《素问·四时刺逆从论》。② 骨痹。邪在肾，肾主骨，故为骨痛，因痛处深，故按不可得。出《灵枢·五邪》。

阴痹(yīn bì) **yin *bi*（Impediment）** Disease syndrome name. ① Refers to cold-*bi*（impediment）syndrome due to local pain and loss of warmth. See *Su Wen* chapter 64. ② Bone-*bi*（Impediment）. The kidney governs the bones, thus if the evil attacks the kidney, it will cause bone pain. As the pain is deep inside the body, it cannot be palpated. See *Ling Shu* chapter 20.

阴痿　痿通萎，阴痿即阳痿。出《素问·阴阳应象大论》。

阴痿（yīn wěi）　**yin limpness** "痿" is the same as "萎". Yin limpness is also called yang decadence. See *Su Wen* chapter 5.

阴精　① 指西北方的阴气。出《素问·五常政大论》。② 指精气。出《素问·六微旨大论》。③ 指生殖之精液。出《灵枢·刺节真邪》。

阴精（yīn jīng）　① Refers to yin qi from the northwest part. See *Su Wen* chapter 70. ② Refers to essence qi. See *Su Wen* chapter 68. ③ Refers to the seminal fluids for reproduction. See *Ling Shu* chapter 75.

阴缩　阴器内缩。见《灵枢·邪气藏府病形》。

阴缩（yīn suō）　**yin shrinkage** Refers to the shrinkage of the yin

organs. See *Ling Shu* chapter 4.

阴器　前阴，外生殖器。见《灵枢·经筋》。

阴器（yīn qì）　**yin organ** Refers to the anterior yin, namely the external genitalia. See *Ling Shu* chapter 13.

羽　五音之一。五行属水，为北方各水之音。运气学说将五音代表五运，以五音建五运，则羽为水运。见《素问·阴阳应象大论》。

羽（yǔ）　**yu tone** One of the five sounds which pertains to water in the five elements, and refers to the sounds of all kinds of water in the north. In the theory of the five circuits and six qi, the five sounds represent and strengthen the five evolutive phases. *Yǔ* refers to the water phase. See *Su Wen* chapter 5.

约方　将医道中的许多诊治方法，提纲挈领地归纳起来，称为约方。见《灵枢·禁服》。

约方（yuē fāng）　**synthesize the theory** To synthesize the theory means to summarize the diagnosis and treatment methods of medical knowledge telegraphically. See *Ling Shu* chapter 48.

约束　指眼胞。又名眼睑，俗称眼皮。因其能开能合，故以为

六画

名。见《灵枢·大惑论》。

约束（yuē shù）　**blepharon** Refers to the pelpebra, and also called blepharon, or commonly known as the eyelid. It is named for the fact that it can both open and close. See *Ling Shu* chapter 80.

纪　① 一年为一纪。见《素问·六元正纪大论》。② 四年为一纪。见《素问·六微旨大论》。③ 三十年为一纪。见《素问·天元纪大论》。④ 纲纪、法则。见《素问·阴阳应象大论》。

纪（jì）　① One arrangement equals to one year. See *Su Wen* chapter 71. ② One arrangement refers to four years. See *Su Wen* chapter 68. ③ One arrangement refers to thirty years. See *Su Wen* chapter 66. ④ Refers to the rules, social orders and laws. See *Su Wen* chapter 5.

七 画

寿夭刚柔　《灵枢》篇名。寿夭，即指寿命的长短。刚柔，在此泛指阴阳各种不同的体质。此篇主要讨论形体的缓急、六气的盛衰及皮肤、肌肉、骨骼、脉搏等方面的差异，分析阴阳刚柔的不同体质类型以及与生命长短的关系，故名。

寿夭刚柔（shòu yāo gāng róu）**Discussion on Long life, Short life, Sturdiness and Softness** Chapter name in *Ling Shu*. *Shòu* and *yāo* refer to longevity and early death respectively. *Gāng róu* refers to different yin and yang constitutions. This chapter discusses the differences between relaxed and tense physiques, the wax and wane of the six qi, and the differences among the skin, muscles, bones and pulses. Also, it analyzes the relationship between the constitutions and life spans. Hence the name.

形　① 泛指在地之万物。出《素问·五运行大论》。② 身体形肉。出《素问·上古天真论》《素问·阴阳应象大论》。③ 身孕。出《素问·奇病论》。④ 病状。出《素问·举痛论》。⑤ 脉象。出《素问·玉机真藏论》⑥ 指针刺的方法和发病的部位。出《灵枢·九针十二原》《灵枢注证发微》。⑦ 指木火土金水。出《素问·六元正纪大论》。

形（xíng）　① Everything on Earth. See *Su Wen* chapter 67. ② The human body，physique and flesh. See *Su Wen* chapter 1 and chapter 5. ③ Pregnancy. See *Su Wen* chapter 47. ④ Symptoms. See *Su Wen* chapter 39. ⑤ Pulse manifestation. See *Su Wen* chapter 19. ⑥ Acupuncture techniques and disease locations. See *Ling Shu* chapter 1，and see *Annotation and Elaboration on Ling Shu*. ⑦ Wood，fire，earth，metal and water. See *Su Wen* chapter 71.

形与神俱　形，指形体。神，指精神。俱，偕同之意。形体与精神的统一协调。此乃健康长寿的基本保证。出《素问·上古天真论》。

形与神俱（xíng yǔ shén jù）　**the**

unity and coordination of physique and spirit *Xíng* means physique, *shén* refers to spirit. *Jù* means both. This term means unity and coordination of physique and spirit, which is the basic guarantee for health and longevity. See *Su Wen* chapter 1.

形气相得者生　形体与气相协调,谓之形气相得。生,指预后好。该句是承上文"形盛脉细,少气不足以息者危;形瘦脉大,胸中多气者死"而言,可见形气相失则预后差。出《素问·三部九候论》。

形气相得者生（xíng qì xiāng dé zhě shēng）**Agreement between physique and qi indicates survival.** Describes the coordination between physique and qi. Survival here refers to a good prognosis. This sentence is based on the above "When the physique abounds, while the vessels are fine and when one is short of qi to a degree that there is not enough for breathing, this indicates danger. When the physique is lean, while the vessels are big and when there is much qi in the chest, this indicates death".

Thus, when physique and qi do not agree, the prognosis is poor. See *Su Wen* chapter 20.

形气绝　形气,这里作"气血"解,指因大怒导致的气血壅遏,阻绝不通的病理。见《素问·生气通天论》《太素·阴阳》。

形气绝（xíng qì jué）**the repression of physique** Physique here refers to qi and blood, indicating the repression and stasis of qi and blood due to great anger. See *Su Wen* chapter 3. See *Tai Su* (*Classified Study on Huang Di Nei Jing*) "Yin and Yang".

形色相得　形,指木火土金水五形之人。色,指五色。本形与本色相配。如土形之人,其色黄,木形之人其色青等,是形色相得,气质和调,康泰的表现。出《灵枢·阴阳二十五人》。

形色相得（xíng sè xiāng dé）**Physique and complexion are matched.** Physique here refers to people's constitutions according to the five elements (metal, wood, water, fire and earth). Complexion refers to the five colors of the five complexions. When physique matches complexion, this indicates the coordination of physique and complexion, and qi and constitution.

七画

For example，people of earth constitution have the yellow complexion，people of wood constitution have green complexion. See *Ling Shu* chapter 64.

形法 古医籍名，已佚。内容可能是关于观察形色变化的方法。见《素问·解精微论》。

形法（xíng fǎ） **The natural approach and the patterns of physique** An ancient medical book which has been lost in history. It most probably discussed the techniques of observing changes in people's physiques and complexions. See *Su Wen* chapter 81.

形独居 气血亏虚，与形体相离，唯留形体独在的病理。见《素问·八正神明论》。

形独居（xíng dú jū） **physique exists alone** Qi and blood are deficient and separate themselves from the physique，thus the physique exists by itself pathologically. See *Su Wen* chapter 26.

形度 形，形体；度，度数。指形体的长短度数。见《素问·通评虚实论》。

形度（xíng dù） **measures of the physique** *Xíng* means physique；*dù* means measures，and this term refers to the size of the physique. See *Su Wen* chapter 28.

形能 能，通态。形能，即形态。出《素问·阴阳应象大论》。

形能（xíng néng） **manifestations** "能" is the same as "态". *Xíng néng* here refers to manifestations. See *Su Wen* chapter 5.

形寒寒饮则伤肺 形寒，寒邪从皮毛入于形体，与肺相合而受邪；寒饮，寒冷的饮食入胃，寒从手太阴肺脉影响到肺。内外两寒相迫于肺，肺气失于宣肃，发生咳嗽。出《灵枢·邪气藏府病形》。

形寒寒饮则伤肺（xíng hán hán yǐn zé shāng fèi） **Physical cold and cold food cause lung injury** *Xíng hán* means that the cold pathogen gets inside into the body and hurts the lung. *Hán yǐn* means that the cold pathogen consumed into the cold body affects the lung along the lung meridian of hand *taiyin* meridian. The internal and external coldness leads to the malfunction of lung in diffusing and sending downwards，and finally causes cough. See *Ling Shu* chapter 4.

形藏四 《素问·六节藏象论》。（1）指传导有形之物的脏器，胃、大肠、小肠、膀胱四腑。见《素问集注》。（2）如器外张之形有四，指头角、耳目、口齿和胸中。见《素问》王冰注。

形藏四（xíng zàng sì） **four physical viscus** See *Su Wen* chapter 9. (1) Refers to viscera which transfer substances，including the stomach，large intestine，small intestine and bladder. See *Su Wen Ji Zhu* (*Collected Annotation of Su Wen*). (2) The four categories of relatively protruding parts on the body，including the head，ears and eyes，mouth，teeth，and chest. See *Su Wen* annotated by Wang Bing.

远死而近生 指遵循四时养生之道，则能远离死亡而能长生久视。出《素问·移精变气论》。

远死而近生（yuǎn sǐ ér jìn sheng） **away from death and close to longevity** This term refers to cultivating life by following the four seasons' health preservation ways，in order to stay away from death and enjoy a long healthy life. See *Su Wen* chapter 13.

远者偶之 病位在下部，远于胃的，属阴，用偶方治疗。出《素问·至真要大论》。

远者偶之（yuǎn zhě ǒu zhī） **to treat diseases located far away below the stomach with even-numbered formulas** For diseases located at the lower part of the body far from the stomach and pertaining to yin，treat with even-numbered formulas. See *Su Wen* chapter 74.

远道刺 九刺法之一。是上病下取，循经远道取穴的一种刺法。从广义看，凡头面、躯干、脏腑的病症，刺四肢肘膝关节以下的穴位都可以称远道刺。见《灵枢·官针》。

远道刺（yuǎn dào cì） **distant needling** One of the nine needling methods. For the diseases located at the upper part of the body，needling the acupoints along the meridians from afar. In a broad sense，distant needling refers to selecting acupoints below the joints，of the four limbs，to treat diseases of the head and face，trunk and viscera. See *Ling Shu* chapter 7.

远痹 邪深病久之痹证。见《灵枢·九针论》。

远痹（yuǎn bì） **prolonged impediment** Long lasting impediment caused by deep pathogens. See *Ling Shu* chapter 78.

运 指木、火、土、金、水五运。出《素问·六元正纪大论》。

运（yùn） **circuits** Refers to the five phases wood, fire, earth, metal and water. See *Su Wen* chapter 71.

运气 即五运六气。参该条。出《素问·气交变大论》。

运气（yùn qì） **circuits and qi** The five circuits and six qi. See *Su Wen* chapter 69.

运星 与岁运相应之星。如木运木星，火运火星之类。出《素问·气交变大论》。

运星（yùn xīng） **the star of year circuit** The star relevant to the circuit of the year, for example, Jupiter is relevant to the wood circuit, and Mars to the fire circuit, etc. See *Su Wen* chapter 69.

扶突 经穴名。属手阳明大肠经，又名水穴，在人迎后一寸五分，与喉结平齐。出《灵枢·寒热病》。

扶突（fú tū） **Fu Tu (LI 18)** It pertains to the large intestine meridian of hand *yangming*. It is also called the water acupoint (*shuǐ xuè*). It is located at one and a half inches behind acupoint Ren Ying (ST 9), and is flush with the Adam's apple.

See *Ling Shu* chapter 21.

坏府 出《素问·宝命全形论》。坏，败坏。"府"字有不同见解。（1）胸府。（2）形体。见《类经·针刺九》。（3）五脏六腑，血气皮肉。见《素问集注》。（4）中宫。

坏府（huài fǔ） **deterioration of the viscera** See *Su Wen* chapter 25. *Huài* means deterioration, while *fǔ* has several meanings. (1) Chest. (2) Physique and body. See *Lei Jing* (*Classified Classic*) "Needling Chapter 9". (3) Five viscera and six bowels, and blood, qi, skin and flesh. See *Su Wen Ji Zhu*(*Collected Annotation of Su Wen*). (4) The middle palace.

走缓 病名。发于内踝部之痈肿。肿处皮色不变。又名内踝疽。出《灵枢·痈疽》。

走缓（zǒu huǎn） **slow walk** Disease name. Carbuncle and swelling in the medial malleolus. The skin color of the swollen part does not change. Also known as carbuncle the medial malleolus. See *Ling Shu* chapter 81.

赤气 五运中之火气。出《素问·气交变大论》。

赤气（chì qì） **the red qi** It refers to fire qi, one of the five cir-

七画

cuits. See *Su Wen* chapter 69.

赤风瞳翳 指火眼云翳目疾。出《素问·本病论》。

赤风瞳翳(chì fēng tóng yì) **red wind shield eyes** It refers to fire eyes and nebulous eye screens. See *Su Wen* chapter 73.

赤沃 大小便下血。出《素问·至真要大论》。

赤沃(chì wò) **red downpour** Hematuria and hematochezia. See *Su Wen* chapter 74.

赤甚者为血 皮肤深赤常提示有瘀血内停。出《灵枢·五色》。

赤甚者为血(chì shèn zhě wéi xuè) **crimson indicates static blood** Crimson skin often indicates blood stasis. See *Ling Shu* chapter 49.

赤脉 ① 目眦内血络。出《灵枢·大惑论》。② 心脉,赤为心之色,故称。出《素问·五藏生成》。

赤脉(chì mài) ① Blood vessels in the canthus. See *Ling Shu* chapter 80. ② Heart meridian. *Chì* (red) is the color of heart, hence the name. See *Su Wen* chapter 10.

赤施 病名。发于大腿内侧的痈疽。出《灵枢·痈疽》。

赤施(chì shī) **red imposition** Disease name. It refers to car-

buncles on the medial thigh. See *Ling Shu* chapter 81.

折风 八风之一。指由西北方刮来的风。出《灵枢·九宫八风》。

折风(shé fēng) **She wind** One of the eight winds, coming from the northwest. See *Ling Shu* chapter 77.

折关败枢 关,开阖,这里的关枢,即三阳三阴的开阖枢。出《灵枢·根结》。(1)指三阳三阴开阖枢失守的病机。(2)指三阳三阴开阖枢失守的病证,如三阳折关败枢则肉节败、骨动摇;三阴折关败枢则水谷不输纳、悲、脉不通等病证。

折关败枢(shé guān bài shū) **to lose the guard of the opening and closing pivot** *Guān* means to open and close. By *guān shū*, here it refers to the opening and closing pivot of the three yin and three yang meridians. See *Ling Shu* chapter 5. (1) It refers to the pathogenesis of the malfunction of the opening and closing pivot. (2) It refers to the symptoms caused by the malfunction of the opening and closing pivot, such as the functional decline of the joints and bones caused by the pivots of the three yang meridians failing to open and close，and the symptoms caused by the pivot of three yin meridians failing to open and close，such as hindered transformation and digestion of water and grains，sorrow，and stagnated meridians，etc.

折收 收气减折。指金运不及，火胜克金，木来反侮，使秋金之收气减折。出《素问·五常政大论》。

折收（shé shōu） **diminished gathering qi** The gathering qi is diminished. It refers to deficient metal phase restrained by fire phase，and then rebelled by wood phase that causes the gathering autumn gold qi to diminish. See *Su Wen* chapter 70.

折郁扶运 指根据五运之气变化而采用的针刺治疗原则，即运气太过治其所胜，使郁气折服；运气不及扶助其本气之衰，以避虚邪。出《素问·刺法论》。

折郁扶运（shé yù fú yùn） **to inhibit the depression and support the circuit-qi** It refers to acupuncture principles according to the change of qi in the five circuits，namely，to inhibit the depression by reducing the excess，supporting the qi and

avoiding deficiency pathogens by tonifying the insufficiency. See *Su Wen* chapter 72.

折脊 病名，腰脊疼痛似折之病。出《灵枢·邪气藏府病形》。

折脊（shé jǐ） **back pain as if there were a fracture** Severe back pain as if there were a fracture. See *Ling Shu* chapter 4.

折髀 出《素问·脉要精微论》。(1) 大腿部如折断而不利动作。见《素问》王冰注。(2) 髀骨折伤。见《素问》吴崑注。

折髀（shé bì） **a broken thigh bone** See *Su Wen* chapter 17. （1） The patient can barely walk as if his thigh was broken. See *Su Wen* annotated by Wang Bing. （2） Broken thigh-bone. See *Su Wen* annotated by Wu Kun.

抑者散之 治法。凡气机抑郁的用疏解散郁的方法治疗。出《素问·至真要大论》。

抑者散之（yì zhě sàn zhī） **to treat inhibition with dispersing methods** A treatment method. The stasis of circuits and qi is treated by the dispersing method. See *Su Wen* chapter 74.

志 ① 在意念的基础上形成的概念称志。志受肾所主，以精为物质基础。出《灵枢·本神》。

七画

② 神志，意识。出《灵枢·热病》。③ 记识。出《素问·宝命全形论》。

志（zhì）　① Will power. *Zhì* is dominated by the kidney, with essence as its material basis. See *Ling Shu* chapter 8. ② Mind and consciousness. See *Ling Shu* chapter 23. ③ To memorize. See *Su Wen* chapter 25.

志发乎四野　指个人的志意、想法不加约束地广传四方，是"太阳之人"心妄好强的表现。出《灵枢·通天》。

志发乎四野（zhì fā hū sì yě）　**mind reaches the four regions** It is a kind of aggressive manifestation of *taiyang*-type people who spread their will and thoughts everywhere without restraint. See *Ling Shu* chapter 72.

志闲而少欲　指心志闲静平和无贪欲，为精神养生之法。出《素问·上古天真论》。

志闲而少欲（zhì xián ér shǎo yù）　**unburdened mind with contentment** To keep one's mind relaxed and at peace with no greediness. It is one of the ways of mental preservation. See *Su Wen* chapter 1.

志意　① 泛指精神意识。赅括神、魂、魄、意、志五种。出《灵枢·本神》。② 机体统帅精神，调节情志，适应外界环境的一种功能。出《灵枢·本藏》。

志意（zhì yì）　① In a broad sense, it refers to spirit and consciousness, mainly including *shen* (spirit), *hun* (part of the mental activity having a close relationship with the liver), *po* (part of the mental activity pertaining to instinctive sense and actions), *yi* (thinking) and *zhi* (emotions). See *Ling Shu* chapter 8. ② The body's function of governing the spirit, adjusting emotions and adapting to the external environment. See *Ling Shu* chapter 47.

报气　报复之气，即复气。出《素问·至真要大论》。参"复气"条。

报气（bào qì）　**retributing qi** This is another name for revenge qi. See *Su Wen* chapter 74. Refer to the term "复气".

报刺　十二刺法之一。出《灵枢·官针》。

报刺（bào cì）　**successive trigger needling** One of the twelve needling methods. See *Ling Shu* chapter 7.

报息　报，重复或接续；息，呼吸。指平顺的呼吸规律。出《素问·藏气法时论》。

报息(bào xī)　**breathe consecutively** *Bào* means repetitive or continous. *Xī* means to breathe. *Bào xī* refers to smooth breathing. See *Su Wen* chapter 22.

苍天之气　① 古代天文学家在危、室、柳、鬼诸宿间看到青色之气。《内经》以此说明"天干纪运"的方法，即青属木，故木运主治丁壬年。出《素问·五运行大论》。② 自然界的天气。出《素问·六节藏象论》。

苍天之气(cāng tiān zhī qì)　① the greenish colour of heaven seen by ancient astronomers among the stars of *wei* and *shi*, *liu* and *gui*. *Nei Jing* (*Internal Classic*) explains the method representing phases by the Heavenly Stems, that is, greenish pertains to the wood phase, so the wood phase governs the year of *ding ren*. See *Su Wen* chapter 67. ② Weather. See *Su Wen* chapter 9.

芳草　即芳香之类药草，其气多走窜。出《素问·腹中论》。

芳草(fāng cǎo)　**Aromatic herbs** Fragrant herbs，with mobility and penetrating qi as its nature. See *Su Wen* chapter 40.

劳风　病名。如风热蕴肺一类病证。症见头项强急，目眩不明，恶风振寒，呼吸困难，涕痰黄稠等。病起于因劳致虚，伤于风邪，故名。出《素问·评热病论》。

劳风(láo fēng)　**taxation wind** Disease name. It mainly refers to the syndrome of wind-heat lingering in the lung，which manifests as stiff neck，headache，dizziness，aversion to wind，dyspnea，yellow phlegm and thick snivel，etc. It is caused by deficiency due to fatigue，allowing the wind pathogen to do harm to the body. See *Su Wen* chapter 33.

劳则气耗　劳则喘息汗出，正气亏耗。出《素问·举痛论》。

劳则气耗(láo zé qì hào)　**overexertion leads to qi consumption** Overexertion leads to wheezing and sweating，thus the loss of healthy qi. See *Su Wen* chapter 39.

劳者温之　治法。劳，劳损。因过度操劳而引起的虚损之病，应用温补法治疗。出《素问·至真要大论》。

劳者温之(láo zhě wēn zhī)　**to treat overstrain with warming methods** Treatment method. *Láo* means overstrain. This principle indicates that diseases of deficiency，caused by overstrain, should be treated by warming and tonifying methods. See *Su Wen* chapter 74.

劳宫 经穴名。手厥阴心包经的荥穴。位于掌中央,中指本节内间,即第二、三掌骨之间。出《灵枢·本输》。

劳宫(láo gōng) **Lao Gong (PC 8).** The brook acupoint of the pericardium meridian of hand *jueyin*. It is located in the middle of the palm, between the second and third metacarpal. See *Ling Shu* chapter 2.

束骨 ① 横骨之一。出《素问·骨空论》。② 穴位名。足太阳膀胱经之腧穴,位于足外侧,小趾本节后下方赤白肉际处。出《灵枢·本输》。

束骨(shù gǔ) ① One of the transverse bones. See *Su Wen* chapter 60. ② The name of acupoint BL 65, which is on the bladder meridian of foot *taiyang*. It is located on the outside of the foot and at the red white flesh border of the lower part of the small toe. See *Ling Shu* chapter 2.

束脉 指地机穴。出《素问·刺腰痛》。地机穴在膝眼下五寸,阴陵泉直下三寸处。

束脉(shù mài) **binding vessel** It refers to acupoint Di Ji (SP 8). See *Su Wen* chapter 41. It is located at 5 inches below the acupoint Xi Yan (ST 35), and 3 inches below the acupoint Yin Ling Quan (SP 9).

两阳 ① 指三四月所主之左、右足阳明经。《灵枢·阴阳系月》。② 指少阳、太阳。出《素问·至真要大论》。

两阳(liǎng yáng) ① *Yangming* meridians of the left and right foot which are dominated by the third and fourth month respectively. See *Ling Shu* chapter 41. ② *Shaoyang* and *taiyang*. See *Su Wen* chapter 74.

两阳合明 出《素问·至真要大论》。(1) 指三四月份,上半年阳气最盛之时。见《类经·经络三十四》。(2) 指合于太阳、少阳之中之阳明。见《素问直解》。

两阳合明(liǎng yáng hé míng) **Two yang qi combine their brightness.** See *Su Wen* chapter 74. (1) March and April, the first half of the year when yang qi is at its peak. See *Lei Jing* (*Classified Classic*) "Meridians and Collaterals Chapter 34". (2) *Yangming* that combines with *shaoyang* and *taiyang*. See *Su Wen Zhi Jie* (*Direct Interpretation* on *Su Wen*).

两阴交尽 出《素问·至真要大论》。(1)指九、十月份下半年阴气极尽转衰之时。见《类经·经络三十四》。(2)指交于太阴，少阴间之厥阴。见《素问直解》。

两阴交尽(liǎng yīn jiāo jìn) **two yin qi are equally exhausted** See *Su Wen* chapter 74. (1) The time when the yin qi in September and October turns to decline. See *Lei Jing*（*Classified Classic*）"Meridians and Collaterals Chapter 34". (2) Reverting yin between *taiyin* and *shaoyin*. See *Su Wen Zhi Jie*（*Direct Interpretation on Su Wen*).

两感 表里两经同时受邪而发病。如太阳与少阴俱病。阳明与太阴俱病，少阳与厥阴俱病之类。邪盛正虚，起病急，发展快，病情重，预后差。出《素问·热论》。

两感(liǎng gǎn) **double contraction** Both exterior and interior meridians contract pathogenic factors at the same time. For example, simultaneously, the pathogen invades the *taiyang* and *shaoyin* meridians, the *yangming* and *taiyin* meridians, and the *shaoyang* and *jueyin* meridians. Excessive pathogenic factors and the deficiency of healthy qi leads to acute onset，rapid developments，severe conditions and poor prognosis. See *Su Wen* chapter 31.

辰戌之纪 指纪年地支是辰、戌之年，为太阳寒水司天。纪，纪年。出《素问·六元正纪大论》。

辰戌之纪(chén xū zhī jì) **arrangements including *chen* and *xu* earth branches** It means that in all the years with *chen* and *xu* earth branches，the greater yang qi，the qi of cold and water，controls heaven. *Jì* refers to the way of numbering the years. See *Su Wen* chapter 71.

辰砂 药名。又称朱砂，性味甘寒，有镇心安神、清热解毒的作用。是小金丹方组成之一。出《素问·刺法论》。

辰砂(chén shā) **cinnabar** A TCM medicine，also named *zhū shā*. Cold in nature and sweet in flavor，it tranquilizes the heart and quiets the spirit，clears heat and removes toxins. It is one of the components of a famous ancient prescription named Xiao Jin Dan Formula. See *Su Wen* chapter 72.

辰星 水星，为五大行星之一，与

七画

五行中的水、五脏中的肾相通应。出《素问·金匮真言论》。

辰星（chén xīng） **Mercury** One of the five planets, corresponding to water in the five elements, and to the kidney in the five viscera. See *Su Wen* chapter 4.

豕膏 指炼净的猪油。用于痈疽生在结喉已化脓者，在排脓时，可配合猪油冷食。出《灵枢·痈疽》。

豕膏（shǐ gāo） **lard** Refined lard, which can be used to treat carbuncles and abscesses in the case of a suppurated throat. It can be eaten for drainage of pus. See *Ling Shu* chapter 81.

步 运气术语。六气以 60.875 日为一步，六步 365.25 日为一年。出《素问·六微旨大论》。

步（bù） **step** A term of circuits and qi. According to the six qi, every 60.875 days are one step, and six steps (365.25 days) account for one year. See *Su Wen* chapter 68.

坚者耎之 治法。耎，即软。病气坚实的，应用软坚的方法治疗。出《素问·至真要大论》。

坚者耎之（jiān zhě ruǎn zhī） **to treat hardness with softening methods** A treatment method.

Ruǎn means to soften. The hard pathogenic qi of some diseases should be treated with softening methods. See *Su Wen* chapter 74.

坚者削之 治法。病属坚硬有形之块物者，如癥块、结石、瘰疬等，要用软坚削积的方法渐消缓散。出《素问·至真要大论》。

坚者削之（jiān zhě xuē zhī） **to treat hardness with whittling methods** A treatment method. For patients with lumps, such as lithiasis, scrofula, etc., it is necessary to treat by gradual softening and whittling. See *Su Wen* chapter 74.

足太阳 十二经脉之一。即足太阳膀胱经。出《素问·血气形志》。

足太阳（zú tài yáng） **foot *taiyang* meridian** id est the bladder meridian of foot taiyang One of the twelve regular meridians. See *Su Wen* chapter 24.

足太阳之正 足太阳别出之正经，又称足太阳经别，为十二经别之一，与足少阴经别相合。其入腘中，当骶下五寸处分出，进入肛门部，归属于膀胱，散络于肾，沿脊旁筋肉上行向内散布于心；直行者一直沿脊旁筋肉上行，出于项，又复合于足太阳经。出《灵枢·经别》。

足太阳之正（zú tài yáng zhī zhèng）**divergent regular from foot** *taiyang* A regular branch meridian departing from foot *taiyang*, also called the divergent branch of foot *taiyang* merdian. As one of the twelve divergent meridians, it joins the divergent meridian of foot *taiyin*. The main course of the meridians diverging from the foot *taiyang* enters the hollow of the knee. One of its paths descends to five *cun* below the buttocks, a diverging meridian enters the anus and links up with the urinary bladder, dissipates in the kidney and follows the flesh beside the spine to the heart where it enters. The straight course ascends from the flesh beside the spine and appears in the nape where it links up again with the foot *taiyang* meridian. See *Ling Shu* chapter 11.

足太阳之别 十五别络之一,穴名飞扬。其络从外踝上七寸处分出后走向足少阴经。出《灵枢·经脉》。

足太阳之别（zú tài yáng zhī bié）**divergent meridian of the foot** *taiyang* One of the fifteen connecting collaterals, also called Fei Yang（BL 58）. It diverges a distance of seven *cun* from the lateral malleolus, and extends separately towards the foot meridian of *shaoyin*. See *Ling Shu* chapter 10.

足太阳之疟 足六经疟之一。症见先寒后热,腰痛,头重等。出《素问·刺疟》。

足太阳之疟（zú tài yáng zhī nüè）**malaria of the foot** *taiyang* **meridian** It is one of the six malarias of the foot meridians, and the main symptoms include cold first and hot afterwards, lower back pain, and a heavy head, etc. See *Su Wen* chapter 36.

足太阳之筋 即足太阳经筋。为十二经筋之一。出《灵枢·经筋》。

足太阳之筋（zú tài yáng zhī jīn）**meridian sinew of foot** *taiyin*. It is one of the twelve meridian sinews. See *Ling Shu* chapter 13.

足太阴 十二经脉之一。即足太阴脾经。出《素问·太阴阳明论》。

足太阴（zú tài yīn）**meridian of foot** *taiyin* It is one of the twelve regular meridians, and it refers to the spleen meridian of foot *taiyin*. See *Su Wen*

七画

chapter 29.

足太阴之正　足太阴别出之正经，又称足太阴经别，为十二经别之一，与足阳明经别相合。其在膝上部别出后至大腿前面，会合足阳明经别，一起上行，络于咽，通贯舌中。出《灵枢·经别》。

足太阴之正(zú tài yīn zhī zhèng) **regular divergent meridian of foot** *taiyin* It is the regular divergent meridian of foot *taiyin* meridian，and is also called the divergent meridian of foot *taiyin*. As one of the twelve divergent meridians，it links up to the meridian of foot *yangming*. It diverges from the knees to the front of the thighs，meeting divergent meridian of the foot *yangming*. Both go up to the throat and link to the tongue. See *Ling Shu* chapter 11.

足太阴之别　十五别络之一。其络从大趾本节后一寸处分出，走向足阳明经，一支上入腹部，散络肠胃。出《灵枢·经脉》。

足太阴之别(zú tài yīn zhī bié) **divergent meridian of foot** *taiyin* It is one of the fifteen connecting collaterals. It starts at one *cun* behind the basic joint of the big toe and extends sepa-rately from the *yangming* meridian. A branch goes up into the abdomen and extends into the intestines and the stomach. See *Ling Shu* chapter 10.

足太阴之疟　足六经疟之一。症见寒热、汗出、不欲食，太息等。出《素问·刺疟》。

足太阴之疟(zú tài yīn zhī nüè) **malaria of the foot** *taiyin* It is one of the six malarias of the foot meridians，in which the main symptoms include feeling cold and hot，sweating，no appetite，and sighing，etc. See *Su Wen* chapter 36.

足太阴之筋　即足太阴经筋，为十二经筋之一。起于大足趾内侧端，向上结于内踝；直行者，络于膝内辅骨（胫骨内踝部），向上沿大腿内侧，结于股骨前，聚集于阴部，上向腹部，结于脐，沿腹内，结于肋骨。散布于胸中；其在里者，附着于脊椎。出《灵枢·经筋》。

足太阴之筋(zú tài yīn zhī jīn) **meridian sinew of foot** *taiyin* It is one of the twelve meridian sinews. It starts from the medial side of the big toe，goes along the medial side of the ankles，knees，thighs，pubic region，ribs，and ends at the spine. See *Ling Shu* chapter 13.

足少阳　十二经脉之一。即足少阳胆经。出《灵枢·本输》。

足少阳（zú shào yáng）　**meridian of foot *shaoyang*** It is one of the twelve regular meridians, referring to the gallbladder meridian of foot *shaoyang*. See *Ling Shu* chapter 2.

足少阳之正　足少阳别出之正经，又称足少阳经别，为十二经别之一，与足厥阴经别相合。其从膝上部别出后，绕行髋部，进入毛际，会合足厥阴经；分支进入季肋部，沿胸里归属于胆，散布于肝，通过心，向上挟咽旁，出于下颔中，散布面部，联系目系，在外眦处与足少阳经相合。出《灵枢·经别》。

足少阳之正（zú shào yáng zhī zhèng）　**regular divergent meridian of foot *shaoyang*** It is the regular divergent meridian of foot *shaoyang*. As one of the twelve divergent meridians, it joins the divergent meridian of foot *jueyin*. It winds around the thigh, enters the pubic hair line, links up with the *jueyin* meridian and extends separately into the lower flanks. Following the inner side of the chest, it links up with the gallbladder. It

dissipates there and ascends to the liver, penetrates the heart and ascends further to the side of the throat. Then it appears at the jaws, dissipates in the face, connects with the eye, and links up with the shao yang meridian at the exterior corner of the eye. See *Ling Shu* chapter 11.

足少阳之别　十五别络之一，穴名光明。其络于外踝上五寸处分出，走向足厥阴，下边散络足背。出《灵枢·经脉》。

足少阳之别（zú shào yáng zhī bié）　**divergent meridian of the foot *shaoyang*** It is one of the fifteen connecting collaterals, and is also called Guang Ming (GB 37). It diverges at the lateral malleolus at a distance of five inches, extends separately along the foot *jueyin* meridian, and descends to wrap the instep. See *Ling Shu* chapter 10.

足少阳之疟　足六经疟之一。症见倦怠乏力，稍有寒热怕见人等。出《素问·刺疟》。

足少阳之疟（zú shào yáng zhī nüè）　**malaria of the meridian of foot *shaoyang*** It is one of the six malarias of the foot meridians. The main symptoms include a lack of vitality, feeling slightly cold or hot, and being afraid to see people. See *Su Wen* chapter 36.

足少阳之筋　即足少阳经筋，为十二经筋之一。起于第四趾，出《灵枢·经筋》。

足少阳之筋(zú shào yáng zhī jīn) **meridian sinew of foot *shaoyang*** It is one of the twelve meridian sinews starting from the fourth toe. See *Ling Shu* chapter 13.

足少阴　十二经脉之一。即足少阴肾经。《灵枢·动输》。

足少阴(zú shào yīn)　**meridian of foot *shaoyin*** It is one of the twelve regular meridians. See *Ling Shu* chapter 62.

足少阴之正　足少阴别出之正经，又称足少阴经别，为十二经别之一，与足太阳经别相合。其在腘中分出上行，并入足太阳经别，上行至肾，当十四椎处出，属带脉；直行者，从肾上行，系于舌本，又出于项，与足太阳经相合。出《灵枢·经别》。

足少阴之正(zú shào yīn zhī zhèng)　**regular divergent meridian of foot *shaoyin*** It refers to the main course of the meridians diverging from foot *shaoyin*, and is also called the divergent channel of the foot *shaoyin* meridian, which is one

of the twelve divergent meridians, and joins the divergent meridian of foot *taiyang*. It enters the popliteal of the knee and extends separately to the *taiyang* meridian with which it eventually links up to. It further ascends to the kidney and appears at the 14th vertebra where it links up with the belt vessel. The straight course links up with the basis of the tongue, reappears at the nape, and links up with the foot *taiyang* meridian. See *Ling Shu* chapter 11.

足少阴之别　十五别络之一，穴名大钟。其络当踝后绕行跟部，分支走向足太阳经，另一支同经脉并行，走向心包下，并通过腰脊。出《灵枢·经脉》。

足少阴之别(zú shào yīn zhī bié) **divergent meridian of foot *shaoyin*** It is one of the fifteen connecting collaterals, and is also called Da Zhong (KI 4). It originates from exactly behind the ankle, wraps around the heel and extends separately from the *taiyang* meridian. Its branch extends along the meridian and reaches upward to below the pericardium. Externally it penetrates the lower back and the spine. See *Ling Shu* chapter 10.

足少阴之疟 足六经疟之一。症见呕吐，热多寒少等。出《素问·刺疟》。

足少阴之疟(zú shào yīn zhī nüè) **malaria of the meridian of foot** *shaoyin* It is one of the six malarias of the foot meridians. The main symptoms include vomiting, and more heat than cold. See *Su Wen* chapter 36.

足少阴之筋 即足少阴经筋，为十二经筋之一。起于足小趾的下边，同足太阴经筋并斜行内踝下方，结于足跟，与足太阳经筋会合，向上结于胫骨内踝下，同足太阴经筋一起向上，沿大腿内侧，结于阴部，沿脊里，挟膂，向上至项，结于枕骨，与足太阳经筋会合。出《灵枢·经筋》。

足少阴之筋(zú shào yīn zhī jīn) **the meridian sinew of foot** *shaoyin* It is one of the twelve meridian sinews. It originates from the lower side of the little toe, runs obliquely under the medial malleolus with the meridian sinew of foot *taiyin*, converges at the meridian sinew of foot *taiyang* at the heel, ascends the medial malleolus of the foot upward, converges at the meridian sinew of foot *taiyin* at the medial aspect of the tibia, and ascends upward along the inner thigh, to the pudendum, along the spine and up to the neck, to the occipital bone, and joins the meridian sinew of foot *taiyang*. See *Ling Shu* chapter 13.

足阳明 十二经脉之一。即足阳明胃经。出《灵枢·经水》。

足阳明(zú yáng míng) **meridian of foot** *yangming* It is one of the twelve regular meridians, namely, stomach meridian of foot yangming. See *Ling Shu* chapter 12.

足阳明之正 足阳明别出之正经，又称足阳明经别，为十二经别之一，与足太阴经别相合，其从大腿前面别出，进入腹内，归属于胃，散布于脾，向上通过心，上沿咽旁出于口腔，上鼻根及目眶下，联系目系，与足阳明本经相合。出《灵枢·经别》。

足阳明之正(zú yáng míng zhī zhèng) **regular divergent meridian of foot** *yangming* It is one of the twelve divergent meridians, converging with the divergent meridian of foot *taiyin*. It originates from the front side of the thigh and goes into the belly, connecting with the stomach and then scattering in the spleen, it continues going upward to the heart and out to the oral cavity along the throat, and finally reaches the root of the nose as well as the eye socket inferiorly that connects with the meridian of foot *yangming*. See *Ling Shu* chapter 11.

足阳明之别　十五别络之一,穴名丰隆。其络于外踝上八寸处分出,走向足太阴经;一支沿胫骨外侧,向上散络头顶,会合各经之气,下边散络喉头部。出《灵枢·经脉》。

足阳明之别(zú yáng míng zhī bié) **divergent meridian of foot yangming** One of the fifteen connecting collaterals, also called Feng Long (ST 40). It is located eight *cun* above the lateral malleolus and runs towards the foot *taiyin* meridian. One branch is along the lateral side of the tibia, dispersing the collaterals upward on the top of the head to meet the qi of each meridian and dispersing the collaterals on the throat below. See *Ling Shu* chapter 10.

足阳明之疟　为足六经疟之一。症见先寒后热,热退汗出等。出《素问·刺疟》。

足阳明之疟(zú yáng míng zhī nüè) **malaria of the meridian of foot yangming** It is one of the six malarias of the foot meridians. The main symptoms include feeling cold first and hot afterwards, sweating after the heat disappears. See *Su Wen* chapter 36.

足阳明之筋　即足阳明经筋,为十二经筋之一。起于第二、三、四趾,出《灵枢·经筋》。

足阳明之筋(zú yáng míng zhī jīn) **meridian sinew of foot yangming** It is one of the twelve meridian sinews, originating at the second, third, and fourth toes. See *Ling Shu* chapter 13.

足悗　因寒所致的下肢筋肉骨节酸痛不利。出《灵枢·百病始生》。

足悗(zú mán) **numb feet** It refers to the soreness and pain of the sinews, bones and joints in the lower limbs usually caused by cold. See *Ling Shu* chapter 66.

足厥阴　十二经脉之一。即足厥阴肝经。出《灵枢·经水》。

足厥阴(zú jué yīn) **foot jueyin** It is one of the twelve regular meridians, namely, liver meridian of foot jueyin. See *Ling*

Shu chapter 12.

足厥阴之正 足厥阴别行之正经，又称足厥阴经别，为十二经别之一，与足少阳经别相合。其从足背部分出，上至毛际，会合足少阳经别后一起上行。出《灵枢·经别》。

足厥阴之正（zú jué yīn zhī zhèng）**divergent regular meridian of foot** *jueyin* It refers to the divergent branch of foot *jueyin* meridian，one of the twelve divergent meridians. It joins the divergent meridian of foot *shaoyang*，extends separately on the instep and ascends to the pubic hair line where it joins the upstream of the divergent meridian of foot *shaoyang*. See *Ling Shu* chapter 11.

足厥阴之别 十五别络之一，穴名蠡沟。其络从内踝上五寸处分出，走向足少阳经；一支沿经脉上行至睾丸，结于阴茎部。出《灵枢·经脉》。

足厥阴之别（zú jué yīn zhī bié）**divergent meridian of foot** *jueyin* It is one of the fifteen connecting collaterals，and is also called Li Gou（LR 5）. It starts at a distance of five *cun* from the medial malleolus and extends separately at the meridian of foot *shaoyang*，leaving a branch extending along the shins，ascending into the testicles and linking up with the penis. See *Ling Shu* chapter 10.

足厥阴之疟 足六经疟之一。症见腰痛、少腹满、小便频数不畅等。出《素问·刺疟》。

足厥阴之疟（zú jué yīn zhī nüè）**malaria of foot** *jueyin* **meridian** It is one of the six malarias of the foot meridians. The main symptoms include lower back pain，fullness of the lower abdomen，frequent and poor urination，etc. See *Su Wen* chapter 36.

足厥阴之筋 即足厥阴经筋，为十二经筋之一。起于足大趾上边，联络各经筋。出《灵枢·经筋》。

足厥阴之筋（zú jué yīn zhī jīn）**meridian sinew of foot** *jueyin* It is one of the twelve meridian sinews，orginating from the top of the big foot toe and connecting to other sinews. See *Ling Shu* chapter 13.

足跗 足背。见《灵枢·本输》。

足跗（zú fū）**instep** It refers to the instep. See *Ling Shu* chapter 2.

足痹 气血衰少，不能荣养下肢皮肉筋脉所致之痹证。出《灵枢·阴阳二十五人》。

足痹（zú bì）　**foot impediment** Impediment syndrome caused by deficiency of qi and blood that are unable to nourish the skin and muscles of the lower limbs. See *Ling Shu* chapter 64.

员针　九针之一。长一寸六分，针身圆柱形，针尖圆钝，后人有称为"圆头针"，可作按摩之用，既可疏泄分肉之间的气血，又不损伤肌肉。出《灵枢·九针十二原》。

员针（yuán zhēn）　**rounded needle** One of the nine needles. It is 1.6 *cun* long with a cylindrical needle body and blunt needle tip, thus later generations also called it the round headed needle. It can be used in massage to rub in partings of the muscles without harming the muscles; it also serves to drain qi from the partings of the muscles. See *Ling Shu* chapter 1.

员利针　"九针"之一，针长一寸六分，针身细小，针尖中部稍大而员利，用治暴痹，急性病症。出《灵枢·九针论》《灵枢·九针十二原》。

员利针（yuán lì zhēn）　**sharp-round needle** One of the nine needles. This needle is 1.6 *cun* long, with a tiny needle body, and with the middle part of the needle tip slightly big and sharp. It can be used to treat violent impediment and acute diseases. See *Ling Shu* chapter 78, and *Ling Shu* chapter 1.

听宫　经穴名。属手太阳小肠经。在耳屏前方，下颌骨髁乳突后缘，张口时呈凹陷处。出《灵枢·刺节真邪》。

听宫（tīng gōng）　**Ting Gong (SI 19)** Acupoint name. It pertains to the small intestine meridian of hand *taiyang* and is located in front of the tragus, at the posterior margin of the mandibular condyle and mastoid process, at the concave part when opening the mouth. See *Ling Shu* chapter 75.

别阳　臂臑穴之古称。在曲池直上七寸处。属手阳明经。出《灵枢·卫气》。

别阳（bié yáng）　**divergent yang** The ancient name of acupoint LI 14, which is 7 *cun* above Qu Chi（LI 11）, pertaining to the large intestine meridian of hand *yangming*. See *Ling Shu* chapter 52.

别络　络脉之较大者，为本经别走邻经之络脉。十二经脉在四肢部各分出一支别络，再加上躯干部的任脉之络、督脉之络及脾之大络，合为十五别络。别络能沟通表里两经的联系，并补充经脉循行分布的不足。出《灵枢·逆顺肥瘦》。

别络（bié luò）　**divergent collaterals** The fifteen main collaterals are made up of twelve collaterals which branch out from the twelve regular channels at the limbs，plus one collateral each for the conception vessel at the front and the governor vessel at the back，and the major collateral of the spleen at the lateral side of the trunk. Connecting collaterals can strengthen the connection between the internally-externally paired meridians and reach areas of the body not supplied or interconnected by the regular meridians. See *Ling Shu* chapter 38.

岐伯　又称天师。为传说中上古时代医家。相传黄帝与岐伯等人讨论医药而创医药学。《黄帝内经》中多以黄帝问、岐伯答的形式撰写，故后人将"岐黄"并称，作为祖国医学的代名词。如《素问·上古天真论》："岐伯对曰。"

岐伯（qí bó）　**Qi Bo** Also called the Heavenly teacher. A leg-endary doctor in early ancient era. It is said that by discussing with Qi Bo and other experts，Huang Di established TCM. *Huang Di Nei Jing*（*Huang Di's Internal Classic*）is mostly written in the form of Huang Di's questions and Qi Bo's answers，so Qihuang is another name for TCM in later generations. For example，"Qi Bo answered" in *Su Wen* chapter 1.

岐骨　泛指骨骼连接成角之处。出《灵枢·经脉》。

岐骨（qí gǔ）　**forking bone** It refers to the body part where bones are connected into angles. See *Ling Shu* chapter 10.

针石　即砭石。是一些经过磨制而成的锥形或楔形的石针，为古代针刺及外科用具。出《素问·移精变气论》。

针石（zhēn shí）　**needling stone** Also named stone needle. It is a kind of ancient stone needle used as a surgical instrument that has been grinded into a cone or wedge-shape. See *Su Wen* chapter 13.

针论　古医籍名。从书名推测当与针刺有关、已佚。出《灵枢·官能》。

针论（zhēn lùn）　***The discourse***

on needles An ancient medical book, which has been lost in history. From the name, it can be deduced that the book was about acupuncture. See *Ling Shu* chapter 73.

针空 空,通孔。即今之所谓针孔。出《素问·刺志论》。

针空(zhēn kōng) **needle hole** "空" is the same as "孔", refers to hole. *Zhēn kōng* refers to pinhole or needle hole. See *Su Wen* chapter 53.

针经 古医籍名,是一部关于针刺疗法的专著。《灵枢》在流传过程中,曾一度名为《针经》,但是否为同一本书,尚待考证。见《素问·八正神明论》。

针经(zhēn jīng) *Needle classic* It is the title of an ancient monograph on acupuncture therapy. In the process of its circulation, *Ling Shu* was once called *Zhen Jing* (*Needle Classic*), but whether the two are the same is yet to be verified. See *Su Wen* chapter 26.

针解 《素问》篇名。针解,即解释用针的方法。此篇主要论述了针刺的补泻手法及用针的要点,解释九针上应天地四时阴阳的道理。故名。

针解(zhēn jiě) **Explanation of Acupuncture** Chapter name in *Su Wen*. *Zhēn jiě* literally means the explanation of acupuncture techniques. This chapter mainly discusses the tonifying and draining methods of acupuncture, and the key points on manipulations. It also explains the principle that the nine needles should correspond to the four seasons, heaven and earth, and yin and yang. Hence the name.

牡藏 阳脏。牡(mǔ 母),雄性鸟兽,与牝相对,引申为阳性。阴阳中又可分阴阳,五脏为阴,心、肝为阴中之阳脏,故为牡藏。出《灵枢·顺气一日分为四时》。

牡藏(mǔ zàng) **male viscera** *Mǔ* refers to male birds and beasts, which is the opposite of *Pìn* (female birds and beasts). Here it refers to yang, an extended meaning. The five viscera pertains to yin, but in further divisions, the heart and the liver pertain to yang, so they are yang viscera in yin, hence the name. See *Ling Shu* chapter 44.

伸欠 症状名。伸,伸动肢体。欠,呵欠。其机理为疟邪发动,阴阳相引。出《素问·疟论》。

伸欠（shēn qiàn）　**yawning and stretching** Symptom name. *Shēn* means to stretch, and *qiàn* here means to yawn. The symptoms are caused by the onset of pathogenic malaria，with the interaction of yin and yang. See *Su Wen* chapter 35.

作强之官　指肾。出《素问·灵兰秘典论》。

作强之官（zuò qiáng zhī guān）　**The organ of strenuous work** Refers to the kidney. See *Su Wen* chapter 8.

伯高　传说中上古时代的医家。为黄帝之臣，精于针灸术。出《灵枢·寿夭刚柔》。

伯高（bó gāo）　**Bo Gao** A legendary doctor in ancient times. He was a minister of Huang Di（Yellow Emperor）and excelled in acupuncture. See *Ling Shu* chapter 6.

身有病而无邪脉　此论怀孕之体征及脉象，其身虽有经断恶阻等不适之象，但脉来和滑，不见病脉，乃是怀子之征兆。出《素问·腹中论》。

身有病而无邪脉（shēn yǒu bìng ér wú xié mài）　**Poor health when no symptom can be felt in the pulse.** It discusses the signs and pulse manifestations of pregnant women，who have symptoms like amenorrhea，nausea，vomiting，dizziness，fatigue，etc.，but their pulses are harmonious and slippery，with no abnormal pulse manifestations，and all of these are signs of pregnancy. See *Su Wen* chapter 40.

近气　针刺时的已至之气。出《素问·调经论》。

近气（jìn qì）　**qi arrival** The qi which has arrived during acupuncture. See *Su Wen* chapter 62.

近者奇之　病位在上部，近于胃的，属阳，用奇方治疗。出《素问·至真要大论》。

近者奇之（jìn zhě qí zhī）　**Proximally located diseases should be treated with odd formulas.** For diseases located in the upper part of the body（close to the stomach），their nature pertains to yang，thus they should be treated with odd formulas. See *Su Wen* chapter 74.

彻衣　刺五节法之一，主要治疗阳气有余，阴气不足的发热病。取天府、大杼、中膂俞以去热，补足手太阴穴以出汗。言其效验，有如去掉衣服之快，故名。出《灵枢·刺节真邪》。

彻衣（chè yī）　**to undress** One of

the five major needling methods, which is mainly employed to treat fever caused by excessive yang qi and deficient yin qi. By needling acupoint Tian Fu (LU 3), Da Zhu (BL 11) and Zhong LYU Shu (BL 29), it disperses the heat, and tonifies the hand *taiyin* acupoints to promote sweating. It works as fast as to undress, hence the name. See *Ling Shu* chapter 75.

谷气 出《灵枢·终始》。① 水谷精气。见《类经·针刺二十八》。② 指胃气。见《类经·针刺八》。

谷气（gǔ qì） See *Ling Shu* chapter 9. ① Essence of water and grain. See *Lei Jing*（Classified Classic）"Needling Chapter 28". ② Stomach qi. See *Lei Jing*（Classified Classic）"Needling Chapter 8".

谷气通于脾 五谷之气属土，脾为土脏，故相通应。出《素问·阴阳应象大论》。

谷气通于脾（gǔ qì tōng yú pí）**Grain qi communicates with the spleen.** Both grain qi and spleen pertain to the earth element, and thus are interconnected. See *Su Wen* chapter 5.

肝 ① 五脏之一。居于膈下，经脉布于两胁。具有藏血、调节血液及升发条达，疏畅气机，调节情志的作用。其经脉为足厥阴肝经，与足少阳胆经相表里。五行配属为木，主时于春。其在体为筋，在志为怒，在液为泪，在窍为目，在味为酸，病理特征为风。出《素问·调经论》《素问·六节藏象论》。② 肝的精气。出《素问·阴阳应象大论》。③ 足厥阴肝经的经气。出《灵枢·本输》。④ 肝病。出《素问·阴阳别论》。⑤ 肝的气化。出《素问·刺禁论》。⑥ 肝的脉象。出《素问·玉机真藏论》。⑦ 肝在面部的望诊部位（鼻柱）。出《灵枢·五色》。

肝（gān） ① One of the five viscera. Located under the diaphragm, and its meridian runs in the costal regions. Liver stores and regulates blood, soothes circuits and qi, and regulates emotions. The liver meridian of foot *jueyin* is interiorly-exteriorly related to the foot *shaoyang* gallbladder meridian. According to five elements, liver pertains to wood, and dominates spring. In the body it is sinews; among the states of mind it is anger; among liquids it is tears; among the orifices it is the eye; among the flavors it is sour. Wind is the pathological characteristic of the liver. See *Su Wen* chapter 9 and chapter 62. ② The essence qi of the liver. See *Su Wen* chapter 5. ③ The qi of the liver meridian of foot *jueyin*. See *Ling Shu* chapter 2. ④ Liver diseases. See *Su Wen* chapter 7. ⑤ The transformation of liver qi. See *Su Wen* chapter 52. ⑥ The pulse manifestation of the liver. See *Su Wen* chapter 19. ⑦ The area on the face showing the condition of the liver (nasal column). See *Ling Shu* chapter 49.

肝气　① 肝的精气。有养筋濡目的生理作用。《灵枢·脉度》。② 指肝的病气。出《素问·玉机真藏论》《灵枢·淫邪发梦》。

肝气(gān qì)　① The essence qi of liver, which physiologically nourishes sinews and eyes. See *Ling Shu* chapter 17. ② The disease qi of liver. See *Su Wen* chapter 19 and *Ling Shu* chapter 43.

肝气内变　即肝气内病。出《素问·四气调神大论》。

肝气内变(gān qì nèi biàn)　**Liver qi changes internally.** It refers to the pathogenic changes of liver qi. See *Su Wen* chapter 2.

肝风　病名。五脏风之一。病起于肝之俞穴，为风邪所中。症候所见与肝的病理特点有关，故名。出《素问·风论》。

肝风(gān fēng)　**liver wind Disease name.** One of the wind syndromes of the five viscera. It is caused by pathogenic wind invading acupoint BL 18. Its symptoms are related to the pathological features of the liver，hence the name. See *Su Wen* chapter 42.

肝风疝　疝病之由风邪侵袭肝脉所致者。出《素问·四时刺逆从论》。

肝风疝(gān fēng shàn)　**liver-wind hernia** Liver-wind hernia is caused by the wind pathogen invading the liver meridian. See *Su Wen* chapter 64.

肝为阴中之少阳　阴阳之中又有阴阳可分。肝为阳脏，而居于膈下阴位，为阴中之阳。由于肝气旺于春，阳气生发而未盛，故曰少阳。出《灵枢·顺气一日分为四时》《素问·金匮真言论》《灵枢·阴阳系日月》。《素问·六节藏象论》作"阳中之少阳"。参该条。

肝为阴中之少阳(gān wéi yīn zhōng zhī shào yáng)　**Liver**

七画

is the *shaoyang* of yin. Yin and yang respectively include a further division of yin and yang. The liver is a yang viscera, but it is located under the diaphragm, pertaining to yin, hence it is yang in yin. The liver qi flourishes in spring, during which yang qi is being generated but not thriving, hence it is called *shaoyang*. See *Ling Shu* chapter 44, *Su Wen* chapter 4, *Ling Shu* chapter 41 and *Su Wen* chapter 9. See "阳中之少阳"。

肝为泪　眼泪为五液之一,出于目,目为肝之窍,故云。出《素问·宣明五气》。

肝为泪（gān wéi lèi）　**liver forms tears** Tears are one of the five kinds of fluids generated by the eye. The eye is the orifice of the liver, thus the liver forms tears. See *Su Wen* chapter 23.

肝心痛　病证名。厥心痛之一。由肝气厥逆犯心所效,症见心痛面色青暗如死灰,常欲太息,然碍于心痛而不能。出《灵枢·厥病》。

肝心痛（gān xīn tòng）　**reversal heartache caused by liver disorder** Disease name. It is one of the reversal heartaches. It is caused by reversal liver qi invading the heart, leading to reversal heart pain, and a pale face like a corpse. The patients tend to sigh, but are always hindered by heart pain. See *Ling Shu* chapter 24.

肝生于左　言肝脏脏气之主治。生,生发之意。人身面南,左东右西。肝主春生之气,位居东方,故生于左。出《素问·刺禁论》。

肝生于左（gān shēng yú zuǒ）　**Liver qi begins circulating from the left.** It refers to the major functions of liver qi. *Shēng* means to generate. When facing south, on the left is the east, and on the right is the west. Liver governs the generating qi of spring, which is located in the east, thus its qi begins circulating from the left. See *Su Wen* chapter 52.

肝生筋　肝主筋,肝的精气有生养筋的作用。见《素问·阴阳应象大论》《素问·经脉别论》。

肝生筋（gān shēng jīn）　**Liver nourishes the sinews.** Liver governs the sinews, and the essence qi of liver generates and nourishes the sinews. See *Su Wen* chapter 5 and *Su Wen* chapter 21.

肝主目　目为肝之窍。出《素问·阴阳应象大论》《灵枢·脉度》。

肝主目（gān zhǔ mù）　**Liver governs the eyes.** The eyes are the orifices of the liver. See *Su Wen* chapter 5, and *Ling Shu* chapter 17.

肝主身之筋膜　出《素问·痿论》。

肝主身之筋膜（gān zhǔ shēn zhī jīn mó）　**Liver governs the sinews and the ligaments.** See *Su Wen* chapter 44.

肝主泣　泣，泪之属。义同"肝为泪"。参该条。出《灵枢·九针论》。

肝主泣（gān zhǔ qì）　**Liver governs tears.** *Qì* literally means to cry, or generating tears. Refer to the term "肝为泪", which shares the same meaning. See *Ling Shu* chapter 78.

肝主春　此以五行学说归纳脏腑与季节时日的关系及治法。春季主要属东方。足厥阴肝是木脏，为乙木、阴木；足少阳胆与肝相表里，为甲木、阳木，故治法相同。出《素问·藏气法时论》。

肝主春（gān zhǔ chūn）　**Liver pertains to spring.** According to five-element theory, spring pertains to the east. This is a term for TCM treatment based on the relationship between the five-element theory and the season. Spring pertains to the east and the liver meridian of foot *jueyin* pertains to wood, which is *yi* wood, or yin wood; the gallbladder meridian of foot *shaoyang*, which is interiorly and exteriorly related with the liver, is *jia* wood, namely yang wood, hence the diseases of these two are treated in the same way. See *Su Wen* chapter 22.

肝主语　语，多言之意。言肝之病。肝病郁，多语以畅之。出《灵枢·九针论》。

肝主语（gān zhǔ yǔ）　**Liver disease causes polylogia.** *Yǔ* means talking much. It refers to liver diseases. Liver diseases are characterized by stagnation and depression, which can be unobstructed and smoothened out by talking more. See *Ling Shu* chapter 78.

肝主筋　主，主持、掌管之意。肝藏血，血养筋而柔，故肝所主之外合为筋。见《素问·宣明五气》。

肝主筋（gān zhǔ jīn）　**Liver governs the sinews.** *Zhǔ* means to govern or dominate. Liver stores blood, which nourishes and softens the sinews, thus liver governs the sinews. See *Su Wen* chapter 23.

肝合胆　合，配合之意。足少阳胆经与足厥阴肝经相表里，胆附于肝，两者功能上有密切的联系。出《灵枢·本输》。

肝合胆（gān hé dǎn）　**Liver is united with the gallbladder.** *Hé* means to cooperate. There is an interior-exterior relationship between the gallbladder meridian of foot *shaoyang* and liver meridian of foot *jueyin*, and the gallbladder is attached to the liver, thus they are closely related functionally. See *Ling Shu* chapter 2.

肝合筋　合，配合之意。义同"肝主筋"，参该条。出《灵枢·五色》。

肝合筋（gān hé jīn）　**Liver and gallbladder are paired.** *Hé* means to cooperate. Refer to the term "肝主筋"，which shares the same meaning. See *Ling Shu* chapter 49.

肝足厥阴之脉　即足厥阴肝经，为十二经脉之一。其循行路线从足大趾丛毛的边缘开始，沿足背上至内踝前一寸处，向上沿胫骨内缘，在内踝上八寸处，交叉到足太阴经之后，上行过膝内侧，沿大腿内侧，入阴毛中，环绕阴器，至少腹与胃经并行，属于肝，络于胆，穿过横膈，分布于胁肋，沿喉咙之后，进入鼻咽部，上行连于目系，上出额部，直达头顶，与督脉交合于巅顶百会穴。一支从目系下行于颊里，环行唇内。再一支从肝穿过膈肌，向上注于肺中（接手太阴肺经）。出《灵枢·经脉》。

肝足厥阴之脉（gān zú jué yīn zhī mài）　**liver meridian of foot** *jueyin* One of the twelve meridians. It starts from the verge of the hair on the big toe and goes along the back of the foot to one *cun* in front of the inner ankle. Then it goes upward along the inner side of the shin bone to the pubic hair and goes around the genitals, after that, it goes to the belly and parallels the stomach meridian, pertaining to liver and connecting to the muscles. Then it penetrates the diaphragm and scatters in the rib area until it arrives at the throat. After that, it goes upward into the nasopharynx nasalis, and then arrives at the eyes, exits from the forehead and finally reaches the top of the head to meet the governor vessel at Bai Hui (DU 20) acupoint. There are two branches, one going downward from the eyes to the inner cheek and then going around the inner side of the lips; another going upward, penetrating the liver and the diaphragm muscles to enter the lung (connecting lung meridian of hand *taiyin*). See *Ling Shu* chapter 10.

肝系　肝连系于胆的脉络。出《灵枢·论勇》。

肝系（gān xì）　**liver connection** The meridian and collaterals connecting the liver to the gallbladder. See *Ling Shu* chapter 50.

肝应爪　应，应合之意。爪为反映肝脏脏气盛衰之处。后世有"爪为筋之余"之说。出《灵枢·本藏》。

肝应爪（gān yìng zhǎo）　**Liver corresponds to the finger/toe nails.** *Yìng* means to correspond. *Zhǎo* (finger/toe nails) reveals the status of the liver qi, and there is a saying by later generations "Nails are the surplus of the sinews". See *Ling Shu* chapter 47.

肝者主为将　义同"将军之官"。《灵枢·五癃津液别》作"肝为之将"。见"将军之官"条。出《灵枢·师传》。

肝者主为将（gān zhě zhǔ wéi jiāng）　**Liver rules as a general.** It refers to the term "The official functioning as a general", which shares the same meaning. In *Ling Shu* chapter 36, it is expressed as "The liver is his general". See "将军之官". See *Ling Shu* chapter 29.

肝胀　病证名。五脏胀之一。症见胁下满痛，波及小腹。《灵枢·胀论》。

肝胀（gān zhàng）　**liver distention** Disease name. It pertains to visceral distension. Liver distention is manifested as fullness and pain in hypochondrium which spreads to lower abdomen. See *Ling Shu* chapter 35.

肝疟　五脏疟之一。症见面色青灰，太息等。出《素问·刺疟篇》。

肝疟（gān nüè）　**liver malaria** Disease name. One out the five visceral malarias. The main symptoms include a greenish complexion, and deep breathing, etc. See *Su Wen* chapter 36.

肝咳　五脏咳之一。证候特点为咳而两胁疼痛。肢胁为肝经分野，该部痛胀，故名肝咳。出《素问·咳论》。

肝咳（gān ké）　**liver cough** Disease

name. One kind of visceral cough with the main symptoms of coughing, and pain in both hypochondriums, etc. The hypochondrium is the division of the liver meridian, hence the pain and swelling in this area caused by the coughing, is considered to be caused by liver. See *Su Wen* chapter 38

肝脉弦　指应指端直而长,如按琴弦的脉象,为肝之正常脉。参"弦"条。出《素问·宣明五气》。

肝脉弦(gān mài xián)　**Liver pulse is string-like.** A straight, long and taut pulse, feeling like a musical string. A string-like pulse is the normal manifestation of the liver. Refer to the term "弦". See *Su Wen* chapter 23.

肝恶风　恶(wù 误),厌憎之意。肝属木,与风相应,感风易伤筋而见瘛疭挛急等病,故恶风。出《素问·宣明五气》。

肝恶风(gān wù fēng)　**Liver is averse to wind.** *Wù* means to dislike or loathe. Liver pertains to the wood element and corresponds to wind, thus it is susceptible to wind pathogens, which undermine the sinews and lead to symptoms like convul-sions, contractures and spasms, etc. Therefore the liver is averse to wind. See *Su Wen* chapter 23.

肝腧　经穴名。属足太阳膀胱经穴名,在第九椎下两旁一寸五分处。出《灵枢·背俞》。

肝腧(gān shù)　**Gan Shu (BL 18)** Acupoint name, which is located one and a half *cun* below the ninth vertebra, and pertains to the bladder meridian of foot *taiyang*. See *Ling Shu* chapter 51.

肝痹　病证名。五脏痹之一。内外感风邪不解,邪阻肝脉,或筋痹日久,反复感受风寒湿邪发展而来。症见胁痛、呕吐,易惊等。出《素问·痹论》《素问·玉机真藏论》。

肝痹(gān bì)　**liver impediment** Disease name. It pertains to visceral impediment. Liver impediment is caused by wind pathogens invading the body and blocking the liver meridian; or caused by the prolonged impediment of sinews caused by the repeated invasion of wind pathogens, cold and dampness. The main symptoms include hypochondriac pain, vomiting and vulnerability to shock, etc.

See *Su Wen* chapter 43 and *Su Wen* chapter 19.

肝雍　雍同壅。出《素问·大奇论》。(1)指肝气壅滞。见《素问注证发微》。(2)指肝气满而外壅于肝之经络。见《素问集注》。

肝雍（gān yōng）　**liver congestion** "雍" equals to "壅". See *Su Wen* chapter 48. (1) The congestion of liver qi. See *Su Wen Zhu Zheng Fa Wei*（*Annotation and Elaboration on Su Wen*）. (2) Excessive liver qi congesting the liver meridian. See *Su Wen Ji Zhu*（*Collected Annotation of Su Wen*）.

肝藏血　肝有贮藏血液和调节血量的功能。见《素问·调经论》《灵枢·本神》。

肝藏血（gān cáng xiě）　**Liver stores blood.** The liver has the function of storing and regulating blood. See *Su Wen* chapter 62, and *Ling Shu* chapter 8.

肝藏魂　肝与人体精神活动有一定关系。魂属精神活动之一,其随神往来,为附气之神,即意识知觉之类,属阳。肝为阴中之阳脏,故魂藏于肝。出《素问·宣明五气》。

肝藏魂（gān cáng hún）　**Liver stores soul.** There is a certain relationship between the liver and human spiritual activities. The changing of the soul is one of the spiritual activities. It travels with spirit and goes with qi, pertaining to yang. Liver is the yang of yin viscera, thus the soul is stored in liver. See *Su Wen* chapter 23.

肘　指前臂与上臂交接处能屈伸的部位。见《素问·刺禁论》。

肘（zhǒu）　**elbow** It refers to the area where the forearm and upper arm meet and can flex. See *Su Wen* chapter 52.

肘网　谓臂肘部犹如网罗之牵急感。《灵枢·经筋》。

肘网（zhǒu wǎng）　**elbow net-contraction** It refers to the tightening feeling in the elbow as if a net is contracting. See *Ling Shu* chapter 13.

肠风　病名。主症为泄泻完谷不化,由病风日久传里,或反复感受风邪入中而致。出《素问·风论》。

肠风（cháng fēng）　**intestinal wind** Disease name in which the main symptom is diarrhea with undigested food. It is caused by the prolonged invasion of wind pathogens, which enter into the interior, or by contracting a wind pathogen repeatedly，which enters into the interior. See *Su Wen* chapter 42.

肠胃　① 泛指大肠、小肠与胃。出《素问·阴阳应象大论》。②《灵枢》篇名。此篇主要介绍肠胃的大小、长短、部位和容量，故名。

肠胃（cháng wèi）　① The large intestine，small intestine and stomach. See *Su Wen* chapter 5. ② A chapter name in *Ling Shu*. This chapter mainly introduces the size，length，location and capacity of the stomach，hence the name.

肠痈　病名。发于肠之痈疡，因热毒内结所致。出《素问·厥论》。

肠痈（cháng yōng）　**intestinal abscess** Disease name，refers to abscesses and ulcers of the intestines，which is caused by the accumulation of heat toxin in the intestines. See *Su Wen* chapter 45.

肠覃　覃同蕈，附木而生之菌类。覃，病名。为附肠而生之肿物。症见腹大如怀子之状，按之坚硬。出《灵枢·水胀》。

肠覃（cháng xùn）　**lower abdominal mass** "覃" equals to "蕈"，refers to fungi that attaches to wood. *Xùn* refers to lumps attached to the intestines which manifests

with a big abdomen as if pregnant，and is hard when pressing. See *Ling Shu* chapter 57.

肠痹　病证名。症见饮水多而小便少，腹中有气攻冲，肠鸣，经常泄泻，完谷不化。出《素问·痹论》。

肠痹（cháng bì）　**intestinal impediment** Disease name. The main symptoms include drinking more water and urinating less，flatulence，rumbling intestines，frequent diarrhea，and undigested food in stools. See *Su Wen* chapter 43.

肠溜　病名。溜亦作瘤。肠间结聚之肿块。由于邪留肠间，卫气凑聚，日久则津液不行，互相结聚而成。出《灵枢·刺节真邪》。

肠溜（cháng liū）　**intestinal tumors** Disease name，referring to lumps accumulated in the intestines. "溜" is also written as "瘤". Due to the retention of pathogens in the intestines，the defense qi accumulates so as to get rid of it. However，the prolonged accumulation of defensive qi blocks the circulation of fluids，thus causing lumps. See *Ling Shu* chapter 75.

肠澼　即肠澼。见该条。出《素问·阴阳别论》。

肠辟（cháng pì）　**dysentery** The same as "肠澼". See *Su Wen* chapter 7.

肠癀　病证名。出《灵枢·邪气藏府病形》。(1) 直肠脱出之脱肛症。癀同癫，通颓。见《太素·五藏脉诊》。(2) 便下脓血。见《灵枢集注》。(3) 疝漏一类病证。见《类经·脉色十九》。(4) 癫病之一。见《灵枢识》。

肠癀（cháng tuí）　**intestinal prominence-illness** Disease name. See *Ling Shu* chapter 4. (1) Rectocele. "癀" is the same as "癫" or "颓". See *Tai Su* "Five viscera pulse diagnosis". (2) Hematochezia. See *Ling Shu Ji Zhu*（*Collected Annotation of Ling Shu*). (3) Symptoms similar to those of hernias and fistulas. See *Lei Jing*（*Classified Classic*）"Pulse and Color Chapter 19". (4) Acute pain from the penis to the paunch. See *Ling Shu Zhi*（*Understanding Ling Shu*).

肠澼　即痢疾。出《素问·生气通天论》。

肠澼（cháng pì）　**intestinal afflux dysentery** See *Su Wen* chapter 3.

狂　病证名。神志失常，躁扰不宁。多为阳盛扰乱神明所致。出《素问·生气通天论》《灵枢·癫狂》。

狂（kuáng）　**madness** Disease name，with symptoms such as insanity，irritability and restlessness，and usually caused by excessive yang disturbing spirit brilliance. See *Su Wen* chapter 3 and *Ling Shu* chapter 22.

狂巅　病证名。出《素问·脉解》。(1) 指狂与癫两种神志病。见《太素·经脉病解》。(2) 狂躁而兼头顶痛。见《素问》吴崑注。(3) 指狂及头顶部疾患。见《素问经注节解》。

狂巅（kuáng diān）　**mania and epilepsy** Disease name. See *Su Wen* chapter 49. (1) Two kinds of mental diseases：mania and epilepsy. See *Tai Su*（*Classified Study on Huang Di Nei Jing*）"Treatment of Meridian Diseases". (2) Manic with headache. See *Su Wen* annotated by Wu Kun. (3) Madness and head diseases. See *Su Wen Jing Zhu Jie Jie*（*Annotation and Explanation of Su Wen*).

角　① jué。五音之一。五行属木，为东方春木之音。运气学说将五音代表五运，以五音建运，则角为木运。出《素问·阴阳应象大论》② jiáo。额角。出《灵枢·经筋》。③ 星宿名。角宿，二十八宿之一。出《素

七画

问·五运行大论》。④ 耳上角。出《灵枢·五阅五使》。

角（jué） ① One of the five tones. *Jué*, the tone of the east, spring and wood，pertains to the wood element. In the theory of five circuits and six qi，the five tones represent the five circuits. *Jué* represents wood. See *Su Wen* chapter 5. ② Pronounced as *Jiáo*，refers to the temporal aspect. See *Ling Shu* chapter 13. ③ The name of a constellation in one of the twenty eight constellations. See *Su Wen* chapter 67. ④ The tip of the upper ear. See *Ling Shu* chapter 37.

角孙　角，jiǎo。经穴名。属手少阳三焦经，在侧头部，当耳尖直上之发际处。出《灵枢·寒热病》。

角孙（jiǎo sūn）　**Jiao Sun（TB 20）**Acupoint name, pertaining to the triple *jiao* meridian of hand *shaoyang*，located at the side of the head，where the tip of the ear meets the hairline. See *Ling Shu* chapter 21.

鸠尾　① 骨骼名。指胸骨剑突。出《灵枢·经脉》。② 经穴名。别名尾翳，属任脉络穴，为膏之原穴。在腹正中线剑突下方，当脐上七寸处。出《灵枢·九

针十二原》。

鸠尾（jiū wěi）　① Bone name. Xiphoid process. See *Ling Shu* chapter 10. ② Acupoint name. Jiu Wei（CV 15）acupoint，also called Wei Yi. It pertains to the conception vessel and is located below the xiphoid process，seven inches above the belly button. See *Ling Shu* chapter 1.

卵　即睾丸。出《灵枢·五色》。

卵（luǎn）　**testicles** See *Ling Shu* chapter 49.

灸　用艾叶做成的艾炷，在穴位上点燃熏灼，以防治疾病的一种方法。出《素问·异法方宜论》。

灸（jiǔ）　**moxibustion** A burning moxa cone is used to cauterize certain acupoints，so as to prevent or treat diseases. See *Su Wen* chapter 12.

灸刺　灸法和刺法，古书中泛指针灸。出《灵枢·四时气》《素问·血气形志》。

灸刺（jiǔ cì）　**moxibustion and acupuncture** See *Ling Shu* chapter 19 and *Su Wen* chapter 24.

灸焫　用艾火烧灼的一种治法。出《素问·异法方宜论》。

灸焫（jiǔ ruò）　**moxibustion with moxafire** The treatment to cauterize certain acupoints with a burning moxa cone. See *Su Wen* chapter 12.

迎　① 针刺方法之一。即迎随补泻法中的泻法,针刺时针尖方向与经脉走向相反。出《灵枢·小针解》。② 受纳。出《灵枢·师传》。

迎 (yíng)　① An acupuncture technique. It refers to a draining method of directional tonification. When needling, the tip of the needle is against the flow direction of the meridian. See *Ling Shu* chapter 3.② To receive. See *Ling Shu* chapter 29.

饮　① 痰饮。出《素问·六元正纪大论》。② 药物煎剂。出《素问·病能论》。③ 喝饮。出《素问·痹论》。

饮 (yǐn)　① Phlegm-fluid retention. See *Su Wen* chapter 71. ② Decoction. See *Su Wen* chapter 46. ③ To drink. See *Su Wen* chapter 43.

饮中热　病证名。出《素问·刺志论》。(1)指痰饮。痰饮留于脾胃之中而发热。见《素问》王冰注。(2)指饮酒。因经常饮酒而导致内热之证。见《素问直解》。

饮中热 (yǐn zhōng rè)　**heat in beverages** Disease name. See *Su Wen* chapter 53. (1) Phlegm-fluid retention, retained in the spleen and stomach, causing heat. See *Su Wen* annotated by Wang Bing. (2) Drinking alcohol. Frequent drinking will cause internal heat syndrome. See *Su Wen Zhi Jie* (*Direct Interpretation on Su Wen*).

辛入肺　与"辛生肺"同理。出《素问·宣明五气》。

辛入肺 (xīn rù fèi)　**Pungency corresponds to the lung.** The same as "辛生肺"(pungency nourishes the lung). See *Su Wen* chapter 23.

辛頞　辛,酸辛。頞(è 遏),鼻梁。辛頞即鼻部感到酸辛。为鼻渊主症之一。出《素问·气厥论》。

辛頞(xīn è)　**irritating sensation in the nose** *Xīn* refers to pungent. *È* refers to the bridge of the nose. This term refers to a sour nose, which is the main symptom of nasosinusitis. See *Su Wen* chapter 37.

肓　① 心下膈上的部位。出《素问·刺禁论》。② 脏腑之间的膈膜,又称肓膜。出《素问·腹中论》。

肓(huāng)　① Cardiodiaphragmatic interspace. See *Su Wen* chapter 52. ② Membranes between viscera and bowels, and

七画

also called huang-membranes. See *Su Wen* chapter 40.

肓之原　亦称肓原，为肓之原穴，在脐下脖胦（即气海穴）处。出《素问·腹中论》《灵枢·九针十二原》。

肓之原（huāng zhī yuán）**Original huang acupoints.** With the name of acupoint CV 6. See *Su Wen* chapter 40 and *Ling Shu* chapter 1.

肓原　在脖胦处（脐下一寸五分）。出《灵枢·四时气》。

肓原（huāng yuán）**original huang acupoints** Located one and a half inches below the navel. See *Ling Shu* chapter 19.

肓膜　肓与膜的合称。指胸腹五脏之间隔的脂膜。出《素问·痹论》。

肓膜（huāng mó）**huang membrane** It is the combination of *huang* and membranes, refers to the membranes among the five viscera. See *Su Wen* chapter 43.

间气　（间，jiān），运气术语。出《素问·至真要大论》。参见"左间""右间"条。

间气（jiān qì）**intermediate qi** It is a term of the five circuits and six qi. See *Su Wen* chapter 74. See "左间" and "右间".

间谷　（间，jiān），出《素问·六元正纪大论》。（1）岁气六步中左右四间气所主时令化成的谷物。见《类经·运气十七》。（2）司天及其左右间气所化之谷物。见《新校正》。（3）邪气所化之谷。间，反间之意。见《新校正》。

间谷（jiān gǔ）**intermediate grain** See *Su Wen* chapter 71. (1) The grains that are produced in the seasons governed by the four intermediate qi of the six steps of annual qi. See *Lei Jing* (*Classified Classic*) "Circuits and Qi Chapter 17". (2) Grains that are produced by celestial control and its left and right intermediate qi. See *Xin Jiao Zheng* (*New Revisions of Su Wen*). (3) The grains produced by pathogenic qi. *Jiān* here means discord or distrust. See *Xin Jiao Zheng* (*New Revisions of Su Wen*).

间使　（间，jiān），经穴名。手厥阴心包经之经穴。在掌后三寸，两筋间。出《灵枢·本输》。

间使（jiān shǐ）**Jian Shi (PC 5)** Acupoint name, pertaining to the pericadium meridian of hand jueyin, which is located between the two sinews three inches posterior to the palm.

See *Ling Shu* chapter 2.

判角　体质名。阴阳二十五人中木形人之一种。

判角（pàn jué）　*pan jue* Name of constitution among one of the twenty-five people of yin and yang，and pertains to the physique of wood.

判角之人　体质名。判，半；角，五音之一，五行属木。判角，角音之一，此代表阴阳二十五人中木形人之一种。其特征是正直不阿。出《灵枢·阴阳二十五人》。参"木形之人"。

判角之人（pàn jué zhī rén）　*panjue*-type people Name of constitution，and is one of the twenty-five people of yin and yang. *Pàn* means half；*jué* is among the five tones，and pertains to the wood element. *Pàn jué* is one of the tones of *jue*，and here refers to one kind of people of the physique of "wood". People of this kind are characterized by integrity. See *Ling Shu* chapter 64. See "木形之人".

判商　运气术语。商，金运。见《素问·五常政大论》。参"商"条。

判商（pàn shāng）　*pan shang* A term of circuits and qi. *Shāng* means metal circuit. See *Su Wen* chapter 70. See "商".

判徵　体质名。又称质判。判，半也；徵（zhǐ 指），五音之一，五行属火。判徵，徵音之一，此代表阴阳二十五人中火形人之一种。出《灵枢·五音五味》。见"质判之人"。

判徵（pàn zhǐ）　*pan zhi* Name of constitution. *Pàn* means half；*zhǐ* is one of the five tones and pertains to the fire element. *Pàn zhǐ* is one of the tones of *zhǐ*，and here refers to people of the physique of "fire". See *Ling Shu* chapter 65. See "质判之人".

沉　① 指沉伏于里，重按乃得的一种脉象，主里证。见《素问·脉要精微论》《素问·平人气象论》。② 指枯晦的色泽。见《灵枢·五色》。③ 指深层部位。见《灵枢·卫气失常》。④ 重着，沉重。见《灵枢·杂病》。⑤ 消沉。见《素问·四气调神大论》。

沉（chén）　① Sunken pulse，indicating an interior syndrome. See *Su Wen* chapter 17 and 18. ② Dull and pale in color. See *Ling Shu* chapter 49. ③ Deep layer part. See *Ling Shu* chapter 59. ④ A depression. See *Ling Shu* chapter 26. ⑤ To sink in the depth. See *Su Wen* chapter 2.

七画

沉痔 病名。出《灵枢·邪气藏府病形》。（1）内痔之谓。见《太素·五藏脉诊》。（2）沉久难愈之痔。见《灵枢识》。

沉痔（chén zhì） **deep hemorrhoid** Disease name. See *Ling Shu* chapter 4.（1）Internal hemorrhoids. *Tai Su*（*Classified Study on Huang Di Nei Jing*）"Pulse Diagnosis based on Five Viscera".（2）Prolonged hemorrhoids. See *Ling Shu Zhi*（*Understanding Ling Shu*）.

沉厥 两足沉滞厥冷。出《灵枢·邪气藏府病形》。

沉厥（chén jué） **deep reversal** It refers to a cold and heavy sensation in the feet. See *Ling Shu* chapter 4.

忧伤肺 肺主气，愁忧过度，肺气抑郁不畅，宣肃之令不行，故谓伤肺。见《素问·阴阳应象大论》《素问·五运行大论》。

忧伤肺（yōu shāng fèi） **Anxiety damages the lung.** Lung governs qi. Excessive anxiety may depress and block lung qi, and in turn, the lung fails to diffuse and descend qi, hence the name. See *Su Wen* chapter 5 and *Su Wen* chapter 67.

忧恚无言 《灵枢》篇名，恚（huì 汇），《说文》："恨也。"忧恚，忧愁愤恨之意；无言，失音。此篇主要论述因忧愁愤恨引起的失音的病机与治疗。故名。

忧恚无言（yōu huì wú yán） **Loss of Voice due to Anxiety and Rage** Chapter name in *Ling Shu*. *Huì* refers to rage. *Yōu huì* means anxiety and rage. *Wú yán* means loss of voice. This article mainly discusses the pathogenesis and treatment of loss of voice caused by anxiety and rage, hence the name.

完骨 ① 骨名。耳后颞骨乳突。出《灵枢·骨度》。② 穴位名。位于颞骨乳突后下方凹陷中，属足少阳胆经。出《素问·气穴论》。

完骨（wán gǔ） ① Bone name. Mastoid process behind the ear. See *Ling Shu* chapter 14. ② The name of acupoint GB 12，which is on the gallbladder meridian of foot *shaoyang*. See *Su Wen* chapter 58.

穷骨 即尾骶骨，又名尻骨、橛骨，俗称尾椎。位于脊椎骨末端。出《灵枢·癫狂》。

穷骨（qióng gǔ） **coccyx** It is also named Kao bone or Jue bone, commonly known as tailbone, located a the lower end of spine. See *Ling Shu* chapter 22.

良工　即良医。出《素问·汤液醪醴论》《灵枢·五色》。

良工（liáng gōng）　**proficient practitioner** Good doctors. See *Su Wen* chapter 14 and *Ling Shu* chapter 49.

评热病论　《素问》篇名。评，评论、评述。此篇评述了阴阳交、风厥、劳风、肾风等四种热病的病因病机、症状及预后。故名。

评热病论（píng rè bìng lùn）　**Comments on Febrile Diseases** Chapter name in Su Wen. *Píng* means to comment. This chapter discusses the etiology, pathogenesis, symptoms and prognosis of febrile diseases including yin yang interaction, wind-recession, exhaustion wind, and kidney wind etc., hence the name.

补　① 服用五谷、五果、五畜、五菜以充养形体，补益精气。出《素问·藏气法时论》。② 药物治疗中顺从脏腑的特性谓补。出《素问·阴阳应象大论》《素问·藏气法时论》。③ 针刺手法中，呼气进针、吸气出针为补。出《素问·八正神明论》。④ 针刺入皮肤后，针尖顺其经脉所去的方向为补。出《灵枢·小针解》。

补（bǔ）　① To nourish the body and tonify the essence and qi by ingesting the five grains，five fruits，five livestock and five fruits. See *Su Wen* chapter 22. ② Refers to the features of medicine that are in compliance with the characteristics of the viscera and bowels. See *Su Wen* chapter 5 and 22. ③ In acupuncture manipulation，inserting the needle when exhaling and withdrawing the needle when inhaling is called tonifying. See *Su Wen* chapter 26. ④ Inserting the needle into the skin with the tip entering along the direction of the meridians which is considered as tonifying. See *Ling Shu* chapter 3.

补必用方　指针刺的手法。运用补法时，手法必须端静从容而和缓，使经气流通，真气自内而不外泄。出《灵枢·官能》。

补必用方（bǔ bì yòng fāng）　**to employ slow-gentle needling for tonifying** Refers to needling techniques. When using the technique of tonifying，manipulations are slow and gentle，in order to sooth the flow of meridian qi，and to ensure there is no leaking of true qi. See *Ling Shu* chapter 73.

七画

补必用员　言针刺行补的作用，在于使经气圆活，周行内外，以导其滞而使真气隆盛而至。员，圆活流利之意。出《素问·八正神明论》。

补必用员(bǔ bì yòng yuán)　**to employ flexible needling for tonifying** To tonify with acupuncture, the key is to promote the circulation of meridian qi that diminishes stasis and ensures that true qi flourishes. *Yuán* refers to being flexible and smooth. See *Su Wen* chapter 26.

初中　运气术语。初，即初气；中，即中气。运气学说中六气的每一步又分为二段，前段为初气，后段为中气。初气，地气受天的作用而升腾；中气，天气受地的作用而下降。出《素问·六微旨大论》。

初中(chū zhōng)　**initial qi and middle qi** A term of the five circuits and six qi. According to the theory of five circuits and six qi, each step of the six qi consists of two sections, the first refers to initial qi and the second is middle qi. The initial qi is the qi of the earth that is lifted up by the sky and the middle qi is the qi of the sky that descends because of the power of the earth. See *Su Wen* chapter 68.

诊法常以平旦　言诊脉的最佳时间是清晨，此时人体的阴阳、气血、脏腑、经络等功能活动均未受到外界影响，其脉象能反映人体的真实情况。临床应用时，可不必拘泥于平旦，但使病人处于安静状态即可。出《素问·脉要精微论》。

诊法常以平旦(zhěn fǎ cháng yǐ píng dàn)　**The best time for taking pulse is dawn.** It means that the best time for pulse diagnosis is in the early morning, when the body's yin and yang, qi and blood, viscera, meridians and other functional activities are not affected by the outside world, and the pulse manifestation can reflect the real situation of the body. In clinical applications, keeping the patient in a quiet state will be enough, as it is not necessary to seek an exact time. See *Su Wen* chapter 17.

诊要经终论　《素问》篇名。诊要，诊病的要旨；经终，十二经脉之气的终绝。

诊要经终论(zhěn yào jīng zhōng lùn)　**Discussion on the Essentials of Diagnosis and the Ex-**

haustion of the Twelve Channels Chapter name in *Su Wen*. *Zhěn yào* refers to the key of diagnosis. *Jīng zhōng* refers to the extinction of qi in the twelve meridians.

诊络脉　诊视手鱼际络脉之色以察病的方法。出《灵枢·经脉》。

诊络脉（zhěn luò mò）　**to diagnose the collateral vessels** Method of examining the color of the thenar collaterals on the hand to diagnose. See *Ling Shu* chapter 10.

君一臣二　指奇方的方剂组方原则。君，君药，主病谓之君。臣，臣药，佐君谓之臣。君药一，臣药二，为奇数，故为奇方。参见"奇方"条。出《素问·至真要大论》。

君一臣二（jūn yī chén èr）　**one sovereign, two ministers** It is the principle for formulating an odd prescription. *Jūn* refers to the sovereign medicinal, the core of the prescription. *Chén* refers to the minister medicinal, which assists the sovereign medicinal. One sovereign and two ministers add up to an odd number, hence it is an uneven prescription. Refer to "奇方". See *Su Wen* chapter 74.

君二臣四　指偶方的方剂组方原则。君，君药，主病谓之君。臣，臣药，佐君谓之臣。君药二，臣药四，为偶数，故为偶方。参见"偶方"条。出《素问·至真要大论》。

君二臣四（jūn èr chén sì）　**two sovereigns, four ministers** It is the principle for formulating an even prescription. *Jūn* refers to the sovereign medicinal, the core of the prescription. *Chén* refers to the minister medicinal, which assists the sovereign medicinal. Two sovereigns and four ministers add up to an even number, hence it is an even prescription. Refer to "偶方". See *Su Wen* chapter 74.

君火　运气术语。君，君主。君火，与相火相对而言，为六气之一，属少阴，主司春分节到小满节，相当于二月中到四月中这一阶段的气候变化。出《素问·天元纪大论》。

君火（jūn huǒ）　**sovereign fire** It is a term of the five circuits and six qi. Sovereign fire, which is a counterpart of the ministerial fire, is one of the six qi that pertains to *shaoyin*. It dominates weather from the Spring Equinox to the full grain period，namely，the period between February and April. See *Su Wen* chapter 66.

君主之官   指心。心为五脏六腑之大主，出《素问·灵兰秘典论》。

君主之官（jūn zhǔ zhī guān） **the monarch organ** It refers to the heart，which is the dominator of the five viscera and six bowels. See *Su Wen* chapter 8.

君臣   君药与臣药，为方剂组成中君、臣、佐、使的配伍原则。出《素问·至真要大论》。

君臣（jūn chén） **the sovereign and the minister** *Jūn*，the sovereign，refers to the medicine which rules the disease. *Chén*，the minister，refers to the medicine which assists the sovereign. This is the principle to formulate a prescription in TCM，namely，*jūn*，*chén*，*zuǒ* and *shǐ*. See *Su Wen* chapter 74.

灵兰秘典论   《素问》篇名。灵兰，即灵台兰室，为古代帝王藏书之所。秘典，经典的秘藏书籍。为强调此篇的重要性，故冠以"灵兰秘典"之名。其主要论述人体脏腑的生理功能及相互关系，着重强调了心的主宰作用。

灵兰秘典论（líng lán mì diǎn lùn） **Discussion on the Secret Cannons Stored in Royal Library** Chapter name in *Su Wen*. In ancient times，*Líng lán* was the royal library. *Mì diǎn* refers to the secret collection of classics. To emphasize the importance of this chapter，it was named *líng lán mì diǎn*. It mainly discusses the physiological functions and interrelations of the viscera，and emphasizes the dominant role of the heart.

灵枢   又称《黄帝内经灵枢经》。是《黄帝内经》的一部分，作者不详，成书年代不晚于东汉。全书八十一篇，内容主要论述人体经络腧穴、针刺治法、精神营卫等。

灵枢（líng shū） *Ling Shu* Also named *Huang Di Nei Jing: Ling Shu*（*Huang Di's Internal Classic: The Spiritual Pivot*）. It is a part of *Huang Di Nei Jing*（*Yellow Emperor's Internal Classic*），the author of which remains unknown. It was written no later than the Eastern Han dynasty. There is a total of 81 chapters discussing the meridians and collaterals，acupoints，acupuncture，mental，spirit，and nutrient-defense.

尾骶   尾骶骨，为脊骨之末节。出《灵枢·骨度》。

尾骶（wěi dǐ）　**tailbone** Sacrum and coccyx，the last segment of the spine. See *Ling Shu* chapter 14.

尾翳　经穴名。鸠尾别名。出《灵枢·经脉》。

尾翳（wěi yì）　**Wei Yi（CV 15）** See *Ling Shu* chapter 10.

迟　迟脉，脉来迟缓，一息二至，常提示正气衰竭。出《素问·三部九候论》。

迟（chí）　**slow pulse** A pulse with less than four beats to one cycle of the physician's respiration，indicating the deficiency of healthy qi. See *Su Wen* chapter 20.

鸡矢醴　矢，同屎。醴，酒也。《内经》十三方之一。以鸡矢白，晒干、焙黄一两，米酒三碗，煎后过滤澄清，服清汁。用以治疗鼓胀病。出《素问·腹中论》。

鸡矢醴（jī shǐ lǐ）　**vinum of chicken droppings** *Shǐ* refers to droppings. *Lǐ* refers to alcohol. It is one of the thirteen formulas in *Huang Di Nei Jing*. Take white chicken's droppings，sun dry and bake until lightly golden. Take 1 *liang* of the baked white chicken's droppings，put in a pot containing 3 bowls of rice wine and decoct. Filter and settle the decoction. Drink the clear liquid. It is used to treat tympanites. See *Su Wen* chapter 40.

鸡足　刺法。正入一针，左右斜入二针，形如鸡爪。出《灵枢·卫气失常》。

鸡足（jī zú）　**chicken's claw needling** A needling method，in which one needle is inserted vertically and two needles are inserted left and right obliquely，in the shape of chickens claws. See *Ling Shu* chapter 59.

鸡鸣　（1）夜半子时。出《素问·金匮真言论》。（2）丑时，即凌晨 1 点至 3 点。出《素问·标本病传论》。

鸡鸣（jī míng）　（1）11 p.m. to 1 a.m.，namely midnight. See *Su Wen* chapter 4.（2）*Chǒu shí*，that is，1 a.m. to 3 a.m. See *Su Wen* chapter 65.

八　画

环谷　出《灵枢·四时气》。(1)脐。见《太素·杂刺》。(2)手足肌肉。见《灵枢集注》。

环谷（huán gǔ）　See *Ling Shu* chapter 19.（1）Umbilicus. See *Tai Su*（*Classified Study on Huang Di Nei Jing*）"Collected Acupuncture Methods".（2）Muscles of the limbs. See *Ling Shu Ji Zhu*（*Collected Annotation of Ling Shu*）.

青尸鬼　指木疫之邪。出《素问·本病论》。

青尸鬼（qīng shī guǐ）　**wood-pestilence** Wood pathogen that causes pestilence. See *Su Wen* chapter 73.

青黑为痛　凡肤色青黑,多为血瘀气滞所致,不通则痛,故青黑主痛。出《素问·举痛论》《灵枢·五色》。

青黑为痛（qīng hēi wéi tòng）　**Green-blue indicates pain.** The green-blue skin color generally indicates blood stasis and qi stagnation，which causes pain. So green and black are associated with pain. See *Su Wen* chapter

39 and *Ling Shu* chapter 49.

耵聍　耵（dīng 丁）聍（níng 咛）,亦称"耳垢",为外耳道正常的油脂分泌物,有保护作用,干耵聍若积聚过多,堵塞耳道,会妨碍听力。出《灵枢·厥病》。

耵聍（dīng níng）　**cerumen** In Chinese，it is also called *ěr gòu*（耳垢），referring to the protective oil secretion of the external auditory canal. Too much cerumen will block the ear canal and hinder hearing. See *Ling Shu* chapter 24.

其高者因而越之　治法。高,指胸膈之上。越之,指吐法。言邪在胸膈之上者,可以涌吐法治疗。此为因势利导之法。出《素问·阴阳应象大论》。

其高者因而越之（qí gāo zhě yīn ér yuè zhī）　**to relieve disease in the upper by emetic therapy** Treatment method. *Gāo* refers to the upper part of the body above the diaphragm. *Yuè zhī* refers to the emetic therapy. When the pathogenic factors are above the diaphragm, the emetic therapy is employed. This is to cure the disease in the light of its general trend. See *Su Wen* chapter 5.

苦入心　心主火，火味苦，故云。出《素问·宣明五气》。

苦入心（kǔ rù xīn）　**Bitterness enters the heart.** The heart dominates fire，and bitterness is the flavor of fire，hence the name. See *Su Wen* chapter 23.

苦伤气　指苦味伤气。出《素问·阴阳应象大论》。

苦伤气（kǔ shāng qì）　**Bitterness harms qi.** See *Su Wen* chapter 5.

苦走血　五行相属，苦属火，心亦属火而主血脉，故苦味入心而走血。出《灵枢·九针论》。

苦走血（kǔ zǒu xuè）　**Bitterness moves with blood.** Bitterness pertains to the fire element，and the heart pertains to fire as well. The heart dominates the blood and vessels，thus bitterness enters the heart and moves with the blood. See *Ling Shu* chapter 78.

苦走骨　指多食苦伤骨。出《素问·宣明五气》《灵枢·五味论》。

苦走骨（kǔ zǒu gǔ）　**Bitterness moves to the bones.** Having too much bitter food does harm to the bones. See *Su Wen* chapter

23 and *Ling Shu* chapter 63.

昔瘤　病名。《说文》："昔，干肉也。"昔与腊同，肉干则坚。昔瘤，谓坚硬之瘤。由卫气津液与邪气搏结日久发展而成。出《灵枢·刺节真邪》。

昔瘤（xī liú）　**long-lasting tumors** Disease name. According to *Elucidations of Script and Explications of Characters*，*xī* means dried meat. "昔" equals to "腊"；when flesh becomes dry，it becomes hard，which is "腊". *Xī liú* means hard tumors，which is the result of prolonged confrontation of defensive qi and fluids against pathogenic qi. See *Ling Shu* chapter 75.

苛毒　剧烈的邪毒。出《素问·生气通天论》。

苛毒（kē dú）　**violent poison** Violent pathogen and toxics. See *Su Wen* chapter 3.

苛轸鼻　症状名。出《灵枢·热病》。（1）身体颓重，鼻上生疹。见《灵枢注证发微》。（2）形容鼻塞较甚。见《类经·针刺四十》。（3）鼻生小疹。见《灵枢识》。

苛轸鼻（kē zhěn bí）　**Small pustules on the nose.** Symptom name. See *Ling Shu* chapter 23. （1）Sense of heaviness with a rash on the nose. See *Su Wen*

Zhu Zheng Fa Wei（*Annotation and Elaboration on Su Wen*）.（2）Severe nasal obstruction. See *Lei Jing*（*Classified Classic*）"Needling Chapter 40". (3) Small rashes on the nose. See *Su Wen Zhi*（*Understanding Su Wen*）.

苛疾　严重之病。出《素问·六元正纪大论》。

苛疾（kē jí）　**violent diseases** Serious diseases. See *Su Wen* chapter 71.

直针刺　刺法之一。言用手捏起穴位处的皮肤，将针沿皮直刺，以治寒气较浅的病症，近代多称作沿皮刺或横刺。这种刺法，进针较浅。出《灵枢·官针》。

直针刺（zhí zhēn cì）　**direct subcutaneous needling** A needling method involving pinching the skin at the acupoint and straight needling along the skin. It is used for symptoms caused by the cold in shallow areas of the body. In modern times, it is often called needling along the skin or transverse needling. This kind of needling is relatively shallow. See *Ling Shu* chapter 7.

茎垂　男子生殖器官阴茎、睾丸阴囊的合称。出《灵枢·邪客》。

茎垂（jīng chuí）　**male genitalia** It refers to the penis and testicular scrotum. See *Ling Shu* chapter 71.

茎痛　茎，阴茎。阴茎疼痛。出《灵枢·五色》。

茎痛（jīng tòng）　**penis pain** *Jīng* refers to the penis. This term refers to pain in the penis. See *Ling Shu* chapter 49.

林钟　六阴吕之一，为商音，即金音。出《素问·刺法论》。

林钟（lín zhōng）　**lin zhong** One of the six yin *lǚ*（吕）that pertains to the *shāng* tone and the metal element. See *Su Wen* chapter 72.

枢中　髀枢之中，环跳穴处。出《素问·缪刺论》。

枢中（shū zhōng）　**Shu Zhong（GB 30）** In the pit along the lateral side of femur，or named Huan Tiao. See *Su Wen* chapter 63.

枢合　指足少阳胆经之环跳穴。出《灵枢·厥病》。

枢合（shū hé）　**pivot union** It refers to Huan Tiao（GB 30），which is on the gallbladder meridian of foot *shaoyang*. See *Ling Shu* chapter 24.

枢折挈　枢，关节。折，折断。出《素问·痿论》。（1）挈作瘈，痉挛、抽搐。见《针灸甲乙经·热在五脏发痿》。（2）挈，提举。

形容关节弛缓,不能提举活动,犹如枢轴折断不能活动一般。见《素问》王冰注。

枢折挈(shū shé qiè)　**broken pivot** *Shū* refers to joints. *Shé* means being broken. See *Su Wen* chapter 44.（1）"挈" can be written as "瘛", which means cramp. See *Zhen Jiu Jia Yi Jing*（*Classic of Acupuncture and Moxibustion*）"Five Viscera Heat Causes Wilting Diseases". （2）*Qiè* means to lift. This term describes the loose joints that are unable to be lifted as if an unmovable broken axis. See *Su Wen* annotated by Wang Bing.

枢持　十二经皮部之一,为少阳经皮部。枢持,转枢、抒轴之意,三阳经主表证,以少阳为枢,故名。出《素问·皮部论》。

枢持(shū chí)　**pivot and axle** The skin section of the *shaoyang* meridian, one of the twelve skin sections. *Shū chí* means pivot. The three yang meridians dominate the exterior syndromes, with *shaoyang* meridian being the pivot, hence the name. See *Su Wen* chapter 56.

枢儒　有转枢、柔软的意思,此指少阴经之皮部。出《素问·皮部论》。

枢儒(shū rú)　**pivot soft** It refers to the pivot, and softness, indicating the skin section of *shaoyin* meridian. See *Su Wen* chapter 56.

枕骨　脑后横骨。出《灵枢·经筋》。

枕骨(zhěn gǔ)　**occipital bone** Transverse bone on the back of the skull. See *Ling Shu* chapter 13.

杼骨　第一胸椎棘突。出《灵枢·背俞》。

杼骨(zhù gǔ)　**shuttle bone** Spinous process of first thoracic vertebra. See *Ling Shu* chapter 51.

刺三变　指三种不同的刺法,即刺营、刺卫、刺寒痹。出《灵枢·寿夭刚柔》。

刺三变(cì sān biàn)　**Triple changes needling.** Three different needling methods, namely, needling the nutrient, the defensive and the cold impediments. See *Ling Shu* chapter 6.

刺五邪　刺治痈邪、实邪、虚邪、热邪、寒邪等五邪的方法。其原则是痈热之邪消灭之,肿聚痈邪消散之,寒痹之邪温其血气,虚者补之使其强壮,邪盛有余者驱除之。出《灵枢·刺节真邪》。

刺五邪(cì wǔ xié)　**to needle five**

pathogens Acupuncture manipulations to treat the five pathogens, namely, abscess pathogens, excess pathogens, deficient pathogens, heat pathogens and cold pathogens. The principle is to eliminate pure heat, dissipate swelling and carbuncles, warm the blood qi in cold pathogens, tonify the deficiencies, and dispel the excesses. See *Ling Shu* chapter 75.

刺节　指刺五节，即振埃、发蒙、去爪、彻衣、解惑等五种针刺方法。出《灵枢·刺节真邪》。

刺节 (cì jié)　**to needle five sections** Five needling methods, namely, to shake off dust, to redeem out of ignorance, to trim the finger/toe nails, to undress and to resolve the doubts. See *Ling Shu* chapter 75.

刺节真邪　《灵枢》篇名。刺节，即刺五节，即振埃、发蒙、去爪、彻衣、解惑等五种针刺方法。真，即真气、正气；邪，邪气。此篇主要论述了刺五节、刺五邪的针刺方法，以及疾病变化过程中邪正胜复的情况，故名。

刺节真邪 (cì jié zhēn xié)　**Discussion on the Five Sections in Needling and Comments on the Genuine Qi and Pathogenic Factors** Chapter name in *Ling Shu*. *Cì jié* refers to the five needling methods, namely, to shake off dust, to redeem out of ignorance, to trim the finger/toe nails, to undress and to resolve the doubts. *Zhēn* means true qi and healthy qi; *xié* refers to pathogenic qi. This chapter mainly discusses the five needling methods, as well as the healthy energy-pathogen struggle in the process of disease.

刺齐论　《素问》篇名。刺，针刺；齐，一致，有常规之意。刺齐，即针刺的浅深要有一定的分寸。此篇主要讨论针刺不可太过不及的道理。强调针刺的正确手法。故名。

刺齐论 (cì qí lùn)　**Discussion on Needling Depth** Chapter name in *Su Wen*. *Cì* refers to needling or acupuncture; *qí* refers to regulation. *Cì qí* means that the depth of the needling is in accordance with certain principles. The principle of proportionality and correct manipulation of acupuncture are stressed in this chapter, hence the name.

刺志论　《素问》篇名。刺，针刺。其内容主要记述气与形、谷与气、脉与血的虚实关系。

刺志论(cì zhì lùn) **Discussion on the Fundamentals of Acupuncture** Chapter name in *Su Wen*. *Cì* refers to needling. This chapter mainly discusses the relationship of excess and deficiency between qi and physique，grains and qi，and pulse and blood.

刺疟 《素问》篇名。刺，针刺；疟，疟疾；刺疟，即对疟疾的针刺方法。此篇主要论述了运用六经和脏腑分证方法对疟疾的归类分型，以及对各类疟疾的治疗方法。故名。

刺疟(cì nüè) **Discussion on Treatment of Malaria by Acupuncture** Chapter name in *Su Wen*. *Cì* refers to needling；*nüè* refers to malaria；*cì nüè* refers to treating malaria with acupuncture. This chapter mainly discusses the classification of malaria by the six meridians，and syndrome differentiation of the five viscera and six bowels，as well as the treatment of various kinds of malaria, hence the name.

刺法 ① 古医籍名。从书名推测可能是一部针刺治疗学专著。见《素问·评热病论》。② 针刺的方法。见《灵枢·海论》。

刺法(cì fǎ) ① The name of an ancient medical book. From the title it is assumed that it is a monograph on acupuncture therapy. See *Su Wen* chapter 33. ② Methods of acupuncture manipulations. See *Ling Shu* chapter 33.

刺法论 《素问》遗篇名。唐王冰注《素问》时已佚，仅目录中存有篇名，并注明"亡"。遗篇主要论述运用针刺为主的方法，以预防和救治因运气失常，气候变异所引发的疫疠问题。

刺法论(cì fǎ lùn) **Discussion on Acupuncture Methods** Chapter name in *Su Wen*. This chapter was lost when Wang Bing of the Tang dynasty annotated *Su Wen*. Only the title remained catalogued，and was termed lost. It mainly discusses the employment of acupuncture as the main method to prevent and cure pestilence caused by the five abnormal circuits and six qi，as well as climate change. See *Su Wen* chapter 72.

刺要论 《素问》篇名。刺，针刺；要，要领。此篇内容主要论述针刺的要领。故名。

刺要论(cì yào lùn) **Discussion on the Essentials of Acupuncture**

Chapter name in *Su Wen*. *Cì* refers to needling. *Yào* refers to essentials. This chapter mainly discusses the essentials of acupuncture，hence the name.

刺热 《素问》篇名。刺，即针刺疗法。热，指五脏热病。此篇内容主要论述五脏热病的症状、预后和针刺治疗的方法，故名。

刺热(cì rè) **Discussion on Acupuncture Treatment of Febrile Diseases** Chapter name in *Su Wen*. *Cì* refers to needling. *Rè* refers to febrile diseases of the five viscera. This chapter is mainly about the symptoms, prognosis and acupuncture treatment of the febrile diseases of the five viscera，hence the name.

刺禁论 《素问》篇名。刺，针刺，禁，禁忌。此篇专论针刺对某些重要脏器、穴位及气血逆乱情况下的禁忌问题，故名。

刺禁论(cì jìn lùn) **Discussion on the Contraindication of Needling Therapy** Chapter name in *Su Wen*. *Cì* refers to needling. *Jìn* means contraindication. This chapter is about the contraindications of needling some important organs, acupoints, and the situation of disordered qi

and blood，hence the name.

刺腰痛 《素问》篇名。刺，即针刺。此篇较全面地论述了十二经脉和奇经八脉等受病后，出现腰痛的特点与针刺方法。故名。

刺腰痛(cì yāo tòng) **Discussion on Treatment of Lumbago with Acupuncture** Chapter name in *Su Wen*. *Cì* refers to needling. This chapter is about the characteristics of lumbago and its treatment with acupuncture，which is caused by the undermined twelve regular meridians and eight extraordinary meridians，etc.，hence the name.

雨气通于肾 出《素问·阴阳应象大论》。(1)雨为水气，肾为水脏，故相通应。(2)通，释为"润"。见《新校正》。

雨气通于肾(yǔ qì tōng yú shèn) **Rain-qi communicates with kidney**. See *Su Wen* chapter 5. (1) The rain and the kidney both pertain to the water element，therefore the two communicate with each other. (2) *Tōng* means to moisten or to nourish. See *Xin Jiao Zheng* (*New Revisions of Su Wen*).

郁乃痤 郁，滞阻。痤，疮疖。邪气不解化热，郁积皮肉，便可成为疮疖。出《素问·生气通天论》。

郁乃痤（yù nǎi cuó）　**Stagnation generates furuncles.** *Yù* refers to stasis. *Cuó* refers to furuncle. Pathogenic factors accumulate in the skin and flesh, and generate heat, thus causing furuncles. See *Su Wen* chapter 3.

郁极乃发　郁，郁遏，抑郁；发，发作。言五运被胜制后，由于抑郁过极，而导致复气发作的现象。例木胜制土，土气抑郁过极，则郁极而发。出《素问·六元正纪大论》。

郁极乃发（yù jí nǎi fā）　**What is restrained to the extreme will break out.** *Yù* means to restrain or control；*fā* means to break out. When the qi of the five elements becomes extremely stagnant, it will burst out. For instance，wood restrains earth，and when earth is extremely restrained by wood qi，earth qi breaks out. See *Su Wen* chapter 71.

奔豚　病名。为肾之积。其症自感有气发于少腹，上冲胸咽，如豚之奔突。故名。出《灵枢·邪气藏府病形》。

奔豚（bēn tún）　**running piglet** Disease name，caused by stagnated kidney qi. Qi rushes up from the abdomen to the chest，like running piglets，hence the name. See *Ling Shu* chapter 4.

奇　即奇方，古之单方或组方药味成单数者。为七方之一。出《素问·至真要大论》。

奇（jī）　**odd formula** The number of ingredients in a formula is odd. It is one of the seven kinds of prescriptions. See *Su Wen* chapter 74.

奇邪　见《素问·三部九候论》。（1）指客于大络之邪，可令生奇病。见《素问集注》。（2）不正之邪。见《素问注证发微》。

奇邪（qí xié）　**uncommon pathogen** See *Su Wen* chapter 20. （1）Intrusive pathogens in the great collateral vessels，which can cause rare diseases. See *Su Wen Ji Zhu*（*Collected Annotation of Su Wen*）. （2）Refers to odd pathogens. See *Su Wen Zhu Zheng Fa Wei*（*Annotation and Elaboration on Su Wen*）.

奇恒　古医籍名，已佚。出《素问·病能论》。

奇恒（qí héng）　*The Strange and The Normal* An ancient medical book，which has been lost in history. See *Su Wen* chapter 46.

奇恒之府　奇，特异；恒，平常，奇恒，异于寻常之意。脑、髓、骨、脉、胆、女子胞六者，因其各具

八画

囊腔,形态与腑相似而为腑,但其功能似脏,贮藏阴精,藏而不泻,与一般的六腑有所不同,故名。出《素问·五藏别论》。

奇恒之府(qí héng zhī fǔ) **extraordinary organs** *Qí* means strange; *héng* means ordinary. *Qí héng* means extraordinary. *Qí héng zhī fǔ* refers to the brain, marrow, bones, vessels, gallbladder, and female uterus. Morphologically, they are all hollow like the six bowels, but functionally, act as the five viscera, and store yin essence without draining. They are named by these characteristics. See *Su Wen* chapter 11.

奇病 异于寻常的奇特之病。见《素问·奇病论》。

奇病(qí bìng) **special diseases** Rare and strange diseases. See *Su Wen* chapter 47.

奇病论 《素问》篇名。奇病,不寻常之病。此篇论述了息积、疹筋、厥逆、脾瘅、胆瘅、厥、胎病、肾风等不寻常之病的病因病机、治法及预后。故名。

奇病论(qí bìng lùn) **Discussion on Special Diseases** Chapter name in *Su Wen*. This chapter discusses the pathogenesis, treatment and prognosis of some special diseases, such as *xi ji* (breath accumulation), *zhen jin* (bellyache with upper limbs cramping), *jue ni* (headache and toothache), *pi dan* (pure spleen heat), *dan dan* (pure gallbladder heat), *jue* (lung-qi reversion), *tai bing* (fetal disease), and *shen feng* (kidney wind), etc. Hence the name.

奇输 手足三阳经脉之别络。出《灵枢·刺节真邪》。

奇输(qí shū) **special collaterals** Connecting collaterals of the three hand yang and three foot yang meridians. See *Ling Shu* chapter 75.

转筋 局部筋肉抽掣挛缩扭曲。出《灵枢·经筋》。

转筋(zhuǎn jīn) **spasm** See *Ling Shu* chapter 13.

软 ① 脉象。其来软弱而和缓,为脾有胃气的正常脉象,应于长夏。见《素问·平人气象论》。② 软弱。见《灵枢·经脉》。

软(ruǎn) ① Normal pulse manifestation in late summer. It is soft and mild, indicating the spleen is supported by the stomach qi. See *Su Wen* chapter 18. ② Weakness. See *Ling Shu* chapter 10.

齿更发长 乳齿更换,头发茂盛。

出《素问·上古天真论》。

齿更发长(chǐ gēng fà zhǎng) **dental transition and hair growth** The deciduous teeth are replaced by permanent teeth and the hair is lush. See *Su Wen* chapter 1.

齿寒　牙齿寒冷的症状。出《素问·缪刺》。

齿寒(chǐ hán)　**tooth cold** Symptoms of cold teeth. See *Su Wen* chapter 63.

齿噤龄　症状名。齿噤，亦称口噤。牙关紧闭不开。龄（xiè泻），磨牙。《灵枢·热病》。

齿噤龄(chǐ jìn xiè)　**gnashing of teeth** Symptom name of tightly locked jaws. *Xiè* means to grind one's teeth in sleep. See *Ling Shu* chapter 23.

齿龋　病名。即蛀齿，牙齿被蛀蚀成孔，时时作痛。出《素问·缪刺论》。

齿龋(chǐ qǔ)　**dental caries** Decayed teeth, in which holes are formed by erosion, causing constant pain. See *Su Wen* chapter 63.

肾　① 五脏之一。位于下焦，具有藏精，促进生长、发育、生殖的功能，为封藏之本。见《素问·上古天真论》《素问·逆调论》《素问·灵兰秘典论》。② 肾的精气。见《素问·阴阳应象大论》。③ 指肾在面部相应的望诊部位（两颊下方）。见《灵枢·五色》。④ 肾之脉象。见《素问·玉机真藏论》。

肾(shèn)　① The kidney is one of the five viscera located in the lower *jiao*. Kidney stores essence, promotes growth, development and reproduction, and dominates essence storage. See *Su Wen* chapter 1, *Su Wen* chapter 34 and chapter 8. ② Kidney essence. See *Su Wen* chapter 5. ③ The area beneath the cheeks, through which by inspection, the condition of the kidney can be observed. See *Ling Shu* chapter 49. ④ Pulse manifestation of the kidney. See *Su Wen* chapter 19.

肾之府　指腰。出《素问·脉要精微论》。见"腰者肾之府"条。

肾之府(shèn zhī fǔ)　**house of kidney** The waist is the house of the kidney. See *Su Wen* chapter 17. See "腰者肾之府".

肾之街　肾气的通道。街，指通道。在此指俞穴。出《素问·水热穴》。

肾之街(shèn zhī jiē)　**pathways of the kidney** Pathways of kidney qi. *Jiē* refers to the meridian, and here refers to acupoints.

八画

See *Su Wen* chapter 61.

肾水 即肾。肾主水，为水脏，故称。出《素问·气交变大论》。

肾水（shèn shuǐ） **kidney water** Refers to the kidney. The kidney governs water，and pertains to the water element，hence the name. See *Su Wen* chapter 69.

肾气 肾之精气，来源于先天，并得到后天的培养，具有促进生长发育及生殖等作用。其与耳相通。出《素问·上古天真论》《灵枢·脉度》。

肾气（shèn qì） **kidney qi** The essence qi of kidney，which comes into being before birth and is nourished and tonified after birth by food and drinks. It connects with the ears and promotes growth，development and reproduction，etc. See *Su Wen* chapter 1 and *Ling Shu* chapter 17.

肾气独沉 出《素问·四气调神大论》。(1) 指肾气不藏而独见注泄等寒气沉于下的病证。见《类经·摄生类》。(2) 独沉，《太素》作"浊沉"，指肾气受邪，浊沉不能营运的病理。

肾气独沉（shèn qì dú chén） **sinking of kidney qi** See *Su Wen* chapter 2. (1) Instead of being stored，the kidney qi is drained most likely due to deep pathogenic cold qi. See *Lei Jing* "Health Preservation". (2) In *Tai Su*（*Classified Study on Huang Di Nei Jing*），"独沉" is written as "浊沉"，which means the kidney qi is turbid and its circulation is hindered.

肾风 病名。症见面肿、发热、身痛、恶风、脉大而紧等。因肾病水肿又见发热、身痛、恶风等风邪表症，故名为肾风。肾风与风水病同为水肿病的初起或急性发作阶段。可与"风水"条互参。出《素问·风论》。

肾风（shèn fēng） **kidney wind** Disease name. The main symptoms include facial swelling，fever，body pains，aversion to wind，and large and tight pulses，etc. Furthermore，because the swelling caused by kidney diseases often comes with exterior symptoms due to pathogenic wind，such as fever，body pains，aversion to wind etc.，hence it is called kidney wind. Kidney wind，the same as wind-water diseases，is the early stage or urgent occurence of swelling diseases. See "风水". See *Su Wen* chapter 42.

肾风疝 疝病之一。由风寒之邪

入肾,以少腹、阴器疼痛为主证的疾病。出《素问·四时刺逆从论》。

肾风疝(shèn fēng shàn) **kidney wind hernia** It is one of the hernias, caused by the invasion of pathogenic wind and cold into the kidney, with symptoms including pain in the lower lateral abdomen and genital organs. See *Su Wen* chapter 64.

肾为欠为嚏　欠,呵欠。嚏,喷嚏。均言肾之病。出《素问·宣明五气》。

肾为欠为嚏(shèn wéi qiàn wéi tì) **Kidney disease causes yawning and sneezing.** *Qiàn* means to yawn, and *tì* means to sneeze. Both refer to the symptoms of kidney diseases. See *Su Wen* chapter 23.

肾为阴中之太阴　根据阴阳五行原理,阴阳之中又有阴阳可分。肾主水,属阴,又居下焦阴位,肾气旺于冬为阴之盛,故为阴中之太阴。出《灵枢·阴阳系日月》。

肾为阴中之太阴(shèn wéi yīn zhōng zhī tài yīn) **Kidney pertains to *taiyin* within yin.** According to the theories of yin-yang and the five elements, *yin* and *yang* respectively can further be divided into *yin* and *yang* respectively. The kidney governs water, and pertains to yin. It is located at the lower *jiao* which is considered a *yin* region. Kidney *qi* is exuberant in winter, hence considered to be the *taiyin* within yin. See *Ling Shu* chapter 41.

肾为唾　唾,唾沫,五液之一,生于舌下。足少阴肾脉循喉咙,挟舌本,故唾为肾之液。出《素问·宣明五气》。《灵枢·九针论》作"肾主唾"。

肾为唾(shèn wéi tuò) **Kidney forms spittle.** *Tuò* refers to spittle, one of five kinds of fluids. which is generated under the tongue. The kidney meridian of foot *shaoyin* follows the throat, running around the root of the tongue, hence spittle pertains to the kidney. See *Su Wen* chapter 23. In *Ling Shu* chapter 78, it is expressed as the kidney controls the spittle.

肾心痛　厥心痛之一种。病由肾气上逆,邪干于心而痛,有心痛胸背相引,背曲不能伸等征象。出《灵枢·厥病》。

肾心痛(shèn xīn tòng) **reversal heartache caused by kidney disease** It is one of the reversal heartaches. The reversing kidney qi invades the heart，which sometimes manifests as heart pain which echoes in the back，with pain and stiffness and difficulty bending. See *Ling Shu* chapter 24.

肾生骨髓 肾主骨，藏精气，有壮骨生髓的生理功能。见《素问·阴阳应象大论》。

肾生骨髓（shèn shēng gǔ suǐ）**Kidney generates bone and marrow.** The kidney governs the bones，stores the essence qi and has the physiological function of strengthening bones and generating marrow. See *Su Wen* chapter 5.

肾主欠 言肾之病。出《灵枢·九针论》《素问·宣明五气》。

肾主欠（shèn zhǔ qiàn）**Kidney disease causes yawning.** See *Ling Shu* chapter 78 and *Su Wen* chapter 23.

肾主冬 此以五行学说归纳脏腑与季节的关系。肾五行属水，冬季五行属水，故肾主冬季。出《素问·藏气法时论》。

肾主冬（shèn zhǔ dōng）**Kidney governs winter.** It is an example that induces the relationship between the viscera and the seasons based on the five ele-ment theory. The kidney pertains to the water element，the same as winter，hence it is said that kidney governs winter. See *Su Wen* chapter 22.

肾主耳 耳为肾窍，足少阴肾络会于耳中。出《灵枢·脉度》《素问·阴阳应象大论》。

肾主耳（shèn zhǔ ěr）**Kidney governs the ears.** The kidney opens into the ears，and the kidney collateral of foot *shaoyin* meets in the ears. See *Ling Shu* chapter 17 and *Su Wen* chapter 5.

肾主身之骨髓 见《素问·痿论》《素问·阴阳应象大论》。

肾主身之骨髓（shèn zhǔ shēn zhī gǔ suǐ）**Kidney governs bone and marrow.** See *Su Wen* chapter 44 and chapter 5.

肾主骨 主，主持、掌管之意。肾为精之处，其精髓注于骨，故肾所主之外合为骨。见《素问·宣明五气》。

肾主骨（shèn zhǔ gǔ）**Kidney governs the bones.** *Zhǔ* here means to govern. Kidney stores essence，and the essence infuses into the bones，thus the kidney governs the bones. See *Su Wen* chapter 23.

肾主唾 义同"肾为唾"。参该条。出《灵枢·九针论》。

肾主唾（shèn zhǔ tuò）　**Kidney forms spittle.** Refer to "肾为唾"，which shares the same meaning. See *Ling Shu* chapter 78.

肾合三焦膀胱　合，应合之意。足太阳膀胱与足少阴肾相表里，肾为水藏，主全身水液代谢，而膀胱为津液之府，三焦为决渎之官，二者相属，皆关乎水液之输布排泄，故与肾相应合。出《灵枢·本藏》

肾合三焦膀胱（shèn hé sān jiāo páng guāng）　**Kidney is connected to the triple *jiao* and bladder.** *Hé* means to be connected with. There is an interior and exterior relationship between the bladder meridian of foot *taiyang* and the kidney meridian of foot *shaoyin*. The kidney pertains to the water element，and rules the fluid metabolism of the body. The bladder is the dwelling of fluids，and the triple *jiao* has the official function of opening the channels，the two are interiorly-exteriorly related， and they both play a role in the transportation and excretion of liquids，thus they are related to the kidney. See *Ling Shu* chapter 47.

肾合骨　合，配合之意。出《灵枢·五色》。义同"肾主骨"。参该条。

肾合骨（shèn hé gǔ）　**Kidney is connected with the bones.** *Hé* here means to be connected with. See *Ling Shu* chapter 49. Refer to the term "肾主骨"，which shares the same meaning.

肾合膀胱　合，配合之意。足太阳膀胱经与足少阴肾经相表里，肾与膀胱功能上密切相关。出《灵枢·本输》。

肾合膀胱（shèn hé páng guāng）　**Kidney is connected with the bladder.** *Hé* here means to be connected with. There is an interior and exterior relationship between the bladder meridian of foot *taiyang* and the kidney meridian of foot *shaoyin*，thus functionally the kidney is closely connected with the bladder. See *Ling Shu* chapter 2.

肾足少阴之脉　即足少阴肾经，为十二经脉之一。其循行路线从足小趾之下开始，斜行于足心（涌泉穴），出内踝前大骨下陷中，沿内踝后，转走足跟，由此上腿肚内侧，至腘内侧，上股内侧后缘通过脊柱，属于肾，络于膀胱。一支从肾上行，穿过

八画

横膈和肝,进入肺中,沿喉咙,挟舌本。再一支从肺出来,络于心,注于胸中(接手厥阴心包经)。出《灵枢·经脉》。

肾足少阴之脉（shèn zú shào yīn zhī mài）　**Kidney meridian of foot *shaoyin*.** It is one of the twelve regular meridians. It originates from below the little toe and extends diagonally through the sole of the foot（acupoint KI 1）and goes out from the depression of the large bone in front of the medial malleolus. Then it extends along the posterior side of the inner ankle，and diverts into the heel，from where it ascends into the calf. It appears at the inner edge of the hollow of the knee，ascends along the posterior edge of the inner side of the thigh，and passes through the spine. It connects with the kidney and wraps the urinary bladder. There are two branches，one ascending from the kidney upward，penetrating the liver and the diaphragm，entering into the lung，following the throat and moving along the basis of the tongue. The other one originates from the lung and wraps the heart，before it pours into the chest（connecting the pericardium meridian of hand *jueyin*）. See *Ling Shu* chapter 10.

肾应骨　应,应合之意。出《灵枢·本藏》。与"肾主骨"义同,见该条。

肾应骨（shèn yīng gǔ）　**Kidney corresponds to the bones.** *Yīng* here means to correspond to. See *Ling Shu* chapter 47. Refer to the term "肾主骨"，which shares the same meaning.

肾者主为外　外,有发露于外的形象、灌输津液于外及感知外界的音声等含义。肾为作强之官,伎巧所出,并开窍于耳,肾精充足则髓足而骨强,故体强才力过人,智巧而多能,听力敏锐;肾藏津液能灌注濡润空窍。出《素问·灵兰秘典论》。

肾者主为外（shèn zhě zhǔ wéi wài）　**Kidney governs the exterior.** *Wài* refers to outward forms，transporting liquid to the exterior，and perceiving the sound of the outside world. The kidney is an official with great power and is responsible for skills and opens into the ears. Sufficient kidney essence maintains abundant marrow and strong bones，thus the body is tough，talented，smart and versatile with sharp hearing. In addition，the empty orifices can be infused and moistened by fluid stored in the kidney. See *Su Wen* chapter 8.

肾和则耳能闻五音矣 出《灵枢·脉度》。

肾和则耳能闻五音矣（shèn hé zé ěr néng wén wǔ yīn yǐ）**The ears can identify the five tones due to the harmony of kidney qi.** See *Ling Shu* chapter 17.

肾胀 病症名。五脏胀之一。症见腰髀痛，腹满引背。出《灵枢·胀论》。

肾胀（shèn zhàng）**kidney distention** Disease name. It pertains to visceral distension. The main symptoms include back pain due to abdominal fullness，and lower back and thigh pain. See *Ling Shu* chapter 35.

肾疟 五脏疟之一。症见恶寒、腰脊痛，大便难，目眩等。出《素问·刺疟》。

肾疟（shèn nüè）**kidney malaria** Disease name. It pertains to visceral malaria. The main symptoms include aversion to cold，pain along the spinal column，constipation，and dizziness etc. See *Su Wen* chapter 36.

肾治于里 指肾的功能，与心相对而言。肾位于下焦，为阴中之阴，肾主水而藏精，为生长发育之根本，故肾气主治于里。治，内治之意。出《素问·刺禁论》。

肾治于里（shèn zhì yú lǐ）**Kidney governs the interior.** Refers to the functions of the kidney，which is a counterpart of the heart that governs the interior. The kidney is in the lower *jiao*，and is the organ pertaining to yin within yin. The kidney governs water and stores essence，which are the foundation of growth and development，hence the name. *Zhì* means to govern the interior. See *Su Wen* chapter 52.

肾咳 五脏咳之一。证候特点为咳而并见腰背疼痛，故名肾咳。出《素问·咳论》。

肾咳（shèn ké）**kidney cough** Disease name. It pertains to visceral cough. The main symptoms include coughing and lower back pain，hence the name. See *Su Wen* chapter 38.

肾俞五十七穴 指治疗水病的五十七穴。肾主水，故又称"水俞五十七穴"。见该条。出《素问·水热穴论》。

八画

肾俞五十七穴(shèn shū wǔ shí qī xué) **fifty-seven acupoints for kidney disorder** Refers to the fifty-seven acupoints for the treatment of diseases related to kidney. Kidney governs water, so it is also expressed as "The fifty-seven water transporter acupoints". Refer to "水俞五十七穴", See *Su Wen* chapter 61.

肾脉 ① 足少阴肾之经脉。出《素问·水热穴论》。② 肾的脉象。其脉沉石,与冬相应。出《素问·宣明五气》。

肾脉(shèn mài) ① Kidney meridian of foot *shaoyin*. See *Su Wen* chapter 61. ② The pulse manifestation of the kidney, which is stone-like, and corresponds to winter. See *Su Wen* chapter 23.

肾脉石 指沉滑坚实如石的脉象,是肾之正常脉。见《素问·宣明五气》。参"石"条。

肾脉石(shèn mài shí) **Kidney pulse is stone-like.** The deep stone-like, smooth and strong pulse, which indicates that the kidney is healthy. See *Su Wen* chapter 23. Refer to the term "石".

肾恶燥 恶(wù 误),厌憎之意。肾为水脏而藏精,燥胜则精伤,故恶燥。出《素问·宣明五气》。

肾恶燥(shèn wù zào) **Kidney is averse to dryness.** *Wù* means to dislike or hate. The kidney pertains to water and stores essence, which could be undermined by dryness, hence the name. See *Su Wen* chapter 23.

肾腧 ① 指肾的背部俞穴。在十四椎下两旁各一寸半处,属足太阳膀胱经。出《灵枢·背俞》。② 指治疗水病的穴位,又称水俞。出《素问·水热穴论》。

肾腧(shèn shū) ① Name of acupoint BL 23, which is located one and a half *cun* on each side of the lower 14th vertebrae, pertaining to the bladder meridian of foot *taiyang*. See *Ling Shu* chapter 51. ② Acupoints for the treatment of diseases caused by the disorders of kidney, which are also named kidney transporter holes. See *Su Wen* chapter 61.

肾痹 病证名。五脏痹之一。由骨痹日久,反复感受风寒湿邪发展而来。症见脘腹易胀,两足挛急,身体踡屈。出《素问·痹论》《素问·五藏生成》。

肾痹(shèn bì) **kidney impediment** Disease name. It is one of the visceral impediments that developed due to chronic bone impediments which repeatedly invaded with pathogenic wind，cold，and dampness. The main symptoms include abdominal distension and spasms in the lower limbs. See *Su Wen* chapter 43 and 10.

肾雍　雍同壅。《素问·大奇论》："肾雍，脚下至少腹满。"(1) 指肾气壅滞。见《素问注证发微》。(2) 指肾气满而外壅于肾之经络。见《素问集注》。

肾雍（shèn yōng）　**kidney obstruction** "雍" equals to "壅". Kidney congestion：the patient experiences fullness from the lower sections of the flanks to the lower abdomen. See *Su Wen* chapter 48. (1) Obstruction of kidney qi. See *Su Wen Zhu Zheng Fa Wei*（*Annotation and Elaboration on Su Wen*）. (2) Excessive kidney qi blocks the kidney meridian. See *Su Wen Ji Zhu*（*Collected Annotation of Su Wen*）.

肾藏志　肾与精神活动有一定关系。志是经验和知识的记存出《素问·宣明五气》。

肾藏志（shèn cáng zhì）　**Kidney stores will.** The kidney is related to metal activities. The memo-

rizing of experience and knowledge is called *zhì*（the will）. See *Su Wen* chapter 23.

肾藏骨髓之气　肾藏精，精生骨髓，故云。出《素问·平人气象论》。

肾藏骨髓之气（shèn cáng gǔ suǐ zhī qì）　**Kidney stores qi of the bone marrow.** The kidney stores essence，which generates marrow，hence the name. See *Su Wen* chapter 18.

肾藏精，精舍志　志舍于精而肾藏之。出《灵枢·本神》。参"肾藏志"条。

肾藏精，精舍志（shèn cáng jīng，jīng shě zhì）　**Kidney stores essence；essence houses will.** The kidney stores essence，which hosts *zhì*（the will）. See *Ling Shu* chapter 8. Refer to "肾藏志".

贤人　古代的养生家。他们以观察天地、日月、星辰、阴阳、四时等自然现象的变化顺逆，作为养生的准则，故可益寿。出《素问·上古天真论》。

贤人（xián rén）　**wise people** Ancient people who were in pursuit of healthy and long lives. By observing the laws of heaven，earth，the sun，the moon，the stars，yin and yang，and the four seasons，they lived in accordance with the rules of nature, thus living a long life. See *Su Wen* chapter 1.

昆仑　经穴名。足太阳膀胱经之经穴,在足外踝后跟骨上陷中。出《灵枢·本输》。

昆仑（kūn lún）　**Kun Lun（BL 60）**. Acupoint name which pertains to the bladder meridian of foot *taiyang*, and is located at the posterior calcaneal depression of the lateral malleolus of the foot. See *Ling Shu* chapter 2.

呿　大张口貌。取上关穴(即客主人)时,须如此方得。出《灵枢·本输》。

呿（kā）　**mouth opening wide** Widely opened mouth. When piercing Shang Guan（GB 3）, the mouth of the patient should be widely opened to determine the exact location of the acupoint. See *Ling Shu* chapter 2.

昌阳之脉　足少阴经在小腿部的支脉。出《素问·刺腰痛》。

昌阳之脉（chāng yáng zhī mài）　**glorious yang meridians** The shank branch of the meridian of foot *shaoyin*. See *Su Wen* chapter 41.

明堂　① 鼻。出《灵枢·五色》。② 古代帝王宣明政教的地方。

出《素问·五运行大论》。

明堂（míng táng）　① Nose. See *Ling Shu* chapter 49. ② Bright hall, the location where in ancient times the emperor and his officials gathered for discussions. See *Su Wen* chapter 67.

炅中　炅(jiǒng 窘),热。炅中,泛指阳热内盛之证。出《素问·调经论》。

炅中（jiǒng zhōng）　**heated center** *Jiǒng* means heat. *Jiǒng zhōng* refers to symptoms of excessive heat and yang. See *Su Wen* chapter 62.

炅气　炅(jiǒng 窘),同炯,热。炅气即热气。出《素问·举痛论》。

炅气（jiǒng qì）　**heat qi** "炅" equals to "炯", which means heat. *Jiǒng qì* refers to heat qi. See *Su Wen* chapter 39.

炅则气泄　炅(jiǒng 窘),即热。热则腠理开,气随汗泄。出《素问·举痛论》。

炅则气泄（jiǒng zé qì xiè）　**Overheat causes qi leakage**. *Jiǒng* means heat. When one is hot, the interstice structures open, and the qi flows out with the sweat. See *Su Wen* chapter 39.

败疵　病名。生于胁部的痈,女子乳痈之类。若病延不愈,则疮面蔓延,长出肉芽如赤小豆。

出《灵枢·痈疽》。

败疵（bài cī）　**costal carbuncle** Disease name. Carbuncles in costal regions，and mastitis，etc. If not treated in time，carbuncles will spread and sprout like red beans. See *Ling Shu* chapter 81.

钛角之人　体质名。钛角，即右角，角音之一，此代表阴阳二十五人中木形人之一种，其特征是努力向前进取。出《灵枢·阴阳二十五人》。

钛角之人（dài jué zhī rén）　*daijue-type people* Name of constitution. It refers to the right *jue*，one of the *jue* tunes. It is one of the twenty five constitutions of yin and yang，pertaining to wood. People of wood always work hard. See *Ling Shu* chapter 64.

钛商之人　体质名。钛，大的意思。钛商，商音之一，此代表阴阳二十五人中金形人之一种，其特征是清廉而洁身自好。出《灵枢·阴阳二十五人》。参"金形之人"。

钛商之人（dài shāng zhī rén）　*daishang-type people* Name of constitution. "钛" means big. *Dai shang* is one of the twenty five constitutions of yin and

yang，pertaining to metal. People of this kind are honest and upright，and always keep their integrity. See *Ling Shu* chapter 64. See "金形之人".

制大　即大方。组方药味数少而量重。出《素问·至真要大论》。参见"大小为制"。

制大（zhì dà）　**large formula** A formula with a small number of medicines but a large quantity of each. See *Su Wen* chapter 74. See "大小为制".

制小　即小方。组方药味数多而量轻。出《素问·至真要大论》。

制小（zhì xiǎo）　**small formula** A formula with a large number of medicines but a small quantity of each. See *Su Wen* chapter 74.

和　① 调和。出《素问·上古天真论》。② 正常和谐状态。出《素问·五运行大论》。③ 指治法中的和法。出《素问·至真要大论》。

和（hé）　① Harmonizing. See *Su Wen* chapter 1. ② A normal，harmonious state. See *Su Wen* chapter 67. ③ Harmonizing method. See *Su Wen* chapter 74.

和于术数　和，调和。术，技也。数，义同"术"。言运用各种养生方法以锻炼身体，如呼吸、按跷、气功疗法等。出《素问·上古天真论》。

和于术数(hé yú shù shù) **adjusting ways to preserve health** To exercise with various health preserving techniques，such as breathing，massage，and *qigong*，etc. See *Su Wen* chapter 1.

季冬痹 季冬，冬季三月之末月，为手少阴经所主之月。季冬痹，即手少阴经筋在季冬所发之痹证。可见转筋、疼痛等症。出《灵枢·经筋》。

季冬痹(jì dōng bì) **impediment in the third month of winter** *Jì dōng* refers to the third month of winter，which is dominated by the meridian of hand *shaoyin*. *Jì dōng bì* refers to the impediment syndrome of the hand *shaoyin* meridian which occurs in the third month of winter，with symptoms such as spasms and pain，etc. See *Ling Shu* chapter 13.

季胁 又名季肋，俗称软肋，为胁下小肋，当十一、十二肋骨处。出《素问·脉要精微论》。

季胁(jì xié) **free ribs** Also called *jì lèi*，or *ruǎn lèi*，and is the area of the eleventh and twelfth ribs. See *Su Wen* chapter 17.

季春痹 季春，春季三月之末月，

为足阳明经所主之月。季春痹，即足阳明经筋在季春所发之痹证。可见转筋、口眼歪斜等症。出《灵枢·经筋》。

季春痹(jì chūn bì) **impediment in the third month of spring** *Jì chūn* refers to the third month of spring，which is dominated by the meridian of foot *yangming*. *Jì chūn bì* refers to the impediment syndrome of the meridian of foot *yangming* which occurs in the third month of spring with symptoms of spasms，and deviation of the mouth and eyes，etc. See *Ling Shu* chapter 13.

季秋痹 季秋，秋季三月之末月，为足厥阴经所主之月。季秋痹，即足厥阴经筋在季秋所发之痹证。可见肢痛、转筋等症。出《灵枢·经筋》。

季秋痹(jì qiū bì) **impediment in the third month of autumn** *Jì qiū* refers to the third month of autumn，which is dominated by the foot *jueyin* meridian. *Jì qiū bì* refers to the impediment syndrome of the foot *jueyin* meridian which occurs in the third month of autumn with symptoms of pain in the limbs，and spasms etc. See *Ling Shu*

八画

chapter 13.

季夏痹 季夏,夏季三月之末月。为手少阳经所主之月。季夏痹,即手少阳经筋在季夏所发之痹证。可见转筋、舌卷等症。出《灵枢·经筋》。

季夏痹(jì xià bì) **impediment in the third month of summer** *Jì xià* refers to the third month of summer，which is dominated by the hand *shaoyang* meridian. *Jì xià bì* refers to the impediment syndrome of the hand *shaoyang* meridian which occurs in the third month of summer with symptoms of spasms，and curled tongue etc. See *Ling Shu* chapter 13.

委中 经穴名。足太阳膀胱经的合穴。在腘窝横纹中央。出《灵枢·本输》。

委中(wěi zhōng) **Wei Zhong (BL 40)** Acupoint name which is the sea acupoint of the bladder meridian of foot *taiyang*，located in the middle of the popliteal line. See *Ling Shu* chapter 2.

委中央 即委中。出《灵枢·邪气藏府病形》。见"委中"条。

委中央(wěi zhōng yāng) **bend center** It refers to *Wei Zhong* acupoint BL 40. See *Ling Shu*

chapter 4. See "委中".

委阳 足太阳膀胱经穴名。是足太阳经的别络,又是三焦的下合穴。在承扶穴下一寸六分,腘窝横纹外侧两筋间。出《灵枢·本输》。

委阳(wěi yáng) **Wei Yang (BL 39)** It is the name of the sea acupoint of the triple *jiao*，and it is also the collateral of foot *taiyang* meridian. It is located 1.6 *cun* under the acupoint BL 36，between the two sinews on the outside of the popliteal stria. See *Ling Shu* chapter 2.

使道 ① 脏腑间气血流行联络之通道。出《素问·灵兰秘典论》。② 指部位。出《灵枢·天年》。(1) 鼻腔。见《太素·寿限》。(2) 人中所在处,即鼻唇沟。见《灵枢注证发微》。

使道(shǐ dào) ① Circulating path of blood，qi. See *Su Wen* chapter 8. ② Body parts. See *Ling Shu* chapter 54.（1）The nasal cavity. See *Tai Su*（*Classified Study on Huang Di Nei Jing*）the Life Span.（2）The nasolabial fold. See *Su Wen Zhu Zheng Fa Wei*（*Annotation and Elaboration on Su Wen*）.

侠脊之脉 伏行于脊里之冲脉,为冲脉之分支,从胞中出,向后

八画

与督脉相通，伏行于脊柱内。出《素问·举痛论》。

侠脊之脉（xiá jǐ zhī mài）　**thoroughfare vessel running on both sides of the spine** A branch of the thoroughfare vessel，which exits the uterus，connecting to the governor vessel and running in the spine. See *Su Wen* chapter 39.

侠溪　经穴名。足少阳胆经之荥穴。在足小趾，次指歧骨间，本节前陷者中。《灵枢·本输》。

侠溪（xiá xī）　**Xia Xi（GB 43）** Acupoint name pertaining to the brook acupoint of the gall-bladder meridian of foot *shaoyang*. It is located at the small pit on the inner side of the small toe，close to the neighbouring toe. See *Ling Shu* chapter 2.

侠瘿　病名。即瘰疬。生于腋下，类似马刀形的称马刀；生于颈部的称侠瘿。一作挟瘿。见《灵枢·经脉》《灵枢·痈疽》。

侠瘿（xiá yǐng）　**Scrofula** Disease name. It is usually found at axilla with the shape of a saber. That found at the neck is named scrofula，sometimes written as "挟瘿". See *Ling Shu* chapter 10 and 81.

质判之人　体质名。此代表阴阳二十五人中火形人之一种，其特征是怡然自得。出《灵枢·阴阳二十五人》。

质判之人（zhì pàn zhī rén）　*zhipan*-**type people** Name of constitution. It is one of the twenty-five people of yin and yang pertaining to the physique of fire. People of this kind are always happy and content. See *Ling Shu* chapter 64.

质徵之人　体质名。此代表阴阳二十五人中火形人之一种，其特征是光明正大而明白事理。出《灵枢·阴阳二十五人》。参"火形之人"。

质徵之人（zhì zhēng zhī rén）　*zhizheng*-**type people** Name of constitution. It is one of the twenty five constitutions of yin and yang，pertaining to fire. This kind of people are fair and honest. See *Ling Shu* chapter 64. See "火形之人".

所不胜　五行生克规律中克我的一行，即我之所不胜。出《素问·五运行大论》。

所不胜（suǒ bú shèng）　**element being un-restrained** In the theory of the five elements，there are relationships of restraining，such as wood restraining earth. While for earth, it is un-restrained by wood. See *Su Wen* chapter 67.

所生 ① 五行中之生我者。出《素问·六节藏象论》。② 五行中之我生者。出《素问·玉机真藏论》。

所生（suǒ shēng） **element being generated** In the theory of the five elements, there are relationships of generating, such as wood generates fire. ① The element that generates, for example, the wood generates fire, here *suǒ shēng* refers to the wood. See *Su Wen* chapter 9. ② The element that is being generated, for example, wood generates fire, here *suǒ shēng* refers to fire. See *Su Wen* chapter 19.

所生病 是指本经经穴所主治的病证。出《灵枢·经脉》。

所生病（suǒ shēng bìng） **Disease of viscera connecting with its meridian** Diseases produced by viscera which connects with their meridians. See *Ling Shu* chapter 10.

所胜 五行生克规律中我克的一行，即为我之所胜。出《素问·五运行大论》。

所胜（suǒ shèng） **element being restrained** In the theory of the five elements, there are relationships of controlling, like fire controls water, and *suǒ shèng* here refers to water. See *Su Wen* chapter 67.

金 五行之一,由自然界"金属"抽象而来。其特性是从革。即变革形态之改变,引申为具有清凉、肃杀、下降、收敛等作用性质的事物。根据五行属性归类的方法,归属于金的在脏为肺,在气候为燥,在季节为秋,在方位为西,在五味为辛,在五色为白等。出《素问·阴阳应象大论》。

金（jīn） **metal** One of the five elements, and a term extracted from the metal occurring in nature. It refers to the substances that have cooling, purifying, downwards-sending, and astringing functions. According to the five element theory, metal refers to the lung as regards to five viscera, dryness to the climate, autumn to the weather, west to the position, spicy taste to the five flavors, and white to the five colors, etc. See *Su Wen* chapter 5.

金曰从革 金气不及曰从革。从,顺从;革,变革。金气不及,不能成坚,则顺从火化而改变形状,故称。出《素问·五常政大论》。

金曰从革(jīn yuē cóng gé)
metal characterized by changing Deficiency of metal qi is called *cóng gé*. *Cóng* means to accept; *gé* means to change. When there is metal qi deficiency, it will not be hard enough, thus its shape will be changed by fire, hence the name. See *Su Wen* chapter 70.

金曰坚成　金运太过曰坚成,是金气有余,坚刚而能成物。出《素问·五常政大论》。

金曰坚成(jīn yuē jiān chéng)
Metal is known as hardness. Excessive metal qi is called hardness. When there is a surplus of metal qi, materials are formed. See *Su Wen* chapter 70.

金曰审平　金运平和曰审平。审平,即审慎平和。金主肃杀,金气平均,则收敛清和,不过杀伐。出《素问·五常政大论》。

金曰审平(jīn yuē shěn píng)
Balance of metal is known as calmness and peace. *Shěn píng* means calmness and peace. Metal is characterized by the functions of clearing and downward promoting, a balanced metal qi will show calmness in-

stead of clearing. See *Su Wen* chapter 70.

金气　运气概念中的六气之一,主气六步中的五之气,主秋分后六十日,其性燥。出《素问·六微旨大论》

金气(jīn qì)　**metal qi** A term of the five circuits and six qi. The fifth qi of the six steps of dominant qi. Metal qi dominates the sixty days after the Autumn Equinox, and has the feature of dryness. See *Su Wen* chapter 68.

金兰之室　出《素问·气穴论》。(1)藏珍贵书籍的处所。见《素问识》《太素·气穴》。(2)指心。见《素问集注》。

金兰之室(jīn lán zhī shì)　**golden fragrant room** See *Su Wen* chapter 58. (1) Places for storing precious books. See *Su Wen Zhi* (*Understanding Su Wen*) and *Tai Su* "Qi Xue" (2) Heart. See *Su Wen Ji Zhu* (*Collected Annotation of Su Wen*).

金形之人　体质名。又称上商。阴阳二十五人之一。出《灵枢·阴阳二十五人》。金形之人在五音属商,分为上商,右商,左商,钛商。其体形多头小、面方,肩背小、腹小、手足少、足跟坚实,突出于外,骨轻、肤色白;其禀性为人清白廉洁,性情急躁刚强。该体质大多能耐于秋冬,不耐于春夏,故春夏易发病。

金形之人（jīn xíng zhī rén）**people pertaining to the metal element** Name of constitution representing one of the twenty-five constitutions of yin and yang that pertains to the physique of metal, also named the *shang shang* tone. See *Ling Shu* chapter 64. People of this kind pertain to *shang* tone, which is further divided into *shang shang*, right *shang*, left *shang*, *dai shang*. People of this kind have small head, square face, small shoulders and back, small abdomen, small hands and feet, firm protruding heels, light bones and white skin; they are normally clean and honest, although can be impatient and tough. They can endure autumn and winter, but not spring and summer, so in spring and summer they are prone to diseases.

金运 五运之一。其时气候凉而干燥、肃杀之气流行,万物成熟结实,树叶凋落,疾病多见伤肺症候等。出《素问·天元纪大论》。

金运（jīn yùn） **metal period** It is one of the five circuits. The dry, harsh and down-sending autumn qi that ripens the fruits and shakes down the leaves easily causes lung diseases. See *Su Wen* chapter 66.

金位 即阳明燥金旺盛所主之时令。出《素问·六微旨大论》。

金位（jīn wèi） **the season of metal** The season that the *yangming* dryness-metal dominates. See *Su Wen* chapter 68.

金郁 金运之令被郁遏。火能克金,若火运太过或金运不及时,会使金气被郁。出《素问·六元正纪大论》。

金郁（jīn yù） **restrained metal** Fire restrains metal. When fire is excess or metal is deficient, metal qi is restrained. See *Su Wen* chapter 71.

金郁泄之 金郁,即金气被郁。从自然气候变化言,秋应燥而反湿,应凉而反热,应收而不收;以人体言,肺气不宣,治节不行,皆称为金郁,应予宣泄疏利。如发汗、利小便等。出《素问·六元正纪大论》。

金郁泄之（jīn yù xiè zhī） **Restrained metal is treated by discharge.** *Jīn yù* refers to the restraining of metal. In nature, wet and hot weather in Autumn, which is expected to be dry and cool，is considered as restraining of metal. In human body，non-diffussion of lung qi and inhibited management and regulation of lung are regarded as restringing of metal. It is necessary to diffuse lung qi，For example，sweat-effusing and urine disin-hibition，etc. See *Su Wen* chapter 71.

金匮　① 藏贵重物品之器具。出《素问·气穴论》。② 古医籍名。出《素问·病能论》。据此其中当包括有关诊断方面的内容,已佚。

金匮(jīn guì)　① Chambers for storing valuables. See *Su Wen* chapter 58. ② The name of an ancient medical book on diagnosis which has been lost in history. See *Su Wen* chapter 46.

金匮真言论　《素问》篇名。匮,同柜;金匮,指古代帝王藏书的处所;真言,至真至要的言论。此篇以阴阳四时五行为中心,说明人体五脏与自然界的收受关系。其之所以冠以"金匮真言"之名,意在强调内容极为珍贵,使读者重视。

金匮真言论(jīn guì zhēn yán lùn)　**Discussion on the Important Ideas in the Golden Chamber**

Chapter name in *Su Wen*. *Guì* (匮) is equivalent to *guì* (柜), refers to the chamber. *Jīn guì* refers to places where ancient emperors collected books. *Zhēn yán* means vital ideas. Based on the theories of yin and yang，the four seasons，and the five elements. This chapter discusses the relationship between the five viscera and nature. By entitling it with golden chamber，the author stresses the value of this chapter，so as to catch the attention of readers.

命门　即目。出《灵枢·根结》《素问·阴阳离合论》。

命门(mìng mén)　**life gate** The eyes. See *Ling Shu* chapter 5 and *Su Wen* chapter 6.

郄中　即委中穴,又名血郄、中郄。为足太阳膀胱经之合穴。在腘窝横纹之中点。出《素问·刺腰痛》。

郄中(xì zhōng)　**Xi Zhong (BL 40)** It is also named Xie Xi, Zhong Xi. The sea acupoint of the bladder meridian of foot *taiyang*. It is located in the middle of the popliteal line. See *Su Wen* chapter 41.

郄阳　经穴名。即委阳穴。属足太阳膀胱经,是三焦下合穴。

在胭中外廉两筋间，屈膝取穴。出《素问・刺腰痛》。

郄阳（xì yáng）　**Xi Yang（BL 53）** Name of acupoint BL 39. It is the lower sea acupoint of the triple *jiao*, which is on the bladder meridian of foot *taiyang*. It is located between the center of the popliteal fossa and the lateral margin, and can be found by bending the knees. See *Su Wen* chapter 41.

受盛之府　指小肠，其功能为受盛由胃而来之物。出《灵枢・本输》。

受盛之府（shòu shèng zhī fǔ）　**the bowel of receiving bounties** Refers to the small intestine, which receives digested food from the stomach. See *Ling Shu* chapter 2.

受盛之官　指小肠。出《素问・灵兰秘典论》。

受盛之官（shòu shèng zhī guān）　**office of receiving bounties** The small intestine. See *Su Wen* chapter 8.

乳子　出《素问・通评虚实论》："乳子而病热，脉悬小者何如？岐伯曰：手足温者生，寒则死。"（1）婴儿。见《素问识》。（2）为婴儿哺乳。见《张氏医通・妇人门下》《素问绍识》。（3）产

子。见《素问绍识》。

乳子（rǔ zǐ）　See *Su Wen* chapter 28, "When a feeding mother suffers from heat with her vessels being suspended and small, how is that? Qi Bo said, When her hands and feet are warm, then she will survive. When they are cold, she will die".（1）Babies. See *Su Wen Zhi*（*Understanding Su Wen*）.（2）Breastfeeding a baby. *Zhang's Medical Book* "Women's Diseases" and Su Wen Shao Zhi（*Continuation of Understanding Su Wen*）.（3）Giving birth to a child. *Su Wen Shao Zhi*（*Continuation of Understanding Su Wen*）.

肤胀　病名。由感受寒邪，气机郁滞所导致的全身肿胀，症见腹大、皮厚，按其腹，窅而不起等。出《灵枢・水胀》《灵枢・胀论》。

肤胀（fū zhàng）　**cutaneous distension** A disease name of a swollen body caused by cold pathogens and stagnation of circuits and qi. It manifests as an enlarged abdomen with thick skin; when abdomen is pressed, it does not rise by itself. See *Ling Shu* chapter 57, and *Ling Shu* chapter 35.

肺 ① 五脏之一。位居胸中，与鼻相通，为脏腑之最高者，主治节，具有宣发与肃降的功能；其司呼吸，布卫气，主一身之气，为气之本；全身百脉皆朝于肺，有协助心推动血行的作用；参与人体水液代谢，有通调水道之功。出《素问·经脉别论》。其经脉为手太阴肺经，与手阳明大肠经相表里。五行配属为金，主时于秋。其在体为皮毛，在志为悲，在液为涕，在窍为鼻，在味为辛，病理特征为燥。《素问·灵兰秘典论》。② 肺的精气。出《素问·阴阳应象大论》。③ 肺病。出《素问·咳论》。④ 肺之脉象。出《素问·玉机真藏论》。⑤ 肺在面部相应的望诊部位（两眉之间）。出《灵枢·五色》。

肺（fèi） ① Lung. One of the five viscera. It is located in the chest on the top of five viscera and six bowels, and is connected to the nose. The lung governs the management and regulation of the body, as well as functions like diffusion, purification and downwards-sending. It dominates qi, controls breathing, distributes the defensive qi, and also is the root of qi. All meridians converge in the lung, assisting the heart to circulate the blood. The lung participates in the metabolism of the body fluids, and regulates the waterways. See *Su Wen* chapter 21. Its meridian is the lung meridian of hand *taiyin*, which is exteriorly-interiorly related to the large intestine meridian of hand *yangming*. In the five element theory, the lung pertains to the metal element, and rules in autumn. It is the skin and body hair on the human body; among the states of mind it is sorrow; among the fluid and humors it is snivel; among the orifices it is the nose; among the flavors it is acrid; and its pathological feature is dryness. See *Su Wen* chapter 8. ② Essence qi of the lung. See *Su Wen* chapter 5. ③ Lung diseases. See *Su Wen* chapter 38. ④ Pulse manifestation of the lung. See *Su Wen* chapter 19. ⑤ The facial inspection area corresponding to the lung (between the eyebrows). See *Ling Shu* chapter 49.

肺手太阴之脉 即手太阴肺经，为十二经脉之一。出《灵枢·

经脉》10。

肺手太阴之脉(fèi shǒu tài yīn zhī mài) **lung meridian of hand taiyin** It is one of the twelve regular meridians. See *Ling Shu* chapter 10.

肺气 ①肺的精气，维系着肺的宣发与肃降等功能活动。"肺气清"是其功能特点，失常则胀满而喘。肺气与鼻相通。出《灵枢·脉度》。②指肺。出《素问·四气调神大论》。

肺气(fèi qì) ① Essence qi of the lung, which maintains the functions of the lung, such as dispersing, diffusing and downwards-bearing of qi, etc. Normally lung qi is clear and light, if not so, there will be fullness and panting. Lung qi is connected to the nose (The qi of the lung passes through the nose). See *Ling Shu* chapter 17. ② Lung. See *Su Wen* chapter 2.

肺气焦满 焦，指肺热叶焦，满，肺气胀满。出《素问·四气调神大论》。

肺气焦满(fèi qì jiāo mǎn) **Lung qi burns with fullness.** *Jiāo* here means lung heat that scorches the lobes. *Mǎn* here means that there is excessive lung qi

that causes fullness in the chest. See *Su Wen* chapter 2.

肺风 病名。五脏风之一。病起于肺之俞穴被风邪所中。症候特点与肺的病理特点有关，故名。出《素问·风论》。

肺风(fèi fēng) **lung wind** Disease name of one of the wind syndromes of the five viscera. It is caused by pathogenic wind undermining the back transport acupoint of the lung, where lung qi is infused, and the symptoms of lung wind show the pathological features of the lung, hence the name. See *Su Wen* chapter 42.

肺风疝 病名。外邪由肾入肺而成之气病。出《素问·四时刺逆从论》。

肺风疝(fèi fēng shàn) **lung wind hernia** Disease name. A qi disease caused by external pathogens entering the lung from the kidney. See *Su Wen* chapter 64.

肺为之相 相，辅助。义同"相傅之官"。出《灵枢·五癃津液别》。见"相傅之官"条。

肺为之相(fèi wéi zhī xiàng) **the lung as officer of assistant** *Xiàng* means to assist. See *Ling Shu* chapter 36. This term shares the same meaning with the term

八画

"相傅之官"，refer to that.

肺为阳中之少阴　根据阴阳、五行原理，阴阳之中又有阴阳可分。肺为阴脏，位居膈上为阳，肺气通于秋，秋气为阴之渐，故以阳中之少阴称之。出《灵枢·阴阳系日月》。《素问·六节藏象论》作"阳中之太阴"。参该条。

肺为阳中之少阴（fèi wéi yáng zhōng zhī shào yīn）　**The lung is the *shaoyin* of yang.** According to the theories of yin and yang, and the five elements, yin and yang can further be divided into yin and yang. The lung is among the five yin viscera as it is located above the diaphragm in the yang section; the lung qi corresponds to autumn, which is yin in nature, hence the name. See *Ling Shu* chapter 41. In *Su Wen* chapter 9 it is expressed as the *taiyin* in the yang（阳中之太阴），refer to this term.

肺为涕　涕，通洟。肺开窍于鼻，肺气燥热，则鼻窍干涩；肺气虚寒，则清涕常流；外邪袭肺，则鼻塞流涕。出《素问·宣明五气》。《灵枢·九针论》作"肺主涕"。

肺为涕（fèi wéi tì）　**The lung forms snivel.** "涕" is the same as "洟".

The lung opens at the nose. If the lung qi is dry and hot, the nasal passages are dry. If the lung qi is deficient and cold, clear nasal discharge will flow frequently. If external pathogens invade the lung, nasal obstruction and runny nose will occur. See *Su Wen* chapter 23. Besides, in *Ling Shu* chapter 78, the term is expressed as the lung controlling nasal mucus.

肺心痛　病证名。厥心痛之一。由肺经受邪所致，症见心痛，静则暂缓，动则加剧，面色不变。出《灵枢·厥病》。

肺心痛（fèi xīn tòng）　**reversal heartache caused by lung disorder** Disease name. It is one of the reversal heartaches, which caused by pathogens invading the lung meridian. The main symptom is heartache, which is temporarily relieved by staying still, and getting worse with movement. See *Ling Shu* chapter 24.

肺生皮毛　肺合皮毛，肺具有生养皮毛的生理功能。出《素问·阴阳应象大论》。

肺生皮毛（fèi shēng pí máo）　**Lung promotes skin and body hair.** The lung is related to skin and body hair, and has the physiological function of promoting skin and body hair. See *Su Wen* chapter 5.

肺主皮　主，掌管、主持之意。肺主气，气行皮毛，故肺所主之外合为皮。见《素问·宣明五气》。

肺主皮（fèi zhǔ pí）　**Lung governs skin and body hair.** *Zhǔ* means to govern. The lung dominates qi，which nourishes and generates the skin and body hair，hence the lung governs skin and body hair. See *Su Wen* chapter 23.

肺主身之皮　出《素问·痿论》。义同"肺生皮毛"。

肺主身之皮（fèi zhǔ shēn zhī pí）　**Lung governs body hair.** The same meaning as "Lung governs skin and body hair". See *Su Wen* chapter 44. It has the same meaning as "肺生皮毛".

肺主咳　言肺之病。肺气宜降，若反上逆则为咳，是咳皆出于肺。出《灵枢·九针论》。

肺主咳（fèi zhǔ ké）　**Lung governs cough.** Refers to a disease of the lung. Naturally lung qi goes downwards，however if lung qi ascends，the counterflow will cause coughing. Thus it is said that all coughs originate from lung. See *Ling Shu* chapter 78.

肺主秋　此以五行学说归纳脏腑与季节的关系，肺五行属金，秋五行属金，故肺主秋季。出《素问·藏气法时论》。

肺主秋（fèi zhǔ qiū）　**Lung is predominant in autumn.** This is to use the theory of the five elements to sum up the relationship between the viscera，the bowels and the seasons. The lung pertains to the metal element，and so does autumn，thus the lung rules in autumn. See *Su Wen* chapter 22.

肺主涕　义同"肺为涕"。参该条。出《灵枢·九针论》。

肺主涕（fèi zhǔ tì）　**Lung governs snivel.** Refer to the term "肺为涕"，which shares the same meaning. See *Ling Shu* chapter 78.

肺主鼻　鼻为肺之窍。出《素问·阴阳应象大论》。

肺主鼻（fèi zhǔ bí）　**Lung governs the nose** The nose is the orifice of the lung. See *Su Wen* chapter 5.

肺合大肠　合，配合之意。手阳明大肠经与手太阴肺经相为表里，肺与大肠在功能上具有相应关系。出《灵枢·本藏》。

肺合大肠（fèi hé dà cháng）　**Lung is connected with large in-**

八画

testine. *Hé* means being connected with. Due to the exterior-interior relationship between the large intestine meridian of hand *yangming* and the lung meridian of hand *taiyin*, the lung is functionally related to the large intestine. See *Ling Shu* chapter 47.

肺合皮　合，配合之意。出《灵枢·五色》。义同"肺主皮"，参该条。

肺合皮（fèi hé pí）　**Lung is connected with skin and body hair.** *Hé* means be connected with. See *Ling Shu* chapter 49. Read the term "肺主皮" for reference，for the two terms share the same meaning.

肺系　与肺连属的气管、喉咙等组织。出《灵枢·经脉》。

肺系（fèi xì）　**lung connection** The trachea，throat and other tissues associated with lung. See *Ling Shu* chapter 10.

肺应皮　应，应合之意。出《灵枢·本藏》。与"肺主皮"义同，见该条。

肺应皮（fèi yīng pí）　**Lung corresponds to the skin.** *Yīng* means to correspond to. See *Ling Shu* chapter 47. Refer to "肺主皮" which shares the same mean-

ing.

肺鸣　喘息有声。症因肺藏气，气郁不利而喘。出《素问·痿论》。

肺鸣（fèi míng）　**lung ringing** The sound when breathing in disease. Asthma is due to lung qi accumulation and qi depression. See *Su Wen* chapter 44.

肺胀　病证名。五脏胀之一。症见胸满咳喘。出《灵枢·胀论》。

肺胀（fèi zhàng）　**lung distension** Disease name and one of the visceral distensions. The main symptoms include fullness in the lung，panting and coughing. See *Ling Shu* chapter 35.

肺疟　五脏疟之一。症见寒热，发热时伴有惊吓和幻视等。《素问·刺疟》。

肺疟（fèi nüè）　**lung malaria** One kind of visceral malaria. The main symptoms include cold，hot，fear and illusion，etc. See *Su Wen* chapter 36.

肺疝　病名。疝之一种。由寒邪挟肝犯肺所致，脉见沉搏。出《素问·大奇论》。

肺疝（fèi shàn）　**lung hernia** Disease name. One kind of hernia caused by cold pathogens，and attack by the liver invading the lung，with a sunken pulse. See *Su Wen* chapter 48.

八画

肺咳　五脏咳之一。喘息有音为肺气上逆，故名肺咳。出《素问·咳论》。

肺咳（fèi ké）　**lung cough** One kind of visceral cough. Wheezing with the sound being caused by the counterflow ascent of lung qi，hence the name. See *Su Wen* chapter 38.

肺俞　经穴名。属足太阳膀胱经。在第三椎下两旁各一寸五分处。出《灵枢·背俞》。

肺俞（fèi shū）　**Fei Shu（BL 13）.** Acupoint name pertaining to the bladder meridian of foot *taiyang*，and is located 1.5 *cun* on each side of the third vertebra. See *Ling Shu* chapter 51.

肺脉　① 手太阴肺之经脉。出《素问·咳论》。② 肺的脉象。其肺来轻虚如毛，与秋相应。出《素问·宣明五气》。

肺脉（fèi mài）　① Lung meridian of hand *taiyin*. See *Su Wen* chapter 38. ② The pulse of the lung，which manifests as a floating feather，and corresponds to autumn. See *Su Wen* chapter 23.

肺脉毛　指脉来轻虚以浮，如按于羽毛之上的一种脉象，属肺的正常脉。出《素问·宣明五气》。

肺脉毛（fèi mài máo）　**Lung pulse is hair-like.** Light and floating pulse of the lung，which feels as if touching a feather. It is the normal pulse of the lung. See *Su Wen* chapter 23.

肺热叶焦　肺脏有热，热灼津伤，这是引起痿证的重要病机。叶焦，形容肺叶受热灼津的病理现象。出《素问·痿论》。

肺热叶焦（fèi rè yè jiāo）　**Lung heat scorches the lobes.** Lung heat burns and consumes body fluid，which is an important pathogenesis of wilting syndrome. *Yè jiāo* refers to the pathological phenomenon of lobes scorched by lung heat. See *Su Wen* chapter 44.

肺恶寒　恶（wù 误），厌憎之意。肺合皮毛，寒气易入而伤肺。《素问·宣明五气》。

肺恶寒（fèi wù hán）　**The lung is averse to cold.** *Wù* means averse. The lung is related to body hair which can easily be invaded by cold pathogens. See *Su Wen* chapter 23.

肺消　病证名。消渴欲饮，小便反多于饮水之证。因心移寒于肺。致水精不能四布，惟下泄膀胱。出《素问·气厥论》。

肺消（fèi xiāo）　**lung wasting** Disease name. Patients with

this syndrome long for water, however, they drink one portion and urinate two. The heart passes cold to the lung, hindering the distribution of water and essence, which have nowhere to go but to go down to the bladder. See *Su Wen* chapter 37.

肺朝百脉　朝（cháo 潮），朝会。百脉朝会于肺，全身血液通过经脉聚会于肺，经肺的呼吸进行体内外清浊之气的交换，将富含清气的血液经经脉输至全身。出《素问·经脉别论》。

肺朝百脉（fèi cháo bǎi mài）**The lung links with all vessels.** *Cháo* means to meet. All vessels meet at the lung, and the blood of the whole body gathers in the lung through those vessels. Inhaling brings clear qi into the body, and exhaling takes turbid qi out. Through the inhalation and exhalation of the lung, blood full of clear qi is transported to the whole body. See *Su Wen* chapter 21.

肺痹　病证名。五脏痹之一。由外感风邪不解，邪气痹肺，或由皮痹日久，反复感受风寒湿邪，发展而来。症见咳嗽气逆，烦满而呕等。出《素问·痹论》《素问·五藏生成》。

肺痹（fèi bì）**lung impediment** Disease name and one kind of visceral impediment. Lung impediment is caused by the invasion of pathogenic wind or the repeated invasion of wind, cold and damp pathogens due to skin impediment for a long time. The main symptoms include coughing with adverse qi, vexation and vomiting. See *Su Wen* chapter 43 and 10.

肺藏于右　言肺脏脏气之主治。藏，收之意。人身面南，左东右西。肺主秋收之气，位居西方，故藏于右。出《素问·刺禁论》。

肺藏于右（fèi cáng yú yòu）**The lung is stored on the right.** The domination of lung qi. *Cáng* means to store. When a person faces south, the east is on his left, and the west is on his right. The lung controls the qi of autumn, which stores and is located in the west, hence the name. See *Su Wen* chapter 52.

肺藏气　肺为一身之气的根本。见《素问·调经论》《灵枢·本神》。

肺藏气（fèi cáng qì）**The lung stores qi.** The lung is the foundation of qi. See *Su Wen* chapter 62, *Ling Shu* chapter 8.

肺藏气,气舍魄　魄舍于气而肺藏之。出《灵枢·本神》《素问·六节藏象论》参"肺藏魄"条。

肺藏气,气舍魄(fèi cáng qì, qì shě pò)　**The lung stores qi and qi houses corporeal soul.** This means that the *qi* is the house of the corporeal soul, and the lung is that of the *qi*. See *Ling Shu* chapter 8 and *Su Wen* chapter 9, and refer to the term "肺藏魄".

肺藏魄　肺与人体精神活动有一定关系。魄属精神活动之一,依附于形体而显现,属阴。肺为阳中之阴脏,故魄藏于肺。出《灵枢·九针论》。

肺藏魄(fèi cáng pò)　**The lung stores the corporeal soul.** The lung has a certain relationship with human mental activities, and the corporeal soul is a kind of mental activity, which manifests depending on the physique and the body, and pertains to yin. The lung is the yin viscera in yang, thus the corporeal soul is stored in the lung. See *Ling Shu* chapter 78.

肱　手臂从肘至腕的部分。亦泛指手臂。出《灵枢·九针论》。

肱(gōng)　**upper arm** The upper part of the arm from the elbow to the wrist. It also refers to the arms. See *Ling Shu* chapter 78.

肬　肬同疣,为皮肤所生之赘肉。出《灵枢·经脉》。

肬(yóu)　**verruca** "肬" equals to "疣". It refers to verruca, the extra flesh generated by the skin. See *Ling Shu* chapter 10.

胁　季胁下空软处。出《素问·骨空论》。

胁(miǎo)　**soft parts around acupoint EX B2.** See *Su Wen* chapter 60.

胁络　挟脊两旁空软处的络脉。出《素问·骨空论》。

胁络(miǎo luò)　**meridians and collaterals on both soft parts of the EX B2** See *Su Wen* chapter 60.

胂　病证名。出《素问·大奇论》。(1)浮肿病。见《类经·脉色类二十四》。(2)痈肿。见《素问》王冰注。

胂(zhǒng)　**swelling** Disease name. See *Su Wen* chapter 48. (1) Edema. See *Lei Jing* (*Classified Classic*) "Pulse and Color Chapter 24". (2) Swollen welling abscesses. See *Su Wen* annotated by Wang Bing.

肿根蚀　因针刺误中乳房,引起乳房脓肿,侵蚀肤肌的病证。出《素问·刺禁论》。

八画

肿根蚀（zhǒng gēn shí）　**swelling and ulceration** Symptoms of breast abscesses and erosion of the skin and muscles. The main cause of this condition is that acupuncture accidentally hit the breast. See *Su Wen* chapter 52.

胀　① 病证名。胀病之总称,可发于身体各部位,深可至胸廓腹腔,浅可在皮肤。由气、血、水等不化或潴留引起。然胀之根源则在脏腑营卫,有五脏六腑胀、脉胀、肤胀、水胀、鼓胀等名。出《灵枢·胀论》。② 症状。指胸腹、胁的胀满。出《素问·阴阳别论》。

胀（zhàng）　① The general name of distension syndromes, which can be found in all parts of the body, deep at the thorax and abdomen, shallow at the skin. It is caused by the failure of transportation and transformation of qi, blood and water, etc., or by their retention. Nevertheless, the root of distension syndromes lies in the viscera and bowels, and the nutrient qi and the defensive qi. It is categorized into five-viscera-six-bowel distension, pulse distension, skin distension, water distension, bulge distension, etc. See *Ling Shu* chapter 35. ② Symptoms. Refers to the fullness of the chest, abdomen and flank. See *Su Wen* chapter 7.

胀论　《灵枢》篇名。胀,指胸腹胀大,皮肤浮肿一类病证。此篇主要论述各种胀病的病因病机、临床表现、治疗方法等,故名。

胀论（zhàng lùn）　**Discussion on Distension** Chapter name in *Ling Shu*. Distention refers to swelling of chest and abdomen with swollen skin. This chapter mainly discusses the etiology, pathogenesis, clinical manifestations and treatment of various kinds of distensions, hence the name.

股骨　大腿骨。出《素问·骨空论》。

股骨（gǔ gǔ）　**thigh bone** The thigh bone. See *Su Wen* chapter 60.

股胫疽　病名。发于大腿、足胫,毒盛脓深搏骨的疽。《灵枢·痈疽》。

股胫疽（gǔ jìng jū）　**thigh or shin flat abscess** Abscesses in the thigh, foot and shin, where pathogens accumulate, generating pus and undermining bones. See *Ling Shu* chapter 81.

肥人　体质名,指肌肉坚实、体形

壮大者。出《灵枢·逆顺肥瘦》。

肥人（féi rén）　**well-nourished people** Name of constitution. Refers to people who are big and strong, and with tough muscles. See *Ling Shu* chapter 38.

肥气　病名。为肝之积，其症见胁下结块如覆杯状。出《灵枢·邪气藏府病形》。

肥气（féi qì）　**liver amassment** Disease name. Amassment of the liver which is caused by the blockage of liver qi. See *Ling Shu* chapter 4.

周痹　①《灵枢》篇名。周，遍也。周痹，指痛处遍及全身的痹证。此篇主要论述了周痹与众痹的病机特点、症候鉴别、治疗方法。② 病证名。呈周身游走性疼痛，由风寒湿之邪侵入血脉所致。见《灵枢·周痹》。

周痹（zhōu bì）　① General Migratory Obstruction Syndrome, a chapter name in *Ling Shu*. *Zhōu* means general. *Zhōu bì* means that there is pain everywhere. This chapter mainly discusses the pathogenesis, syndrome differentiations and treatments of generalized impediments. ② Disease name. Wandering pain all over the body, which is caused by the invasion of pathogenic wind, cold and dampness into the blood and meridians. See *Ling Shu* chapter 27.

烦颧　出《灵枢·经筋》。

烦颧（qiú quán）　**cheek bone** See *Ling Shu* chapter 13.

鱼际　① 部位名。统指手足掌两侧肌肉丰厚处的边缘赤白肉际。见《灵枢·经脉》。② 穴位名。为手太阴经之荥穴。在手掌鱼际部，第一掌骨中点，赤白肉际处。见《灵枢·本输》。

鱼际（yú jì）　① Fish's margin, or the red and white flesh border of the thick muscular areas on both sides of the hand and foot. *Jì* means the margin. See *Ling Shu* chapter 10. ② The name of acupoint LU 10, the brook acupoint of the hand *taiyin* meridian, which is in the thenar of the palm, at the midpoint of the first metacarpal bone between the red and white flesh. See *Ling Shu* chapter 2.

鱼络　手鱼际部之脉络。出《灵枢·邪气藏府病形》。

鱼络（yú luò）　**fish network meridians and collaterals** The meridians and collaterals at the thenar of the hand. See *Ling Shu* chapter 4.

鱼腹　小腿肚，又称腓、腨、腨肠。

八画

出《素问·刺腰痛》。

鱼腹(yú fù) **fish belly** Calf. It is also named Fei（腓）, Shuan（腨）, Shuan Chang（腨肠）. See *Su Wen* chapter 41.

兔啮 病名。发于足胫部的痈肿。啮(niè 聂)，咬之义。其状赤色，如兔所咬，故名。出《灵枢·痈疽》。

兔啮(tù niè) **hare bite** Disease name for an abscess at the lower leg. *Niè* means to bite. This kind of abscess is red, like a rabbit bite, hence the name. See *Ling Shu* chapter 81.

狐疝 病名。疝之一种。腹、腹股沟、阴囊等处，局部内容物向外突出。常伴气痛，时有时无，如狐之出没不定。《灵枢·经脉》。

狐疝(hú shàn) **inguinal hernia** Disease name of one kind of hernia, presenting with a protruding abdomen, groin, and scrotum etc. It is often accompanied with sporadic pain, which is unpredictable like foxes. See *Ling Shu* chapter 10.

狐疝风 疝之一种。疝在厥阴经，其上下出入不定，如狐之出没不常，故曰狐疝。称风者，因脉滑之故。出《素问·四时刺逆从论》。

狐疝风(hú shàn fēng) **inguinal hernia wind** A hernia in the *jueyin* meridian, which goes up and down, unpredictable like foxes, hence the name *hú shàn*. *Fēng* here refers to its slippery pulse manifestation. See *Su Wen* chapter 64.

京骨 经穴名。足太阳膀胱经之原穴。在足外侧大骨下，赤白肉际陷者中。出《灵枢·本输》。

京骨(jīng gǔ) **Jing Gu (BL 64)** Acupoint name of the source acupoint of the bladder meridian of foot *taiyang*, which is located at the lateral aspect of the foot, below the big bone, in the depression between the red and white flesh. See *Ling Shu* chapter 2.

府俞 府，是大肠、小肠、胃、膀胱、三焦、胆六府之经脉。俞，是井、荥、俞、原、经、合六种俞穴，计三十六穴，左右合而言之，共七十二穴。见表3。出《素问·气穴论》。

表3　府　俞

俞别 府别	井(金)	荥(水)	俞(木)	原	经(火)	合(土)
大肠	商阳	二间	三间	合谷	阳溪	曲池
小肠	少泽	前谷	后溪	腕骨	阳谷	小海
胃	厉兑	内庭	陷谷	冲阳	解溪	三里
膀胱	至阴	通谷	束骨	京骨	昆仑	委中
三焦	关冲	液门	中渚	阳池	支沟	天井
胆	窍阴	侠溪	临泣	丘墟	阳辅	阳陵泉

府俞（fǔ shū）　**viscera and acupoint** *Fǔ* refers to the meridians of the large intestine, small intestine, stomach, bladder and triple *jiao*. *Shū* refers to the six groups of acupoints, namely, the well acupoints, brook acupoints, transport acupoints, source acupoints, meridian acupoints and sea acupoints, which equal to 36 acupoints on one side of the body. On both sides, there are 72 acupoints. See Table 3. Also see *Su Wen* chapter 58.

Table 3　Fu Shu

Meridians Viscera	well point (meta)	brook point (water)	transport point (wood)	source point	meridian point (fire)	sea point (earth)
Large Intestine	Shang Yang (LI 1)	Er Jian (LI 2)	San Jian (LI 3)	He Gu (LI 4)	Yang Xi (LI 5)	Qu Chi (LI 11)
Small Intestine	Shao Ze (SI 1)	Qian Gu (SI 2)	Hou Xi (SI 3)	Wan Gu (SI 4)	Yang Gu (SI 5)	Xiao Hai (SI 8)
Stomach	Li Dui (ST 45)	Nei Ting (ST 44)	Xian Gu (ST 43)	Chong Yang (ST 42)	Jie Xi (ST 41)	San Li (ST 36)
blader	Zhi Yin (BL 67)	Tong Gu (BL 66)	Shu Gu (BL 65)	Jing Gu (BL 64)	Kun Lun (BL 60)	Wei Zhong (BL 40)

八画

续 表

Merdians / Viscera	well point (meta)	brook point (water)	transport point (wood)	source point	meridian point (fire)	sea point (earth)
Triple Jiao	Guan Chong (SJ 1)	Ye Men (SJ 2)	Zhong Zhu (SJ 3)	Yang Chi (SJ 4)	Zhi Gou (SJ 6)	Tian Jing (SJ 10)
gallbladder	Qiao Yin (GB 44)	Xia Xi (GB 43)	Lin Qi (GB 41)	Qiu Xu (GB 40)	Yang Fu (GB 38)	Yanglingquan (GB 34)

疟 由风寒等邪引起周期性寒热交替发作的疾病。出《素问·疟论》。

疟（nüè） **malaria** A disease manifested as cyclically alternating coldness and heat, which is caused by the invasion of pathogenic wind, and coldness, etc. See *Su Wen* chapter 35.

疟论 《素问》篇名。疟，疟疾。此篇论述了疟疾的病因、病机、症候、诊断和治疗原则。故名。

疟论（nüè lùn） **Discourse on Malaria** Chapter name in *Su Wen*. This chapter discusses the cause, pathogenesis, symptoms, diagnosis and therapeutic principles of malaria, hence the name.

疠 病名。① 即疠风，亦称大风，即今之麻风，详"疠风"条。见《素问·脉要精微论》。② 为木、火、土、金、水疠，温疠等之统称，属烈性传染性疾病，感受天时不正之气而发。见《素

问·刺法论》《素问·本病论》。

疠（lì） ① Leprosy, which is also called *li*-wind or *da*-wind. Refer to the term "疠风". See *Su Wen* chapter 17. ② Pestilent qi. It refers to various kinds of pestilence, including wood, fire, earth, metal, water and febrile pestilence, etc. It is a deadly infectious epidemic due to the evil qi. See *Su Wen* chapter 72 and 73.

疠风 病名。又名疠，大风，即今称之麻风病。主症皮肤溃烂，鼻柱腐败，骨节重痛，须眉坠落。病由感受风邪，客于经脉，致营气郁热，气血不清。出《素问·风论》。

疠风（lì fēng） **leprosy** Disease name. *Lì fēng* is also abbreviated to *Li*, or named heavy-wind. The main symptoms include skin ulcers, decay of nasal column, sense of heaviness, pain

八画

on the joints, and loss of beard and eyebrows. It is caused by the invasion and retention of pathogenic wind in the meridians, leading to the stasis of nutrient qi, generation of heat and disturbance of qi and blood. See *Su Wen* chapter 42.

疝　病证名。① 疝气。气聚腹痛之病，多与太阴经脉有关。出《素问·大奇论》。② 诸疝之总称。出《素问·骨空论》。参"七疝"条。

疝（shàn）　Disease name. ① Hernia. A disease of qi retention and abdominal pain, which is mainly related to the *taiyin* meridians. See *Su Wen* chapter 48. ② A collective name for all kinds of hernias. See *Su Wen* chapter 60. See "七疝".

疝气　气积腹痛一类疾病。出《灵枢·邪气藏府病形》。

疝气（shàn qì）　**hernia** Disease of qi retention and abdominal pain. See *Ling Shu* chapter 4.

疝瘕　病名。① 即疝与瘕两种疾病。详各条。出《素问·平人气象论》。② 即蛊。以少腹闷热而痛，溺出白液为主证。出《素问·玉机真藏论》。

疝瘕（shàn jiǎ）　Disease name. ① It refers to *Shàn* (lower ab-

dominal colic) and *Jiǎ* (abdominal mass). Check each term for details. See *Su Wen* chapter 18. ② Parasitic tympanites. The main symptoms include sensations of pressure in the lower abdomen, heat and pain, and the main symptom is white discharge. See *Su Wen* chapter 19.

疡　指皮肤溃烂疮痈。出《素问·风论》。

疡（yáng）　**ulcers** Ulcerations and carbuncles of the skin. See *Su Wen* chapter 42.

卒口僻　卒同猝，突然。僻，歪斜。指突然口角歪斜。出《灵枢·经筋》。

卒口僻（cù kǒu pì）　**sudden deviation of the mouth** *Cù* means all of a sudden. *Pì* means deviation. This term refers to the sudden deviation of the mouth. See *Ling Shu* chapter 13.

卒中　病名。猝然中（zhòng 种）于天时不正之风，以猝然口眼歪斜、舌强语謇，甚至昏仆为主症。卒（cù 促）通猝，急遽、突然。出《素问·刺法论》。

卒中（cù zhòng）　**sudden stroke** Disease name, which is caused by the sudden invasion of pathogenic wind, presenting with sudden distortions of the eyes

八画

and mouth，a stiff tongue and blurred speech，even syncope. "卒" is the same as "猝"，means all of sudden. See *Su Wen* chapter 72.

卒心痛　猝然心痛。出《素问·刺热》。

卒心痛（cù xīn tong）　**sudden heart pain** Sudden heartache. See *Su Wen* chapter 32.

卒死　卒通猝。突然死亡。出《灵枢·五色》。

卒死（cù sǐ）　**sudden death** "卒" is the same as "猝". Refers to sudden death. See *Ling Shu* chapter 49.

卒疝　肝脉气血凝滞，少腹睾丸猝然疼痛之病。出《素问·缪刺论》。

卒疝（cù shàn）　**sudden hernia** Sudden and violent pain in the lateral aspect of the lower abdomen and testes，which is caused by stasis of qi and blood in the liver meridian. See *Su Wen* chapter 63.

法于阴阳　法，即效法，遵循。即遵循自然界的阴阳变化规律来调节人体阴阳以达养生的目的。出《素问·上古天真论》。

法于阴阳（fǎ yú yīn yáng）　**following the rule of yin and yang** *Fǎ* means to follow. This term means to follow the rule of yin

and yang in nature to regulate the yin and yang in the human body，in order to maintain health. See *Su Wen* chapter 1.

泄　① 腹泻。见《素问·阴阳别论》。② 汗泄。见《素问·举痛论》。③ 发散。见《素问·四气调神大论》。④ 治法中的泻法。见《素问·至真要大论》。⑤ 渗出。见《素问·宝命全形论》。⑥ 泄露机密。见《素问·三部九候论》。

泄（xiè）　① Diarrhea. See *Su Wen* chapter 7. ② Sweating. See *Su Wen* chapter 39. ③ To disperse. See *Su Wen* chapter 2. ④ Draining method. See *Su Wen* chapter 74. ⑤ To exudate. See *Su Wen* chapter 25. ⑥ Divulging secrets. See *Su Wen* chapter 20.

泄风　病名，由风客腠理所致。因汗出甚多如泄，故名。出《素问·风论》。

泄风（xiè fēng）　**sweat discharging** Disease name，caused by the wind invading the *Còu Lǐ* (a term refers to the striae of the skin，muscles and viscera，and also to the tissue between the skin and muscles). Patients may have excessive sweat，thus the name. See *Su Wen* chapter 42.

泄注　大便泄泻如水注。出《素问·玉机真藏论》。

泄注（xiè zhù）　**outpour diarrhea** Watery diarrhea. See *Su Wen* chapter 19.

泆饮　泆同溢。泆饮即水饮不化之病。出《灵枢·论疾诊尺》。

泆饮（yì yǐn）　**subcutaneous fluid retention** *Yì* means subcutaneous. *Yì yǐn* refers to the disease of fluid retention. See *Ling Shu* chapter 74.

注下赤白　注下，大便泄泻。赤白，指大便中夹有赤色白色之冻状物。出《素问·六元正纪大论》。

注下赤白（zhù xià chì bái）　**red and white in downpour diarrhea** *Zhù xià* refers to diarrhea. *Chì bái* refers to the red and white viscous substances in the stool. See *Su Wen* chapter 71.

泣　① 即泪。出《素问·阴阳应象大论》《灵枢·口问》。② 哭。出《素问·解精微论》。③ 音义并同涩，不滑利之谓。出《素问·举痛论》《素问·调经论》。

泣（qì）　① Tears. See *Su Wen* chapter 5 and *Ling Shu* chapter 28. ② To cry. See *Su Wen* chapter 81. ③ It shares the same pronunciation and meaning as *sè*（涩）, which means stop-page. See *Su Wen* chapter 39 and 62.

泻　① 治疗中的泻法。用药物或针、砭等方法去其实邪。出《素问·三部九候论》。② 泄泻。出《素问·阴阳应象大论》。

泻（xiè）　① The draining method, which means to drain the excess pathogens with medications, and acupuncture by metal needles or stone needles, etc. See *Su Wen* chapter 20. ② Diarrhea. See *Su Wen* chapter 5.

泻必用方　方，犹正也，即正当之意。此言运用泻法的恰当时机。出《素问·八正神明论》。

泻必用方（xiè bì yòng fāng）　**drainage at appropriate time** *Fāng* means good timing. See *Su Wen* chapter 26.

泻必用员　指针刺的手法。运用泻法时，必须圆活流利，使经气通畅，邪气很快外散。《灵枢·官能》。

泻必用员（xiè bì yòng yuán）　**drainage with flexible manipulation** Drainage with nimble and smooth acupuncture manipulations that enable the meridian qi to move unobstructedly while the pathogen qi is dissipated quickly. See *Ling Shu* chapter 73.

泥丸宫 出《素问·本病论》。（1）指脑部。见《黄庭内景经》。（2）指百会穴。见《普济本事方》。

泥丸宫（ní wán gōng） **mud ball palace** See *Su Wen* chapter 73. (1) Brain. See *Huang Ting Nei Jing Jing*（*Taoist Cannon of Health Preservation*）. (2) The name of acupoint GV 20. See *Pu Ji Ben Shi Fang*（*Experiential Prescriptions for Universal Relief*）.

泽泻 药名。味甘淡，性微寒，能渗利湿热。与白术、麋衔组成方剂，为《内经》十三方之一。《圣济总录》名泽泻汤，《三因极一病证方论》名麋衔汤。主治酒后中风，有发热、倦怠，汗出如浴，恶风少气等症者。出《素问·病能论》。

泽泻（zé xiè） **Ze Xie**（*Rhizoma Alismatis*） Medicine name, with a light taste and slightly cold in character that can percolate and disinhibit dampheat. The decoction made from *Rhizoma Alismatis* along with *Rhizoma Atractylodis Macrocephalae* and *Herba Pyrolae* as the major components is one of the thirteen decoctions recorded in *Nei Jing*, and is named Ze Xie Decoction in *Sheng Ji Zong Lu Comprehensive Recording of Sage-like Benefit*（*short form of Comprehensive Recording of Sage-like Benefit from the Zhenghe Reign*）and Mi Xian Decoction in *San Yin Ji Yi Bing Zheng Fang Lun*（*Treatise on Diseases, Patterns, and Prescriptions Related to Unification of the Three Etiologies*）. The decoction cures strokes by alcohol with the symptoms of fever, fatigue, excessive sweating, aversion to wind and shortage of qi. See *Su Wen* chapter 46.

泾溲 见《素问·厥论》《素问·调经论》《灵枢·本神》。（1）泾，指大便。溲，指小便。见《素问》王冰注。（2）泾，指妇女月经。溲指大小便。见《新校正》。（3）泾，即经常之意。溲，指小便。（4）小便。见《素问识》。

泾溲（jīng sōu） **frequent urination** See *Su Wen* chapter 45, chapter 62 and *Ling Shu* chapter 8. (1) *Jīng* refers to stool and *sōu* refers to urine. See *Su Wen* annotated by Wang Bing. (2) *Jīng* refers to menstruation and *sōu* refers to urine. See *Xin Jiao Zheng*（*New Revisions of Su Wen*）. (3) *Jīng* means usually, and *sōu* refers to urine.

（4）Urine. See *Su Wen Zhi* (*Understanding Su Wen*).

治上补上制以缓 治疗上部疾病,宜循缓方之制。缓方气味薄,药性上行而不下迫,有利于药至上部病所。出《素问·至真要大论》。

治上补上制以缓（zhì shàng bǔ shàng zhì yǐ huǎn） **to tonify and treat the upper with mild formula** Mild formulas usually have a light flavor in order to enable the drug's property to ascend instead of descend to the focus. See *Su Wen* chapter 74.

治未病 ① 指未病先防,防患于未然。出《素问·四气调神大论》。② 指已病早治,防微杜渐。出《素问·刺热》。

治未病（zhì wèi bìng） ① Precaution before onset of disease. See *Su Wen* chapter 2. ② To treat a disease at an early stage. See *Su Wen* chapter 32.

治节 治,治理;节,节度、调节。治理事物井然有序之义,专喻肺的功能,如肺主一身之气,有调节呼吸及气的宣发、肃降作用。通调水道,则能调节水液的流行与排泄。百脉会于肺,更有协助心调节血行的作用。出《素问·灵兰秘典论》。

治节（zhì jié） **management and regulation** To manage things in order, specifically refers to the function of the lung. The lung governs qi in the human body by breath regulation, diffusion and disputative downbearing of qi, and controlling the waterways to ensure the smooth movement and excretion of fluids. All the vessels are assembled in the lung, which enables the lung to assist the heart in regulating the circulation of blood. See *Su Wen* chapter 8.

治有缓急 缓急指方制之缓与急。缓是用量轻、气味薄,作用较平和之方制。一般治疗上部不足等轻症。急是用量重、气味厚,作用较峻烈之方制,一般治疗下部不足等较重病症。制方治病,应根据病情而有缓、急之分。出《素问·至真要大论》。

治有缓急（zhì yǒu huǎn jí） **Treatment is either drastic or mild.** Mild formulas are of light dosage and flavor, and usually for minor diseases of the upper part of the body. Drastic formulas are of heavy dosage and flavor, and usually for severe diseases of the lower part of the body. Formulas are prescribed according to the degree

八画

of urgency of the disease. See *Su Wen* chapter 74.

治身 治理身体，即养生。出《素问·阴阳应象大论》。

治身（zhì shēn） **manage body** Life nurturing. See *Su Wen* chapter 5.

治病必求于本 本，指阴阳。阴阳为天地万物之根本，人体疾病的形成也不外乎阴阳失调，故治病要在探求阴阳失调之本。这是中医治疗学中最基本的原则。出《素问·阴阳应象大论》。

治病必求于本（zhì bìng bì qiú yú běn） **Treating disease should focus on the root.** Yin and yang are the basic laws of everything in nature，including human life. According to TCM therapeutic theory，diseases are basically caused by the disorder of yin and yang，which must be taken into consideration as the essential pathogenic factor of disease. See *Su Wen* chapter 5.

治痿者独取阳明 独，注重。痿证的主要病机是五脏气热导致精血津液耗伤，以致筋骨痿废不用。而阳明是五脏六腑之大源，主润宗筋，宗筋主束骨而利机关。阳明虚则宗筋弛纵，带脉不引，故是痿不用。所以在治痿时，除治疗受病之经、脏

外，还必须同时着重治疗阳明。出《素问·痿论》。

治痿者独取阳明（zhì wěi zhě dú qǔ yáng míng） **Treating flaccidity mainly takes *yangming*.** *Dú* means emphasis. The pathogenesis of wilting syndrome is the consumption and damage of essence，blood and fluids because of heat in five viscera，which ends in flaccidity of the sinews and bones. The *yangming* meridian，the energy source of the five viscera and six bowels，is responsible for nourishing the sinews that controls the bones and ensures the joints to be flexible. Deficiency of *yangming* leads to looseness of the sinews and weakness of the belt vessel，hence resulting in the feet flaccid syndrome. The treatment must focus on the related meridians and organs，along with the *yangming* meridian simultaneously. See *Su Wen* chapter 44.

怯士 为体质的一种类型，与勇士相对。其人外貌特征是眼睛大而无神，其内脏特点是三焦纹理竖直，胸骨剑突短少，肝系松弛，胆汁不盈而弛纵，肠胃直少弯曲，胁下空虚，发怒时，气势

不盛,不能充满胸廓。肝肺虽然上举,但随即因气衰而降下,故不能久怒。出《灵枢·论勇》。

怯士(qiè shì) **cowardly male** A type of body constitution, opposite to that of a courageous male. A cowardly male has large eyes but with no focus. His viscera are characterized by a vertical texture in the triple *jiao*, a short and small xiphoid process of the sternum, a lax liver system, insufficient bile, less bending stomach and intestine system, empty flank, etc. Even when angry, this person is not full of momentum to fill his thorax. Although the liver and the lung are raised, they are lowered immediately due to the falling qi, thus he can not remain angry for a long time. See *Ling Shu* chapter 50.

宝命全形论 《素问》篇名。宝,珍视;全形,形神统一的形体。宝命全形,意指要珍视神与形俱的生命。此篇主要讨论人体生命与自然界的关系,强调只有法天则地,针刺才能取得效果,并着重论述了针刺方法的几个关键问题。

宝命全形论(bǎo mìng quán xíng lùn) **Discussion on Preserving Health and Protecting Life** Chapter name in *Su Wen*. *Bǎo* means to cherish, *quán xíng* means the unified human body, physically and mentally. *Bǎo mìng quán xíng* means to cherish a physically and mentally unified body. This chapter discusses the relationship between human life and nature, emphasizes that acupuncture works when abiding by the laws of nature, and focuses on some key issues of acupuncture methods.

宗气 由肺吸入的自然界清气和脾胃化生的营卫之气相互结合而成,积于胸中气海。主要功能有二:一是出于肺,循喉咙以行呼吸,并关系到声音之强弱。二是贯心脉而行气血,与心动及脉搏有直接联系。出《灵枢·邪客》。

宗气(zōng qì) **pectoral qi** A combination of clear qi breathed into the lung from nature, and nutrient and defensive qi transformed by the stomach and spleen that is assembled in Qi Hai (CV6). It has two major functions, that is, to promote breathing and control voice level when the qi comes out of the lung along the throat; the second function is to promote the qi and blood，and govern the heart beat and pulse when the qi goes through the heart vessels. See *Ling Shu* chapter 71.

宗司　运气术语。出《素问·六元正纪大论》。（1）总管一年之中岁运岁气与分别职司各时令的运和气。见《类经·运气十七》。（2）六气之宗与三阴三阳之司岁。见《素问直解》。

宗司（zōng sī）　**governor of circuits and qi** A term of the five circuits and six qi. See *Su Wen* chapter 71. (1) Dominating the circuit qi and the yearly qi. See *Lei Jing*（*Classified Classic*）"Circuits and Qi Chapter 17". (2) The origin of the six qi，and the governor of the triple yin and triple yang. See *Su Wen Zhi Jie*（*Direct Interpretation on Su Wen*）.

宗脉　指汇聚于目部和耳部的众多经脉。出《灵枢·口问》。

宗脉（zōng mài）　**gathering place of the ancestral vessels** Multiple vessels gather around the eyes and ears. See *Ling Shu* chapter 28.

宗筋　① 众多的筋。出《素问·痿论》。② 前阴部之筋。出《素问·厥论》《灵枢·五音五味》。

宗筋（zōng jīn）　① Multiple sinews. See *Su Wen* chapter 44. ② Anterior pudendum. See *Su Wen* chapter 45.

宗精　肾所主之津液。出《素问·解精微论》。

宗精（zōng jīng）　**body fluid dominated by the kidney** See *Su Wen* chapter 81.

官五色　官，主之意。官五色，即五色各有所主的证候。出《灵枢·五色》。

官五色（guān wǔ sè）　**diagnostic significance of the five colors** *Guān* means governing. This term means that the five colours all indicate specific symptoms. See *Ling Shu* chapter 49.

官针　① 大众所公认的针刺常规和常法。出《灵枢·官针》。②《灵枢》篇名。主要论述正确使用九针的重要性，以及九针的不同性能和它的适应证。

官针（guān zhēn）　① Common methods accepted by the majority of the people. See *Ling Shu* chapter 7. ② Chapter name in *Ling Shu*（*Application of Needles*）. This chapter mainly states the importance of utilizing the nine needles, and the respective functions and applications of each kind of needle.

官能　《灵枢》篇名。官,任也。能,技能。根据人的不同技能和特点,给予不同的工作,称之为官能。此篇主要讨论针刺治疗的原则和具体方法,强调早期治疗的重要性,指出针刺技术传授后人必须量才取用。

官能(guān néng)　**Qualifications of Acupuncturists** Chapter name in *Ling Shu*. *Guān* means allocating; *néng*, technique. As a whole, it means allocating different work to people according to their abilities and characteristics. This chapter mainly discusses the principles and methods of acupuncture, highly stresses the importance of treatment in the early stages of disease, and specially points out that acupuncture techniques must be passed down to those who are talented and engrossed in this field.

空窍　① (空,kǒng)即孔窍。指七窍。出《灵枢·动输》。见《太素·脉行同异》。② (空,kòng)泛指体内空隙处。出《素问·四气调神大论》。见《素问注证发微》。

空窍(kǒng/kòng qiào)　① Orifice. Seven orifices of the human body. See *Ling Shu* chapter 62.

See *Tai Su*(*Classified Study on Huang Di Nei Jing*)"The Similarities and Differences of Pulse". ② The interspaces in the human body. See *Su Wen* chapter 2. See *Su Wen Zhu Zheng Fa Wei*(*Annotation and Elaboration on Su Wen*).

宛陈则除之　宛(yù郁),同菀,通郁,积滞的意思。陈,陈旧。积留于血脉之中的瘀血等宛陈之物,当驱除之。出《素问·针解》。

宛陈则除之(yù chén zé chú zhī)　**to eliminate stagnation** "宛" is the same as "菀" or "郁",which means accumulation and stagnation. *Chén* refers to chronic accumulated stagnations. This terms mean that chronic accumulated stagnations in the meridians and collaterals must be eliminated. See *Su Wen* chapter 54.

实　① 邪气有余的实证。出《素问·通评虚实论》《灵枢·刺节真邪》。② 气血有余。出《素问·调经论》。③ 针刺中的补法。出《灵枢·小针解》,指慢进针,快出针的补法。出《灵枢·热病》。④ 实物结果。出《素问·气交变大论》。⑤ 充实。出《素问·上古天真论》。⑥ 指脉象。脉来举按有力充实。出《素问·通评虚实论》。

⑦ 指天时之实。出《灵枢·岁露论》。

实（shí）　① Excess syndrome that manifests as excessive pathogenic qi. See *Su Wen* chapter 28 and *Ling Shu* chapter 75. ② Excessive qi and blood. See *Su Wen* chapter 62. ③ Tonifying method in acupuncture. See *Ling Shu* chapter 3. It usually refers to the method of slow insertion of the needle and fast withdrawing of the needle. See *Ling Shu* chapter 23. ④ Fructification. In *Su Wen* chapter 69. ⑤ Replete. See *Su Wen* chapter 1. ⑥ Pulse manifestation. It feels powerful and replete. See *Su Wen* chapter 1. ⑦ Good timing. See *Ling Shu* chapter 79.

实风　指每一季节中所出现的当令风向，即指有利于万物生长的正常气候。如春多东风、夏多南风等。出《灵枢·九宫八风》。

实风（shí fēng）　**excess wind** Seasonal wind which is beneficial to the growth of all living things. For example, there is more easterly wind in spring, and more southerly wind in summer. See *Ling Shu* chapter 77.

肩甲　即肩胛，背部肩胛骨部位。

出《素问·藏气法时论》。

肩甲（jiān jiǎ）　**scapular** The dorsal scapular region. See *Su Wen* chapter 22.

肩贞　经穴名。属手太阳小肠经。在肩曲胛下两骨解间，肩髃后陷者中。出《素问·气穴论》《素问·气府论》。

肩贞（jiān zhēn）　**Jian Zhen** The name of acupoint SI 9. It pertains to the small intestine meridian of hand *taiyang* and is located between the two joints under the scapular curvature and the posterior depression of the shoulder. See *Su Wen* chapter 58 and 59.

肩胛　即肩甲，胳膊上边靠颈脖的部分。又称肩髆。出《灵枢·经脉》。

肩胛（jiān jiǎ）　**Scapular** The part of the upper arm near the neck. The part close to neck above the shoulder, similar to scapular. See *Ling Shu* chapter 10.

肩息　症状名。抬肩呼吸，因呼吸困难之故。出《素问·通评虚实论》。

肩息（jiān xī）　**raised-shoulder breathing** Symptom name. Refers to the lifting of the shoulders due to difficulty in breathing.

See *Su Wen* chapter 28.

肩解　① 部位名。指肩关节。出
《灵枢·经脉》。② 经穴名。指
肩井穴。属足少阳胆经,在大
椎与肩峰连线的中点上。出
《素问·气穴论》。③ 经穴名。
指秉风穴。属手太阳小肠经,
在天宗穴直上,肩胛冈上窝正
中。出《素问·气府论》。

肩解（jiān jiě）　① Shoulder
joints. See *Ling Shu* chapter
10. ② Name of acupoint GB 21
which belongs to the gallbladder
meridian of foot *shaoyang*,
and is located at the midpoint
of the line connecting GV 14
and the acromion. See *Su Wen*
chapter 58. ③ Name of acupoint
SI 12, pertaining to the small
intestine meridian of hand *taiyang* and located at the center
of the pit of scapula spine
above Tian Zong (SI 11). See
Su Wen chapter 59.

肩膊　泛指肩膀部位。《灵枢·
终始》。

肩膊（jiān bó）　shoulder area See
Ling Shu chapter 9.

肩髃　手阳明大肠经之穴名,在
肩峰与肱骨大结节之间,上臂
平举时,肩前凹陷处是穴。出
《灵枢·经筋》。

肩髃（jiān yú）　**Jian Yu (LI 15)**

Pertaining to the large intestine
meridian of hand *yangming*,
and located between the shoulder
peak and the trochiter. When
stretching the arms horizontally,
the pitting at the shoulder is the
acupoint. See *Ling Shu* chapter
13.

肩髆　即肩膊、肩胛。出《灵枢·
经脉》。

肩髆（jiān bó）　**shoulder girdle**
See *Ling Shu* chapter 10.

肩髓　出《灵枢·四时气》。(1) 大
椎处之骨髓。见《素问集注》。
(2) 疑为骨髓之误。见《素问
释义》。

肩髓（jiān suǐ）　**shoulder marrow**
See *Ling Shu* chapter 19.
(1) The bone marrow of Da
Zhui (GV14). See *Su Wen Ji
Zhu* (*Collected Annotation of
Su Wen*). (2) Probably a mistake
of "骨髓" (bone marrow). See
Elaboration of Su Wen.

视岁南北　南北,即南政与北政。
政,有主令、掌管的意思。运气
学说将甲子六十年中各主事年
份分别归属于南政之岁与北政
之岁,并根据南政北政之年与
太阴、少阴、厥阴的司天在泉的
关系变化来讨论寸口脉象的变
化。出《素问·至真要大论》。
对于南北政的划分,历代意见

分歧：（1）五运中除甲己土运为南政，其余木、火、金、水运为北政。甲子六十年中，南政十二年，北政四十八年。见《类经·运气五》。（2）戊癸火运为南政，其他木、金、水、土运为北政。见《素问集注》。（3）岁支的亥子丑寅卯辰属于南政，巳午未申酉戌属于北政。所谓政，即指司天、在泉居于南纬或北纬的主令。见《运气辨·辨南北政》。

视岁南北（shì suì nán běi）　**to judge by south-dominating or north-dominating years** According to the doctrine of the five circuits and six qi, the sixty-year cycle can be divided into south-dominating years and north-dominating years. The *cun kou* pulse changes based on the celestial control and terrestrial effect in the *taiyin*, *shaoyin*, *jueyin* meridians in the south-dominating or north-dominating years. See *Su Wen* chapter 74. There have been more than one way in dividing south-dominating and north dominating years in history. (1) Earth pertains to a south-dominating year, while wood, fire, metal, and water pertain to the north. There are 12 years pertaining to south-dominating years, and 48 years to north-dominating years. See *Lei Jing* (*Classified Classic*) "Circuits and Qi Chapter 5". (2) Fire pertains to south-dominating years, while the other four pertain to north dominating years. See *Su Wen Ji Zhu* (*Collected Annotation of Su Wen*). (3) The terrestrial branches, *hai*, *zi*, *chou*, *yin*, *mao*, *chen* pertain to south-dominating years, while *si*, *wu*, *wei*, *shen*, *you*, *xu* pertain to north-dominating years. *Zheng* (dominating) refers to the governing power of celestial control and terrestrial effect in the southern latitude or the northern latitude. See *Differentiating Circuits and qi* "Differentiating South and North Dominating Years".

弦　①脉象。正常的弦脉端直而长，柔和滑利，按之如琴弦，为春季脉象，属于肝。若弦劲如竿，则提示肝有病变；若弦急强劲，如新张弓弦，毫无冲和之象，则说明肝之真气败露，无胃气之真藏脉，预后凶险。出《素问·玉机真藏论》。②弓弦。出《素问·平人气象论》。

弦（xián）　① Pulse manifestation. The normal string pulse is straight and long，soft and smooth，as of the string of a musical instrument. It is the typical pulse of spring，pertaining to the liver. If the pulse feels as stiff as a bamboo stick，disease may occur in liver；if the pulse feels as stretched and strong as a full bow，the genuine qi might be leaking from the stomach and the patient is in danger. See *Su Wen* chapter 19. ② Bowstring. See *Su Wen* chapter 18.

承山　经穴名。属足太阳膀胱经。又名鱼腹、肉柱。在腓肠肌两肌腹交界下端。出《灵枢·卫气》。

承山（chéng shān）　**Cheng Shan （BL 57）** Acupoint name pertaining to the urinary bladder meridian of foot *taiyang* and located at the lower end of the gastrocnemius. It is also named *yú fù*（鱼腹）or *ròu zhù*（肉柱）. See *Ling Shu* chapter 52.

承岁　承，一致之意。运气推算中，如主运与该年年支的五行属性相同，即为承岁，又称岁直，亦称岁会，如丁卯、戊午等年。出《素问·天元纪大论》。

承岁（chéng suì）　**annual congru-**ence *Chéng* means unity. According to the doctrine of the five circuits and the six qi，if the main circuit of one year is exactly the same as the five element qi of the year it pertains to，this year is named *cheng sui*，or *sui zhi*，or *sui hui*，for example，the *ding mao* year and *wu wu* year. See *Su Wen* chapter 66.

承浆　经穴名。属任脉经穴名。为足阳明、任脉之会，在面部正中线，当颏唇沟中央。出《灵枢·经脉》。

承浆（chéng jiāng）　**Cheng Jiang （CV 24）** Acupoint name pertaining to the conception vessel and located in the middle of the chinolabial sulcus where the meridian of foot *yangming* and the conception vessel meet. See *Ling Shu* chapter 13.

孟冬痹　孟冬，冬季三月之首月，为手心主（厥阴）经所主。孟冬痹，即手心主经筋在孟冬所发之痹证。可见转筋、胸痛等症。《灵枢·经筋》。

孟冬痹（mèng dōng bì）　**early winter impediment** *Mèng dōng* refers to the first month of the three months in winter，which is governed by the hand *jueyin*

八画

meridian. *Mèng dōng bì* is the impediment syndrome occurring along the hand *jueyin* meridian in the first month of winter, usually manifested as spasms, and chest pain, etc. See *Ling Shu* chapter 13.

孟春痹 孟春,春季三月之首月,为足少阳经所主。孟春痹,即足少阳经筋在孟春所发之痹证。可见转筋,不可屈伸,疼痛等症。出《灵枢·经筋》。

孟春痹 (mèng chūn bì) **early spring impediment** *Mèng chūn* refers to the first month of the three months in spring, governed by the foot *shaoyang* meridian. *Mèng chūn bì* is the impediment syndrome occurring along the foot *shaoyang* meridian in the first month of autumn, and usually manifests as spasms, the disability to flex and stretch the extremities, and pain, etc. See *Ling Shu* chapter 13.

孟秋痹 孟秋,秋季三月之首月,为足少阴经所主。孟秋痹,即足少阴经筋在孟秋所发之痹证。可见转筋、内踝痛等症。出《灵枢·经筋》。

孟秋痹 (mèng qiū bì) **early autumn impediment** *Mèng qiū* re-

fers to the first month of the three months in autumn, governed by the foot *shaoyin* meridian. *Mèng qiū bì* is the impediment syndrome occurring along the foot *shaoyin* meridian in the first month of autumn, it usually manifests as spasms, and inner-ankle pain, etc. See *Ling Shu* chapter 13.

孟夏痹 孟夏,夏季三月之首月,为手阳明经所主。孟夏痹,即手阳明经筋在孟夏所发之痹证。可见转筋、肩不举、颈强等症。出《灵枢·经筋》。

孟夏痹 (mèng xià bì) **early summer impediment** *Mèng xià* refers to the first month of the three months in summer, governed by the hand *yangming* meridian. *Mèng xià bì* is the impediment syndrome occurring along the hand *yangming* meridian in the first month of summer, and usually manifests as spasms, the disability to raise the shoulders, and a stiff neck, etc. See *Ling Shu* chapter 13.

孤之府 指三焦。六腑中胃、大肠、小肠、膀胱、胆五脏分别与五腑相应合,惟三焦无配,故称。出《灵枢·本输》。

孤之府 (gū zhī fǔ) **solitary bowel**

八画

Triple *jiao*. No bowels coordinate with the triple jiao, as opposed to the stomach, large intestine, small intestine, bladder, and gallbladder which coordinate with the five bowels, hence named the solitary bowel. See *Ling Shu* chapter 2.

孤精于内　出《素问·汤液醪醴论》。（1）指精中无气。见《类经·论治类十五》。（2）指阴精于机体内部耗损。见《素问》王冰注。

孤精于内（gū jīng yú nèi）　**internal stagnation of essence** See *Su Wen* chapter 14.（1）Within the essence there is no qi. See *Lei Jing*（*Classified Classic*）"On Treatment Chapter 15". （2）Consumption of yin essence in the body. See *Su Wen* annotated by Wang Bing.

孤藏　孤，孤独，独特之意。① 脾。出《素问·玉机真藏论》。脾属土，为万物之母，运行水谷，化津液以溉心、肺、肝、肾四脏，其气分旺于四季而无定位，故为孤脏。② 肾。出《素问·逆调论》。

孤藏（gū zàng）　**solitary viscera** *Gū* means solitary or unique. ① Spleen. See *Su Wen* chapter 19. Spleen pertains to the earth element, the mother of all, and regulates the water and grains. It generates body fluids to nourish the heart, lung, liver and kidney, and pertains to all four seasons, hence called the solitary viscera. ② Kidney. See *Su Wen* chapter 34.

姑洗　阳六律之一，为商音，即金音。出《素问·本病论》。

姑洗（gū xǐ）　*gu xi* One of the six yang tones of ancient Chinese music, also named *shang* tone or metal tone. See *Su Wen* chapter 73.

参伍不调者病　言全身上中下三部九候的脉象相互不协调一致为病脉。参伍，谓相互比较参照。调，协调。出《素问·三部九候论》。

参伍不调者病（cān wǔ bú tiáo zhě bìng）　**Irregular pulse indicates disease.** *Cān wǔ* refers to comparison and contrast. *Tiáo* means regular. See *Su Wen* chapter 20.

细　脉象。指脉来细如丝线，主气虚。出《素问·脉要精微论》。

细（xì）　**fine** Pulse manifestation. Weak pulse feeling like a silk thread, and caused by qi deficiency. See *Su Wen* chapter 17.

细子　雷公的自谦之称。出《灵枢·禁服》。

细子(xì zǐ) The name Lei Gong humbly called himself. See *Ling Shu* chapter 48.

细则气少 细,即细脉,其脉形细如丝线,为气血虚少之象,多见于虚证。出《素问·脉要精微论》。

细则气少(xì zé qì shǎo) **Thin pulse indicates shortage of qi.** A pulse manifestation of blood and qi deficiency always found in deficiency syndromes. See *Su Wen* chapter 17.

终始 ①《灵枢》篇名。终,终结;始,开始。此篇主要论述脏腑阴阳,经脉气血运行的始末及脉象的变化,以制定适当的针刺方法。还说明了针刺十二禁及各经所见死证。故名。②指病史。出《素问·疏五过论》。

终始(zhōng shǐ) ① Chapter name in *Ling Shu*. *Zhōng* means the end; *shǐ* means the beginning. This chapter mainly discusses yin and yang, the beginning and ending of the meridians, qi and blood, and the variation of pulse manifestation, which are all essential for acupuncture. It also mentions the 12 contraindications for acupuncture and some vital conditions. ② A patient's medical history. See *Su Wen* chapter 77.

经 ① 经脉。包括十二经脉的正经、经别和奇经八脉,是气血运行的主要干道。出《素问·经络论》。② 五输穴之一。十二经脉各有一经穴,多位于腕踝或前臂小腿部。因脉气流注至此,如畅流之水,行经通过,故称。出《灵枢·九针十二原》。③ 经典书籍。出《素问·疟论》。④ 与纬相对。天文地理中称通过南北两极而与赤道垂直之线为经。出《灵枢·卫气行》。⑤ 经过,通过。出《素问·五运行大论》。⑥ 人身排泄物之一。出《灵枢·本神》。〈1〉通"泾"。(i)借指小便。见《素问识》。(ii)大便。见《素问》王冰注。〈2〉月经。见《太素·藏府》。

经(jīng) ① Meridians, including the twelve meridians, divergent meridians and eight extraordinary meridians, and are the main path of qi and blood. See *Su Wen* chapter 57. ② One of the five transport acupoints. Each of the twelve meridians has one transport acupoint, usually located at the wrist, ankle, forearms or lower legs. As qi passes these acupoints as the flow of water, hence its name as transport acupoint. See

八画

Ling Shu chapter 1. ③ Classics. See *Su Wen* chapter 35. ④ Opposite to latitude. In archeology and geology，the lines which go through two polars are named longitude，and meet the latitude lines at right angles. See *Ling Shu* chapter 76. ⑤ Pass through. See *Su Wen* chapter 8. ⑥ Human excrement. See *Ling Shu* chapter 8.〈1〉"经" is the same as the other chinese word "泾". (i) Urine. See *Su Wen Zhi* (*Understanding Su Wen*). (ii) Stool. See *Su Wen* annotated by Wang Bing.〈2〉 Menstruation. See *Tai Su*（*Classified Study on Huang Di Nei Jing*）"Viscera and Bowels".

经水 ① 指古代清、渭、海、湖、汝、渑、淮、漯、江、河、济、漳十二经水。出《素问・离合真邪论》。②《灵枢》篇名。此篇根据天人相应理论，以自然界十二经水的大小、深浅、远近来说明人体十二经气的多少和循行内外、营灌全身的作用。

经水（jīng shuǐ） ① Refers to the 12 rivers that were named Qing River，Wei River，Hai River，Hu River，Ru River，Sheng River，Huai River，Luo River，Jiang River，He River，Ji River and Zhang River. See *Su Wen* chapter 27. ② Chapter name in *Ling Shu*. This chapter，according to the theory of correspondence between man and nature，discusses the 12 rivers in natural world，to explain the amount of qi in the 12 meridians，and the way it circulates through，and nourishes the body.

经气 ① 经脉之气。来源与饮食，与肺之清气相结合而成。出《素问・经脉别论》。② 真气。出《素问・离合真邪论》。

经气（jīng qì） ① Meridian qi, a combination of the grains and the clear qi in the lung. See *Su Wen* chapter 21. ② Genuine qi. See *Su Wen* chapter 27.

经分 本经经脉循行的分部。出《灵枢・官针》。

经分（jīng fēn） **meridian section** The sections along the main meridians. See *Ling Shu* chapter 7.

经月之病 即月经之病。出《素问・三部九候论》。

经月之病（jīng yuè zhī bìng） **menstrual disease** See *Su Wen* chapter 20.

经风 侵袭五脏经脉的风。出《素问・金匮真言论》。

经风（jīng fēng） **meridian wind**

The wind which invades the five viscera and the meridians. See *Su Wen* chapter 4.

经别　① 别行的正经，即从十二经脉四肢部别行分出，进入胸腹深处，再浅出体表、头项等部的重要支脉。出《灵枢·经别》。十二经别中，六阳经的经别复注入原来的阳经；六阴经的经别则注入与其表里相合的阳经，组成六合。足太阳，足少阴经别为一合；足少阳，足厥阴经别为二合；足阳明，足太阴经别为三合；手太阳，手少阴经别为四合；手少阳，手厥阴经别为五合；手阳明，手太阴经别为六合。十二经别的循行特点，表现为"离"（分别，别出），"合"（会合，相合），"出"（浅出），"入"（深入）的关系。从而加强了十二经脉中表里两经的联系，以及十二经脉与头面部，体表与体内，四肢与躯干的联系，扩大了十二经脉的循行范围。② 《灵枢》篇名。该篇主要论述十二经别的循行路线以及表里相应的阴经与阳经离合出入的配合关系。

经别（jīng bié）　① Divergent meridians, namely those important branches diverging from the twelve meridians along the four limbs, going deep into the breast and abdomen and then out to the surface of the body and the area of the head and neck. See *Ling Shu* chapter 11. Among the twelve divergent meridians, the six yang divergent meridians will go back to the original yang meridians, while the six yin divergent meridians flow into the the exterior-interior related yang meridians and form the six pairs. The foot *taiyang* and foot *shaoyin* meridians form the first pair; the foot *shaoyang* and foot *jueyin* meridians form the second pair; the foot *yangming* and foot *taiyin* meridians form the third pair; the hand *taiyang* and hand *shaoyin* meridians form the fourth pair; the hand *shaoyang* and hand *jueyin* meridians form the fifth pair; the hand *yangming* and hand *taiyin* meridians form the sixth pair. The characteristics of the twelve divergent meridians manifest as parting (separating or divergent) and converging (joining and fusion); coming out (superficially) and going into (deeply), thus to strengthen the exterior-interior relationship

八画

of the twelve meridians as well as the relationship between the twelve meridians and the head-face area; the outer and inner body; the four limbs and the trunk and expand the area where the meridians circulate. ② Chapter name in *Ling Shu*. This chapter mainly discusses the course of the meridians and the exterior-interior coordination of the yin and yang meridians.

经刺　① 按经取穴以刺之。出《灵枢·禁服》。② 刺大经，与络刺相对，属九刺之一。出《灵枢·官针》。③ 即巨刺。左病取右，右病取左，刺其大经，调其经气。出《素问·缪刺论》。

经刺（jīng cì）　① Meridian needling. To needle the acupoints along the meridians. See *Ling Shu* chapter 48. ② To needle the major meridians（opposite to the minor collaterals）, with one of the nine needling methods. See *Ling Shu* chapter 7. ③ Counterlateral channel needling. Needling the left when the ailment occurs on the right side of the body and vice versa. Needling the main meridians to regulate the meridian qi. See *Su Wen* chapter 63.

经治　指针刺、服药等常规治疗方法。出《灵枢·禁服》。

经治（jīng zhì）　**common treatment** Common treatment with acupuncture or medicine. See *Ling Shu* chapter 48.

经俞　即经输。参该条。见《素问·缪刺论》。

经俞（jīng shū）　See "经输". See *Su Wen* chapter 63.

经脉　① 指经络系统。遍布于全身，为气血的通道。有十二经脉、奇经八脉等。出《灵枢·本藏》。② 指经脉系统中直行的干线。出《灵枢·脉度》。③《灵枢》篇名。该篇主要论述十二经脉、十五络脉的名称，起止点，循行路线，发病，症候及治疗原则等，是经络学说的重要篇章。

经脉（jīng mài）　① Meridian system spread all over the body and serves as a channel for qi and blood. There are twelve meridians, eight extra meridians, etc. See *Ling Shu* chapter 47. ② Major meridians that circulate straight. See *Ling Shu* chapter 17. ③ Chapter name in *Ling Shu*. This is an important chapter that discusses the name, the beginning and ending, the course and onset, the

八画

syndromes and treatments of the twelve meridians and fifteen collaterals.

经脉二十八会　会，交会。全身左右手足三阴三阳二十四脉，加任、督、阴阳两跷脉的交会之处。出《灵枢·玉版》。

经脉二十八会（jīng mài èr shí bā huì）　**twenty eight joints of meridians and vessels** *Huì* means joints. It refers to the joints of the twenty four hand and foot meridians along with the conception vessel，governor vessel，and the yin and yang heel vessel. See *Ling Shu* chapter 60.

经脉别论　《素问》篇名。别，区别。其主要阐述惊、恐、恚、劳等原因致经脉失常，五脏失调的喘、汗等病变；说明饮食在人体通过经脉输布全身的过程；并且论述了三阴三阳脉气独至的症治，因内容都涉及区别经脉的常与变，故名。

经脉别论（jīng mài bié lùn）　**Special Discussion on Channels and Vessels** Chapter name in *Su Wen*. *Bié* means differentiation. This chapter focuses on the panting and sweating diseases caused by the disorder of the meridians and five viscera which are usually triggered by fright，

horror，anxiety and fatigue，and explains the whole procedure of the vessels transporting food，and discusses the treatment of the symptoms caused by vessel qi prevailing，either one of the three yang vessels and three yin vessels. Hence，this chapter is entitled according to its contents.

经络　① 指人体经络系统。出《灵枢·邪气藏府病形》。② 指经络之气。出《灵枢·口问》。③ 指经穴和络穴。出《素问·经脉别论》。

经络（jīng luò）　① Meridian and collateral system. See *Ling Shu* chapter 4. ② Qi of the meridians and collaterals. See *Ling Shu* chapter 28. ③ Meridian points and collateral points. See *Su Wen* chapter 21.

经络论　《素问》篇名。该篇主要讨论经络色泽与五脏之色的相应关系。说明根据五色的变化，诊察人体内部病变的道理。

经络论（jīng luò lùn）　**Discussion on Channels and Collaterals** Chapter name in *Su Wen*. This chapter mainly discusses how the color of the meridians corresponds to the color of the five viscera and how to diagnose diseases according to changes

八画

in the five colors.

经渠　手太阴肺经之经穴，在腕横纹桡侧端上一寸处。出《灵枢·本输》。

经渠（jīng qú）　**Jing Qu（LU 8）** One of the meridian points along the lung meridian of hand *taiyin* at the region one inch above the radial end of the transverse crease on the wrist. See *Ling Shu* chapter 2.

经筋　① 十二经脉连属于肢体外周筋肉的体系。《灵枢·经筋》依照十二经脉，全身筋肉按部位分为十二经筋。经筋在周身的分布，一般都在浅部，起于四肢末端，走向头身，多结聚于关节和骨骼附近；有的进入胸腹腔，但不络属于脏腑。其功能是约束骨骼，有利于关节的屈伸运动。②《灵枢》篇名。该篇主要介绍了十二经筋的循行部位和病证等。

经筋（jīng jīn）　① It refers to meridian sinews，the twelve meridians connecting the sinews and flesh on the surface of the body. According to *Ling Shu* chapter 13，the twelve meridians divide the sinews of whole body into twelve parts. The meridian sinews start from the surface of the end of the four limbs，move to the head and trunk，and usually gather at the joints and bones. Some may penetrate into the chest and abdomen，but pertain to no viscus. The function of this system is to constrain the skeleton for movements of the joints. ② Chapter name in *Ling Shu*. This chapter introduces the area the twelve meridians circulate，and the diseases occuring on these meridians.

经溲　出《灵枢·本神》。（1）经，指月经。溲，指大小便。见《太素·藏府》。（2）泾溲。见该条。

经溲（jīng sōu）　See *Ling Shu* chapter 8. （1）*Jīng* refers to menstruate，*sōu* to urine and excrement. See *Tai Su*（*Classified Study on Huang Di Nei Jing*）Viscera. （2）See term "泾溲".

经输　经脉之腧穴。出《灵枢·寒热病》。

经输（jīng shū）　**meridian point** See *Ling Shu* chapter 21.

经腧　即经输。参该条。见《灵枢·四时气》。

经腧（jīng shū）　See "经输". See *Ling Shu* chapter 19.

经隧　即经脉。《素问·调经论》。

经隧（jīng suì）　**meridian** See *Su Wen* chapter 62.

九 画

春气 ① 春天生发之气，其性温和。出《素问·六元正纪大论》。② 肝气，与春相应，故云。出《素问·金匮真言论》。③ 春季之人体精气，其在经脉。出《素问·四时刺逆从论》。④ 春季中人的病气。出《灵枢·终始》。

春气(chūn qì) ① Spring qi. The mild generating qi in spring. See *Su Wen* chapter 71. ② Liver qi, corresponding to spring. ③ In spring, the essence qi of the human body flows in the meridians. See *Su Wen* chapter 64. ④ The pathogenic qi in spring. See *Ling Shu* chapter 9.

春分 ① 二十四节气之一。在春三月之中，立春后四十五日，太阳直射赤道之时，昼夜等长。出《灵枢·九宫八风》。② 指经脉。是春时人体精气相对集中的部分，与五脏之肝相应。出《素问·诊要经终论》。

春分(chūn fēn) ① Spring divide. One of the twenty four solar terms. In the three months of spring, the forty-fifth day after the Beginning of Spring (1st solar term) has the same length of day and night because the sunshine goes vertically on the equator. See *Ling Shu* chapter 77. ② A meridian where, in spring, the essence qi of the human body concentrates at. See *Su Wen* chapter 16.

春脉 春季应时之弦脉，属肝。出《素问·玉机真藏论》。

春脉(chūn mài) **spring pulse** A taut pulse complying with spring and pertaining to the liver. See *Su Wen* chapter 19.

春脉如弦 春气主肝，五行属东方木，春令万物生发，人体脉气与之相应，脉来轻虚柔和滑利，端直以长，似弓弦之状，故云。出《素问·玉机真藏论》。

春脉如弦(chūn mài rú xián) **Spring pulse feels like strings** Spring qi governs the liver and pertains to wood in the east. Spring generates liver, hence the spring pulse complies with the season and feels light, soft, smooth, straight and long as in the strings of a bow. See

Su Wen chapter 19.

毒　①作用峻烈的药物。出《素问·五常政大论》。②毒性物质。出《素问·徵四失论》。

毒(dú)　① Drastic medicine. See *Su Wen* chapter 70. ② Poisonous substances. See *Su Wen* chapter 78.

毒气　即疫毒之气，指有强烈传染和伤害作用的致病因子。出《素问·刺法论》。

毒气(dú qì)　Refers to epidemic qi, or toxic qi that contains severely infectious and harmful pathogenic factors. See *Su Wen* chapter 72.

毒药　泛指治病的药物。出《素问·异法方宜论》。

毒药(dú yào)　**toxic** Medicine in the broad sense. See *Su Wen* chapter 12.

持针纵舍　①用针之法。出《灵枢·邪客》。(1) 根据病情轻重用针，或从缓治，或舍而勿针。见《类经·针刺二十三》。(2) 用针时的进止留退补泻之道。见《类经·针刺二十三》。②《灵枢》曾有之篇名。见《素问·三部九候论》中王冰注。

持针纵舍(chí zhēn zòng shě)　① One of the needling methods. See *Ling Shu* chapter 71. (1) To needle according to the condi-

tion. If necessary, postpone the needling or give it up. See *Lei Jing*（*Classified Classic*）"Needling Chapter 23". (2) The specific method of needling, like entering, stopping, retaining, retreating, nourishing and reducing. See *Lei Jing*（*Classified Classic*）"Needling Chapter 23". ② Chapter name in *Ling Shu*. See *Su Wen* chapter 20 annotated by Wang Bing.

贲　①贲门。出《灵枢·本藏》。②膈。出《灵枢·经筋》。③通"坟"，高起来的意思。出《灵枢·邪气藏府病形》。

贲(bēn)　① Rushing Gate (cardia). See *Ling Shu* chapter 47. ② Diaphragm. See *Ling Shu* chapter 13. ③ "贲" is the same as "坟", refers to an uplift. See *Ling Shu* chapter 4.

按跷　又称按摩、乔摩。是古代用来保健和治病的方法。出《素问·异法方宜论》。

按跷(àn qiāo)　**massage** The same as *àn mó* or *qiáo mó*. An ancient method for health preservation and treatment of diseases. See *Su Wen* chapter 12.

按摩　以一定的手法，如推、按、捏、揉，施于人体特定的部位，以防治疾病的方法。也称乔摩、按跷，后世称推拿。有疏通经络，滑利关节，促进气血运行，调节脏腑功能，增强人体抗病能力的作用。出《素问·血气形志》。

按摩（àn mó）　massage The manipulations such as push, press, pinch, rub, etc. on specific parts of the body to prevent or treat diseases. It was also named *qiáo mó*（乔摩）or *àn qiāo*（按跷）previously, and Tui Na manipulation later. This is a treatment that can dredge meridians, soften joints, promote qi and blood, regulate the viscera, and boost body resistance. See *Su Wen* chapter 24.

甚则从之　治法之一。病势重，病情复杂，症候表现与病机不相符者，如真寒假热，真热假寒，治疗可顺从症状之假象，用性质相同的方法治之。如以寒治寒，以热治热，属于反治法。出《素问·至真要大论》。

甚则从之（shèn zé cóng zhī）　**to treat the severe case in compliance with the pseudo-symptom** One of the treatment methods used for those severe and complicated diseases with syndromes and pathogenesis contradictory to each other, such as true heat and false coldness or true coldness and false heat, and using routine treatment, for example, treating coldness with coldness, treating heat with heat, etc. That is named paradoxical treatment. See *Su Wen* chapter 74.

带脉　① 奇经八脉之一。起于季胁下，围绕腰腹一周，腰背部与督脉、足太阳、足少阳经相联系，前方与腰腹部各经相联系。能约束全身直行的各条经脉，以调节脉气，并主司妇人带下。出《灵枢·经别》。② 经穴名。在腰侧部，第十一肋游离章门穴直下，与脐相平处，属足少阳胆经。出《灵枢·癫狂》。

带脉（dài mài）　① Belt vessel. One of the eight extraordinary meridians. It starts from the free rib (region) and goes around the waist. On the back it meets the governor vessel, the foot *taiyang* meridian, and the foot *shaoyang* meridian; on the front it meets with all the meridians going across the waist and abdomen. It regulates the qi of all the meridians and corresponds to vaginal discharge. See *Ling Shu* chapter 11. ② An acupoint name located at the side of the waist under the 11th rib near the acupoint Zhang Men（LR 13）, at the same level with the navel, and pertaining to the gallbladder meridian of foot *shaoyang*. See *Ling Shu* chapter 22.

荣　① 营气。出《素问·痹论》。② 通荥,指荥穴。出《素问·八正神明论》。③ 荣华,五脏精气表现于外的华光、色泽。出《素问·五藏生成》。④ 濡养。出《灵枢·邪客》。⑤ 茂盛。出《素问·四气调神大论》。

荣（róng）　① Nutrient qi. See *Su Wen* chapter 43. ② "荣" is the same as "荥", the name of an acupoint. See *Su Wen* chapter 26. ③ The luster and color manifested by the essence qi stored in the five viscera. See *Su Wen* chapter 10. ④ To nourish. See *Ling Shu* chapter 71. ⑤ Prosperity. See *Su Wen* chapter 2.

荣气　即营气。参该条。出《素问·逆调论》。

荣气（róng qì）　nutrient qi See "营气". See *Su Wen* chapter 34.

荥　（xíng 形；又读 yíng 营）,五腧穴之一。其穴多在指（趾）掌（跖）附近。十二经各有一个荥穴。出《灵枢·九针十二原》《灵枢·顺气一日分为四时》。

荥（yíng）　brook acupoint There are two pronunciations, *xíng*（形）, or *yíng*（营）, which is one of the five transport acupoints. Ying acupoints are usually located close to the fingers, toes, or palms. Every one of the twelve meridians contains a brook acupoint. See *Ling Shu* chapter 1 and *Ling Shu* chapter 44.

荧惑星　火星,为五大行星之一,与五行中的火、五脏中的心相通应。出《素问·金匮真言论》。

荧惑星（yíng huò xīng）　Mars One of the five major planets, corresponding to the fire element, and related to the heart in the five viscera. See *Su Wen* chapter 4.

南政　出《素问·至真要大论》。见"视岁南北"条。

南政（nán zhèng）　southern policy See *Su Wen* chapter 74. See "视岁南北".

药熨　将药物烧热,布包后热熨患处,或以辛热之药敷熨病处,功能散寒止痛,多用于痹症。见《素问·调经论》。

药熨（yào yùn）　hot medicinal compress To dissipate coldness and relieve pain through applying a cloth bag of heated herbal medicine to the affected area of the body. It is usually used for impediment diseases. See *Su Wen* chapter 62.

标本 标,原指树木之枝末;本,指树木之根。《内经》引申为一种相对概念,含主次关系。① 病人的正气为本,医生的治疗措施为标。出《素问·汤液醪醴论》。② 先病为本,后病为标。出《素问·标本病传论》。③ 运气学说中,风、寒、暑、湿、燥、火为六气变化之本;太阴、少阴、厥阴、太阳、阳明、少阳三阴三阳为六气之标象。出《素问·至真要大论》。④ 十二经脉之所起和所止。本是经气汇聚的中心,标是经气扩散的区域。人体十二经脉之标都在头面脑背等上部,本在四肢下部,出《灵枢·卫气》。⑤ 水肿病,肺为标,肾为本。出《素问·水热穴论》。

标本（biāo běn） **tip and root** *Biāo* refers to the tree branches, while *běn* refers to the roots. In *Internal Classic*, it is a pair of concepts with a primary-secondary relationship. ① The healthy qi is the root while the treatment is the branch. See *Su Wen* chapter 14. ② The former disease is the root while the latter one is the branch. See *Su Wen* chapter 65. ③ According to the doctrine of the five circuits and the six qi, wind, cold, heat, dampness, dryness, and fire are the root of the changes of the six qi; *taiyin*, *shaoyin*, *jueyin*, *taiyang*, *yangming*, *shaoyang*, are the branches of the changes of the six qi. See *Su Wen* chapter 74. ④ The beginning and end of the twelve meridians. The region where the meridian qi gathers is the root while where meridian qi disperses is the branch. The branches of the twelve meridians are located at the upper part of the head, face and back, while the roots are located at the bottom of the four limbs. See *Ling Shu* chapter 52. ⑤ For edema disease, the lung is the branch while kidney is the root. See *Su Wen* chapter 61.

标本相移 标病与本病的治疗,其先后次序没有固定,如标病重则先治标,本病重则先治本,视具体情况,可以相互转移。出《素问·标本病传论》。

标本相移（biāo běn xiāng yí） **flexible treatment of branch and root of diseases** There is no fixed order to treat the branch-disease and root-disease. The severe disease should be treated first depending on the specific conditions. See *Su Wen* chapter 65.

标本病传论 《素问》篇名。标本,先病为本,后病为标。病传,疾病的传变。此篇主要论述病有标本,治有逆从以及疾病的传变及预后转归,故名。

标本病传论(biāo běn bìng chuán lùn) **Discussion on the Transmission of Biao and Ben** Chapter name in *Su Wen*. The earlier condition is the root, and the latter one is the branch. *Bìng chuán* refers to the progress of the diseases. This chapter mainly discusses the symptoms and root causes of the disease, the reversal of treatment, and the transmission and prognosis of the disease.

相火 运气术语。相,辅助。相火,与君火相对而言,为六气之一,属少阳,为主气中的第三气,主司小满节到大暑节,相当于四月中至六月中这一阶段的气候变化。出《素问·天元纪大论》。

相火(xiàng huǒ) **ministerial fire** A term in the five circuits and six qi. *Xiàng* means assis-

tance. Ministerial fire is a term with the meaning opposite to sovereign fire. It is one of the six qi, the third qi of dominant qi, pertaining to *shaoyang* and governing the climate changes between Grain Full (the 8th solar term) and Great Heat (12th solar term) (from the middle of April to the middle of June). See *Su Wen* chapter 66.

相傅之官 指肺。出《素问·灵兰秘典论》。

相傅之官(xiàng fù zhī guān) **the official functioning as chancellor and mentor** Refers to the lung. See *Su Wen* chapter 8.

柱骨 第七颈椎隆起处,大椎穴在其下方。出《灵枢·骨度》。

柱骨(zhù gǔ) **pillar bone** The protrusion at the seventh cervical vertebra, above Da Zhui acupoint (DU14). See *Ling Shu* chapter 14.

咸入肾 出《素问·宣明五气》。与"咸生肾"同理。《素问·至真要大论》作"咸先入肾"。

咸入肾(xián rù shèn) **salt enters the kidney** See "咸生肾", See *Su Wen* chapter 23. *Su Wen* chapter 74 recorded it as "咸先入肾".

咸生肾 咸为五味之一,根据五

行理论,咸与肾同属水行,故咸味入口,先入肾而滋养肾水。《素问·至真要大论》:"咸先入肾"。出《素问·阴阳应象大论》。

咸生肾(xián shēng shèn) **salt nourishes the kidney** Salt is one of the five tastes. According to the five viscera theory, salt, the same as kidney, pertains to water. Hence, after salt is taken, it first goes into the kidney and nourishes the kidney water, therefore *Su Wen* chapter 74 recorded it as "咸先入肾". See *Su Wen* chapter 5.

咸伤血 咸属水,心生血而属火,水能胜火,故咸伤血。出《素问·阴阳应象大论》。

咸伤血(xián shāng xuè) **salt pertains to water** The heart that generates blood pertains to fire. Water restrains fire. Thus it can be said that salt harms the blood. See *Su Wen* chapter 5.

咸走血 血味咸,同气相求故尔。多食咸则伤血。出《素问·宣明五气》《灵枢·五味论》。

咸走血(xián zǒu xuè) **salt enters blood** Blood tastes salty, hence to eat too much salt harms the blood. See *Su Wen* chapter 23 and *Ling Shu* chapter 63.

咸走骨 五行中咸属水,肾亦属水而主骨,故咸味入肾而走骨。出《灵枢·九针论》。

咸走骨(xián zǒu gǔ) **salt governs bones** Salt pertains to water, and the kidney pertains to water, as well. The kidney governs the bones, hence after eating salt it is absorbed by the kidney and governs the bones. See *Ling Shu* chapter 78.

砭石 古代的一种石制医疗工具,由锥形或楔形的石块制成,用于刺体表穴位以治疗病痛,或作排脓、放血之用。出《素问·宝命全形论》《素问·异法方宜论》。

砭石(biān shí) **stone needle** An ancient medical tool made of stone. The stone is ground into the shape of a cone or wedge with a sharp end, so as to be able to needle the acupoint and relieve the pain or discharge the pus and blood. See *Su Wen* chapter 12 and chapter 25.

面王 指鼻尖,又称鼻准。出《灵枢·五色》。

面王(miàn wáng) **king of face** Tip of nose. See *Ling Shu* chapter 49.

面中 指面部中央,鼻唇之间部位,即人中沟。出《素问·气府论》。

面中(miàn zhōng) **philtrum** The

center of the face between the nose and lips. See *Su Wen* chapter 59.

面脱 指面部大肉脱削，为真气将竭之象。出《素问·玉版论要》。

面脱(miàn tuō) **bony face** Indicates the exhaustion of genuine qi. See *Su Wen* chapter 15.

面頄骨 即頄骨。出《素问·气府论》。

面頄骨(miàn qiú gǔ) **zygomatic bone** See *Su Wen* chapter 59.

背俞 ① 即五脏之俞，因均在背部的足太阳经，故称。见《素问·血气形志》。② 足太阳经在背部的腧穴。见《素问·刺疟》。

背俞(bèi shū) ① Back transport acupoints. Transport acupoints of the five viscera that are all on the back pertaining to the foot *taiyang* meridian. See *Su Wen* chapter 24. ② The points of the foot *taiyang* meridian that are on the back of the body. See *Su Wen* chapter 36.

背俞之脉 指足太阳膀胱经脉，其脉行于背部，为脏腑俞穴分布之处。出《素问·举痛论》。

背俞之脉(bèi shū zhī mài) **foot taiyang meridian** The foot *taiyang* meridian circulates along the back of the body and mainly contains the acupoints of the

viscera. See *Su Wen* chapter 39.

背腧 ①《灵枢》篇名。腧，古通俞。背腧，指五脏所主的背部俞穴。此篇讨论了背部五脏俞的部位及其临床意义，指出应根据病证的虚实分别采用艾灸补泻法，故名。② 泛指背部各经的腧穴。出《灵枢·终始》。

背腧(bèi shū) ① Chapter name in *Ling Shu*. "腧" is the same as "俞" in ancient Chinese. This term refers to the acupoints on the back of the body governed by the five viscera. This chapter mainly discusses the locations and clinical applications of the back transport acupoints, especially the usage of moxibustion to tonify deficiency or reduce excess according to the conditions. ② Generally refers to all the acupoints on the back. See *Ling Shu* chapter 9.

背膂筋 附着脊椎的筋肉。出《素问·标本病传论》。

背膂筋(bèi lǚ jīn) **the sinews and flesh that adhere to spine** See *Su Wen* chapter 65.

临泣 经穴名。指足临泣穴，为足少阳胆经之输穴。在侠溪上一寸半凹陷处，足小趾、次趾本节后间陷者中。出《灵枢·本输》。

临泣(lín qì) **lin qi** The name of

acupoint GB 41. It pertains to the gallbladder meridian of foot *shaoyang* and is located on the foot at one and a half *cun* above Xia Xi (GB 43), namely the small depression on the dorsal aspect of the foot between the little toe and the forth toe. See *Ling Shu* chapter 2.

临御之化 运气术语。临，来临。御，统御。寒暑燥湿风火六气有主气、客气之分。主气统御一岁四时之气，客气有司天、在泉的不断变化，运气学说通过客气加临于主气的变化，来推演运气的变化，以了解气象物候及疾病的发生等情况。出《素问·六元正纪大论》。

临御之化（lín yù zhī huà） **changing of dominating qi** A term of the circuits and qi. *Lín* means befalling, and *yù* means governing. The six qi, coldness, heat, dryness, dampness, wind and fire, can be categorized into two groups, dominant qi and guest qi. The dominant qi governs the four seasons, while the guest qi adjusts to the yearly changes of the four seasons, specifically named *si tian* (celestial control, governing the first half year) and *zai quan* (terrestrial effect, governing the latter or second half year). The five circuits and six qi predicts the changes of the seasons as well as the weather, phenology, and diseases according to the way the guest qi affects the dominant qi. See *Su Wen* chapter 71.

削 ① 治法。即软坚削积，属于消法，主治癥积痰核等病证。出《素问·至真要大论》。② 削弱。出《素问·生气通天论》。

削（xuē） ① Treatment method, namely to soften the toughness and reduce the stagnation. As one of the dispersion treatments, it treats accumulation and phlegm. See *Su Wen* chapter 74. ② Reduction. See *Su Wen* chapter 3.

是动则病 指本经络脉变动所现病证。是，此，指示代词。动，变动，异常。病，患，作动词。出《灵枢·经脉》。

是动则病（shì dòng zé bìng） **disease transmitted by meridian** *Shì* is a pronoun meaning "this"; *dòng* means changes and abnormal conditions; *bìng* is always used as a verb in ancient Chinese, meaning "to fall ill". See *Ling Shu* chapter 10.

胃 ① 六腑之一，又称太仓。位

于中焦，与脾相连，为曲屈状囊形器官。主要功能是受纳和腐熟水谷。出《灵枢·海论》。② 指胃的脉象。出《素问·大奇论》。③ 脉之胃气。有胃气之脉，其来从容和缓，具冲和之象。出《素问·平人气象论》。④ 星宿名。二十八宿中西方七宿之一。运气推演中属辛，主水。出《素问·五运行大论》。

胃（wèi）　① Stomach. One of the six bowls, also named *tai cang*. It is a curved organ as if it were a bag located at the middle *jiao* and connected with spleen. It receives and digests food. See *Ling Shu* chapter 33. ② The stomach pulse. See *Su Wen* chapter 48. ③ Stomach qi manifested in pulse. The pulse with stomach qi usually feels peaceful with a harmonious flow. See *Su Wen* chapter 18. ④ The name of a constellation. It refers to the seven constellations on the west among all the twenty eight constellations. According to the doctrine of the five circuits and six qi, they pertain to *xin* (the eighth one of totally 10 Heavenly Stems) and govern water. See *Su Wen* chapter 67.

胃口　① 指胃脘部。出《素问·病能论》。② 单指或统指胃之上口贲门与下口幽门。出《灵枢·经脉》。

胃口（wèi kǒu）　① Stomach duct. See *Su Wen* chapter 46. ② Rushing gate (cardia) or dark gate（pylorus），or both. See *Ling Shu* chapter 10.

胃之大络　由胃直接分出之络脉，不同于别络。其始自胃上行贯膈，络于肺，出于左乳之下的虚里，即心尖搏动处，是测候宗气的部位。出《素问·平人气象论》。

胃之大络（wèi zhī dà luò）　**the large collateral of the stomach** The collateral derived directly from the stomach meridian, different from the divergent collateral. It starts from the stomach, goes upwards to penetrate the diaphragm, connects with the lung, and finally exits from *Xu Li*, namely, the heart apex under the left breast, where pectoral qi is usually assessed. See *Su Wen* chapter 18.

胃之五窍　指咽门、贲门、幽门、阑门、魄门。食道、胃、肠皆胃气上下所行之地，此五门为其孔窍门户。出《灵枢·胀论》。

胃之五窍（wèi zhī wǔ qiào）　**the**

five gates of the stomach Namely, the Throat Gate, Rushing Gate, Dark Gate, Screen Gate, and Corporeal Soul Gate. Stomach qi goes up and down through the five gates in the esophagus, stomach and intestines. See *Ling Shu* chapter 35.

胃不和则卧不安　胃的功能失调,不能顺降,或出现睡卧不安的症状。出《素问·逆调论》《素问·评热病论》。

胃不和则卧不安(wèi bú hé zé wò bú ān)　**The malfunction of the stomach may lead to restless sleeping or insomnia.** See *Su Wen* chapter 33 and 34.

胃气　① 胃的精气。出《素问·平人气象论》。② 正常的脉气,即脉来时无太过,无不及,自有一种雍容和缓之状。胃为五脏之本,故正常之脉必含胃气。出《素问·玉机真藏论》《素问·平人气象论》《素问·经脉别论》《灵枢·四时气》。

胃气(wèi qì)　① The essence qi in the stomach. See *Su Wen* chapter 18. ② Normal qi in the pulse, both moderate and peaceful. The stomach is the root of the five viscera; hence, a normal pulse contains stomach qi. See *Su Wen* chapter 18，19

and 21，and *Lin Shu* chapter 19.

胃风　病名。见多汗恶风及脘痞腹满、泄泻不食等症。出《素问·风论》。

胃风(wèi fēng)　**stomach wind** Disease name, with the symptoms of profuse sweeting, aversion to wind, distention in the stomach duct, abdominal fullness, diarrhea, and the inability to eat. See *Su Wen* chapter 42.

胃为之市　胃主受纳五谷,如市之聚散。出《素问·刺禁论》。

胃为之市(wèi wéi zhī shì)　**stomach as the market** The stomach receives all kinds of food, just as a market which contains various kinds of things. See *Su Wen* chapter 52.

胃为之海　胃主受纳,容纳水液五谷,如海之集容盛大。出《灵枢·师传》。

胃为之海(wèi wéi zhī hǎi)　**stomach as the ocean** The stomach receives water and grain, as if it were the ocean with a vast capacity. See *Ling Shu* chapter 29.

胃心痛　病证名。厥心痛之一。由胃气上逆犯心所致,症见胸腹闷胀,心痛尤烈。出《灵枢·厥病》。

胃心痛(wèi xīn tòng)　**reversal**

heartache caused by stomach disorder Disease name. It is one of the reversal heartaches, and caused by the reversal of stomach qi that attacks the heart and manifests as oppression in the chest and abdomen, along with fierce heart pain. See *Ling Shu* chapter 24.

胃足阳明之脉　即足阳明胃经，为十二经脉之一。出《灵枢·经脉》。其循行路线从鼻翼两侧迎香穴，挟鼻上行至鼻根部，下循鼻外，入上齿龈内，复出环绕口唇交叉于唇下沟的承浆穴处，再向后沿着下颌骨后下缘出大迎穴，沿颊车，上行耳前，过客主人穴处，沿发际，到达额前（头维穴）。一支从大迎穴下行到人迎穴，沿喉咙入缺盆，穿过横膈，属于胃，络于脾。再一支从缺盆下行沿乳内侧，挟脐两旁，下行至阴毛两侧的气街穴（又名气冲穴）。再一支从胃的下口幽门处，沿腹内，下至气街，与前脉汇合，再由此下行至髀关（大腿前外侧）。直达伏兔，下至膝盖，沿胫骨前外侧至足背，进入足中趾外侧端（厉兑穴）。再一支从膝下三寸处（足三里穴），下行至中趾外侧。再一支从足背走入足大趾，出大趾尖端（隐白穴与足太阴脾经接）。

胃足阳明之脉（wèi zú yáng míng zhī mài）　**stomach meridian of foot *yangming*** One of the twelve regular meridians. See *Ling Shu* chapter 10. It starts from *Ying Xiang*（LI 20）on both sides of the nose, goes upwards to the root of the nose, downwards along the outer sides of the nose into the gums, and then goes out and around the lips from both sides until meeting at Cheng Jiang（CV 24）. After that, it goes backwards along the lower jawbone, penetrates Da Ying（ST 5）, goes upwards along Jia Che（ST 6）to the ears through Ke Zhuren, or Shang Guan（GB 3）acupoint, and then goes along the hair line to Tou Wei（ST 8）on the forehead. It has five branches. One starts from Da Ying（ST 5）, goes downwards to Ren Ying（ST 9）, moves along the throat to penetrate Que Pen（ST 12）, and finally goes through the diaphragm into the stomach and connects with the spleen. Another goes downwards from Que Pen（ST 12）along the inner sides of the breasts and both sides of the navel to

Qi Jie acupoint, the other name of Qi Chong acupoint (ST 30) at both sides of the pubic hair. Another goes downwards from the pylorus of the stomach in the belly to Qi Jie (ST 30), where it meets with the previous-mentioned branch, and then continues to move downwards to Bi Guan (ST 31) at the anterior lateral aspect of the thighs. After that, it goes straight to Fu Tu (ST 32) and then to the knees; then it goes along the anterior lateral aspect of the shin bones to the dorsal aspect of the feet, and finally enters the outer sides of the middle toes, at Li Dui (ST 45). Another branch starts from three *cun* under the knees, where Zu Sanli (ST 36) is located, and goes downwards to the outer sides of the middle toes. Another branch starts from the dorsal aspect of the feet and goes out from the tips of the big toes, where Yin Bai (SP 1) is connected with the spleen meridian of foot *taiyin*.

胃胀 病证名。六腑胀之一,症见腹满、胃脘痛、食少便难。出《灵枢·胀论》。

胃胀(wèi zhàng) **stomach distention** Symptom name. It is one of the six types of bowel distention symptoms manifested as abdominal distention, epigastric pain, poor appetite, and difficulty defecating (dyschezia). See *Ling Shu* chapter 35.

胃疟 六腑疟之一。症见饥而不食,食即腹满胀大。出《素问·刺疟》。

胃疟(wèi nüè) **stomach malaria** Manifested as the inability to eat when hungry, and abdominal distention. See *Su Wen* chapter 36.

胃咳 六腑咳之一。由脾咳不愈传变而成。症候特点为咳而呕,甚则呕蛔,为胃气上逆,故称胃咳。出《素问·咳论》。

胃咳(wèi ké) **stomach cough** It is one of the six types of bowel coughs. It is induced from chronic spleen cough and manifested as cough provoking vomiting, with occasional emetic ascaris. It is named stomach cough because there is obvious reversal of stomach qi. See *Su Wen* chapter 38.

胃脉 ① 经脉。足阳明胃经。出《灵枢·本输》。② 寸口脉。出《素问·病能论》。

胃脉(wèi mài) ① Stomach meridian of foot *yangming*. See *Ling Shu* chapter 2. ② *Cun kou* pulse. See *Su Wen* chapter 46.

胃鬲 胃脘与横膈间部位。出《素问·至真要大论》。

胃鬲(wèi gé) **stomach diaphragm** The region between the stomach duct and the diaphragm. See *Su Wen* chapter 74.

胃病 胃的功能失常所致之病证。诸如脘腹胀满疼痛、呕吐不能食等。出《灵枢·邪气藏府病形》。

胃病(wèi bìng) **stomach disease** The diseases caused by the malfunction of the stomach，for example，stomach pain and distention，vomiting，and difficulty eating，etc. See *Ling Shu* chapter 4.

胃疸 "疸"同"瘅"，热之义。胃热杀谷，故虽食犹饥，是名胃疸。出《素问·平人气象论》。

胃疸(wèi dǎn) **stomach heat** "疸" is also written as "瘅"，which means heat. The heat in the stomach excessively boosts digestion of food，leaving the patient always feeling hungry even after eating. See *Su Wen* chapter 18.

胃脘 ① 胃的内腔，分上、中、下三部，胃上口贲门部，称上脘(wǎn 宛)，中部为中脘，下口幽门部为下脘。出《灵枢·邪气藏府病形》《素问·阴阳别论》。② 指中脘穴。位于腹部正中线脐上四寸，属任脉，为胃经之募穴。出《素问·气穴论》。见《素问集注》。

胃脘(wèi wǎn) ① Stomach duct. The stomach cavity including the upper，middle and lower parts. The upper part close to the Rushing Gate(cardia) is named Stomach Duct；the middle part Central Stomach Duct；while the lower part Lower Stomach Duct. See *Ling Shu* chapter 4 and *Su Wen* chapter 7. ② *Zhong Wan* acupoint (CV 12). As the front-*mu* acupoint of the stomach meridian and also pertaining to the conception vessel, it is located at 4 *cun* above the navel on the central line of abdomen. See *Su Wen* chapter 58. See *Su Wen Ji Zhu* (*Collected Annotation of Su Wen*).

胃脘痈 病名。痈疡发于胃脘。由于阳热聚于胃口，腐败血肉而然。出《素问·病能论》。

胃脘痈(wèi wǎn yōng) **stomach duct abscess** Disease name. It

九画

refers to welling-abscesses and sores occuring at the stomach duct. They are caused by the gathering heat at the stomach duct that rottens the flesh. See *Su Wen* chapter 46.

贵人　运气术语。指太一天符之年,其气最盛,好像贵人一般,暴戾专横。出《素问·六微旨大论》。

贵人(guì rén)　**arrogant person** A term of the five circuits and six qi. It refers to the year of *tai yi tian fu* (heavenly complement) which has a supreme power as if it were a ruthless and tyrannical magnate. See *Su Wen* chapter 68.

贵贱　① 六气于四时中之衰旺变化。出《灵枢·决气》。② 五脏六腑不同的地位和作用。出《素问·灵兰秘典论》。

贵贱(guì jiàn)　① The wax and waning of the six qi in the four seasons. See *Ling Shu* chapter 30. ② The different status and functions of the five viscera and six bowels. See *Su Wen* chapter 8.

思　① 在认识确定目标的基础上反复思考谓思。出《灵枢·本神》。② 过度的思虑。出《素问·阴阳应象大论》《素问·举痛论》。

思(sī)　① Repeated contemplation after setting the goal. See *Ling Shu* chapter 8. ② Excessive thought. See *Su Wen* chapter 5 and chapter 39.

思则气结　思则精神凝聚,正气留结不行,出现胸闷、痞胀、食欲不振等症。出《素问·举痛论》。

思则气结(sī zé qì jié)　**Excessive thought causes qi stagnation.** Manifested as oppression in the chest, stuffiness, loss of appetite, etc. See *Su Wen* chapter 39.

思伤脾　思虑过度,脾气郁结,脾运失畅,出现胸脘痞闷、食欲不振、食谷胀满等症。出《素问·阴阳应象大论》《素问·五运行大论》。《素问·举痛论》有:"思则气结",可参该条。

思伤脾(sī shāng pí)　**Excessive thought damages spleen.** Excessive thought causes stagnation of the spleen qi, which in turn, leads to glomus and oppression in the chest, loss of appetite, distention and fullness in the stomach, etc. See *Su Wen* chapter 5, chapter 39, and See *Su Wen* chapter 67. Also see "思则气结".

思胜恐　思为脾土之志,恐为肾水之志,土能克水,故云思胜

恐。出《素问·阴阳应象大论》
《素问·五运行大论》。

思胜恐(sī shèng kǒng) **Excessive thought restrains panic.** Among the five states of mind, spleen (earth) is pensiveness, while kidney (water) is panic. Since earth restrains water, pensiveness restrains panic. *Su Wen* chapter 5 and See *Su Wen* chapter 67.

思虑而心虚　思虑过度损伤心气导致心气虚弱，为心痹病的内因。出《素问·五藏生成》。

思虑而心虚(sī lǜ ér xīn xū) **Excessive thought weakens heart qi.** Excessive thought damages heart qi, thus weakening the heart and leading to heart impediment. See *Su Wen* chapter 10.

咽门　水谷饮食之门户。出《灵枢·肠胃》。

咽门(yān mén)　**the gate of water and grain** See *Ling Shu* chapter 31.

哕　即呃逆，干呕的症状。为胃气上逆所致，久病见哕为胃气将绝。出《灵枢·口问》。

哕(yuě)　**eructation** A symptom of dry retching caused by the reversal of stomach qi. For chronic patients, hiccups usually indicate deficiency of stomach qi. See *Ling Shu* chapter 28.

咳论　《素问》篇名。咳，咳嗽，此篇专论咳嗽的病因病机、症状、分类、传变及治疗原则。故名。

咳论(ké lùn)　**Discussion on Cough** Chapter name in *Su Wen*. *Ké* means cough. This is a chapter on the etiology, pathogenesis, symptoms, category, transformation and therapeutic principles of coughs. Hence the name.

咳唾　唾，这里指痰液。咳唾指咳嗽有痰的症状。出《素问·玉机真藏论》。

咳唾(ké tuò)　**cough with sputum** *Tuò* refers to sputum. This term refers to the symptom of cough with sputum. See *Su Wen* chapter 19.

骨之精为瞳子　肾主骨，骨之精即肾之精。瞳子，即瞳孔，能反映肾之生理病理状态。出《灵枢·大惑论》。

骨之精为瞳子(gǔ zhī jīng wéi tóng zǐ)　**Kidney essence is reflected in the pupil.** The kidney dominates the bones, which means the essence of the bones is the essence of the kidney. Pupils reflect the physiological and pathological conditions of the kidney. See *Ling Shu*

九画

chapter 80.

骨者髓之府 髓为骨之脂，充养骨骼，故骨为髓之府。若髓减骨弱则不能久立，步履不稳，是骨将衰败的征兆，由于肾主骨髓，实是肾之衰惫。出《素问·脉要精微论》。

骨者髓之府（gǔ zhě suǐ zhī fǔ）**Bone is the house of marrow.** Marrow is the nutrient for bones. Lack of marrow may lead to weakness of the bones. The difficulty in standing for a prolonged period of time and taking staggering steps may indicate the declining condition of the bones. Since the kidney dominates the marrow, it is induced from the exhaustion of kidney. See *Su Wen* chapter 17.

骨空 "空"通"孔"。即骨孔，亦称髓空、髓孔，是骨髓与骨外气血交通之处。多为穴位所在，一般圆形长骨有之，扁平之骨多无。出《素问·骨空论》。

骨空（gǔ kōng） **bone orifice** "空" is the same as "孔", or orifice. *Gǔ kōng* bears the same meaning as *suǐ kōng*（髓空）or *suǐ kǒng*（髓孔），all of which refer to the acupoints, which are usually located to connect with the qi and blood

outside the bones. These acupoints usually exist in long and round bones instead of flat bones. See *Su Wen* chapter 60.

骨空论 《素问》篇名。空，通"孔"，穴也。骨空，即全身骨节交会之俞穴。此篇主要论述风病、水病的针刺方法，以及督、任、冲脉的循行路线和病证的刺法，着重介绍了各种针灸方法所取的俞穴。故名。

骨空论（gǔ kōng lùn） **Discussion on Osseous Orifices** Chapter name in *Su Wen*. "空" is the same as "孔", which means a hole. *Gǔ kōng* is an acupoint where the bones all over the body converge. This chapter mainly states the treatment methods, with acupuncture, for wind and water diseases, the circulation of the thoroughfare vessel, the conception vessel and the governor vessel, and the needling methods for diseases along these vessels, and the acupoints adopted by various needling methods. Hence the name.

骨蚀 病证名。由于虚邪侵入机体深部，寒热相搏，壅滞不散，久则化脓，伤蚀及骨。出《灵枢·刺节真邪》。

骨蚀（gǔ shí） **bone erosion** Disease

name. The vacuity pathogen attacks the inner body deeply which leads to alternate cold (chill) and hot (fever), lingering stagnation, and finally suppuration which rots the bones. See *Ling Shu* chapter 75.

骨度 ① 古代以骨节为标志,定出一定的度数,以测量人体各部的长度和宽度。出《灵枢·骨度》。②《灵枢》篇名。该篇主要通过对骨骼长度、大小的度量来描述头项、四肢、躯干等三十八处体表的长度,以此测知内脏的大小、经脉的长短,以便针灸的取穴。故名。

骨度(gǔ dù) ① Bone degree. Ancient people used the length of bones as the standard to assess the length and width of various parts of the human body. See *Ling Shu* chapter 14. ② Chapter name in *Ling Shu*. This chapter discusses how to use the bones as the standard to assess the length of thirty-eight parts of the human body, including the head, the neck, the four limbs, the trunk, etc. and hence to help calculate the size of the viscera and length of the meridians so as to precisely position the acupoints.

Hence the name.

骨疽 病名。阴疽之生于骨者,肿而不化脓。出《灵枢·刺节真邪》。

骨疽(gǔ jū) **bone abscess** Disease name. Yin abscesses occurring on bones usually swell without suppuration. See *Ling Shu* chapter 75.

骨清 清,寒冷之意。骨清即寒冷彻骨。出《灵枢·癫狂》。

骨清(gǔ qīng) **bone coldness** *Qīng* means coldness. *Gǔ qīng* means chill in the bone. See *Ling Shu* chapter 22.

骨厥 病证名。① 足少阴肾经的病候。肾主骨,因足少阴肾经气逆所致之病证。《灵枢·经脉》:"肾足少阴之脉……是为骨厥。"② 指骨寒而厥。《灵枢·寒热病》:"骨厥亦然。"

骨厥(gǔ jué) Disease name. ① Diseases on the kidney meridian of foot *shaoyin*. The kidney dominates the bones, therefore the reversal qi along the kidney meridian of foot *shaoyin* leads to bone reversal. See *Ling Shu* chapter 10. ② The coldness in the bones leads to reversal. See *Ling Shu* chapter 21.

骨解 骨之关节缝隙。出《灵枢·

九画

九针论》。

骨解（gǔ jiě）　**sutura** The gaps between the joints. See *Ling Shu* chapter 78.

骨痹　病名。①五体痹之一，多发于冬季，症以沉重为特征。出《素问·痹论》。②以身寒至骨，汤火不能热，厚衣不能温，关节拘挛为特征的痹证。多因纵欲过度，肾虚髓枯，骨不能满所致。出《素问·逆调论》。

骨痹（gǔ bì）　Disease name. ① Bone impediment. As one of the five types of body impediments, bone impediment usually occurs in winter and one develops severe symptoms. See *Su Wen* chapter 43. ② An impediment disease with the features of joint constriction and coldness deep into the joints that even are unable to be warmed with hot water, fire and clothes, usually caused by excessive sex that leads to kidney deficiency and vacuity of the marrow. See *Su Wen* chapter 34.

骨痿　病证名。症见腰脊至两下肢不能伸举站立。病起于远行劳倦，动则生热，又逢天气大热，两热相合，热舍于肾，致骨枯髓虚。出《素问·痿论》。

骨痿（gǔ wěi）　**bone wilting** Disease name. It is difficult for the patient to straighten the spine and lower limbs, and stand up straight. It is caused by long hours of walking and taxation fatigue. Heat generated by movements along with the heat of the weather goes into the kidney and ends in desiccation of the bone and vacuity of the marrow. See *Su Wen* chapter 44.

骨骶　即尾骶骨。出《灵枢·癫狂》。

骨骶（gǔ dǐ）　**coccyx** See *Ling Shu* chapter 22.

骨繇　骨节动摇，弛缓不收。出《灵枢·根结》。

骨繇（gǔ yáo）　**bone shaking** Uncontrollable shaking of the body and flaccidity of the bones. See *Ling Shu* chapter 5.

骨癫疾　病证名。癫疾之一种，病较深重，因其骨强之症，故名。出《灵枢·癫狂》。

骨癫疾（gǔ diān jí）　**bone epilepsy** Disease name, and one type of epilepsy usually onset with severe typical symptoms, as the rigidity of the bones. See *Ling Shu* chapter 22.

钩　钩脉。其脉来较充盈，去势较衰，其状如钩，是心的正常脉象，也是夏季的主脉。出《素问·平人气象论》《素问·宣明五气》《素问·玉机真藏论》。若脉来洪大而不滑利，如操带钩，是无胃气的心的真藏脉，则属危候。

钩（gōu）　**hook pulse** This pulse comes with a slightly stronger power，while leaving without much force，thus to feel like a hook. It is the normal manifestation of the heart pulse and the governing pulse in summer. See *Su Wen* chapter 18，chapter 19 and chapter 23. If the pulse feels surging and unsmooth as the handle of a clothing-hook，it is a dying pulse named *Zhen Zang* pulse which contains no stomach qi and indicates an extremely dangerous condition.

秋气　① 秋季的肃降收敛之气，与肺相应。出《素问·四气调神大论》《素问·六节藏象论》。② 秋季人体之精气，在于皮肤。出《素问·四时刺逆从论》。③ 秋季中人之病气。出《灵枢·终始》。

秋气（qiū qì）　① Autumn qi. The downbearing and astringing qi in autumn which corresponds to the lung. See *Su Wen* chapter 2 and chapter 9. ② The essence qi of the human body that is usually on the skin. See *Su*

Wen chapter 64. ③ The pathogenic qi in autumn. See *Ling Shu* chapter 9.

秋脉　秋季应时之脉，其脉浮，属肺。出《素问·玉机真藏论》。

秋脉（qiū mài）　**autumn pulse** It is the pulse that corresponds to autumn，which is floating and pertaining to the lung. See *Su Wen* Chapter 19.

秋脉如浮　秋季阴气微上，阳气微下，但尚在皮毛，且秋气主肺，肺合皮毛，脉气从之，故浮。因其阳气微下而未至沉下，故其脉浮而轻虚，来时稍急，去时略散，与春夏之浮不同。出《素问·玉机真藏论》。

秋脉如浮（qiū mài rú fú）　**autumn pulse feels floating** In autumn，yin qi ascends moderately and yang qi descends slightly，but both are floating on the skin and（body）hair. Autumn qi dominates the lung，which connect with the skin and（body）hair，hence the pulse feels floating. The pulse comes slightly abrupt，while dispersing when leaving，quite different from the pulse in spring and summer. See *Su Wen* chapter 19.

重方　方制名称，奇方偶方迭用之谓。又称复方，为七方之一。

用于病情较复杂者。出《素问·至真要大论》。

重方（chóng fāng） **compound formula** Formula name. As a combination of odd-ingredient prescriptions and even-ingredient prescriptions, it is one of the seven kinds of prescriptions that is applied for severe conditions. See *Su Wen* chapter 74.

重舌 病证名。重（chóng 虫），重叠之意。即舌下生一肿物，状如小舌，故名。出《灵枢·终始》。

重舌（chóng shé） **double tongue** Disease name. *Chóng* means overlapping. It refers to the lump under the tongue that looks like a small tongue. See *Ling Shu* chapter 9.

重阳 两种属于阳的性质重合。① 指日中，阳气隆盛之时。出《灵枢·营卫生会》。② 色诊中男子病色见于左面之谓。男属阳，阳从左，故称。属逆证。出《素问·玉版论要》。③ 示阳盛极。出《灵枢·论疾诊尺》。参"重阳必阴"条。

重阳（chóng yáng） Two kinds of things pertaining to yang overlap. ① Midday, yang qi is overwhelming. See *Ling Shu* chapter 18. ② A symptom of a disease occurring in males manifested on the left side of the face. Males pertain to yang and yang pertains to the left, hence the name. See *Su Wen* chapter 15. ③ Excess of yang. See *Ling Shu* chapter 74. See "重阳必阴".

重阴 两种属于阴的性质重合。① 指夜半，阴气隆盛之时。出《灵枢·营卫生会》。② 色诊中女子病色见于右面之谓。女属阴，阴从右，故称。属逆证。出《素问·玉版论要》。③ 指肺病传肾。出《素问·阴阳别论》。④ 示阴盛极。出《灵枢·论疾诊尺》。

重阴（chóng yīn） Two kinds of things pertaining to yin overlap. ① Midnight. Yin qi is overwhelming at midnight. See *Ling Shu* chapter 18. ② A symptom of a disease occurring in females manifested on the right side of the face. Females pertain to yin and yin pertains to the right, hence the name. It is a kind of unfavorable pattern. See *Su Wen* chapter 15. ③ Lung disease transforms to the kidney. See *Su Wen* chapter 7. ④ Excess of yin. See *Ling Shu* chapter 74.

重身 妊娠怀孕。出《素问·奇病论》。

重身（chóng shēn）　**pregnancy** See *Su Wen* chapter 47.

重言　言语謇塞,俗称口吃。出《灵枢·忧恚无言》。

重言（chóng yán）　**stutter** See *Ling Shu* chapter 69.

重实　①重(chóng 虫),重叠。重实,即实之又实。出《素问·八正神明论》。②热病出现气热脉满之证。出《素问·通评虚实论》。

重实（chóng shí）　① *Chóng* means overlapping. *Chóng shí* refers to overlapping excess. See *Su Wen* chapter 26. ② A symptom of febrile disease, namely heat of qi and fullness in the meridians. See *Su Wen* chapter 28.

重虚　重,复。重虚,虚上加虚,虚之极甚。①指证脉皆虚。出《素问·通评虚实论》。②指精血皆虚。出《素问·刺禁论》。③虚证用泻法针刺。出《灵枢·终始》。

重虚（chóng xū）　*Chóng* means doubled. *Chóng Xū* means doubled deficiency or extreme deficiency. ① Both the syndrome and the pulse are deficient. See *Su Wen* chapter 28. ② Both the essence and the blood are deficient. See *Su Wen* chapter 52. ③ Apply the draining method with needling for deficient syndromes. See *Ling Shu* chapter 9.

重强　①肢体沉重拘僵。强(jiàng 匠),僵硬不柔之意。出《素问·至真要大论》。②病名。指脾病而引起的四肢不举,九窍不利的病证。出《素问·玉机真藏论》。

重强（zhòng jiàng）　① Heavy and stiff body. *Jiàng* refers to stiffness. See *Su Wen* chapter 74. ② Disease name. Stiff limbs and blockage of nine orifices induced from spleen diseases. See *Su Wen* chapter 19.

复　①病愈而复发。出《素问·热论》。②运气术语。即复气。出《素问·至真要大论》。见"复气"条。③返回的意思。出《素问·阴阳应象大论》。④恢复。出《素问·汤液醪醴论》。

复（fù）　① Recrudescence. The disease returns. See *Su Wen* chapter 31. ② A term of the five circuits and six qi. See "复气". See *Su Wen* chapter 74. ③ Return. See *Su Wen* chapter 5. ④ Recover. See *Su Wen* chapter 14.

复气　运气术语。六气变化中对胜气的制约之气称为复气。出《素问·至真要大论》。

复气（fù qì）　**retaliatory qi** A

term of the five circuits and six qi. It refers to the retaliatory qi that restrains the prevailing qi in the changes of the six qi (climate factors). See *Su Wen* chapter 74.

复溜 经穴名。属足少阴肾经，位于足内踝上二寸，在动脉跳动不休。出《灵枢·本输》。

复溜（fù liū) **Fu Liu（KI 7）**It pertains to the kidney meridian of foot *shaoyin* and is located at two *cun* above the medial malleolus，beating endlessly. See *Ling Shu* chapter 2.

顺气一日分为四时 《灵枢》篇名。"一日分为四时"，即一日的阴阳变化，可以用一年春夏秋冬四季的阴阳变化来分析、理解。"顺气"，即治疗疾病时要顺应一日之中人体阴阳之气的盛衰变化。此篇主要讨论了一日分为四时的原因及百病多旦慧、昼安、夕加、夜甚的道理，并以此应用于诊断和治疗。故名。

顺气一日分为四时（shùn qì yī rì fēn wéi sì shí) **Division of the Four Seasons in One Day** Chapter name in *Ling Shu*. Each day has four seasons，therefore，the treatment of disease must comply with the changes of yin and yang in the four seasons.

This chapter discusses the reasons why each day contains four seasons，and why most of the diseases are mild in the morning，light in the daytime，worse in the afternoon and deteriorate in the evening. This can be applied to diagnosis and treatment. Hence the name.

促 促脉。脉来急促有力，时有不规则间歇。主阳热火盛，血气痰食停滞及肿痛。出《素问·平人气象论》。

促（cù) **irregular-rapid pulse** It comes rapid and strong with an irregular pause，indicating excessive yang qi and heat，induced by stagnation of blood，qi，phlegm，and food，and by painful swelling. See *Su Wen* chapter 18.

侮 侮，欺凌。多用于五行相克关系中。或由于五行中的某一行过于强盛而对原来"克我"的一行进行反侮、反克。也可由于某一行的不足，不仅己所不胜之"克我"者进一步相侮，即使原来被我克者，亦起来反侮之。它是五行之间生克制化中不正常的相克现象。出《素问·五运行大论》。

侮（wǔ) **rebellion** It is usually used to describe the restraining relationship of the five elements. One element gains enough strength to restrain the other one which once restrained it; or an element is not only restrained by the stronger one, but even restrained by the once weaker one. This is an abnormal restraining relationship. See *Su Wen* chapter 67.

鬼臾区　一作鬼客区，又称大鸿。为传说中上古时代的医家。出《素问·天元纪大论》。

鬼臾区（guǐ yú qū）　**Gui yuqu** Also written as "鬼客区", the other name *dà hóng*（大鸿）, a doctor of ancient times. See *Su Wen* chapter 66.

侯　为封建时代最高封爵之一。先秦时代将爵位分成公、侯、伯、子、男五个等级。出《素问·著至教论》。

侯（hóu）　**marquis** One of the highest titles in feudal society. In pre-Qin dynasty, there are five titles of nobility, namely, duke, marquis, count, viscount and baron. See *Su Wen* chapter 75.

徇蒙招尤　徇（xùn 训），眩。蒙，通"矇"，视物不清。出《素问·五藏生成》。

徇蒙招尤（xùn méng zhāo yóu）

dizziness, unclear vision, and shaking body *Xùn* means dizziness. "蒙" is the same as "矇", which means unclear vision. See *Ling Shu* chapter 10.

律吕　音律之总称，十二音律分阴阳各六，阳者为律，阴者为吕。六阳律为：黄钟、太簇、姑洗、蕤宾、夷则、无射；六阴吕为：林钟、南吕、应钟、大吕、夹钟、仲吕，合称律吕。出《素问·刺法论》。

律吕（lǜ lǚ）　**temperament** General term for mode or tonality. The twelve temperaments consist of six yin and six yang temperaments, the former named "律" and the latter "吕". The six yang temperaments are *Huangzhong, Taizu, Guxi, Ruibin, Yize, Wushe*; the six yin temperaments are *Linzhong, Nanlv, Yingzhong, Dalv, Jiazhong, Zhonglv*. Collectively, they are named *lǜ lǚ*. See *Su Wen* chapter 72.

俞　俞穴之简称，亦作"腧""输"。是经脉气血输注出入之所，也是针刺治疗的部位。出《素问·气府论》。

俞（shū）　**acupoint** Short for "acupuncture point", and sometimes written as "腧" or "输". It is

九画

the place where meridian qi and blood gather and pass, and the place where acupuncture treatment applies. See *Su Wen* chapter 59.

俞气　经脉传输出入之气。俞通腧，为经脉之气输注出入之处。出《素问·生气通天论》。

俞气（shū qì）　**meridian qi** "俞" is the same as "腧", which refers to the place where meridian qi gather and pass. See *Su Wen* chapter 3.

俞度　俞，俞穴。度，度数。指俞穴的位置度数。出《素问·方盛衰论》。

俞度（shū dù）　**measurement of acupoints** *Shū* refers to acupoints, and *dù* the measurement of the locations of acupoints. See *Su Wen* chapter 80.

俞窍　深近筋骨的俞穴。出《素问·诊要经终》。

俞窍（shū qiào）　**acupoints deep into sinews and bones** See *Su Wen* chapter 16.

俞理　俞穴的穴理。出《素问·疏五过论》。

俞理（shū lǐ）　**the measurement and calculation of acupoints** See *Su Wen* chapter 77.

食亦　亦，易。食亦，即善食易饥而瘦的病证。大肠与胃两热相合，胃热则消谷；消铄肌肉，故瘦。出《素问·气厥论》。

食亦（shí yì）　**eating much while easily being hungry** *Yì*（亦）is the same as *yì*（易）. It is a symptom in which the patient is easy to feel hungry after frequent eating, and always appears thin. The heat in the stomach along with that in the large intestine digests food and consumes flesh and muscle, hence the patient is always thin. See *Su Wen* chapter 37.

食痹　病证名。食后气滞不行，胃脘闷胀，甚则疼痛之证。出《素问·脉要精微论》。

食痹（shí bì）　**digestion impediment** Symptom name, in which food stagnates in the stomach duct and pain due to qi stagnation occurs. See *Su Wen* chapter 17.

胠　指腋下的胁肋部分。出《素问·五藏生成》。

胠（qū）　**the ribs under axilla** See *Su Wen* chapter 10.

胪胀　胪（lú 炉），指腹部。胪胀，即腹胀。出《素问·六元正纪大论》。

胪胀（lú zhàng）　**abdominal distension** *Lú* refers to abdomen. This term refers to abdominal distention. See *Su Wen* chapter

71.

胆　六腑之一，又属奇恒之腑，胆附于肝，贮藏胆汁。出《素问·灵兰秘典论》。其经脉为足少阳胆经，与足厥阴肝经相表里。

胆(dǎn)　**gallbladder** One of the six bowels and extraordinary organs. The gallbladder attaches to the liver and stores bile. See *Su Wen* chapter 8. It pertains to the gallbladder meridian of foot *shaoyang*, which has an interior-exterior relationship with the liver meridian of foot *jueyin*.

胆气　胆中之精气。出《素问·大奇论》。

胆气(dǎn qì)　**gallbladder qi** The essence qi in the gallbladder. See *Su Wen* chapter 48.

胆足少阳之脉　即足少阳胆经，为十二经脉之一。出《灵枢·经脉》。其循行路线从眼外角开始，向上到头角，再向下至耳后，沿颈走手少阳经之前，至肩上，又交叉到手少阳经之后入于缺盆，一支从耳后入耳中，再出走于耳前，至眼外角（目外眦）后方。再一支从眼外角下行至大迎穴，与手少阳经会合至眼眶下，再向下经过下颌角部（颊车穴），下行到颈部，经颈前人迎穴，与前脉会合于缺盆，然后向下入胸腔，穿过横膈，络于肝，属于胆，沿胁里，出少腹两侧气街，绕阴毛处，横向至髋关节的环跳穴处。再一支从缺盆下行至腋，沿胸侧，经过季胁，与前一支脉相会合于髀厌（环跳），再向下沿大腿外侧，膝关节外缘，下行外辅骨（腓骨）之前，直下至外踝上部的骨凹陷处，下出外踝之前，沿足背，行出于足第四趾外侧端（窍阴穴）。再一支从足背，前行至足大趾外侧端，折回穿过爪甲，分布于足大趾爪甲丛毛处（接足厥阴肝经）。

胆足少阳之脉(dǎn zú shào yáng zhī mài)　**gallbladder meridian of foot *shaoyang*** It is one of the twelve regular meridians. See *Ling Shu* chapter 10. It starts from the outer canthus and goes upwards to both sides of the forehead, and then goes downwards to the back of the ears, along the neck to the front of the hand *shaoyang* meridian, and finally goes to the shoulders to cross the hand *shaoyang* meridian again until it goes into Que Pen (ST 12). There are four branches, one of which goes from the back of the ears into the ears and then out to the front of the ears until it ar-

九画

rives at the back of the outer canthus. Another one goes from the outer canthus downwards to Da Ying (ST 5), and then meets the hand *shaoyang* meridian under the rim of the eyes. After that, it goes downwards through *Jia Che* (ST 6) at the lower jaw to the neck, and then goes through Ren Ying (ST 9) to meet the previous branch at Que Pen (ST 12). Then it continues to go downwards into the chest and penetrates the diaphragm, pertaining to the gallbladder and connecting to the liver, and then goes along the rib area out from Qi Jie, or Qi Chong (ST 30) at both sides of the lower belly around the pubic hair, and finally transverses to Huan Tiao (GB 30). Another branch starts from Que Pen (ST 12), goes downwards to the axilla, and then goes across the third rib along the sides of the chest to meet the previous branch at Bi Yan, or Huan Tiao (GB 30). After that, it continues to go downwards along the outer side of the thighs to the outer side of the knees, then downwards

to the front of the shinbones, to the pit on the upper-outer sides of the ankle bones, and then goes along the back of the feet to foot Qiao Yin (GB 44) at the outer sides of the fourth toes. Another branch starts from the back of the feet and goes forward to the outer sides of the big toes, and then retreats backwards through the toe nail to the hair area on the big toe where it meets the liver meridian of foot *jueyin*.

胆胀 病证名。六腑胀之一。症见胁下胀痛、口苦、太息。出《灵枢·胀论》。

胆胀（dǎn zhàng）　**gallbladder distention** Disease name. It is one of the six types of bowl distentions, in which the symptoms manifested are distension and pain in the ribs, and a bitter taste in the mouth and sighing. See *Ling Shu* chapter 35.

胆咳 六腑咳之一。由肝咳不愈传变而成。证候特点为咳呕胆汁，故称胆咳。出《素问·咳论》。

胆咳（dǎn ké）　**gallbladder cough** One of the six types of bowel coughs, and is transformed from chronic liver cough with the typical features of coughing and vomiting bile, hence named gallbladder cough. See *Su Wen* chapter 38.

胆病　胆的疾患。出《灵枢·邪气藏府病形》。

胆病(dǎn bìng)　**gallbladder disease** See *Ling Shu* chapter 4.

胆募俞　指胆的募穴与俞穴。五脏六腑之气聚于胸腹的某些特定腧穴称为募穴,而输注于背部的则称为俞穴,又称背俞穴,皆属足太阳膀胱经。胆的募穴为日月,在第七肋间隙,距腹中线三寸五分处。胆的背俞为胆俞,位于第十胸椎棘突下旁开一寸五分处。出《素问·奇病论》。

胆募俞(dǎn mù shū)　**gallbladder front-*mu* acupoint and transport acupoint** The specific acupoints on the chest and abdomen where the viscera qi gathers are named mustering acupoints, while those on the back are named transport acupoints, or back transport acupoints. All pertain to the urinary bladder meridian of foot *taiyang*. The gallbladder front-*mu* acupoint is Ri Yue (GB 24) located between the seventh and eighth ribs, 3.5 *cun* apart from the central line of the abdomen. The gallbladder has its back transport acupoint which is named gallbladder transport acupoint, located at 1.5 *cun* laterally from the spinous process of the tenth thoracic vertebra. See *Su Wen* chapter 47.

胆瘅　病名。瘅即热。由思虑过度,胆有郁热,胆气上溢而致口苦之病。出《素问·奇病论》。

胆瘅(dǎn dān)　**gallbladder heat** *Dān* means heat. Excessive thought causes heat to stagnate in the gallbladder, and in turn the bile reverses upward to cause a bitter taste. See *Su Wen* chapter 47.

肿　夹脊两侧及腰下髂部丰满隆起的肌肉。出《素问·刺腰痛》。

肿(shèn)　**bulging muscle** Fully bulging muscles on both sides of the spine and on the ilium below the waist. *Su Wen* chapter 41.

胜　①偏盛、偏胜。出《素问·阴阳应象大论》。②克制。出《素问·阴阳应象大论》《素问·金匮真言论》。③战胜。出《素问·评热病论》。④胜任,耐受。出《素问·五常政大论》。⑤运气之胜气,与复气相对而言。一般情况下,各年度的司天在泉之气都是胜气。出《素问·至真要大论》。

胜(shèng)　①Predominance.

See Su Wen chapter 5. ② To restrain. See *Su Wen* chapter 4 and chapter 5. ③ To conquer. See *Su Wen* chapter 33. ④ To endure and tolerate. See *Su Wen* chapter 70. ⑤ Predominant qi, the counter part of retaliatory qi in the theory of the five circuits and six qi. Generally speaking, the celestial-controlling and and terrestrial-controlling qi are both predominant qi. See *Su Wen* chapter 74.

胜复 运气术语。胜,胜气。复,即复气。六气偏胜时,可产生相应之复气来抑制胜气。正常情况下是自然气候的一种自稳调节现象。对维持正常的生态环境有重要意义。在异常情况下则有邪气亢害承制之胜复,而有灾变。出《素问·六微旨大论》。参"胜""复"条。

胜复(shèng fù) **predominant and retaliatory qi** A term of the five circuits and six qi. *Shèng* refers to *Sheng* qi, or predominant qi, and *fù* refers to *fu* qi, or retaliatory qi. When one of the six qi is predominant, there will always be a retaliatory qi coming up to restrain it. Normally, the natural system runs smoothly with the ability of

self-adjustment, which is extremely important for the regular ecological environment. When a pathogen qi does harm to the system and disturbs the order, disaster may occur. See *Su Wen* chapter 68. See "胜" "复".

胕 ① (fú)浮肿。《素问·评热病论》。② (fū)通肤。出《素问·水热穴论》。③ (fǔ)通腐。指发酵腐熟的一类食物。出《素问·异法方宜论》《素问·阴阳类论》。

胕(fú/fū/fǔ) ① (fú), refers to swelling. See *Su Wen* chapter 33. ② (fū) "胕" is the same as "肤", namely skin. See *Su Wen* chapter 61. ③ (fǔ) "胕" is the same as "腐", namely fermented food. See *Su Wen* chapter 12 and chapter 79.

胕肿 ① fú(扶)。为同义复词,即浮肿。出《素问·水热穴论》。② 指局部焮红肿胀。出《素问·至真要大论》。

胕肿(fú zhǒng) ① The same as skin swelling, namely, edema. See *Su Wen* chapter 61. ② Partly red and swollen. See *Su Wen* chapter 74.

胕髓病 (胕,fú)病名。邪气深附于髓而造成的疾病。出《素问·刺疟》。

胕髓病(fù suǐ bìng)　**marrow disease** Disease name. It occurs when pathogenic factors enter deep into the bones and linger in the marrow. See *Su Wen* chapter 36.

胞　① 子宫，又称女子胞。出《灵枢·水胀》。② 同"脬"，指膀胱。出《灵枢·淫邪发梦》。③ 囊皮。出《灵枢·五味论》。

胞（bāo）　① Uterus, also is called *nv zibao*. See *Ling Shu* chapter 57. ② The same as *pāo*（脬）, referring to the bladder. See *Ling Shu*. ③ Pouch skin. See *Ling Shu* chapter 63.

胞气　胞，指膀胱。胞气指膀胱气化功能。出《素问·通评虚实论》。

胞气(bāo qì)　**urinary bladder qi** The qi transformation of the urinary bladder. See *Su Wen* chapter 28.

胞脉　联系子宫（胞宫）的络脉，主要指冲脉。出《素问·评热病论》。

胞脉(bāo mài)　**urinary meridian** The collaterals, especially the thoroughfare vessel，that connect with the uterus. See *Su Wen* chapter 33.

胞络　① 心胞络之脉。出《素问·痿论》。② 子宫的络脉。出《素问·奇病论》。

胞络(bāo luò)　① Collaterals in the pericardium. See *Su Wen* chapter 44. ② Collaterals in the uterus. See *Su Wen* chapter 47.

胞痹　病证名。胞即膀胱。症见膀胱部按之内痛，似灌以热汤的感觉，小便不畅，鼻流清涕等。出《素问·痹论》。

胞痹(bāo bì)　**bladder impediment** Disease name. *Bāo* refers to urinary bladder. It manifests as pain in the urinary bladder when pressed with force, heat inside as if filled with hot water, difficulty in urinating, and a runny nose with clear snivel. See *Su Wen* chapter 43.

脉　① 五体之一，是营运气血的管道。出《灵枢·经脉》《灵枢·决气》《素问·脉要精微论》《素问·痿论》。② 奇恒之腑之一。出《素问·五藏别论》。③ 动脉，切脉诊断之处。出《素问·脉要精微论》。④ 脉象。出《素问·平人气象论》。⑤ 诊察。动词。出《素问·平人气象论》《素问·金匮真言论》。

脉（mài）　① One of the five body constituents, the vessel for the transportation of qi and blood. See *Ling Shu* chapter 21 and 30；*Su Wen* chapter 17 and 44. ② One of the extraordinary organs. See *Su Wen* chapter 11. ③ The pulsating vessel where the pulse taking applies. See *Su Wen* chapter 17. ④ Pulse. See *Su Wen* chapter 18. ⑤ To diagnose. Adverb. See *Su Wen* chapter 4 and chapter 18.

脉口 即寸口，又称气口。因其可切脉之动静，故名。出《灵枢·终始》。参见"寸口"条。

脉口（mài kǒu） **pulse opening** Refers to *cun kou*, or *qi kou* (a small region on the wrist close to the thumb), where the pulse-taking is applied. See *Ling Shu* chapter 9. See "寸口".

脉气 ① 经脉之气，包括经气和络气。出《素问·经脉别论》《素问·气穴论》。② 脉象。出《素问·方盛衰论》。脉象反映正气之盛衰，故脉气有余则生，脉气不足则死。

脉气（mài qì） ① Vessel qi, including meridian qi and collateral qi. See *Su Wen* chapter 21 and chapter 58. ② Pulse manifestation. See *Su Wen* chapter 80. The pulse is the manifestation of qi, hence exuberant qi in the pulse indicates life, while lack of qi indicates death.

脉风 风邪侵袭血脉之病。出《素问·脉要精微论》。

脉风（mài fēng） **vessel wind** The disease caused by wind invading the vessels. See *Su Wen* chapter 17.

脉色 ① 络脉之色。出《灵枢·经脉》。② 脉象与人体外现之五色，用以诊病。出《素问·五藏生成》。

脉色（mài sè） ① The color of the collaterals. See *Ling Shu* chapter 10. ② The pulse and the five colors of the body for the diagnosis of diseases. See *Su Wen* chapter 10.

脉胀 病证名。由于卫气逆行于脉所引起之胀，相对于肤胀而言。出《灵枢·胀论》。

脉胀（mài zhàng） **vessel distention** Disease name. Distention caused by the reversal protective qi, a concept opposite to skin distention. See *Ling Shu* chapter 35.

脉变 古医籍名。从书名推测，可能是一部论脉象变化的专著，已佚。出《素问·玉版论要》。

脉变（mài biàn） *Mai Bian（The Change of Pulse）* An ancient medical classic. Inferring from the title of the book, it is probably a lost monograph on pulse variations. See *Su Wen* chapter 15.

脉法 古医籍名,据书名推测,可能是一种脉学专著,已佚。出《素问·五运行大论》。

脉法(mài fǎ) *Mai Fa(Pulse-taking Methodology)* The name of an ancient medical classic. The title of the book indicates that it is probably a lost monograph on pulse-taking. See *Su Wen* chapter 67.

脉经 古医籍名,已佚。从书名推测当属脉学方面的论著。出《素问·示从容论》。

脉经(mài jīng) *Mai Jing(The Cannon of Pulse-taking)* An ancient medical classic which was lost in history. The name indicates that it is a book on pulse-taking. See *Su Wen* chapter 76.

脉要 古医籍名,据书名推测当是一部脉学专籍,已佚。出《素问·至真要大论》。

脉要(mài yào) *Mai Yao(The Principles of Pulse-taking)* An ancient medical classic,lost in history. See *Su Wen* chapter 74.

脉要精微论 《素问》篇名。其内容主要论述脉诊的原理及方法,并扼要阐述了望、闻、问、切的诊察方法,提出了四诊合参的诊断原则。

脉要精微论(mài yào jīng wēi lùn) **Discussion on the Essentials of Pulse** Chapter name in *Su Wen*. This chapter focuses on the principles and methods of pulse-taking, along with the combined application of diagnostic methods including observing, listening(smelling), inquiring and pulse-taking.

脉度 ①《灵枢》篇名。脉,经脉;度,度量。此篇主要论述了经脉的长度,故名。另外,篇中还简要地讨论了关格病及跷脉的循行路线、功能等内容。② 经脉长短的度数。出《灵枢·骨度》。

脉度(mài dù) ① Length of Channels. Chapter name in *Ling Shu*. *Mài* means meridians and vessels; *dù* is measurement. This chapter discusses the length of the meridians and vessels, hence the name. As well, it briefly introduces the disease name *Guan Ge*(blocking and repulse disease)and the circulation route and function of the springing vessel. ② The length of the meridians and vessels. See *Ling Shu* chapter 14.

脉脱 《素问·方盛衰论》。(1)脉脱略不备。见《素问》王冰注。

（2）指脉虚。见《素问直解》。

（3）指脉不显。见《素问》吴崑注。

脉脱（mài tuō） See *Su Wen* chapter 80.（1）Missing pulse. See *Su Wen* annotated by Wang Bing.（2）Feeble pulse.See *Su Wen Zhi Jie*（*Direct Interpretation on Su Wen*）.（3）Inconspicuous pulse. See annotated *Su Wen* annotated by Wu Kun.

脉解 《素问》篇名。脉，经脉。解，解释。此篇主要内容是解释三阴三阳经脉之气各有主时，以及六经病证的机理，故名。

脉解（mài jiě） **Pulse Explanation** Chapter name in *Su Wen*. *Mài* refers to meridians. *Jiě* means explanation. This chapter mainly explains the specific timing of the three yin and three yang meridians，as well as the mechanism of the six-meridian diseases. Hence the name.

脉痹 病证名。五体痹之一，病发于夏季的痹证。因夏主脉，故名。出《素问·痹论》。

脉痹（mài bì） **vessel impediment** One of the five-body impediments. As summer dominates the vessels，hence，the impediment occurs in summer and is named vessel impediment. See

Su Wen chapter 43.

脉痿 病证名。症见关节不能提挚，下肢纵缓而不能站立。病起于心气热，加之悲哀太甚，阳气内动，致失血而经脉空虚。出《素问·痿论》。

脉痿（mài wěi） **vessel wilting** Disease name. Symptoms include inflexibility of joints，and flaccidity of lower limbs with difficulty to support standing. The reason lies in that heart heat or excessive sadness stirs up abnormal yang qi to cause the loss of blood and empty vessels. See *Su Wen* chapter 44.

脉癫疾 癫疾之邪在血脉者。出《灵枢·癫狂》。参"癫疾"条。

脉癫疾（mài diān jí） **vessel epilepsy** When the pathogenic factors are in the vessels，it is named vessel epilepsy. See *Ling Shu* chapter 22. See "癫疾".

胫 ①泛指小腿。出《素问·骨空论》。②胫骨。出《灵枢·经脉》。

胫（jìng） ① Lower leg (shin). See *Su Wen* chapter 60. ② Lower leg bone (shinbone). See *Ling Shu* chapter 10.

胫纵 胫，小腿，在此指下肢。胫纵，即下肢弛缓不收。出《素问·痿论》。

胫纵（jìng zòng） **lower-limb**

flaccidity *Jing* generally refers to lower leg（shin），but here means lower limbs. This term refers to flaccidity of the lower limbs. See *Su Wen* chapter 44.

胫枯　小腿部肌肉萎缩。出《灵枢·经脉》。

胫枯（jìng kū）　**atrophy of muscles on the shinbone** See *Ling Shu* chapter 10.

胫骨　小腿内侧之长骨。出《灵枢·经脉》。

胫骨（jìng gǔ）　**shinbone** The long bone of the inner side of the shin. See *Ling Shu* chapter 10.

胎孕不育　指五运六气中司天之气与在泉之气对天地间五类生物（毛羽倮鳞介）的胎孕影响。出《素问·五常政大论》。

胎孕不育（tāi yùn bú yù）　**pregnancy and sterility** The celestial qi and terrestrial qi among five circuits and six qi affect the pregnancy and sterility of five types of creatures（beasts, birds, shellfish and bugs, human beings, and insects）. See *Su Wen* chapter 70.

胎病　由胎中所得之病。此指孕妇受惊所造成的先天性癫病。出《素问·奇病论》。

胎病（tāi bìng）　**born disease** It usually refers to epilepsy at birth

caused by fright in pregnant women. See *Su Wen* chapter 47.

急　① 脉象弦急。出《素问·平人气象论》。② 急方。由气味纯厚，作用峻烈的药物组成。出《素问·至真要大论》。③ 筋脉拘急。出《素问·举痛论》。④ 皮肤紧急。出《灵枢·邪气藏府病形》《素问·汤液醪醴论》。⑤ 劲疾。出《素问·四气调神大论》。

急（jí）　① A pulse that is wiry and fast. See *Su Wen* chapter 18. ② Urgent prescription composed of drastic components with heavy tastes. See *Su Wen* chapter 74. ③ Contraction of the meridians. See *Su Wen* chapter 14. ④ Contraction of the skin. See *Ling Shu* chapter 4 and *Su Wen* chapter 14. ⑤ Powerful and fast. See *Su Wen* chapter 2.

急者缓之　治法。言拘急痉挛一类病症，如口噤、项强、手足拘挛、内脏器官痉挛等，应用缓急解痉法治疗。出《素问·至真要大论》。

急者缓之（jí zhě huǎn zhī）　**treating spasms with relaxation** Treatment method for diseases with muscle spasms, such as clenched jaw, stiff neck, cramps of the hand and foot, spasms of the inner organs，etc. See *Su Wen* chapter 74.

急脉　出《素问·气府论》。（1）为睾之系。在阴毛中阴器上两傍,相去同身寸二寸半。厥阴大络通行其中。（2）穴名。属足厥阴肝经,位于大腿内侧,在髂前上棘与耻骨连线下缘中点旁开二寸半处。见《素问注证发微》。

急脉（jí mài）　See *Su Wen* chapter 59. (1) Urgent pulse. It pertains to the testicle system and is located at either side of the genitals in the pubic hair，2.5 *cun* apart from each other. The reverting yin collateral goes through it.（2）The name of acupoint LV 12. It pertains to the liver meridian of foot *jueyin* and is located at the inner side of the thigh，2.5 cun from the midpoint of the line between the anterior superior iliac spine and the pubis. See *Su Wen Zhu Zheng Fa Wei*（*Annotation and Elaboration on Su Wen* ）.

将军之官　指肝。出《素问·灵兰秘典论》。

将军之官（jiāng jūn zhī guān）　**the general organ** It refers to liver. See *Su Wen* chapter 8.

庭　又称颜、额。出《灵枢·五色》。色诊上主候头面部位。

庭（tíng）　**the middle of the forehead** The same as *yán*（颜）and *é*（额）. See *Ling Shu* chapter 49.

疫　指某些发病凶险,传染性极强,能造成大流行的疾病。又名"温疫"。出《素问·刺法论》。

疫（yì）　**plague** Severe diseases that are epidemic and vital，also named *wēn yì*（瘟疫）. See *Su Wen* chapter 72.

养长之道　夏季是自然界万物处于长势旺盛的阶段,根据这个季节及生物发展的特征,来调摄精神情志及生活起居以养生,即为"养长之道"。如夜卧早起,精神愉快,切勿发怒,对外界事物有浓厚的兴趣,使气机宣畅,通泄自如,以适应夏季的长养之气。出《素问·四气调神大论》。

养长之道（yǎng zhǎng zhī dào）　**health preservation of growth in summer** In summer，all lives grow fast and thrive. Hence，health preservation in summer，featuring growth，is attained through regulating emotions，spirit and daily routines according to the features of the season，for example，sleep late and get up early，keep in mood and avoid anger，stay curious to the world，etc. In this way， the qi circulates smoothly to better comply with the seasonal features of summer. See *Su Wen* chapter 2.

养生 又称摄生。采用一定的措施调养身心，以延年益寿。出《素问·灵兰秘典论》。

养生（yǎng shēng） **health preservation** To regulate the mind and body in certain ways for longevity. See *Su Wen* chapter 8.

养生之道 春气生发是自然万物处下推陈出新、生命萌发的阶段，根据这个季节及生物发展的特征，来调摄精神情志及生活起居以养生，即为"养生之道"。如夜卧早起，漫步于庭院，使精神愉快，胸怀开畅，以适应春季的生发之气。出《素问·四气调神大论》。

养生之道（yǎng shēng zhī dào） **health preservation of generating in spring** The qi in spring generates new lives, hence, it is appropriate to preserve health by regulating emotions and daily life according to the features of generating in spring. For example，going to bed late while getting up early；strolling in gardens to keep a good mood

and open-mindedness，etc. See *Su Wen* chapter 2.

养收之道 秋季是自然万物处于肃杀收敛的阶段，根据这个季节及生物发展特征，来调摄精神情志及生活起居以养生，即为"养收之道"。如早睡早起，保持神志安宁，不使神思外驰，以适应秋季的收敛之气。出《素问·四气调神大论》。

养收之道（yǎng shōu zhī dào） **health preservation of convergence in autumn** Autumn is a period when all lives withdraw and converge. According to the characteristics of this season, it is appropriate to preserve health by going to bed early and get up early, too, so as to maintain a tranquil mind and avoiding excessive thoughts. See *Su Wen* chapter 2.

养藏之道 冬季是主闭藏的季节，万物蛰藏，生机潜伏，根据这一季节和生物发展的特征，来调摄精神情志及生活起居以养生，即为"养藏之道"。如早睡晚起，不妄事操劳，神情安静自若，趋暖避寒，不使皮肤开泄，以适应冬季的闭藏之气。出《素问·四气调神大论》。

养藏之道（yǎng cáng zhī dào） **health preservation with storage**

in winter Winter is featured by storage. All lives hibernate and store energy. It is appropriate to preserve health according to the features of winter. For example，going to bed early and getting up late，avoiding to work too hard，keeping calm with a tranquil mind，remaining warm in case of catching a cold，and keeping the pores on the skin closed so as to comply with the characteristic of storage in winter. See *Su Wen* chapter 2.

前阴 又称阴器，即外生殖器。出《素问·厥论》。

前阴（qián yīn） **genitals** See *Su Wen* chapter 45.

前谷 经穴名。手太阳小肠经之荥穴，在手小指外侧本节前陷者中。出《灵枢·本输》。

前谷（qián gǔ） **Qian Gu (SI 2)** The brook acupoint of the small intestine meridian of hand *tai-yang*，located at the small pit on the dorsal aspect of the hand on the little finger laterally. See *Ling Shu* chapter 2.

首风 病名。因沐发而感受风邪的风证。症见多汗恶风，每临刮风则头痛。出《素问·风论》。

首风（shǒu fēng） **head wind** Disease name. It refers to the wind syndrome caused by wind evil after washing the hair. The symptoms include excessive sweating，aversion to wind，and headaches when feeling wind blow on the head. See *Su Wen* chapter 42.

逆治 违背治疗规律，不可治而治之，称为逆治。出《灵枢·玉版》。

逆治（nì zhì） **counteracting treatment** To treat the disease when it seems to be untreatable. See *Ling Shu* chapter 60.

逆顺 ①《灵枢》篇名。逆顺，指反常与正常，包括气行的逆顺和针刺方法运用的逆顺。此篇主要论述人体发生气血逆乱后，针刺方法运用的逆与顺，故名。② 正、反两种治法。出《素问·至真要大论》。③ 偏义复词，指反常状态。见《素问·痿论》。④ 气血之有余、不足。出《灵枢·海论》。⑤ 经脉循行的不同方向。出《灵枢·逆顺肥瘦》。⑥ 疾病的轻重预后的好坏。出《素问·五运行大论》。

逆顺（nì shùn） ① Chapter name in *Ling Shu*. It refers to normal and abnormal qi circulation and the application of acupuncture. ② Routine and counteracting treatment. See *Su Wen* chapter 74. ③ A compound

Chinese word laying the stress on one of the two characters which refers to the abnormal condition. See *Su Wen* chapter 44. ④ Superabundance and deficiency of qi and blood. See *Ling Shu* chapter 33. ⑤ Different directions that the meridians run in. See *Ling Shu* chapter 38. ⑥ The severity and the prognosis of the disease. See *Su Wen* chapter 67.

逆顺肥瘦　《灵枢》篇名。逆顺，指经脉循行走向及气血上下运行的逆顺。肥瘦，言形体之肥壮与瘦小。该篇着重讨论了经脉走向规律，气血滑涩以及形体的肥瘦壮幼，并以此作为施治的依据，故名。

逆顺肥瘦(nì shùn féi shòu)　**Abnormality, Normality, Obesity and Emaciation** Chapter name in *Ling Shu*. *Nì shùn* refers to the circulation route of the meridians, qi and blood. *Féi shòu* refers to a stout and strong or a thin and small stature, which is the basic factor for treatment.

逆调论　《素问》篇名。逆，反也；调，调顺。逆调，即不调顺。人体气血阴阳，和调为顺，逆调则病。本篇论述了由于气血阴阳、脏脉、脏腑失调所致的内热、内寒、骨痹、肉烁、肉苛以及不得卧等病征，故名。

逆调论(nì tiáo lùn)　**Discussion on Disharmony** Chapter name in *Su Wen*. *Nì* means adverse； *tiáo* means harmonious and smooth，hence the term *nì tiáo* means disharmonious or unsmooth，which refers to a condition. This chapter discusses symptoms such as interior heat，interior coldness，bone impediment，emaciation（by interior heat），paralysis，and difficulty in lying down，etc. caused by the disorder of yin and yang，qi and blood，and viscera.

洁净府　治法。利小便，使膀胱洁净，是消除水湿的常用方法。净府，即膀胱。出《素问·汤液醪醴论》。

洁净府(jié jìng fǔ)　**cleaning the bladder** Treatment method，disinhibiting the urine and purging the urinary bladder. Usual treatment method to eliminate dampness. See *Su Wen* chapter 14.

洪　指洪脉。脉来如洪水，滔滔满指，为太阳气盛之象，又主邪热亢盛。出《素问·平人气象论》。

洪(hóng)　**surging pulse** The pulse feels as if flooding，which

九画

is the manifestation of the exuberance of qi in the *taiyang* meridian, and pathogenic heat. See *Su Wen* chapter 18.

浊气 ① 水谷精气中富有营养而浓厚的部分。出《素问·经脉别论》。② 积于气海之宗气。出《灵枢·阴阳清浊》。③ 糟粕。出《灵枢·小针解》《素问·五藏别论》。④ 浊阴之气。出《素问·阴阳应象大论》。见《类经·阴阳一》。⑤ 邪气。出《灵枢·忧恚无言》。⑥ 卫气。出《灵枢·五乱》。见《太素·营卫气行》。

浊气（zhuó qì） ① Turbid qi. The essence and qi from water and grains with rich nutrients. See *Su Wen* chapter 21. ② Ancestral qi that gathers in Qi Hai（CV 6）. See *Ling Shu* chapter 40. ③ Dross. See *Ling Shu* Chapter 3 and *Su Wen* chapter 11. ④ Turbid yin qi. See *Su Wen* chapter 5. See *Lei Jing*（*Classified Classic*）"Yin and Yang Chapter 1". ⑤ Pathogenic qi. See *Ling Shu* chapter 69. ⑥ Defensive qi. See *Ling Shu* chapter 34. See *Tai Su*（*Classified Study on Huang Di Nei Jing*）"Nutrient and Defensive qi Circulation".

浊阴 ① 食物的糟粕和废浊的水液。出《素问·阴阳应象大论》。② 五脏阴精。出《素问·阴阳应象大论》。③ 饮食物。出《素问·阴阳应象大论》。④ 自然界中重浊有形物质。出《素问·阴阳应象大论》。

浊阴（zhuó qì） ① Turbid yin. Food waste matters and waste liquid. See *Su Wen* chapter 5. ② Yin essence of the five viscera. See *Su Wen* chapter 5. ③ Drinks and food. See *Su Wen* chapter 5. ④ All the heavy tangible matter in the nature. See *Su Wen* chapter 5.

洞心 心中空虚感。出《灵枢·五味论》。与"心气内洞"义似，参阅该条。

洞心（dòng xīn） sense of emptiness See *Ling Shu* chapter 56. See "心气内洞".

洞泄 病证名。泄泻无度，如洞之漏下，故名。出《素问·生气通天论》。

洞泄（dòng xiè） through-flux diarrhea Disease name. Through-flux diarrhea is as serious as a leaking cave. See *Su Wen* chapter 3.

涎 口液，五液之一。脾开窍于口，涎（xián 咸）与脾关系密切。出《素问·宣明五气》。

涎（xián）　**saliva** One of the five kinds of fluids. The spleen opens at the mouth，therefore saliva is closely related to the spleen. See *Su Wen* chapter 23.

涎下　口涎流出之症。出《灵枢·口问》。

涎下（xián xià）　**uncontrollable drooling** See *Ling Shu* chapter 28.

津　① 指津液中较清稀，流动性较大的部分。由水谷所化生，布散于皮肤、肌肉、孔窍等组织，有濡养、滋润作用。出《灵枢·五癃津液别》。② 津液。出《灵枢·决气》。③ 淫溢。出《素问·生气通天论》。④ 渗泌出的汁液。出《素问·六元正纪大论》。

津（jīn）　① The thin part of the body fluids with high mobility. It is generated from water and grain，and permeates the skin，muscles and orifices for nourishment and moisture. See *Ling Shu* chapter 36. ② Essence liquid. See *Ling Shu* chapter 30. ③ Surplus. See *Su Wen* chapter 3. ④ Exudated liquid. See *Su Wen* chapter 71.

津脱　津液的突然亡失，多因大汗所致。出《灵枢·决气》。

津脱（jīn tuō）　**fluid collapse** The sudden loss of body fluids，mostly caused by excessive sweating. See *Ling Shu* chapter 30.

津液　① 津与液的合称，包括体内正常体液及分泌物。来源于水谷，由脾胃化生而成。根据其性状、分布部位及功用不同，分为津和液。出《灵枢·五癃津液别》。② 小便。出《灵枢·本输》。③ 病理性水饮。每由阳气阻遏，气化失司，津液失其敷布之常，聚集而成。出《素问·汤液醪醴论》。④ 水谷精气。出《素问·太阴阳明论》。

津液（jīn yè）　① A term combining body fluids and secretions. They are generated from water and grain by the spleen and the stomach. According to their consistency，location and function，they are named body fluids and secretions. See *Ling Shu* chapter 36. See "津" and "液". ② Urine. See *Ling Shu* chapter 2. ③ Water-rheum caused by the disorder of qi transformation induced from the stagnation of yang qi and the malfunction of body fluids and secretions in moisturizing and distributing. See *Su Wen* chapter 14. ④ The essence qi from water and grain. See *Su Wen* chapter 29.

九画

津液之府 指膀胱。膀胱所聚之溺液,是气化过程中的代谢产物,由津液所化,故以津液之府名之。出《灵枢·本输》。

津液之府(jīn yè zhī fǔ) **the house of body fluids** The fluids collected in the urinary bladder is the outcome of qi transformation and originates from body fluids. Hence the name. See *Ling Shu* chapter 2.

恢刺 刺法之一。在患处附近取穴,先直刺入针,再提针于皮下,向前后两旁斜刺,需数次行针,以恢复其气。用治筋脉拘急痹痛之证。

恢刺(huī cì) **lateral needling** One of the needling methods, in which the needling is applied near the affected part. It is performed by needling inside the flesh directly before lifting the needle up until it stops under the skin, and then needling obliquely for several times to regain the qi of the constrained, paralyzed or painful sinews.

恬惔虚无 恬惔,(tiándàn 田旦)安静的意思。言闲静淡泊,没有杂念。出《素问·上古天真论》。

恬惔虚无(tián dàn xū wú) tranquilized mind and empty thoughts See *Su Wen* chapter 1.

举痛论 《素问》篇名。举,列举。篇内列举了十四种痛证的病机和特征,故名。又,林亿、吴崑认为"举"乃"卒"之误,篇中有因寒气入经而引起的卒然而痛,故名。此篇主要讨论寒邪客于脏腑经脉引起多种疼痛的病机与症状,以及鉴别不同痛证的具体方法,阐述了九气为病的病机与症状。

举痛论(jǔ tòng lùn) **Discussion on Pains** Chapter name in *Su Wen*. *Jǔ* means enumeration. This chapter enumerates fourteen pain diseases and their manifestations. *Lin Yi* and *Wu Kun* thought *Jǔ*(举) was a mistake of *Zú*(卒, sudden), for this chapter records the sudden pain caused by cold qi in the meridians. This chapter mainly discusses the mechanism and symptoms of multiple pain diseases caused by pathogenic cold in the viscera and meridians, along with various methods to identify pain diseases and the mechanism and symptoms caused by the nine pathogenic qi.

宣明五气 《素问》篇名。宣明,宣扬阐明;五气,五脏之气。此篇主要阐述五脏的生理、病理活动变化规律，运用五行学说，将病因、脉象、药物性味、饮食等方面加以分类归纳，作为临床辨治的指导原则，故名。

宣明五气（xuān míng wǔ qì）
Discussion on the Elucidation of Five Qi Chapter name in *Su Wen*. *Xuān míng* means to expound and clarify; *wǔ qì* means the qi of the five viscera. This chapter mainly expounds the physiological and pathological movements and the discipline of the five viscera, and collates the clinical guidance based on the five elements theory into categories including causes, pulse manifestations, nature and flavors of medicine, food and drink, etc.

宫　五音之一。五行属木，为中央长夏土之音。运气学说将五音代表五运，以五音建运，则宫为土运。出《素问·阴阳应象大论》。

宫（gōng）　*gong* One of the five musical tones. It pertains to the wood element, and is the tone of the central long-summer. According to the doctrine of the five circuits and six qi, the five tones represent the five circuits, and *gong* refers to the circuit of earth. See *Su Wen* chapter 5.

客　① 运气学说中的客气，与主气相对而言，司值年天气的盛衰变化，包括司天、在泉、四间气，根据值年地支而演变，十二年一轮转，周而复始，如客之往来。见《素问·至真要大论》。参"间气""司天""在泉"诸条。见"司天在泉左右间气位置图"。② 泛指邪气，因其自外而入，故名。见《灵枢·小针解》。③ 后至于寸口部的脉象。三阴三阳之脉来有先后之分，先至脉气为主，后至脉气为客。见《素问·阴阳类论》。④ 寄附、留着的意思。见《素问·风论》。

客（kè）　① Exogenous qi according to the doctrine of the five circuits and six qi, a counterpart of dominant qi. It dominates the changes of the yearly circuit, including celestial control, terrestrial effect, and four interval qi. They come and go regularly every twelve years according to the Earthly Branches as if guests coming and going. See *Su Wen* chapter 80. See "间气""司天""在泉"; and refer to "The position of the interval qi of Celestial control and Terrestrial effect". ② Pathogen qi. It originates from the outside world and enters the body, hence the name. See *Ling Shu* chapter 3. ③ The pulse behind *cun kou*. Among the pulses of the three yin and three yang, some come early, some later. The pulses which come early are dominant pulses, while those which come later are guest pulses. See *Su Wen* chapter 79. ④ To linger in or to reside in. See *Su Wen* chapter 42.

客气 出《素问·标本病传论》。① 指外感邪气,在身犹客之在舍,故称。见《素问直解》。② 运气术语。与主气相对而言,主值年天气的盛衰变化。见《类经·标本五》。

客气(kè qì) See *Su Wen* chapter 65. ① The exogenous pathogen qi, as if it were a guest in the body. See *Su Wen Zhi Jie*(*Direct Interpretation on Su Wen*). ② Guest qi. A term of the five circuits and six qi. Opposite to dominant qi, dominate the yearly circuit. See *Lei Jing*(*Classified Classic*)"Branch and Root Chapter 5".

客主人 经穴名。别名上关,属足少阳胆经。在颧弓上缘,距耳廓前缘约一寸处,与下关直

对。出《素问·刺禁论》。

客主人(kè zhǔ rén) **Ke Zhu Ren(GB 3)** It pertains to the gallbladder meridian of foot *shaoyang*. It is located at the upper rim of the cheekbones, one *cun* apart from the auricle and opposite to Xia Guan(ST 7) vertically. See *Su Wen* chapter 52.

客者除之 治法。客,指自外而入客留的病邪。言外邪侵入人体而留着者,应用驱除病邪的方法。如邪犯体表,用解表发汗法;邪犯于里,用攻里通下法等。出《素问·至真要大论》。

客者除之(kè zhě chú zhī) **exogenous pathogens should be expelled** Treatment method. *Kè* refers to the exogenous pathogens residing in the body. It is appropriate to apply the methods of expelling the exogenous pathogens with the exterior-relieving method if the surface of the body is attacked, and the cathartic and laxative methods if they attack the interior viscera. See *Su Wen* chapter 74.

扁骨 泛指扁平形无骨髓腔的骨骼,如肋骨。出《素问·骨空论》。

扁骨(biǎn gǔ) **flat bone** It refers to the flat-shaped bones without marrow cavities, eg., ribs. See

九画

Su Wen chapter 60.

神　① 自然界阴阳神妙莫测的变化。出《素问·天元纪大论》。② 生命功能活动的总称。出《灵枢·天年》。③ 人的精神活动，包括意识、思维、情感、悟性、智慧等。出《素问·八正神明论》。④ 人体生命活动的外在表现，即神采。出《素问·刺法论》。⑤ 针刺感应。出《素问·诊要经终论》。⑥ 医生的医疗技术高超。出《灵枢·邪气藏府病形》。⑦ 某些维持生命活动的重要物质。如正气、气血、水谷精气等。出《素问·八正神明论》《灵枢·平人绝谷》《灵枢·九针十二原》。⑧ 神灵。出《素问·宝命全形论》。

神（shén）　① The mysterious and unpredictable changes of yin and yang in nature. See *Su Wen* chapter 66. ② A general term for life and activities. See *Ling Shu* chapter 54. ③ Mental activities including mind, thoughts, emotions, comprehension, wisdom, etc. See *Su Wen* chapter 26. ④ Spirit glitter, the manifestation of human lives. See *Su Wen* chapter 72. ⑤ Acupuncture response. See *Su Wen* chapter 16. ⑥ Superb medical techniques. See *Ling Shu* chapter

4. ⑦ Vital substances to sustain life, such as healthy qi, blood, food, liquids, and essence qi, etc. See *Su Wen* chapter 26; *Ling Shu* chapter 1 and chapter 32. ⑧ God. See *Su Wen* chapter 25.

神门　手掌后锐骨之端心经动脉，可诊察心气之盛衰。出《素问·至真要大论》。

神门（shén mén）　spirit gate The stirred heart pulse at the tip of the palm bone where the amount of heart qi can be examined. See *Su Wen* chapter 74.

神不使　神气衰败，不能使针药等发挥治疗作用。出《素问·汤液醪醴论》。

神不使（shén bú shǐ）　the spirit was not employed The deteriorating spirit hinders the function of the medicine and acupuncture. See *Su Wen* chapter 14.

神气　① 心所主的精神意识情志活动。出《灵枢·天年》。② 真气。出《灵枢·九针十二原》。③ 血。血是维持人体生命功能的重要物质，是神的物质基础。出《灵枢·营卫生会》。④ 五脏的阳气。出《素问·生气通天论》。

神气（shén qì）　① The mind activities controlled by the heart. See *Ling Shu* chapter 54. ② Gen-

九画

uine qi. See *Ling Shu* chapter 1. ③ Blood. Blood is a substance of vital importance to maintain life，and it is fundamental to spirit. See *Ling Shu* chapter 18. ④ Yang qi in the five viscera. See *Su Wen* chapter 3.

神机　生命活动之征象。出《素问·五常政大论》。(1) 泛指生命体内在的阴阳变化之机，是生命征象的根本。见《素问直解》《素问集注》。(2) 具体指动物内在的知觉运动之机及生长壮老之变化。见《类经·运气十五》。

神机（shén jī）　**spirit mechanism** See *Su Wen* chapter 70. (1) It generally refers to the changes and exchanges of yin and yang in the body，which is considered the sign of life. See *Su Wen Zhi Jie*（*Direct Interpretation on Su Wen*）. See *Su Wen Ji Zhu*（*Collected Annotation of Su Wen*）. (2) It specifically refers to the mental activities and changes that occur with growth. See *Lei Jing*（*Classified Classic*）"Circuits and Qi Chapter 15".

神光　神明。出《素问·本病论》。

神光（shén guāng）　**spirit brilliance** See *Su Wen* chapter 73.

神农　为传说中的古代帝王，与燧人、伏羲合称"三皇"。出《素问·著至教论》。

神农（shén nóng）　**Shen Nong (the farmer god)** He is the legendary ancient king, the founder of farming and medicine. He is considered one of the Three Kings，the other two being Sui Ren（the god of fire）and Fu Xi（the forebear of human beings）. See *Su Wen* chapter 75.

神明　① 事物内部的变化及其外在的征象。出《素问·阴阳应象大论》。② 人的精神意识聪明智慧。《素问·灵兰秘典论》。③ 形容治疗技术的灵验神妙。见《素问·八正神明论》。

神明（shén míng）　① The interior changes and exterior manifestations. See *Su Wen* chapter 5. ② The mind，thoughts，and wisdom of human beings. See *Su Wen* chapter 8. ③ A description of superb medical techniques. See *Su Wen* chapter 26.

神明之乱　神明，在此指精神意识思维活动，由心所藏守。人的精神思维意识活动发生紊乱，是由于心主神明的功能失常。其时可见衣被不检敛，言语善骂詈，且无论是否亲近或不熟悉，皆不回避等现象。出

《素问·脉要精微论》。

神明之乱（shén míng zhī luàn）
the disorder of spirit brilliance
Spirit brilliance here refers to the mental activities stored by the heart. The disorder of spirit brilliance is caused by the malfunction of the heart which is the governor of the mind. The patients are known to be disheveled, using profanity in their speech, and having no sense of distance between people, farmiliar or not. See *Su Wen* chapter 17.

神藏五 指藏神气的五脏,即肝、心、脾、肺、肾。见《素问·六节藏象论》。

神藏五（shén cáng wǔ） **five viscera storing five Shen (spirit) qi** The five viscera include the liver, heart, spleen, lung, and kidney. See *Su Wen* chapter 9.

祝 即祝由。出《灵枢·贼风》。见"祝由"条。

祝（zhù） **zhu** See *Ling Shu* chapter 58. See "祝由".

祝由 祝,祝说、祝告。由,病由。通过祝说发病的原由,转移患者的精神情志,以达到调整病人的气机,使精神内守以治病的一种方法。古代设有祝由科,专以祝祷治病。祝由疗法

包含有精神疗法的意义。出《素问·移精变气论》。

祝由（zhù yóu） **exorcism therapy** *Zhù* means to invoke; *yóu* refers to the origin of diseases. It is a treatment method that distracts the patient from the suffering through invoking the origin of the disease. It may regulate and smooth the qi circulation and preserve the inner mind, hence to treat the patient. In ancient times, Chinese medicine included it as a specific branch to treat people through invoking the origin of the disease. In modern times, it is considered a kind of psychotherapy. See *Su Wen* chapter 13.

退位 运气术语。指旧岁司天之气退位作右间气,旧年在泉之气退位作右间气。此为客气司天、在泉、四间气转移变化的规律。出《素问·本病论》。

退位（tuì wèi） **qi abdication** A term of the five circuits and six qi. The past celestial qi and terrestrial qi abdicate to be the right-spaced qi. This is a discipline of the exchanges of celestial, terrestrial and four-spaced qi. See *Su Wen* chapter 73.

眉本 穴位名。即攒竹穴。在眉

毛内侧端。出《素问·气穴论》。

眉本(méi běn)　**Mei Ben（BL 2）**
Located at the inner side of the eyebrows. See *Su Wen* chapter 58.

怒　① 七情之一。怒为肝志,大怒易伤肝。出《素问·阴阳应象大论》。② 形容冬季气候寒冷凛冽。出《素问·脉要精微论》。

怒(nù)　① Anger, one of the seven emotions. Anger corresponds to the liver, thus violent anger harms the liver. See *Su Wen* chapter 5. ② A description of coldness in winter. See *Su Wen* chapter 17.

怒则气上　怒则气上逆,症见面红、目赤、头胀头痛,甚则呕血飧泄等。出《素问·举痛论》。

怒则气上(nù zé qì shàng)
Anger causes qi rising. Symptoms include a red face, red eyes, headache, vomiting blood and diarrhea. See *Su Wen* chapter 39.

怒则气逆　大怒伤肝使肝气上逆,出现面红目赤、头痛头晕,甚则呕血;肝气横逆犯脾,出现腹胀纳呆、泄泻等。出《素问·举痛论》。

怒则气逆(nù zé qì nì)　**Anger reverses liver qi.** Violent anger reverses liver qi upwards to cause a red face and eyes, head-aches, dizziness, and sometimes even vomiting blood; violent anger reverses the qi traversely which leads to abdominal distention, loss of appetite, and diarrhea. See *Su Wen* chapter 39.

怒伤肝　怒为肝志,大怒则肝气上逆,可出现面赤头痛、眩晕,甚或血随气逆而吐血等。出《素问·阴阳应象大论》《素问·五运行大论》。

怒伤肝(nù shāng gān)　**Anger damages the liver.** Anger corresponds to the liver. Violent anger reverses the liver qi up-wards to cause a red face and eyes, headaches, dizziness, and sometimes even vomiting blood. See *Su Wen* chapter 5 and chapter 67.

怒胜思　怒为肝木之志,思为脾土之志,木能克土,故云怒胜思。思虑过度而气结,怒可宣泄气机,忘思虑,这是一种“以情制情”的心理现象和治病方法。出《素问·阴阳应象大论》《素问·五运行大论》。

怒胜思(nù shèng sī)　**Anger prevails over thought.** Anger corresponds to liver wood, and thought to spleen earth. Wood restrains earth, hence anger prevails over thought. Excessive thought blocks qi, while anger may unblock the qi and dismiss excessive thought. This is a kind of psychotherapy of using one emotion to restrain another emotion. See *Su Wen* chapter 5 and chapter 67.

勇士　为体质的一种类型，与怯士相对。其人外貌特征是目光深沉而坚定，前额宽阔，发怒时怒目圆睁，毛发竖立，面色青黑，其内脏特点是三焦的纹理横行，心脏端直，肝脏大而坚定，胆汁充盈，发怒时，气势旺盛，胸廓张大，肝脏上举，而胆气横溢。出《灵枢·论勇》。

勇士（yǒng shì）　**brave man** The body constitution opposite to a coward. Brave men have deep and stony gazes, and wide foreheads. When they are angry, their eyes are widely opened, with hair standing straight, and faced darkened. They have clear traversed lines on their triple *jiao*, an upright heart, a big and firm liver, and full bile. When they are angry, they look aggressive with a widened chest, an uplifted liver and overflowing bile. See *Ling Shu* chapter 50.

柔痓　病证名。即柔痉。出《素问·气厥论》。(1)筋柔缓无力。见《素问》王冰注。(2)柔即阴，因肺属太阴，肾属少阴，肺移热于肾，以阴传阴，故称柔痓。见《素问识》。

柔痓（róu chì）　**febrile convulsion without chills** Disease name. See *Su Wen* chapter 37.（1）The sinews are soft and powerless. See *Su Wen* annotated by Wang Bing.（2）*Róu* has the same meaning as yin. The lung pertains to *shaoyin* and the kidney to *shaoyin*, both of which pertain to yin. When the lung transfers heat to the kidney, it is transferred from yin to yin. See *Su Wen Zhi*（*Understanding Su Wen*）.

结　①结脉。脉来迟缓，有不规则歇止。出《素问·平人气象论》。②结滞。出《素问·举痛论》。③结聚之症。出《素问·至真要大论》。④绳结。出《灵枢·九针十二原》。⑤终止。出《灵枢·根结》。

结（jié）　① Knotted pulse. The pulse comes slowly and pauses irregularly. See *Su Wen* chapter 18. ② Block. See *Su Wen* chapter 39. ③ Gathering and binding. See *Ling Shu* chapter

1. ④ Knot. See *Ling Shu* chapter 1. ⑤ Termination. See *Ling Shu* chapter 5.

结阳　阳气郁结。出《素问·阴阳别论》。

结阳（jié yáng）　**knotted yang qi** See *Su Wen* chapter 7.

结阴　阴气内结。出《素问·阴阳别论》。

结阴（jié yīn）　**knotted yin qi** See *Su Wen* chapter 7.

结者散之　治法。体内有气血郁结、津液积聚等症，应用消散法治疗。出《素问·至真要大论》。

结者散之（jié zhě sàn zhī）　**treating pathogenic accumulation with dissipation** Treatment method applied to the symptoms of stagnated qi and blood, with liquid gathering and binding in the human body. See *Su Wen* chapter 74.

结络　结，连结；络，连络。结络，筋肉之间相联系的部分。《素问·皮部论》。

结络（jié luò）　**connecting parts** *Jié* refers to binding, and *luò* to connection. It refers to the part that connects the sinews with the flesh. See *Su Wen* chapter 56.

结喉　喉头软骨隆起处，又称喉结。出《灵枢·骨度》。

结喉（jié hóu）　**Adam's apple** The large protrusion at the front of the neck. See *Ling Shu* chapter 14.

络　① 泛指孙络、浮络、别络等大小不同的各种络脉。由经脉分出，其状如网，遍布全身，沟通表里、经脉、脏器，以流通气血。出《灵枢·脉度》。② 专指较大络脉。出《素问·调经论》。③ 专指血络。出《灵枢·百病始生》《灵枢·血络论》。④ 目眦内的赤色脉络。出《灵枢·大惑论》。⑤ 连络。出《灵枢·经脉》。⑥ 络穴。即十五络脉别出的穴位。出《灵枢·寒热病》。

络（luò）　① All of the collaterals, such as the minute collateral, the floating collateral, and the division collateral, which are branches of the major meridians. They act as nets covering the whole body and connect the interior and exterior of the body, the meridians, and the viscera for the circulation of the blood and qi. See *Ling Shu* chapter 17. ② Major collaterals. See *Su Wen* chapter 62. ③ Blood vessels. See *Ling Shu* chapter 66 and *Ling Shu* chapter 10. ④ The red collateral in the canthus. See *Ling Shu* chapter

80. ⑤ To connect. See *Ling Shu* chapter 10. ⑥ Acupoints along the collaterals. See *Ling Shu* chapter 21.

络气　行于络脉的气，与经气相对而言。出《素问·通评虚实论》。

络气（luò qì）　**collateral qi** That which pairs with the meridian qi. See *Su Wen* chapter 28.

络刺　九刺法之一。刺皮下小络之血脉，以泻其郁血，多用于热证、实证。目前临床上各种浅刺放血法，均属于本法范围。出《灵枢·官针》。

络刺（luò cì）　**collateral needling** One of nine needling methods, which is used to treat heat and excess syndromes by releasing blood from small collaterals under the skin. Many kinds of clinical needling therapies pertain to collateral needling. See *Ling Shu* chapter 7.

络俞　孙络的俞穴。出《素问·诊要经终论》。

络俞（luò shū）　**the acupoints along the minute collaterals** See *Su Wen* chapter 16.

络脉　经脉的分支，是经脉系统的主要组成部分，其循行部位较经脉为浅。络脉有别络、浮络、孙络之分。出《灵枢·经脉》。

络脉（luò mài）　**collateral** Collaterals are the branches of the meridian system running along the relatively superficial area of body. They can be categorized into diverging collaterals, floating collaterals and minute collaterals. See *Ling Shu* chapter 10.

绝汗　症状名。为汗暴出如油、如珠而难收，常见于濒死期。出《素问·诊要经终论》。

绝汗（jué hàn）　**exhausted sweating** Name of syndrome which is manifested as uncontrollable sweating, as if oil or water, and is usually seen among dying patients. See *Su Wen* chapter 16.

绝阳　纯阴无阳之谓。出《素问·阴阳离合论》。

绝阳（jué yáng）　**absolute yin without yang** See *Su Wen* chapter 6.

绝阴　绝，尽也，阴之尽，谓之绝阴，指足厥阴肝经。出《素问·阴阳离合论》。

绝阴（jué yīn）　**the end of the yin meridian** *Jué* refers to the end, and *jué yīn* refers to the end of the liver meridian of foot jueyin. See *Su Wen* chapter 6.

绝骨　① 经穴名。出《素问·刺疟》。(1) 悬钟穴。见《类经·疾病五十》《难经·四十五难》。(2) 阳辅穴。见《素问》王冰注。

九画

② 骨骼部位名。指外踝上方，当腓骨与腓骨长短肌之间的凹陷处。出《灵枢·经脉》。

绝骨（jué gǔ） ① Acupoint name. See *Su Wen* chapter 36. (1) Xuan Zhong（GB 39）. See *Lei Jing* (*Classified Classic*) "On Diseases Chapter 50" and *Nan Jing* (*Classic of Difficult Issues*) "The 45th Difficult Issue". (2) Yang Fu（GB 38）. See *Su Wen* annotated by Wang Bing. ② Specific location on the bone，at the pit between the fibula and the long and short fibula muscles over the lateral malleolus. See *Ling Shu* chapter 10.

十 画

素天之气　古代天文学家在亢、氐、昴、毕诸宿间看到的白色之气。其中亢、氐二宿当东方偏南之乙位；昴、毕二宿当西方偏南之庚位。《内经》以此说明"天干纪运"的方法，即白属金，故金主治乙庚年。出《素问·五运行大论》。

素天之气（sù tiān zhī qì）　**qi of white heaven** The white qi that ancient astronomers saw in the area between amiboshi, root, pleiades, and astarname. Among them, amiboshi and root are at the yi place in the south east; pleiades and astarname are at the geng place in the south west. The *Nei Jing*（*Internal Classic*）used this to explain the "Using the ten Heavenly Stems to record the year" method, that is, white pertains to metal, so metal governs the year of yi geng. See *Su Wen* chapter 67.

素问　又称《黄帝内经素问》。是《黄帝内经》的一部分，作者不详，成书年代不晚于东汉。参"黄帝内经"条。

素问（sù wèn）　*Su Wen* Also named *Huang Di Nei Jing Su Wen*（*Huang Di's Internal Classic: Su Wen*）. Section of *Huang Di's Internal Classic* of which the author is unknown. It was written in no later than the Eastern Han Dynasty. See "黄帝内经" for detail.

振埃　刺五节法之一。主要用于阳气逆于胸中而出现的咳喘胸满、肩息上气等症。取天容穴或廉泉穴。言其效验有如振落尘埃，故名。出《灵枢·刺节真邪》。

振埃（zhèn āi）　**to shake off dust** One of the five needling methods mainly used in yang qi reversing symptoms such as cough, asthma, and raised-shoulder breathing. Using the acupoints Tian Rong（SI 17）or Lian Quan（CV 23）to treat, the effects are obvious like shaking dust off clothes, hence the name. See *Ling Shu* chapter 75.

振栗　振，颤抖。栗因寒冷而发抖。出《素问·六元正纪大论》。

振栗（zhèn lì）　**shake** It usually

refers to shaking due to cold. See *Su Wen* chapter 71.

振掉 颤动摇晃的一类症状。出《素问·脉要精微论》。

振掉(zhèn diào) **tremble** Symptoms of trembling and shaking. See *Su Wen* chapter 17.

振寒 症状名。身躯因畏寒而振栗。多因风寒客于肌腠，阳气遏郁，不能达于体表所致。出《素问·评热病论》。

振寒(zhèn hán) **quivering with cold** Name of symptom where the body shudders from chills, usually due to wind-coldness invading the muscles and restraining yang qi from reaching the body's surface. See *Su Wen* chapter 33.

损者温之 治法。言虚损疾病，如阳虚、阴虚、气虚、血虚等，应用温养补益法治疗。出《素问·至真要大论》。

损者温之(sǔn zhě wēn zhī) **treating impairment with warming method** Treatment method. Deficiency diseases, such as yang deficiency, yin deficiency, qi deficiency, and blood deficiency, should be treated with the method of warming. See *Su Wen* chapter 74.

热中 病证名。由火热内盛，消烁阴津，而见多饮多尿、消谷善饥的病证。出《素问·腹中论》《素问·脉要精微论》《素问·平人气象论》。

热中(rè zhōng) **heat middle** Disease name of which the major cause is fiery inner heat and deficiency yin liquids; symptoms include increased drinking, increased urine and swift digestion with rapid hungering. See *Su Wen* chapter 17, 18, and 40.

热气 ① 自然界炎热之气。出《素问·至真要大论》。② 人体阳热之气。出《灵枢·血络论》。③ 邪热之气。出《素问·调经论》。

热气(rè qì) ① Heat qi in nature. See *Su Wen* chapter 74. ② Yang heat qi in the human body. See *Ling Shu* chapter 39. ③ Pathogenic heat qi. See *Su Wen* chapter 62.

热化 从热而化。① 用热药使病向热的方面转化。出《素问·六元正纪大论》。② 气候从热转化。出《素问·至真要大论》。

热化(rè huà) **Transform from heat.** ① Using heat to transform the disease into heat. See *Su Wen* chapter 71. ② Climate changes from heat. See *Su Wen* chapter 74.

十画

热因寒用　反治法。出《素问·至真要大论》。① 用药反佐。即热性药剂中佐以少量寒凉药作向导，以治大寒证。见《素问注证发微》。② 服药反佐。如热药治寒病用冷服法。见《类经·论治四》。③ 现代一般据下文"塞因塞用，通因通用"迳改为"热因热用"，为反治法，即真寒假热证用热药治疗。

热因寒用（rè yīn hán yòng）**treating with cold** Paradoxical treatment. See *Su Wen* chapter 74. ① Anti-adjuvant medication. In heat therapy, a small amount of cold-natured medicine is used as a guide to treat the great cold syndrome. See *Su Wen Zhu Zheng Fa Wei*（*Annotation and Elaboration on Su Wen*）. ② Take the medicine reversely. Such as taking cold decoctions to treat cold diseases with heat therapy. See *Lei Jing*（*Classified Classic*）"On Treatment Chapter 4". ③ Anti-treatment method, such as using hot-natured medicine to treat true cold with false heat syndrome.

热伤气　热胜则腠理开，气易泄，故伤气。出《素问·阴阳应象大论》《素问·五运行大论》。

热伤气（rè shāng qì）**Heat damages qi.** Pores open easily in hot temperatures，which can easily cause the loss of qi. Hence to say heat hurts qi. See *Su Wen* chapter 5 and 67.

热伤皮毛　热胜则津液亏耗，皮毛失其濡养，可见皮毛憔悴色泽夭然。出《素问·阴阳应象大论》《素问·五运行大论》。

热伤皮毛（rè shāng pí máo）**Heat impairs skin.** In hot temperatures，body fluids are depleted，and the skin cannot be nourished. As a result，the skin is pale in color. See *Su Wen* chapter 5 and 67.

热论　①《素问》篇名。该篇专门讨论热病的概念、主证、传变规律、治疗原则和预后、禁忌等。② 上古时代一部讨论热病的专著。已佚。出《素问·评热病论》。

热论（rè lùn）① Discussion on Heat. Chapter name in *Su Wen*. This chapter discusses the concept of febrile diseases，the main syndromes，the law of transmission，the principles of treatment，the prognosis，and contraindications. ② A monograph in ancient times discussing febrile diseases. It has been lost in history. See *Su Wen* chapter

33.

热者寒之　治法。热病应用寒凉之法治疗。出《素问·至真要大论》。

热者寒之（rè zhě hán zhī）**treating heat with cold** Treatment method. Febrile diseases should be treated with cold methods. See *Su Wen* chapter 74.

热俞　治疗热病的俞穴。有五十九穴。出《素问·气穴论》。

热俞（rè shū）　**heat acupoints** There are 59 acupoints for febrile diseases. See *Su Wen* chapter 58.

热俞五十九穴　出《素问·气穴论》。即"热病五十九俞"，详见该条。

热俞五十九穴（rè shū wǔ shí jiǔ xué）　**fifty nine acupoints for treating febrile diseases**. See *Su Wen* chapter 58. See "热病五十九俞".

热胜则肿　因热邪偏胜，导致皮肉痈肿。见《素问·阴阳应象大论》《素问·六元正纪大论》。

热胜则肿（rè shèng zé zhǒng）**heat swelling** Excessive heat results in swelling of the skin. See *Su Wen* chapter 5 and 71.

热病　①是指以发热为主症的一类外感病证。出《素问·热论》。②《灵枢》篇名。该篇主要讨论热病的病机、症候、治法和预后，同时介绍了五十九个治疗热病的穴位以及偏枯、痱病等的症状，治法。故名。

热病（rè bìng）　① **febrile disease** It refers to a type of exogenous disease with fever as the main symptom. See *Su Wen* chapter 31. ② A chapter name of *Ling Shu*. This chapter mainly discusses the pathogenesis, syndromes, treatment methods and prognosis of febrile disease, and introduces 59 acupoints for treating febrile disease, as well as the symptoms and treatment methods of hemiplegia and stroke. Hence the name.

热病五十九俞　指治疗热病的五十九个俞穴。中行的上星、囟会、前顶、百会、后顶。次两傍二行的五处、承光、通天、络郄、玉枕。又次两傍二行的临泣、目窗、正营、承灵、脑空，五行共二十五穴，可散越诸阳热之逆于上者。大杼、膺俞、缺盆、背俞，此八者，可泻胸中之热。气街、三里、巨虚、上下廉，此八者，可泻胃中之热。云门、髃骨、委中、髓空，此八者可泻四肢之热。五藏俞之傍的魄户、神堂、魂门、意舍、志室共十穴，可泻五脏之热。出《素问·水热穴论》。另《灵枢·热病》载"五十九刺"与此有出入。参见该条。

热病五十九俞（rè bìng wǔ shí jiǔ shū） **fifty nine acupoints for treating febrile disease** It refers to the 59 acupoints for treating febrile disease. Shang Xing (DU 23)，Xin Hui（DU 22），Qian Ding（DU 21），Bai Hui（DU 20），and Hou Ding（DU 19）in the middle of the body；Wu Chu（BL 5），Cheng Guang（BL 6），Tong Tian（BL 8），Luo Xi（BL 8），Yu Zhen（BL 9），Lin Qi（BL 9），Lin Qi（GB 15），Mu Chuang（GB 16），Zheng Ying（GB 17），Cheng Ling（GB 18）and Nao Kong（GB 19）on both sides；The above-mentioned acupoints can dispel reversing yang heat in the upper part. Da Zhu（BL 11），Ying Yu（LU 1），Que Pen（ST 12）on both sides，and back-shu points can dispel the heat in the chest. Qi Jie（ST 30），Zu Sanli（ST 36）on both sides，and Shang Ju Xu（ST 37），Xia Ju Xu（ST 39），Shang Lian（LI 8），Xia Lian（LI 9）can dispel the heat in the stomach. Yun Men（LU

2），Yu Gu（LI 15），Wei Zhong（BL 40），Sui Kong（GB 39）on both sides can dispel the heat in the four limbs. Po Hu（BL 42），Shen Tang（BL 44），Hun Men（BL 47），Yi She（BL 49），Zhi Shi（BL 52）can dispel the heat in the five viscera. See *Su Wen* chapter 61. Noted that *Ling Shu* chapter 23 also recorded "Fifty-nine Needling"，but the details are slightly different from those in *Su Wen*. See "五十九刺" for detail.

热病不可刺者有九 言热病针刺的九种禁忌，这九种症候皆为热病之重症，邪盛正衰，故预后较差，针刺恐亦难以为功。出《灵枢·热病》。

热病不可刺者有九（rè bìng bú kě cì zhě yǒu jiǔ） **nine contraindications of needling for febrile disease** The nine contraindications of febrile disease acupuncture are all for serious syndromes, that is, the pathogen qi is prosperous while the healthy qi is declining，thus the prognosis is poor，and it is difficult for acupuncture to make a difference. See *Ling Shu* chapter 23.

热厥 病证名。主症为手足心

热,小便黄赤。因经常醉饱入房,耗伤肾精,酒热与谷气相搏,热盛于中,转耗肾阴,遂成阴虚热盛之热厥。出《素问·厥论》。

热厥(rè jué)　**heat reversal** Name of disease where patients feel hot in the palms and soles and have yellow urine. It is usually caused by frequent sexual intercourse after drinking which consumes kidney essence. Alcohol's heat and food qi entangle with each other to raise the heat which consumes kidney yin. Finally, it becomes heat reversal caused by yin deficiency and heat excess. See *Su Wen* chapter 45.

热痹　病名。局部红肿热痛之痹证。出《素问·四时刺逆从论》。

热痹(rè bì)　**heat impediment** Disease name. An impediment syndrome of swelling and heat pain. See *Su Wen* chapter 64.

恐　恐惧。为五志之一,为肾之志。出《素问·阴阳应象大论》。

恐(kǒng)　**fear** One of the five emotions, pertaining to the kidney. See *Su Wen* chapter 5.

恐则气下　恐惧伤肾,精气下却,症见大小便失禁,或尿闭少腹急结等。出《素问·举痛论》。

恐则气下(kǒng zé qì xià)　**Fear causes qi sinking.** Fear hurts the kidney and causes the the qi to sink. Fear may cause symptoms like incontinence, anuresis, and hypogastric pain. See *Su Wen* chapter 39.

恐则精却　却(què 确),退缩的意思。肾藏精,恐惧伤肾,肾精下却,脏气失守,临床可见二便失禁等。出《素问·举痛论》。参阅"恐则气下"条。

恐则精却(kǒng zé jīng què)　**Fear leads to loss of essence.** *Que* means to withdraw and downbear (kidney essence). The kidney stores essence, and fear hurts the kidney, forcing kidney essence to withdraw downwards. When the visceral qi fails to contain itself, urinary and fecal incontinence occurs. See *Su Wen* chapter 39. See "恐则气下".

恐伤肾　恐则气下,大恐则肾气陷下,肾主藏精,肾气伤则可见小便失禁、遗精、阳痿等症。出《素问·阴阳应象大论》《素问·五运行大论》。

恐伤肾(kǒng shāng shèn)　**Fear damages kidney.** Fear causes the kidney qi to sink. Since the kidney stores essence, damaging kidney qi may lead to urinary incontinence，nocturnal emissions，impotence，etc. See *Su Wen* chapter 5 and 67.

恐胜喜　恐为肾水之志,喜为心火之志,水能克火,故云恐胜喜。过喜伤心,以事恐之,则可制喜。这是一种“以情制情”的心理现象和治病方法。出《素问·阴阳应象大论》《素问·五运行大论》。

恐胜喜（kǒng shèng xǐ）　**Fear prevails over-joy.** Fear is the emotion of kidney water，and joy is the emotion of the heart fire. Water restrains fire，so fear prevails over joy. Overjoy may hurt the heart，so to frighten the patient may restrain overjoy. This is a psychological treatment method of restraining emotions with emotions. See *Su Wen* chapter 5 and chapter 67.

恶气　① 自然界的有害之气。出《素问·四气调神大论》。② 体内之邪气病气。出《灵枢·水胀》《灵枢·四时气》。

恶气（è qì）　① Harmful qi in nature. See *Su Wen* chapter 2. ② Pathogenic qi in the human body. See *Ling Shu* chapter 19 and chapter 57.

恶风　① 恶疠之邪气。出《素问·脉要精微论》。② 恶(wù 误)风,畏风。出《素问·评热病论》。

恶风（è/wù fēng）　① (è) Pathogenic wind. Pathogenic qi of the plague. See *Su Wen* chapter 17. ② (wù) Aversion to wind. See *Su Wen* chapter 33.

恶血　① 妇女经血。出《灵枢·水胀》。② 瘀血。出《灵枢·贼风》。

恶血（è xuè）　① Menstrual blood. See *Ling Shu* chapter 57. ② Blood stasis. See *Ling Shu* chapter 58.

真人　理想中上古时代的养生家。他们能掌握自然界阴阳的变化规律,通过调息(呼吸精气)、调神(独立守神)、调形(肌肉若一),达到健康长寿的目的。出《素问·上古天真论》。

真人（zhēn rén）　**immortal** Ideal health care experts in ancient times. They mastered the changing laws of yin and yang in nature and achieved the goal of health and longevity by adjusting the breath (breathing essence qi)，spirit (guarding the spirit when alone)，and shape (bones coordinating with muscles). See *Su Wen* chapter 1.

真牙　智齿。即生长最迟的臼

齿,俗称尽头牙。智齿生,表示人身发育成熟。出《素问·上古天真论》。

真牙(zhēn yá)　**wisdom teeth** That is the last growing molar, commonly known as the end tooth. Wisdom teeth indicates that the body is mature. See *Su Wen* chapter 1.

真气　① 亦称正气,由水谷精气及肺吸入的清气结合而成的气,流布全身,无处不到,是人体生命活动的动力,并具有抗病能力。出《灵枢·刺节真邪》《素问·上古天真论》。② 经脉之气。出《素问·离合真邪论》。

真气(zhēn qì)　① Healthy qi, a combination of the essence qi of water and grains as well as the clear air inhaled by the lung. It spreads throughout the body as the driving force of human life and activities, and has the function of resisting disease. See *Ling Shu* chapter 75 and *Su Wen* chapter 1. ② The qi of the meridians and channels. See *Su Wen* chapter 27.

真心脉　心的真脏脉。其来搏急坚硬,毫无和缓之状,是无胃气之象。出《素问·玉机真藏论》.

真心脉(zhēn xīn mài)　**true heart pulse** A pulse which beats quickly and hard, without signs of easing, indicating a lack of stomach qi. See *Su Wen* chapter 19.

真心痛　病证名。乃邪气直犯心而致的心痛。特点为心痛甚剧,手足清冷至肘膝,其死在旦夕之间。出《灵枢·厥病》。

真心痛(zhēn xīn tòng)　**genuine heart pain** Name of the disease Heart pain caused by the invasion of pathogen qi. It is characterized by severe heartache, cold reaching the hands and feet as well as the elbows and knees. This disease easily becomes fatal. See *Ling Shu* chapter 24.

真头痛　病证名。是邪气直犯于脑而致的头痛。特点为头痛剧烈、痛遍满脑、手足冷至肘膝关节。属邪盛正衰,预后欠佳。出《灵枢·厥病》。

真头痛(zhēn tóu tòng)　**true headache** Disease name of a headache caused by pathogen qi directly invading the brain. It is characterized by a severe headache, with pain all over the brain, cold reaching the hands and feet as well as the elbows and knees. This syndrome indicates the strength of pathogen qi and the weakness of healthy qi, as well as poor prognosis. See *Ling Shu* chapter 24.

真邪　真，即正气。真邪，即正气和邪气。出《灵枢·口问》。

真邪（zhēn xié）　**healthy qi and pathogen qi** See *Ling Shu* chapter 28.

真色　五脏安和之正常人反映于外的色泽，即正色。出《灵枢·五色》。

真色（zhēn sè）　**true color** The color of healthy people with normal five viscera reflected by their appearance, that is, the common color. See *Ling Shu* chapter 49.

真肝脉　肝的真脏脉。其来浮沉皆弦细坚急而硬，是无胃气之象。出《素问·玉机真藏论》。

真肝脉（zhēn gān mài）　**true liver pulse** A pulse whose comings and goings are all fast, small, wiry and hard, indicating a lack of stomach qi. See *Su Wen* chapter 19.

真肾脉　肾的真脏脉。脉来坚搏沉实，如指弹石，是无胃气之象。出《素问·玉机真藏论》。

真肾脉（zhēn shèn mài）　**true kidney pulse** A pulse which beats hard as if flicking a stone, indicating a lack of stomach qi.

See *Su Wen* chapter 19.

真肺脉　肺的真脏脉，浮大虚弱无根，是无胃气之象。出《素问·玉机真藏论》。

真肺脉（zhēn fèi mài）　**true lung pulse** The true visceral meridian and channel of the lung with a pulse that beats weak and floating without a root, indicating a lack of stomach qi. See *Su Wen* chapter 19.

真骨　坚固之骨。出《灵枢·逆顺肥瘦》。

真骨（zhēn gǔ）　**true bone** Hard bones. See *Ling Shu* chapter 38.

真脉之藏脉　即真脏之脉。出《素问·阴阳别论》。

真脉之藏脉（zhēn mài zhī zàng mài）　**true pulse of the real viscera** See *Su Wen* chapter 7.

真脾脉　脾的真脏脉。脉来软弱，节律不均，忽快忽慢，是无胃气之象。出《素问·玉机真藏论》。

真脾脉（zhēn pí mài）　**true spleen pulse** The true visceral meridian and channel of the spleen with a weak and uneven pulse, indicating a lack of stomach qi. See *Su Wen* chapter 19.

真藏　①即真脏脉，是毫无胃气冲和，失去柔和从容之态的脉象。包括真肝脉、真心脉、真肺

十画

脉、真肾脉、真脾脉等五脏之真脏脉,是病人垂危时出现的脉象。出《素问·玉机真藏论》《素问·平人气象论》。② 肺脏。出《素问·示从容论》。

真藏(zhēn zàng) ① Genuine-zang pulse of the viscera. It is the pulse indicating a lack of stomach qi which is manifested as the loss of softness and calmness. It can be categorized into true liver pulse, true heart pulse, true lung pulse, true kidney pulse and true spleen pulse. This kind of pulse appears when the patient is critically ill. See *Su Wen* chapter 18 and chapter 19 ② Lung. See *Su Wen* chapter 76.

真藏脉 真脏之气独见,而无丝毫雍容和缓之状,是无胃气之脉,如但弦但石之类,见者垂危。出《素问·平人气象论》。

真藏脉(zhēn zàng mài) **genuine-zang pulse** The unique true visceral qi, without the slightest grace and gentleness, with a pulse manifesting a lack of stomach qi, for example, a pulse beating as a wire or a stone, etc. Seeing this kind of pulse manifestation indicates the patient is in danger. See *Su Wen* chapter 18.

桂 药名,即肉桂。性辛热,功能温经通脉。出《灵枢·经筋》。

桂(guì) **Cinnamon** (*Cortex Cinnamomi*) Name of medicine which is pungent and hot, and which has the function to warm and dredge the meridians. See *Ling Shu* chapter 13.

桎之为人 体质名。又称桎羽。此代表阴阳二十五人中水形人之一种,其特征是很安定,身体活动似被桎梏所束缚。出《灵枢·阴阳二十五人》。

桎之为人(zhì zhī wéi rén) **people of the zhi constitution** Name of constitution, also known as *zhi yu*. This represents one of the twenty-five people divided by yin and yang. It is characterized by stability, as for the *zhi* people, their physical activity seems to be constrained as a puppet's. See *Ling Shu* chapter 64.

桎羽 体质名。简称桎。桎(zhì致),比喻束缚人或事物的东西;羽,五音之一,属水。桎羽,代表阴阳二十五人中水形人之一种。出《灵枢·五音五味》。

桎羽(zhì yǔ) *zhi yu* Name of constitution. *Zhì* means something that binds people or things; *yǔ*, one of the five tones, pertains to the water element. *Zhi* *yu*, representing one of the twenty-five people divided by yin and yang, is a water-shaped person. See *Ling Shu* chapter 65.

格　① 阳气太盛，与阴气不相协调，可出现气逆呕吐等证，亦称"格阳"。出《灵枢·脉度》《素问·至真要大论》。② 格拒不顺应。出《素问·奇病论》。

格（gé）　① The yang qi is too strong, and is not in harmony with the yin qi, thus syndromes such as qi reversing and vomiting will appear. It is also known as "Ge Yang". See *Ling Shu* chapter 17 and *Su Wen* chapter 74. ② Resistance and noncompliance. See *Su Wen* chapter 47.

格阳　气血盛于三阳，与三阴格拒不相交通之病证。简称"格阳"，又名"溢阳""外格"。出《素问·六节藏象论》。

格阳（gé yáng）　*ge yang* The qi and blood are sufficient in triple yang, and refuse to communicate with triple yin. *Gé yáng* is also known as *yì yáng* and *wài gé*. See *Su Wen* chapter 9.

核骨　大趾本节后内侧之圆骨，状如核。出《灵枢·经脉》。

核骨（hé gǔ）　**node bone** The round bone at the postero-medial part of the big toe. It is

shaped like a kernel. See *Ling Shu* chapter 10.

根　① 根本。出《素问·四气调神大论》。② 脉气所起之处。出《灵枢·根结》。

根（gēn）　① Foundation. See *Su Wen* chapter 2. ② The place of origin of the pulse qi. See *Ling Shu* chapter 5.

根结　《灵枢》篇名。根，根本，脉气所起为根；结，终结，脉气所归为结。此篇主要讨论六经根结的部位及穴名，阴阳各经的开、阖、枢的作用及其所主病证、治疗；提出不同的体质，针刺应区别对待。但重点论述根结与治疗的关系。故名。

根结（gēn jié）　**Root and Knot** Chapter name in *Ling Shu*. Root means the foundation, and here it means the root where pulse qi originates; knot means the end, and here it refers to the knot where pulse qi returns. This chapter mainly discusses the root and knot of the six meridians and acupoints, the functions of the opening, closing, and axillary of the yin and yang meridians, as well as their main syndromes and treatments. This chapter also puts forward which acupuncture should be applied according to different constitutions. The key point of this chapter is the relationship between root，knot and treatment. Hence the name.

鬲 通膈，又称膈膜，指胸腔与腹腔之间的肌膜结构。出《素问·平人气象论》。

鬲（gé） **diaphragm** "鬲" is the same as "膈"，also called diaphragm membrane. Refers to the sarcolemma between the thorax and the abdomen. See *Su Wen* chapter 18.

鬲肓 膈与肓的合称。出《素问·刺禁论》。参"鬲"与"肓"条。

鬲肓（gé huāng） **diaphragm and the region between the heart and the diaphragm** See *Su Wen* chapter 52. See "鬲" and "肓" for detail.

鬲消 病证名。"鬲"通"膈"，为心肺间膈膜，通于横膈膜。鬲消为胸膈心肺有热，消渴而多饮，即后世所谓上消证。出《素问·气厥论》。

鬲消（gé xiāo） **diaphragm febrile** Disease name. "鬲" is the same as "膈"，which refers to the diaphragm febrile that connects the heart and lung. The patient with this disease has heat in the chest，diaphragm，

the heart and the lung，and feels thirsty and drinks a lot. It is the so-called upper heat syndrome in later generations. See *Su Wen* chapter 37.

唇四白 唇四周之赤白肉际。出《素问·六节藏象论》。

唇四白（chún sì bái） **lip four white** The pale white flesh around the lips. See *Su Wen* chapter 9.

唇胗 唇部黏膜所生之疱疮。出《灵枢·经脉》。

唇胗（chún zhēn） **dry sore on the lips** Herpes labialis. See *Ling Shu* chapter 10.

唇槁腊 槁、腊同为干枯之义。唇槁腊为口唇干枯萎缩之状。出《灵枢·寒热病》。

唇槁腊（chún gǎo là） **dry lips** Withered lips. See *Ling Shu* chapter 21.

夏气 ① 夏季长养之气，与心相通。出《素问·四气调神大论》《素问·六节藏象论》。② 夏季之人体精气，其在孙络。出《素问·四时刺逆从论》。③ 夏季中人之病气。出《灵枢·终始》。

夏气（xià qì） ① The qi of summer which makes things grow and is interlinked with the heart. See *Su Wen* chapter 2 and chapter 9. ② The essence qi in the minute collaterals of the human body in summer. See *Su Wen* chapter 64. ③ The disease qi of humans in summer. See *Ling Shu* chapter 9.

夏脉　夏季应时之脉,其脉钩,属心。出《素问·玉机真藏论》。参"夏脉如钩"条。

夏脉(xià mài)　**summer pulse** The pulse in summer which feels like a hook and pertains to the heart meridian. See *Su Wen* chapter 19. See "夏脉如钩".

夏脉如钩　夏气主心,五行属南方火,夏令万物盛长,人体脉气与之相应,其脉来时充盛,去势较衰,似"钩"之状。出《素问·玉机真藏论》。

夏脉如钩(xià mài rú gōu)　**Summer pulse feels like a hook.** Summer qi dominates the heart and pertains to the southern fire in the five elements. In summer, all things are prosperous, and the pulse manifestation corresponds to it, which is full when it comes, and fades when it leaves, as if feeling a hook. See *Su Wen* chapter 19.

破䐃脱肉　䐃(jùn 俊),肌肉丰厚突起之处,如臀、腨等部。破,破削。脱,脱失。形容肌肉极度消瘦。出《灵枢·本神》。

破䐃脱肉(pò jùn tuō ròu)　**muscle waning and loss** *Jùn* means the area where the muscles are thick and protruding, such as the buttocks and hips. *Pò* means break and cut. *Tuō* means losing muscle, especially extreme muscle wasting. See *Ling Shu* chapter 8.

原　① 原穴。脏腑原气经过和停留的腧穴,十二经各有一原穴,可主治五脏六腑的疾病。出《灵枢·九针十二原》。② 本源。出《素问·八正神明论》。

原(yuán)　① Source point. The acupoints through which the visceral primordial qi passes and stays, each with twelve meridians, and which can treat the diseases of the five viscera and six bowels. See *Ling Shu* chapter 1. ② Origin. See *Su Wen* chapter 26.

紧　脉象。脉来劲急。如牵绳转索,紧张度较高。多主痛证、寒证。出《灵枢·禁服》《素问·奇病论》。

紧(jǐn)　**tense** Pulse manifestation. The pulse comes fast, as if pulling a string with high tension. It usually indicates pain or cold syndromes. See *Ling Shu* chapter 48 and *Su Wen* chapter 47.

唏　症状名。唏(xī 希)同欷,为

悲泣抽咽。出《灵枢·口问》。

唏（xī）　**weep and sob** Symptom name. "唏" is the same as "欷", refers to sob for sadness. See *Ling Shu* chapter 28.

罷极之本　罷（pí 疲）通疲。出《素问·六节藏象论》。人之运动,在于筋力,肝主筋,司人体运动,故肝为罷极之本。

罷极之本（pí jí zhī běn）　**basis of resistance to extreme fatigue** "罷" is the same as "疲". See *Su Wen* chapter 9. Human movement depends on the strength of the muscles and sinews, and the liver dominates the muscles and sinews as well as the movements of the human body, therefore the liver is the basis of resistance to extreme fatigue.

贼风　① 泛指四时不正之气,能够贼害人体,故名。出《灵枢·岁露论》。②《灵枢》篇名。该篇主要讨论贼风邪伤气伤人为病的问题,批判了鬼神致病的错误认识,体现了朴素唯物主义的发病观。

贼风（zéi fēng）　① It generally refers to the pathogenic qi of the four seasons that can threaten human health, hence the name. See *Ling Shu* chapter 78. ② Chapter name in *Ling Shu*. This chapter mainly discusses the thief wind pathogen causing disease, criticizes the theory of disease caused by ghosts and gods, and reflects the simple materialistic view of pathogenesis.

贼邪　泛指自然界能贼害人体的致病因素。出《素问·生气通天论》。

贼邪（zéi xié）　**thief pathogen** It generally refers to the pathogenic factors that do harm to the body in nature. See *Su Wen* chapter 3.

铍针　九针之一。长四寸,宽二分半,形似剑,后人有称"剑头针"用于切开排脓,治痈肿,脓已成。出《灵枢·九针十二原》。

铍针（pí zhēn）　**stiletto needle** One of the nine needles. It is four inches long, two-and-a-half-inches wide, and shaped like a sword. Later generations called it the sword-shaping needle, which could cut open abscesses and drain pus. People used it to cure swelling and abscesses. See *Ling Shu* chapter 1.

缺盆　① 部位名。在前胸上方,锁骨下凹陷如盆处,即锁骨上窝。出《素问·气府论》。② 经穴名。属足阳明胃经,别名天盖,在锁骨上窝中点处。出《素问·刺禁论》。

缺盆(quē pén) ① Supraclavicular fossa. It is located above the anterior aspect of the chest at the depression below the clavicle. See *Su Wen* chapter 59. ② The name of acupoint ST 12 which pertains to the stomach meridian of foot *yangming*. Que Pen(ST 12)is located at the midpoint of the supraclavicular fossa. See *Su Wen* chapter 52.

乘 ① 欺凌、克贼。指五行的克制太过。从而引起一系列的异常相克反应。引起相乘的原因有二,一是某一行过于强盛,从而欺凌被克的一行使之衰弱,如木过于强盛,则克土太过,造成土的不足,称为木乘土。二是某一行之不足,而使"克我"一行相对增强克制的力量,而其本身就更衰弱。如由于土之不足,以致木克土的力量相对增强,使土更加不足,即称为"土虚木乘"。出《素问·五运行大论》。② 趁,遇。出《灵枢·岁露论》《素问·咳论》。③ 经过。出《灵枢·经脉》。

乘(chéng) ① Overwhelming. It refers to the restraint of the five elements. This will cause a series of abnormal phase reactions. There are two reasons for the overwhelming. One is that a certain element is too strong, and thus the restrained one is weakened. If the wood element is too strong, then the earth element is over-restrained, which causes the lack of earth element. The second is that the deficiency of a certain element leaves the element which restrains it relatively more powerful. For example, due to the lack of earth element, the strength of wood element is relatively strengthened, which makes the earth element more insufficient. See *Su Wen* chapter 67. ② To take advantage of; to meet. See *Ling Shu* chapter 79 and *Su Wen* chapter 38. ③ Pass. See *Ling Shu* chapter 10.

乘袭 承袭的意思。面部色诊中根据五行关系,子脏之色见于母脏之位。出《灵枢·五色》。

乘袭(chéng xí) **inherit** According to the five-element theory, in the facial color inspection, the color of the child-viscera is found in the related facial position of the mother-viscera. See *Ling Shu* chapter 49.

秫米　药名,属谷类。气味甘微寒,能利大肠,疗不眠,与半夏组成半夏汤,为《内经》十三方之一,用以治疗不寐证。出《灵枢·邪客》。

秫米(shú mǐ)　**husked sorghum** Medicine name. A cereal that is sweet in flavor and slightly cold in nature. It helps dredge the large intestine and treat insomnia. Husked sorghum, along with pinellia, forms Pinellia Decoction, which is one of the thirteen prescriptions in the *Nei Jing*(*Internal Classic*)to treat insomnia. See *Ling Shu* chapter 71.

积　① 病名。泛指腹部的包块,其成因为外中于寒邪,内伤于忧怒,起居失节,饮食失调,遂致寒气与痰血互相搏结,日益增大而成。出《灵枢·百病始生》。② 积滞。出《素问·调经论》。

积(jī)　① Accumulation. Disease name. It generally refers to an abdominal mass, which is caused by the cold pathogen invading from the outside, internal damage caused by worry and anger, living and diet disorders that gradually lead to the stagnation of cold qi, sputum and blood. See *Ling Shu* chapter 66. ② To accumulate. See *Su Wen* chapter 62.

积气　出《素问·四时刺逆从论》。(1) 积聚,泛指腹中之结块。见《类经·疾病七十》。(2) 少腹中积气。见《素问直解》。

积气(jī qì)　See *Su Wen* chapter 64.(1) To accumulate. Broadly refers to an abdominal mass. See *Lei Jing*(*Classified Classic*)"On Diseases Chapter 70". (2) Accumulated qi in the lower lateral abdomen. See *Su Wen Zhi Jie*(*Direct Interpretation on Su Wen*).

积聚　病证名。由寒邪、寄生虫、瘀血等凝结而成的腹内积块。出《灵枢·五变》《灵枢·上膈》。

积聚(jī jù)　**aggregation accumulation** Disease name. Intraabdominal mass formed by the coagulation of cold pathogens, parasites, and blood stasis. See *Ling Shu* chapter 46 and chapter 68.

积精全神　即保全精神之意。精为生命之本,神为生命之用,保精、全神是养生的根本原则。出《素问·上古天真论》。

积精全神(jī jīng quán shén)　**to preserve essence and concentrate mind** To preserve the essence and spirit. Essence is the basis of life，spirit is the function of life，and keeping the essence and spirit is the fundamental principle of health. See *Su Wen* chapter 1.

俳 《灵枢·热病》作"痱"，即废之义。指双侧肢体瘫痪，如中风后遗症之类。参"痱"条。出《素问·脉解》。

俳(pái) *pái* See *Ling Shu* chapter 23. It refers to bilateral limb paralysis，such as the sequelae of stroke. See the term "痱" for detail. See *Su Wen* chapter 49.

候 ① 看视。出《灵枢·五癃津液别》。② 待，等。出《素问·六节藏象论》。③ 气候，物候。出《素问·六节藏象论》《素问·六元正纪大论》。④ 诊察。出《灵枢·卫气失常》。⑤ 五日为一候。出《素问·六节藏象论》。⑥ 诊脉部位。出《素问·三部之候》。⑦ 守护。出《灵枢·师传》。⑧ 症候。出《灵枢·决气》。

候(hòu) ① To look. See *Ling Shu* chapter 36. ② To wait. See *Su Wen* chapter 9. ③ Climate；phenology. See *Su Wen* chapter 9 and 71. ④ Inspection. See *Ling Shu* chapter 59. ⑤ Five consecutive days is a pentad. See *Su Wen* chapter 9. ⑥ The

position of pulse-taking. See *Su Wen* chapter 20. ⑦ To guard. See *Ling Shu* chapter 29. ⑧ Symptom. See *Ling Shu* chapter 30.

息 ① 呼吸。出《素问·三部九候论》。② 指一呼一吸。古人以此作为诊脉计时之用。出《素问·平人气象论》。③ 通瘜。指人体上的赘生物。出《灵枢·邪气藏府病形》《素问·病能论》。④ 停止。出《素问·六微旨大论》。

息(xī) ① Breath. See *Su Wen* chapter 20. ② Each breath that the ancients used as time-keeping for pulse-taking. See *Su Wen* chapter 18. ③ "息" is the same as "瘜". Refers to the neoplasms on the human body. See *Ling Shu* chapter 4. ④ To cease. See *Su Wen* chapter 68.

息贲 病症名。息，气息，呼吸。贲，同奔。即呼吸喘急之病证。出《素问·阴阳别论》。

息贲(xī bēn) **rushing respiration** Disease name. *Xī* means breath，*bēn* means rush，the same as "奔（bēn）". *Xī bēn* means shortness of breath. See *Su Wen* chapter 7.

息积 为胁下胀满而呼吸气逆之证，病情顽固，数年不愈。出

《素问·奇病论》。（1）为肺之积，因症见息贲（气息喘促），故名。（2）即积在左胁下之痞证，症见胁胀气逆息难，故名。见《类经·疾病七十四》。（3）息，谓生长。积，谓积而不散，皆作动词。见《素问识》。

息积（xī jī）　**breath accumulation** Insufficiency breathing syndrome due to fullness under the flank. This is a stubborn syndrome that usually lasts for several years. See *Su Wen* chapter 47. (1) The accumulation of lung qi，with symptoms of shortness of breath. Hence the name. (2) The stuffiness accumulated under the left flank，with symptoms of breathing difficulties and qi reversing. Hence the name. See *Lei Jing*（*Classified Classic*）"On Diseases Chapter 74". (3) *Xi* refers to grow and *ji* refers to stagnate，*xi* and *ji* are verbs. See *Su Wen Zhi*（*Understanding Su Wen*）.

胚　出《素问·五藏生成》《灵枢·杂病》《灵枢·水胀》等。义见"胚血"条。

胚（pēi）　*pei* See *Su Wen* chapter 10，*Ling Shu* chapter 26 and chapter 57. See "胚血"

for detail.

胚血　胚（pēi 胚），凝聚败恶之血。胚血，今称瘀血。出《灵枢·杂病》。

胚血（pēi xuè）　*pei* **blood** Coagulated purple-black blood. Today it is called stasis blood. See *Ling Shu* chapter 26.

衄血　机体浅表部位出血之总称。如鼻衄、肌衄、齿衄等，由于阳络伤所致。出《灵枢·百病始生》。

衄血（nǜ xuè）　**spontaneous external bleeding** General term for superficial bleeding in the body. Such as epistaxis，sweat pore bleeding，gum bleeding，etc. It is caused by injuries of the yang collaterals. See *Ling Shu* chapter 66.

徒痫　病证名。徒，仅有。痫，同水。徒水，为有水而无风的水肿病，与有风有水的"风痫"相对而言。出《灵枢·四时气》。

徒痫（tú shuì）　*tu* **water** Disease name. *Tú* means only and *shuì* means water. *Tu* water means edema without wind，in contrast to *fēng shuǐ* which has both wind and water. See *Ling Shu* chapter 19.

豹文刺　五刺法之一，是一种多刺法，刺病变部位的前后左右，

十画

刺中经脉为标准,使之出血,故称豹文刺。此法与"九刺法"中"络刺""十二刺法"中"赞刺"同属浅刺出血的方法。出《灵枢·官针》。

豹文刺(bào wén cì) **leopard-spot needling** One of the five needling methods which is a multi-needling method that needles the front, back, left and right of the treated area. This method is the same as collateral needling in the nine needling methods and repeated shallow needle in the twelve needling methods, and are all shallow needling methods for bleeding. See *Ling Shu* chapter 7.

䯒　同膂。出《素问·气穴论》。见"膂"条。

䯒(lǚ)　**backbone** See *Su Wen* chapter 58. See the term "backbone"(膂) for details.

脆者坚之　治法。脆弱的,应用药使之坚实。出《素问·至真要大论》。

脆者坚之(cuì zhě jiān zhī)　**to treat weakness with strengthening method** It is a treatment method that uses medicine to strengthen the weakness. See *Su Wen* chapter 74.

脂人　体质名,指肌肉坚实而身

形较小者。出《灵枢·卫气失常》。

脂人(zhī rén)　*zhi* **person** Name of constitution of a person with strong muscles and a relatively small stature. See *Ling Shu* chapter 59.

胸中之府　出《素问·脉要精微论》。

胸中之府(xiōng zhōng zhī fǔ)　**depot of chest** See *Su Wen* chapter 17.

胸俞十二穴　指俞府、彧中、神藏、灵墟、神封、步廊,左右共十二穴。属足少阴肾经。出《素问·气穴论》。

胸俞十二穴(xiōng yú shí èr xué)　**12 chest acupoints** It refers to 12 acupoints on the chest(left and right):Shu Fu(KI 27), Yu Zhong(KI 26), Shen Cang(KI 25), Ling Xu(KI 24), Shen Feng(KI 23), and Bu Lang(KI 22), all pertaining to the kidney meridian of foot *shaoyin*. See *Su Wen* chapter 58.

胸痹　病证名。因痰、瘀等邪阻滞胸中,胸中阳气痹阻失宣,可见胸闷疼痛、气促等证。出《灵枢·本藏》。

胸痹(xiōng bì)　**chest impediment** Disease name, caused by sputum, stasis and other pathogens stagnated in the chest, and due to impediment and loss of diffusion of yang qi in the chest. Common symptoms are chest pain and distress as well as shortness of breath. See *Ling Shu* chapter 47.

脑　又称髓海,属奇恒之腑。指颅腔中之髓质,是髓质集中之处。肾生骨髓,与肾有密切关系。出《素问·五藏生成》《灵枢·海论》。

脑(nǎo)　**brain** Also called the sea of marrow and pertains to the extraordinary organs. It refers to the medulla in the cranial cavity, the place where the medulla is concentrated. As the kidney produces bone marrow, thus marrow is closely related to the kidney. See *Su Wen* chapter 10, and *Ling Shu* chapter 33.

脑风　病名。病成于风邪循风府而上入于脑,故名。出《素问·风论》。

脑风(nǎo fēng)　**brain wind** Disease name. It is caused by the wind pathogen invading the upper parts of the body at the brain, hence the name. See *Su Wen* chapter 42.

脑为髓之海　容量极大谓之海。髓质聚于脑,故云。出《灵枢·海论》。参“髓海”条。

脑为髓之海(nǎo wéi suǐ zhī hǎi)　**brain is the sea of marrow** The brain's huge capacity is like that of the sea, with the medulla gathering in the brain, hence the name. See *Ling Shu* chapter 33. See “髓海”.

脑户　经穴名。属督脉经。在枕骨上,强间穴后一寸五分。古人认为此处禁针,针之令哑或有生命危险。出《素问·刺禁论》。

脑户(nǎo hù)　**Nao Hu (DU 17)** An acupoint that pertains to the governor vessel (DU). DU 17 is located on the occipital bone, one *cun* and five *fen* behind DU 18. The ancients believed that acupuncture was forbidden here and needling DU 17 may lead to muteness or be life-threatening. See *Su Wen* chapter 52.

脑烁　病名。烁(shuò 朔),消熔。脑烁,生于项部之痈,热毒炽烈,消烁脑髓,故名。出《灵枢·痈疽》。

脑烁(nǎo shuò)　**brain consuming** Name of a disease in which *shuò* means to consume. Brain consuming refers to an abscess on the neck with strong heat toxins consuming the marrow, hence the name. See *Ling Shu* chapter 81.

十画

脓胕　脓,脓肿。胕,同"腐",腐烂。为外科疮疡之疾。出《素问·阴阳类论》。

脓胕(nóng fū)　**abscess and rot.** "胕" is the same as "腐", meaning to rot. and refers to surgical ulcers and the like. See *Su Wen* chapter 79.

留血　血液渗溢于孙络之外,停留而不能周流。出《素问·调经论》。

留血(liú xuè)　**staying blood** Blood flowing out of the meridians, staying and not circulating. See *Su Wen* chapter 62.

留者攻之　治法。言积滞停留体内的痰饮、宿食、瘀血、水邪等,应用攻逐泻下法治疗。出《素问·至真要大论》。

留者攻之(liú zhě gōng zhī)　**to treat retention with purgation** Name of the treatment method which uses purgation for phlegm, food stagnation, blood stasis, and water pathogens accumulating and staying in the body. See *Su Wen* chapter 74.

挛痹　挛,筋脉拘挛。痹,肢体疼酸麻重。出《素问·异法方宜论》。

挛痹(luán bì)　**contracture impediment** *Luán* means contracture and *bì* means sore and numb limbs. See *Su Wen* chapter 12.

衰者补之　治法。凡衰弱不足的,应用补法治疗。出《素问·至真要大论》。

衰者补之(shuāi zhě bǔ zhī)　**to treat debility with tonifying methods** A treatment method using tonification to treat debility. See *Su Wen* chapter 74.

高者抑之　治法。上盛上逆曰高,治当以降逆之法抑制之。见《素问·至真要大论》。

高者抑之(gāo zhě yì zhī)　**to treat up-reversing with repression** The treatment method used to treat up-reversing diseases with repression. See *Su Wen* chapter 74.

高骨　突起之骨的泛称。出《素问·生气通天论》《灵枢·邪客》。

高骨(gāo gǔ)　**protruding bones** The general term for protruding bones. See *Su Wen* chapter 3 and *Ling Shu* chapter 71.

高梁之疾　高梁即膏梁,肥肉美谷厚味之谓。甘肥贵人多食厚味,久致内热中满,而发为消瘅暴仆等证,故称。出《素问·通评虚实论》。

高梁之疾(gāo liáng zhī jí)　**sorghum disease** Sorghum refers to those foods that are rich or strong in flavor. Overeating these kinds of foods will cause internal central heat fullness, and finally lead to syndromes such as pure-heat dispersion-thirst or sudden syncope. See *Su Wen* chapter 28.

病　① 泛指疾病。出《素问·五藏别论》。② 患病。出《素问·金匮真言论》。③ 危害。出《灵枢·九宫八风》。④ 指女子月水不行。出《素问·腹中论》。⑤ 侵害。出《素问·经脉别论》。

病（bìng）　① It generally refers to disease. See *Su Wen* chapter 11. ② Disease development. See *Su Wen* chapter 4. ③ Detriment. See *Ling Shu* chapter 77. ④ Amenorrhea. See *Su Wen* chapter 40. ⑤ To invade. See *Su Wen* chapter 21.

病气　病邪。出《灵枢·根结》。

病气（bìng qì）　**disease qi** A pathogen. See *Ling Shu* chapter 5.

病心脉　指心之病脉。脉来如喘人之息,喘喘连属,急促之状,而少滑利之象,是缺少胃气之征。出《素问·平人气象论》。

病心脉（bìng xīn mài）　**heart disease pulse** It refers to the pulse manifestation of heart disease, in which the pulse is as fast as hasty panting and lacks smoothness, which indicates a lack of stomach qi. See *Su Wen* chapter 18.

病本　《灵枢》篇名。本,根本,本源。病本,治病求本之意。此篇列举七个先病后病的例子,说明治病必须根据疾病发生的先后及其传变来确定标本,然后依病情的缓急决定标本先后的治疗原则,故名。

病本（bìng běn）　**Root Cause of Diseases** Chapter title in *Ling Shu*. *Běn* means fundamental and origin. *Bìng běn* means treating diseases according to their root. This chapter enumerates seven examples of first disease and second disease, demonstrating that treatment must be based on the sequence of the disease and its transformation in order to determine the root and the symptoms, and then according to the urgency of the disease to choose treating the root first or the symptoms first, hence the name.

病机　指疾病发生、发展、变化和转归的机制。出《素问·至真要大论》。

病机（bìng jī）　**disease mechanism** Refers to the mechanism of occurrence, development, change and outcome of a disease. See *Su Wen* chapter 74.

病传　《灵枢》篇名。病,指外邪

入侵人体引起的病证;传,传变,转移。此篇主要讨论病邪在内脏以五行生克关系,相互转移的传变规律,以及不同传变方式对疾病预后的影响。故名。

病传(bìng chuán) **Transmission of Diseases** Chapter title in *Ling Shu*. *Bìng* refers to the diseases and syndromes caused by the invasion of external pathogens into the human body; *Chuán* refers to transformation. This chapter mainly discusses the transfer of disease in the viscera according to the five elements theory, and the impact of the different modes of transfer on the prognosis of the disease. Hence the name.

病色 疾病时,在体表出现的异常颜色变化。诊察时每以面部色泽变化为主。出《灵枢·五色》。

病色(bìng sè) **abnormal facial coloration in disease** Abnormal color changes on the body's surface during illness with facial coloration being the major indicator. See *Ling Shu* chapter 49.

病形 ① 疾病之形状征象。出《素问·脉要精微论》。② 指疾病。出《素问·移精变气论》。

病形(bìng xíng) ① Condition and symptoms of a disease. See

Su Wen chapter 17. ② Refers to disease. See *Su Wen* chapter 13.

病肝脉 肝脉弦,弦而胃气不足,缺少冲和之象,则为肝之病脉。其脉来满实带滑,如循抚长竿之状。出《素问·平人气象论》。

病肝脉(bìng gān mài) **liver disease pulse** The liver pulse is wiry when there is a deficiency of stomach qi. The pulse lacks harmony indicating liver disease. It is a full and slippery pulse, like touching a long pole. See *Su Wen* chapter 18.

病肾脉 即肾之病脉。其脉来坚搏,犹如牵拉葛藤,按之益坚如石而少胃气冲和之象。出《素问·平人气象论》。

病肾脉(bìng shèn mài) **kidney disease pulse** Refers to the pulse manifestation of kidney disease. This pulse is firm, as if pulling a kudzu vine and pressing on a hard stone, without harmonious stomach qi. See *Su Wen* chapter 18.

病肺脉 指肺的病脉。其脉往来滞涩不畅,轻而虚浮,缺少胃气冲和之象。出《素问·平人气象论》。

病肺脉(bìng fèi mài) **lung disease pulse** Refers to the pulse manifestation of lung disease. This

十画

pulse feels uneven，light and floating without harmonious stomach qi. See *Su Wen* chapter 18.

病能 ① 疾病的状态。出《素问·风论》。见《素问经注节解》。②《素问》篇名。篇中主要讨论了胃脘痛、卧不安、腰痛、颈痛、酒风等证的辨治方法，而诊病当参合病之形，故名。

病能（bìng néng） ① Manifestations of diseases. See *Su Wen* chapter 42. See *Su Wen Jing Zhu Jie Jie*（*Collected and Revised Annotation of Su Wen*）. ② Chapter title in *Su Wen*. This chapter mainly discusses the methods of differentiating and treating the syndromes of epigastric pain， restlessness， lower-back pain， neck pain， and alcohol wind. The diagnosis refers to the manifestations of the disease，hence the name.

病脾脉 指脾之病脉。其来满实而数，缺少和缓之意，是胃气不足失却冲和之象。出《素问·平人气象论》。

病脾脉（bìng pí mài） **spleen disease pulse** Refers to the pulse manifestation of spleen disease. This pulse feels full，fast，and uneasy，indicating a deficiency

of stomach qi. See *Su Wen* chapter 18.

疽 病名。泛指属于阴证的外科疮疡疾患。一般病变部位热象不明显，皮色不变，或漫肿或不肿，脓疡位于深部，溃后脓液清稀或冷稠秽臭，疮口难敛，易内陷，而耗伤五脏精血。出《灵枢·痈疽》。

疽（jū） **subcutaneous ulcer** Name of a disease. Refers to a surgical sore pertaining to the yin syndrome. In general，the heat manifestation of the disease part is not obvious，as the skin color may remain normal，while others may be swollen and others not. The abscess is located in the deeper layers and after ulceration，the pus is thin，cold or stinky. The sore converges with difficulty，and sinks in easily，consuming the essence and blood of the five viscera. See *Ling Shu* chapter 81.

疾 ① 迅速。出《素问·阴阳应象大论》。针刺手法中以此示进针出针之快者。出《灵枢·小针解》。② 疾病。出《灵枢·官针》。③ 通"嫉"。出《灵枢·通天》。

疾（jí） ① Fast. See *Su Wen* chapter 5. Refers to acupuncture techniques，*jí* means entering and exiting the needle with speed. See *Ling Shu* chapter 3. ② Disease. See *Ling Shu* chapter 7. ③ "疾" is the same as "嫉". See *Ling Shu* chapter 72.

疹　疹，疾病。出《素问·奇病论》。

疹（zhěn）　**rash** Disease. See *Su Wen* chapter 46.

疹筋　病名。疹（zhěn 诊），病之义。即筋拘急之病。症见尺肤绷急，四肢与腹筋挛急。出《素问·奇病论》。

疹筋（zhěn jīn）　**sinew disease** *Zhěn* means disease. *Zhěn jīn* refers to diseases of sinew contractures. Symptoms include cubit skin tension，and cramps in the limbs and abdomen. See *Su Wen* chapter 46.

痈　① 病名。泛指属于阳证的外科疮疡疾患。一般病变部位红肿焮热疼痛，表皮薄而光泽，范围较大，较浅、溃后易收口，不易内陷，不伤五脏精血，预后较好。出《灵枢·痈疽》。② 症状名。即肿大。出《灵枢·痈疽》。

痈（yōng）　① Disease name. Generally refers to surgical sores that pertain to yang syndromes. They manifest with disease parts that are red，swollen，hot and painful，with thin and shiny epidermis，and which are large in scope. As the diseased part is shallow，it closes easily after ulceration，without invading or hurting the essence and blood of the five viscera. Furthermore，the prognosis is good. See *Ling Shu* chapter 81. ② Symptom name. Swelling. See *Ling Shu* chapter 81.

痈肿　病证名。泛指一切疮疡肿毒。由于外受邪气，内伤情志饮食等而致局部郁热凝蓄，营卫不通，肿毒积聚，腐肉化脓，甚至烂筋伤骨。此证外可生于皮肉筋骨，内可发于肺、胃、肝、肠等脏器。出《灵枢·痈疽》等篇。

痈肿（yōng zhǒng）　**swollen welling abscess** Disease name Generally refers to all sores，swellings and poisons which are caused by external pathogens. Internal injuries due to mental disease and diet will cause local stagnation of heat pathogens，which obstructs the circulation of nutrient and defensive qi，the accumulation of swelling poison，slough and pus，and even rotten the sinews and hurt the bones. This syndrome can arise either outside the flesh，bones，and muscles，or inside the internal organs such as the lung, stomach，liver, and intestines. See *Ling Shu* chapter 81.

痈疡 泛指痈肿疮疡,为外科疾患之总称。出《素问·异法方宜论》。

痈疡（yōng yáng）　**abscess and ulcer** Broadly refers to abscesses and ulcers，and is a general term for surgical diseases. See *Su Wen* chapter 12.

痈疽 《灵枢》篇名。痈疽,为外科疮疡类病证。此篇论述了痈与疽的概念,病机及鉴别诊断,并简介了猛疽等十八种痈疽的概况,是《内经》中关于外科学方面的重要篇章。

痈疽（yōng jū）　**Carbuncles and Gangrene** Chapter title in *Ling Shu*. Gangrene is a syndrome involving surgical sores. This chapter discusses the concept, pathogenesis，and differential diagnosis of carbuncles and gangrene，and introduces an overview of eighteen kinds of gangrene，including abscesses on the prominentia laryngea，which is an important chapter on surgery in the *Nei Jing*（*Internal Classic*）.

疰　疰(zhù 住),深部脓疡,以其随

处可生,流窜无定,故亦名"流注"。出《素问·五常政大论》。

疰（zhù）　**infixation** Infectatious abscesses，also known as "deep multiple abscesses" because they can grow everywhere and flow without certainty. See *Su Wen* chapter 70.

痂疥 痂,疮面所结之壳。疥,小疮小癣之类的皮肤病。出《灵枢·经脉》。

痂疥（jiā jiè）　**scabs and scabies** Scabs，or the covers of sores. Scabies，skin diseases such as small sores and ringworms. See *Ling Shu* chapter 10.

痉 《素问·至真要大论》:"诸痉项强,皆属于湿。"(1)痉,病名。见《类经·疾病一》。(2)症状名。筋强直不柔之谓,可见颈项强直、四肢抽搐、角弓反张等状。见《素问注证发微》。

痉（jìng）　**spasm** *Su Wen* chapter 74 recorded that，"All cases of tetany and stiff nape, without exception，are associated with dampness". (1) Spasm. Disease name. See *Lei Jing*（*Classified Classic*）"On Diseases Chapter 71". (2) Symptom name. Having symptoms such as stiff neck，twitching of the limbs，and opisthotonos. See *Su Wen Zhu*

Zheng Fa Wei（*Annotation and Elaboration on Su Wen*）.

离合真邪论　《素问》篇名。真，正气；邪，邪气。离合。此篇论述了针刺的宜忌和操作方法，强调了治疗要顺应四时阴阳的重要性，以及三部九候脉诊法对治疗的指导作用。

离合真邪论（lí hé zhēn xié lùn）**Discussion on the Separation and Combination of Zhen Qi（Genuine Qi）and Xie Qi（Pathogen Qi）** Chapter title in *Su Wen*. *Zhēn* means healthy qi and *xié* means pathogenic qi. This chapter discusses the contraindications and operation methods of acupuncture, emphasizing the importance of treatment complying with the four seasons as well as with yin and yang, and the guiding role of the three sections and nine indicators.

颃颡　出《灵枢·忧恚无言》。（1）腭上之窍，与鼻相通。见《灵枢集注》。（2）咽喉。见《灵枢识》。

颃颡（háng sǎng）**nasopharynx** See *Ling Shu* chapter 69. (1) The aperture on the palate which is connected with the nose. See *Su Wen Ji Zhu*（*Collected An-*

notation of *Su Wen*）. (2) Throat. See *Ling Shu Zhi*（*Understanding Ling Shu*）.

畜门　鼻内通脑之处，位于颃颡之上。出《灵枢·营气》。

畜门（chù mén）**Nostril** The area above the nasopharynx connecting with the brain. See *Ling Shu* chapter 16.

酒风　病证名。症见身热怠惰，少气恶风，汗出如浴。如饮酒腠理疏松，风邪乘虚入侵所致。又名漏风。出《素问·病能论》。

酒风（jiǔ fēng）**alcohol wind** Name of a disease with symptoms of body heat and laziness, deficient breath and aversion to wind, and sweating as if when having a bath. Drinking alcohol makes the pores and the texture of subcutaneous flesh loose, so that wind pathogens invade the human body. This disease is also called leaking wind. See *Su Wen* chapter 46.

酒悖　悖（bó 勃）通勃，盛貌。酒悖指胆怯之人酒后冲动，胆大妄为。出《灵枢·论勇》。

酒悖（jiǔ bó）**roaring drunk** "悖" is the same as "勃", which meas roaring. Refers to a timid person who is impulsive and bold after drinking. See *Ling*

Shu chapter 53.

消 ① 治法中的消法。即用消导化积的药物去除积滞。出《素问·五常政大论》。② 消损。出《素问·举痛论》。③ 消渴病。出《素问·阴阳别论》。④ 消化。出《灵枢·五癃津液别》。⑤ 消瘦。出《素问·疟论》。

消（xiāo） ① Resolving method. Using the method of abductive dispersion and transforming accumulations to resolve indigestion. See *Su Wen* chapter 70. ② Consuming. See *Su Wen* chapter 39. ③ Diabetes. See *Su Wen* chapter 7. ④ Digestion. See *Ling Shu* chapter 36. ⑤ Emaciation. See *See Wen* chapter 35.

消中 病证名。以善食而瘦为主症的病证，由热盛所致。出《素问·脉要精微论》。

消中（xiāo zhōng） center wasting Disease name in which the main symptoms are emaciation with polyphagia. This disease is caused by the domination of heat. See *Su Wen* chapter 17.

消气 体内的阴阳之气消亡。出《素问·玉版论要》。

消气（xiāo qì） loss of qi The elimination of yin and yang qi in the body. See *Su Wen* chapter 15.

消谷善饥 消烁水谷，容易饥饿。出《灵枢·经脉》。

消谷善饥（xiāo gǔ shàn jī） swift digestion with rapid hungering Digesting water and grain quickly with the tendency to feel hungry easily. See *Ling Shu* chapter 10.

消渴 病名。消，有消瘦、消食、消水之义。以多饮、多食、多尿为主要临床特点。后世又分为三消。出《素问·奇病论》。

消渴（xiāo kě） drinking and urinating Name of a disease，in which x*iāo* has the meaning of emaciation，digestion and eliminating water. The main clinical features are polydipsia，polyphagia and polyuria. Later generations divided it into three eliminations. See *Su Wen* chapter 47.

消瘅 病名。消，内消。瘅，热。因内热而致多饮、多食、多尿的消渴病证。出《灵枢·五变》。

消瘅（xiāo dān） pure-heat dispersion-thirst Name of a disease，in which *xiāo* means elimination and *dān* means heat. The syndrome manifests as pure-heat and dispersion-thirst with symptoms of polydipsia，polyphagia and polyuria due to internal heat. See *Ling Shu* chapter 46.

海论　《灵枢》篇名。此篇将自然界之海的汇聚、充盈以喻称胃、冲脉、膻中、脑为人体之海。同时论述了人体四海逆顺、有余不足的病变及治疗原则,故名。

海论（hǎi lùn）　**Discussion on Seas** Chapter name in *Ling Shu*. In this chapter, the convergence and filling of the seas in nature is used as a metaphor, and the stomach, the thoroughfare vessel, the acupoint CV 17 and the brain are called the seas of the human body. At the same time, the pathological changes and the treatment principles of the four seas in the human body, such as deficiency or excess and good or poor, are discussed, hence the name.

浮　① 脉象。脉来轻虚,轻取即得。为秋季脉象。又主病在表及新病。出《素问·玉机真藏论》《素问·脉要精微论》。② 形容比较明润的色泽。出《素问·玉机真藏论》。③ 浅表的部位。出《灵枢·卫气失常》《灵枢·经脉》。④ 浮越。出《素问·生气通天论》。

浮（fú）　① A pulse manifestation in which the pulse feels weak and can be taken easily. It is the pulse in autumn, and indicates a neopathic or exterior disease. See *Su Wen* chapter 17, and Chapter 19. ② Describing a bright color. See *Su Wen* chapter 19. ③ Superficial part. See *Su Wen* chapter 3, *Ling Shu* chapter 10 and 59. ④ Outward dispersion. See *Su Wen* chapter 3.

浮气　① 指经脉浮于头部巅顶之气。出《素问·气府论》。② 指卫气。出《灵枢·卫气》。

浮气（fú qì）　① The qi of the meridians floating on top of the head. See *Su Wen* chapter 59. ② Defensive qi. See *Ling Shu* chapter 52.

浮白　经穴名。属足少阳胆经。在耳后入发际一寸。出《素问·气穴论》。

浮白（fú bái）　**Fu Bai（GB 10）** The acupoint pertaining to the gallbladder meridian of foot *shaoyang*. GB 10 is located one inch into the hairline behind the ear. See *Su Wen* chapter 58.

浮刺　刺法之一。是斜而浅的一种刺法,以治肌肉寒热。近代应用皮内针法,就是本法的演变。浮刺和毛刺、扬刺同属浅刺法,但毛刺为少针而浅刺,扬刺是多针而浅刺,与本法均有

十画

所不同。出《灵枢·官针》。

浮刺（fú cì） **superficial needling** A needling method in which oblique and superficial needles are inserted to cure cold or heat syndromes in the muscles. The application of the intra-dermal needling method in modern times evolved from this method. Superficial nee-dling, skin needling, and dis-semination needling are all shallow acupuncturing methods, however skin needling uses fewer needles and less shallow needles. Dissemination needling uses multiple and shallow nee-dles，which is different from this method. See *Ling Shu* chapter 7.

浮络 浮现于人体浅表部位的络脉。见《素问·皮部论》等篇。

浮络（fú luò） **superficial meridians and channels** The meridians and channels appearing in the superficial parts of the human body. See *Su Wen* chapter 56.

浮痹 痹证中属邪在浅表皮肤的一种。出《灵枢·官针》。

浮痹（fú bì） **superficial impediment** One of the impediment syndromes caused by pathogens in superficial skin areas. See *Ling Shu* chapter 7.

涕 ① 鼻涕。为肺所化之液，有滋润鼻孔的作用。出《素问·宣明五气》。② 指痰液。出《素问·评热病论》。

涕（tì） ① Nasal mucus. The fluid transformed and produced by the lung，has the function of nourishing the nostrils. See *Su Wen* chapter 23. ② Sputa-mentum. See *Su Wen* chapter 33.

浸淫 出《素问·玉机真藏论》。（1）疾病发展蔓延之谓。见《素问》王冰注。（2）浸淫疮。疮疡浸淫成片。见《素问集注》。

浸淫（jìn yín） See *Su Wen* chapter 19.（1）The development of a disease. See *Su Wen* annotated by Wang Bing.（2）Acute ecze-ma. Sores spread around the body. See *Su Wen Ji Zhu*（*Col-lected Annotation of Su Wen*）.

涩 ① 脉象。其脉往来艰涩，不滑利，如轻刀刮竹之象。提示气滞、血瘀、水停、气虚。多见于积聚，心痛，腹满，溢饮，气虚等证。见《灵枢·邪气藏府病形》《素问·四时刺逆从论》《素问·脉要精微论》。② 凝涩不利。出《素问·五藏生成》《灵枢·论疾诊尺》。

涩（sè） ① Pulse manifestation in which the pulse feels hesitant and not slippery，like a knife scraping bamboo. This pulse manifestation indicates qi stagnation，blood stasis，retention of water，and qi deficiency. These symptoms are commonly seen in syndromes such as accumulation，cardiodynia，abdominal fullness，anasarcous fluid retention，and qi deficiency. See *Ling Shu* chapter 4，*Su Wen* chapter 17 and 64. ② Not smooth nor slippery. See *Su Wen* chapter 10，and *Ling Shu* chapter 74.

涩则心痛　涩,涩脉。脉来艰涩，不流利,如轻刀刮竹,为气血凝滞痹阻之象。不通则痛,故可见于心痛等病证。出《素问·脉要精微论》。

涩则心痛（sè zé xīn tòng）　**hesitant pulse indicating precordial pain** *Sè* means hesitant pulse which manifests as hesitant and not slippery，like a knife scraping bamboo，and indicates the stagnation and obstruction of qi and blood. As it is the obstruction causing the pain，thus syndromes like cardiodynia can be seen. See *Su Wen* chapter 17.

涌水　病证名,水病之一。肺移寒于肾,肾不化水,水气客于大肠之间,如囊中之水濯濯有声，似水之涌,故名。出《素问·气厥论》。

涌水（yǒng shuǐ）　**surge water** Disease name of one of the water diseases，in which the lung transports coldness to the kidney，and the kidney cannot transform water，therefore water and qi are detained in the large intestine. It triggers abdominal sounds like water flowing in a bag about to surge out，hence the name. See *Su Wen* chapter 37.

涌泉　经穴名。足少阴肾经之井穴。在足心屈趾所出现凹陷中。出《灵枢·本输》。

涌泉（yǒng quán）　**Yong Quan (KI 1)** An acupoint pertaining to the kidney meridian of foot *shaoyin* and located in the depression of the foot at the center of the sole easily seen when flexing the toes. See *Ling Shu* chapter 2.

害肩　十二经皮部之一,为手足厥阴经皮部。害,同阖,厥阴为三阴之阖,其脉上抵腋肩,故名害肩。出《素问·皮部论》。

害肩（hài jiān）　***hai* shoulder** One of the twelve skin zones，refers to that of the hand and foot reverting yin meridians.

The position of the reverting yin is close to that of the triple yin and its meridian reaches the axillary shoulders, hence named *hai* shoulder. See *Su Wen* chapter 56.

害蜚 十二经皮部之一,为手足阳明经皮部。出《素问·皮部论》。

害蜚(hài fēi) *hai fei* One of the twelve skin zones, refers to that of the hand and foot *yangming* meridians. See *Su Wen* chapter 56.

窍阴 经穴名。足少阳胆经之井穴。在足小趾次趾的外侧。出《灵枢·本输》。

窍阴(qiào yīn) **Qiao Yin (GB 44)** An acupoint pertaining to the gallbladder meridian of foot *shaoyang*. GB 44 is located on the outside of the fourth toe. See *Ling Shu* chapter 2.

诸血者皆属于心 心主身之血脉,全身血液的生成与运行均与心的功能有关。出《素问·五藏生成》。

诸血者皆属于心(zhū xuè zhě jiē shǔ yú xīn) **All blood pertains to the heart.** The heart dominates the blood of whole body. The generation and operation of the blood throughout the body are all related to the

function of the heart. See *Su Wen* chapter 10.

诸脉者皆属于目 脉,周身脉道,运行气血者,内连五脏,外行全身。而脏腑之精华皆上注于目,故诸脉皆与目相通而属于目。出《素问·五藏生成》。

诸脉者皆属于目(zhū mài zhě jiē shǔ yú mù) **All meridians and channels pertains to the eyes.** *Mai* refers to the meridians and channels of the whole body that move the qi and blood, connect the five internal viscera, and circulate all over the body. The viscera essence goes upwards to the eyes, thus all meridians and channels relate and pertain to the eyes. See *Su Wen* chapter 10.

诸筋者皆属于节 筋有连属骨节、肌肉的作用,与骨节曲伸活动有直接关系。出《素问·五藏生成》。

诸筋者皆属于节(zhū jīn zhě jiē shǔ yú jié) **All sinews pertains to the joints.** The sinews have the function of connecting the joints and muscles, and are directly related to the flexion and extension of the joints. See *Su Wen* chapter 10.

诸髓者皆属于脑 肾主骨,骨生

髓,髓质汇聚于颅腔之中而成脑,故脑与肾有密切关系。出《灵枢·海论》《素问·五藏生成》。

诸髓者皆属于脑(zhū suǐ zhě jiē shǔ yú nǎo) **All marrow pertains to the brain.** The kidney dominates the bones, the bones produce marrow, and the marrow converges in the cranial cavity to form the brain, so the brain and the kidney are closely related. See *Su Wen* chapter 10, *Ling Shu* chapter 33.

调经论　《素问》篇名。此篇阐述经脉在人体生理病理等方面重要性的同时,着重讨论了外感六淫,内伤情志引起经脉气血失调所出现的各种虚实病证,以及针刺调理经脉的方法和意义,故名。

调经论(tiáo jīng lùn) **Discussion on the Regulation of Channels** Chapter title in *Su Wen*. This chapter explains the physiological and pathological importance of the meridians in the human body, and focuses on the deficiency and excess syndromes that arise from qi and blood disorders of meridian vessels which are caused by the six evils and emotional injuries. It also discusses the method and meaning

of acupuncture in regulating meridian vessels. Hence the name.

弱　① 正常人和软柔弱的脉象。出《素问·玉机真藏论》。② 虚弱之脉。中气不足或久病之人,脉软弱无神。出《素问·平人气象论》。③ 婴幼时期。出《素问·上古天真论》。④ 虚弱。出《素问·生气通天论》。

弱(ruò) ① The mild, soft, and weak pulse manifestation of a normal person. See *Su Wen* chapter 19. ② Weak pulse. A person who lacks middle qi or suffers from a chronic disease and has a weak and lifeless pulse. See *Su Wen* chapter 18. ③ The period of infancy and childhood. See *Su Wen* chapter 1. ④ Weakness. See *Su Wen* chapter 3.

弱风　八风之一,指由东南方刮来的风。出《灵枢·九宫八风》。

弱风(ruò fēng) *ruo* wind One of the eight winds coming from the South-East. See *Ling Shu* chapter 77.

陷谷　经穴名。属足阳明胃经之输穴。在足中趾,次趾间,在内庭上二寸凹陷中。出《灵枢·本输》。

陷谷(xiàn gǔ) **Xian Gu (43)**

An acupoint pertaining to the stomach meridian of foot *yangming*, and located between the middle and second toe, in the indentation two inches above Nei Ting (ST 44). See *Ling Shu* chapter 2.

通天　《灵枢》篇名。通,通应。天,自然界。此篇依据天人相通应的观点,将人划分为太阴、少阴、太阳、少阳、阴阳和平等五种体质类型,来指导疾病的辨治。是古代研究体质的重要文献之一。

通天(tōng tiān)　**Celestial Connection** Chapter title in *Ling Shu*. *Tōng* means to connect, and *tiān* refers to heaven, or nature. In this chapter, people are divided into five categories according to their constitution and perspective of correspondence between human and nature: *taiyin* type persons, *shaoyin* type persons, *taiyang* type persons, *shaoyang* type persons, and persons with yin-yang balance. This categorization can guide the diagnosis and treatment of disease, thus "Celestial Connection" is one of the important ancient literatures on human constitution.

通因通用　反治法。如通泻泄利之属于邪实于内的病证,应用攻下通利之法治之。出《素问·至真要大论》。

通因通用(tōng yīn tōng yòng)　**treating diarrhea with purgative methods** A paradoxical treatment which treats the unstoppable by unstopping, such as using purgation to treat diarrhea and dysentery. See *Su Wen* chapter 74.

通里　经穴名。手少阴心经络穴,在腕横纹内侧上一寸处。出《灵枢·经脉》。

通里(tōng lǐ)　**Tong Li (HT 5)** Acupoint name. An acupoint pertaining to the heart meridian of hand *shaoyin*, and which is located at the medial side of the wrist, one inch above the wristband. See *Ling Shu* chapter 10.

通谷　经穴名。足太阳膀胱经之荥穴。在足小趾外侧,本节前陷者中。出《灵枢·本输》。

通谷(tōng gǔ)　**Tong Gu (BL 66)** An acupoint pertaining to the bladder meridian of foot *taiyang*. It is located at the indentation of the first joint on the lateral of the little toes. See *Ling Shu* chapter 2.

通评虚实论　《素问》篇名。此篇以"邪气盛则实,精气夺则虚"

为纲，全面地评述五脏、四时、气血、经络、脉象等各种虚实。简要地介绍了痈肿、霍乱、惊风等证针刺治疗的方法。故名。

通评虚实论（tōng píng xū shí lùn）**General Discussion on Xu (Deficiency) and Shi (Excess)** Chapter name in *Su Wen*. This chapter，based on the theory "exuberance of pathogens causing excess，lack of essential qi causing deficiency"，comprehensively reviews deficiency and excess of the five viscera，four seasons，qi and blood，meridians，and pulse manifestations，and briefly introduces the acupuncture treatment for swollen welling abscesses，cholera，and infantile convulsion. Hence the name.

通脉 经过之脉，指手阳明经脉之通过耳前者。出《素问·缪刺论》。

通脉（tōng mài） **tong meridians** Meridians that pass by，refers to the large intestine meridian of hand *yangming* that passes by the front of the ear. See *Su Wen* chapter 63.

通髯 通连鬓角之髯，俗称连鬓须。出《灵枢·阴阳二十五人》。

通髯（tōng rán） **a full beard** A beard that links the temples，commonly known as sideburns. See *Ling Shu* chapter 64.

十
画

十一画

排针　引针,俗称出针。排,去除之意。出《素问·八正神明论》。

排针(pái zhēn)　**needle removal** *Pái* means to remove. See *Su Wen* chapter 26.

掉眩　掉,动摇。眩,眩晕。掉眩,泛指一切肢体振颤抽掣、头目昏晕一类病证。出《素问·六元正纪大论》。

掉眩(diào xuàn)　**tremble and dizziness** *Diào* means tremble;*xuàn* means dizziness. *Diào xuàn*, generally refers to all the syndromes manifested as limb tremor and dizziness. See *Su Wen* chapter 71.

推而休之　出《灵枢·阴阳二十五人》。① 指推针并留针休息,等候气至的针法。见《灵枢注证发微》。② 凡是上部正气不足的,用推而扬之的针法,催其气以上行。

推而休之(tuī ér xiū zhī)　See *Ling Shu* chapter 64. ① Pushing and waiting. The method of inserting a needle and leaving it in until the arrival of qi. See

Ling Shu Zhu Zheng Fa Wei (*Annotation and Elaboration on Ling Shu*). ② Using the pushing method of acupuncture to force the healthy qi upward, in order to treat those who lack healthy qi in the upper part of the body.

掖　即腋。肩关节下方窝状部。出《素问·至真要大论》。参"腋"。

掖(yè)　**armpit** The fossa below the shoulder joint. See *Su Wen* chapter 74. See "腋".

掖痈　掖,《太素》《针灸甲乙经》均作腋。掖痈,痈发于腋下。出《素问·通评虚实论》。

掖痈(yè yōng)　**Armpit abscess** in *Tai Su* (*Classified Study on Huang Di Nei Jing*) and *Zhen Jiu Jia Yi Jing* (*Classic of Acupuncture and Moxibustion*), "掖" is written as "腋" which refers to armpit. This term refers to the abscess under the armpit. See *Su Wen* chapter 28.

基墙　基指下巴,墙指面部四旁。面部外周轮廓统称基墙。《内经》用以判断寿命长短。出《灵枢·天年》。

基墙（jī qiáng）　**base wall** *Jī* refers to the chin，and *qiáng* refers to the area around the face. The facial contours are collectively referred to as the base wall. *Nei Jing*（*Internal Classic*）uses it to judge the length of life. See *Ling Shu* chapter 54.

著至教论　《素问》篇名。此篇内容主要讨论学医的方法和理论，并举三阳病为例，加以说明。其文是以雷公问黄帝的形式进行讨论，因黄帝被尊为圣人，故名。

著至教论（zhù zhì jiāo lùn）　**Discussion on the Abstruse and Profound Theory of Medicine** Chapter name in *Su Wen*. This chapter mainly discusses the methods and theories of learning medicine. It uses triple yang disease as an example，and the text takes the form of a conversation between Lei Gong and Huang Di，the latter revered as a saint，hence the name.

黄尸鬼　指土疫之邪。出《素问·本病论》。

黄尸鬼（huáng shī guǐ）　**yellow corpse ghost** Refers to the pathogen that comes from Earth-Pesti-

lence. See *Su Wen* chapter 73.

黄而膏润为脓　局部表皮色黄如油膏之润泽，提示痈疡已化脓。见《灵枢·五色》。

黄而膏润为脓（huáng ér gāo rùn wéi nóng）　**yellow and moist indicates pus** Local skin is yellow and moist like ointment，suggesting that the ulcer is purulent. See *Ling Shu* chapter 49.

黄赤为热　凡面部或局部见黄赤之色，多为有热之象。见《素问·举痛论》《灵枢·五色》等篇。

黄赤为热（huáng chì wéi rè）　**Yellow and red indicate heat.** When the face or a body part is seen as yellow and red，it usually indicates heat. See *Su Wen* chapter 39，and *Ling Shu* chapter 49.

黄钟　阳六律之一，为宫音。出《素问·本病论》。

黄钟（huáng zhōng）　**huang zhong** One of the six yang tonalities of ancient Chinese music，also named *gong* tone. See *Su Wen* chapter 73.

黄脉　即脾脉。黄为脾之色，故称。出《素问·五藏生成》。

黄脉（huáng mài）　**yellow pulse** It is the pulse of the spleen，because yellow is the color of the spleen. See *Su Wen* chapter 10.

黄帝 为《内经》作者的托名。见《黄帝内经》书名条。

黄帝（huáng dì） **Huang Di（Yellow Emperor）** The name borrowed for the author of *Nei Jing*（*Internal Classic*）. See "黄帝内经" for detail.

黄帝内经 简称《内经》。我国现存最早的较为完整的医学典籍，由《素问》和《灵枢》两部分组成，初步确立了中医学理论体系。作者不详，黄帝乃伪托，实为春秋战国至秦汉间医学理论的总结，非一时一人之作。成书年代不晚于东汉。参见"素问""灵枢"。

黄帝内经（huáng dì nèi jīng） *Huang Di's Internal Classic* Abbreviated into *Nei Jing*, and the earliest and most complete medical book of China, consists of two parts, *Su Wen* and *Ling Shu*. This book has been the theoretical foundation of traditional Chinese medicine. The author is unknown and Huang Di is a borrowed figure. It is a summary of the medical theory from the Spring and Autumn Periods to the Qin and Han Dynasties. It was written by collective wisdom and came into being no later than the Eastern Han Dynasty. See term *Su Wen* and *Ling Shu*.

黄疸 病名。又名黄瘅。以目黄、身黄、小便黄、乏力等为主症。多由感受时邪，饮食不节，湿热或寒湿中阻，迫使胆汁外溃所致。出《素问·平人气象论》。

黄疸（huáng dǎn） **jaundice** Name of disease in which the main symptoms consist of yellow eyes, yellow skin, yellow urine, and fatigue. It causes bile to overflow resulting from pathogenic qi, inadequate diet, heat or cold damp resistance. See *Su Wen* chapter 18.

黄瘅 即黄疸。出《素问·六元正纪大论》。

黄瘅（huáng dǎn） **jaundice** Refers to 黄疸. See *Su Wen* chapter 71.

营 ①指营气。出《灵枢·营卫生会》。②营养。出《灵枢·五味论》。③营运。出《灵枢·本藏》《灵枢·营气》。④营垒。借喻脉搏沉实之象。出《素问·玉机真藏论》。

营（yíng） ① Nutrient qi. See *Ling Shu* chapter 18. ② Nutrition. See *Ling Shu* chapter 56. ③ Transportation. See *Ling Shu* chapter 47 and 16. ④ Army camp. Used to describe a calm and solid pulse manifestation.

See *Su Wen* chapter 19.

营卫生会　《灵枢》篇名。营,营气;卫,卫气;生会,即生成与会合。此篇主要论述营卫之气的生成布敷与会合的规律,还介绍了三焦的划分、功能及其与营卫的关系。

营卫生会(yíng wèi shēng huì)

The Production and Convergence of Ying Qi (Nutrient Qi) and Wei Qi (Defensive Qi) Chapter name in *Ling Shu*. *Yíng*, nutrient qi; *wèi*, defensive qi; *shēng huì* means generating and meeting. This chapter mainly discusses the law of formation, deployment, and convergence of the nourishing and defensive qi, as well as introduces the division, function, and relationship between the triple *jiao* and the nourishing and defensive qi.

营气　① 营运于脉中的精气,由水谷化生而来,循脉运行全身,内入脏腑,外达肢节,具有营养全身、化生血液等功能。出《灵枢·邪客》。②《灵枢》篇名。此篇系统论述了营气的来源、性质和运行规律。

营气(yíng qì)　① The essence qi running in the meridians and channels coming from water and grains. It circulates in the whole body along the meridians and channels, enters the internal organs, and reaches the limbs. It has the function of nourishing the whole body as well as transforming and generating blood. See *Ling Shu* chapter 71. ② Chapter name in *Ling Shu*. This chapter systematically discusses the source, nature, and operation laws of the nutrient qi.

营出中焦　营,指营气。营气源于中焦脾胃所化生的水谷精气转化而成;且营气之运行始于手太阴肺经,而肺经起始于中焦,故称。出《灵枢·营卫生会》。

营出中焦(yíng chū zhōng jiāo)

Nutrient qi comes from the middle jiao. *Yíng* means nutrient qi. Nutrient qi originates from essence qi that is transformed and generated by the spleen and stomach which both pertain to the middle *jiao*; and nutrient qi starts operating from the lung meridian of hand *taiyin*, which starts from the middle *jiao*. See *Ling Shu* chapter 18.

盛水　① 指农历正月雨水较多的时节。出《素问·阴阳类论》。② 指人体的水液。出《素问·水热穴论》。

十一画

盛水（shèng shuǐ） ① Abundant water. The first month of the lunar year with abundant rain. See *Su Wen* chapter 79. ② Body fluids. See *Su Wen* chapter 61.

盛火 火属阳，心肝两脏为阳脏，盛火，指心肝之火亢盛。出《素问·逆调论》。

盛火（shèng huǒ） **abundant fire** Fire pertains to yang, and the heart and liver are yang viscera. Abundant fire refers to the hyperactive fire of the heart and liver. See *Su Wen* chapter 34.

盛血 脉中满盛之血。出《素问·离合真邪论》。

盛血（shèng xuè） **abundant blood** Sufficient blood in the meridians and channels. See *Su Wen* chapter 27.

盛经 指阳经经脉。出《素问·水热穴论》。

盛经（shèng jīng） **predominant meridian** Refers to the yang meridian. See *Su Wen* chapter 61.

辅针导气 用辅助行针的手法，以引导正气。出《灵枢·邪客》。

辅针导气（fǔ zhēn dǎo qì） **Auxiliary needling guides the healthy qi.** Using auxiliary needling technique to guide the healthy qi. See *Ling Shu* chapter 71.

辅骨 大骨之傍骨。① 膝旁股骨下端内外侧髁及胫骨上端内外侧髁形成的骨突。出《素问·骨空论》。② 桡骨与肱骨接合处的骨突，在肘外侧。出《灵枢·本输》。

辅骨（fǔ gǔ） **auxiliary bone** Bones beside the large bones. ① The catapophysis formed by the medial and lateral condyles of the lower end femur as well as the medial and lateral condyles of the upper tibia. See *Su Wen* chapter 60. ② The catapophysis at the junction of the radius and humerus, located at the exterior aspect of the elbow. See *Ling Shu* chapter 2.

颅 头盖骨。出《素问·骨空论》。

颅（lú） **cranium** See *Su Wen* chapter 60.

虚 ① 亏虚、不足。出《素问·通评虚实论》《灵枢·刺节真邪》。② 祛除。出《素问·调经论》。③ 虚邪，即四时不正之气。出《素问·八正神明论》。④ 证候名。虚证，以正气不足为主的证候。出《灵枢·禁服》。⑤ 通嘘，即呼气。出《素问·经脉别论》。⑥ 快进针、慢出针的针刺泻法。出《灵枢·小针解》。⑦ 空虚。出《素问·五藏别论》《素问·五藏生成》。⑧ 指脉体空虚。见《素问·五藏生成》。

⑨ 太虚,天空。出《素问·五运行大论》。⑩ 星宿名。二十八宿之一,即虚宿,位居北方。出《灵枢·卫气行》。⑪ 指(月廓)亏缺。出《素问·八正神明论》。⑫ 指(岁运或岁气)不及。出《素问·至真要大论》。

虚(xū) ① Deficiency or insufficiency. See *Su Wen* chapter 28 and *Ling Shu* chapter 75. ② Dispelling. See *Su Wen* chapter 62. ③ Deficient pathogen qi of the four seasons. See *Su Wen* chapter 26. ④ Name of a deficiency syndrome. Refers to those syndromes characterized by lack of healthy qi. See *Ling Shu* chapter 48. ⑤ Expiration. "虚" is the same as "嘘", which means exhale. See *Su Wen* chapter 7. ⑥ The fast-forward and slow-out acupuncture method for purging. See *Ling Shu* chapter 3. ⑦ Emptiness. See *Su Wen* chapter 11. ⑧ The emptiness of pulse manifestation. See *Su Wen* chapter 10. ⑨ Sky. See *Su Wen* chapter 67. ⑩ The name of the constellation, Emptiness, which is one of the lunar mansions located in the north. See *Ling Shu* chapter 76. ⑪ The waning of the moon phase. See *Su Wen* chapter 26. ⑫ The deficiency of a year's evolutive phase. See *Su Wen* chapter 74.

虚之乡　与当令季节所主方向相对的方位。如春属木,主东方,则西方为虚乡。凡从虚乡来之风,易贼害人体。出《灵枢·九宫八风》。

虚之乡(xū zhī xiāng)　**home of deficiency** Orientation opposite to the direction of the season. For example, spring pertains to wood and governs the east, so the west which is opposite to the east is the home of deficiency. Winds coming from the home of deficiency are prone to cause diseases. See *Ling Shu* chapter 77.

虚风　泛指能伤害人体的四时不正之气,包括风、寒、暑、湿、燥、火六淫邪气。出《灵枢·刺节真邪》《灵枢·九宫八风》。

虚风(xū fēng)　**deficient wind** Generally refers to the six kinds of pathogenic qi that harm the human body, including wind, cold, summer-heat, dampness, dryness, and fire. See *Ling Shu* chapter 75 and chapter 77.

虚邪　指来自自然界八方的非时之气。能乘虚而入,致人于病,故名。出《素问·八正神明论》。

十二画

虚邪（xū xié）　**deficient pathogen** Refers to the non-seasonal qi from all directions in nature that enters human body to cause diseases. Hence the name. See *Su Wen* chapter 26.

虚邪贼风　泛指一切不正常的气候及自然界的致病因素。出《素问·上古天真论》。

虚邪贼风（xū xié zéi fēng）　**pathogenic exogenous factors** Generally refers to all abnormal climates and natural pathogenic factors. See *Su Wen* chapter 1.

虚里　胃之大络，出于左乳下心尖搏动处。为十二经脉气之所宗，宗气汇聚之地。测虚里动势可知宗气、胃气之盛衰。出《素问·平人气象论》。

虚里（xū lǐ）　**apical pulse** The large channel of the stomach comes from the apex of the left lower breast. It is the place where the pectoral qi of twelve meridians gathers. Apical impulse examination shows the rise and fall of pectoral and stomach qi. See *Su Wen* chapter 18.

虚者实之　治疗原则。正气虚者，当用补法治疗，使正气充实。原指针刺而言，亦适用于其他各种疗法。出《素问·宝命全形论》。

虚者实之（xū zhě shí zhī）　**to treat deficiency with tonification** Treatment principles. Those who are deficient in healthy qi should be treated with tonification to enrich the healthy qi. This is an acupuncture treatment method which is also used in other therapies. See *Su Wen* chapter 25.

虚实　①指虚证和实证。出《素问·玉机真藏论》。②人体阴阳的消长变化。出《素问·宝命全形论》。

虚实（xū shí）　① Excess syndrome and deficiency syndrome. See *Su Wen* chapter 19. ② Changes in yin and yang in the human body. See *Su Wen* chapter 25.

慮瘕　慮，通伏，深伏隐匿之谓。瘕，为腹中结块而隐现不常，多为水、气、血、虫等积聚而成。伏瘕为深伏之瘕，因小肠之热下移大肠，热结不散，致气血留伏而成。出《素问·气厥论》。

慮瘕（fú jiǎ）　**hiding abdominal mass** "慮" is the same as "伏", means deep hiding. *Jiǎ* means abdominal mass, mostly caused by the accumulating of water, qi, blood, worms, etc. *Fú jiǎ* means deep hiding abdominal mass, which is caused by the heat of the small intestine that moves down to the large intestine and finally leads to the stagnation of qi and blood. See *Su Wen* chapter 37.

雀卵　麻雀之卵。气味甘温，功能助阳补精益血。出《素问·腹中论》。

雀卵（què luǎn）　**sparrow eggs** Sweet in flavor，and warm in nature，it tonifies the yang as well as essence and blood. See *Su Wen* chapter 40.

眦　① 眼角。上下眼睑连结处，有内外之分；鼻侧为内眦；颞侧为外眦，又称锐眦。出《灵枢·经脉》。② 视觉。出《素问·脉要精微论》。

眦（zì）　① Corner of the eye. The junction of the upper and lower eyelid is divided into internal and external. The nasal side is the internal canthus；the temporal side is the external canthus，also known as the acute canthus. See *Ling Shu* chapter 10. ② Vision. See *Su Wen* chapter 17.

眴仆　眴，音义同眩，头晕目眩。仆，突然昏仆。出《素问·脉要精微论》。

眴仆（xuàn pú）　**dizziness and fainting suddenly** *Xuàn* means

dizziness. *Pú* means sudden syncope. See *Su Wen* chapter 17.

眼系　眼内连于脑的脉络。又名目系。出《灵枢·寒热病》。

眼系（yǎn xì）　**eye connection** Meridian in the eye connected to the brain. See *Ling Shu* chapter 21.

眸子　即瞳子。出《灵枢·刺节真邪》。

眸子（móu zǐ）　**pupil** Refers to the pupil of the eye. See *Ling Shu* chapter 75.

悬阳　出《灵枢·九针十二原》。① 悬。提举之意；阳，神气。意谓提举患者之神气。② 指心。

悬阳（xuán yáng）　See *Ling Shu* chapter 1. ① *Xuán* means to lift. *Yáng* means spirit. *Xuán yáng* means to lift the patient's spirit. ② Refers to the heart.

悬颅　经穴名。属足少阳胆经，在头维与曲鬓穴之间。出《灵枢·寒热病》。

悬颅（xuán lú）　**Xuan Lu（GB 5）** An acupoint pertaining to the gallbladder meridian of foot *shaoyang* and located between acupoint Tou Wei（ST 8）and Qu Bin（GB 7）. See *Ling Shu* chapter 21.

悬雍垂　口腔内中央由软腭游离缘向下突出之"小舌"。出《灵枢·忧恚无言》。

悬雍垂（xuán yōng chuí）　**uvula** The little tongue protruding downwards from the free edge in the center of the mouth. See *Ling Shu* chapter 69.

啮舌　啮（niè 聂），义同咬。啮舌为自咬其舌的症状。出《灵枢·口问》。

啮舌（niè shé）　**to bit one's tongue** *Niè* means to bite. *Niè shé* is the symptom of biting one's own tongue. See *Ling Shu* chapter 28.

啮齿　咬牙，多因热病所引起。出《灵枢·热病》。

啮齿（niè chǐ）　**to grind one's teeth** It is mostly caused by febrile diseases. See *Ling Shu* chapter 23.

啮唇　啮（niè 聂），义同咬。啮唇为自咬其唇的症状。出《灵枢·口问》。

啮唇（niè chún）　**to bit one's own lips** *Niè*, to bite; *niè chún*, the symptom of biting one's own lips. See *Ling Shu* chapter 28.

啮颊　啮（niè 聂），义同咬。啮颊为咬牙鼓颊。出《灵枢·口问》。

啮颊（niè jiá）　**to grind one's teeth and bulge one's cheeks** *Niè* means to bite; *Niè jiá*, to grind one's teeth and bulge one's cheeks.

See *Ling Shu* chapter 28.

蛊　因虫食内积所致之臌胀。出《素问·玉机真藏论》。

蛊（gǔ）　**tympanitis** Caused by the accumulation of worms and food. See *Su Wen* chapter 19.

唾　①唾液，五液之一。唾生于舌本舌下，足少阴肾脉循喉咙挟舌本，故与肾关系密切。出《素问·宣明五气》。②吐痰沫水液。出《素问·评热病论》。

唾（tuò）　① Saliva，one of the five kinds of fluids. Saliva is secreted under the tongue，and the kidney meridian of foot *shaoyin* runs along the throat and the tongue，thus it is closely related to the kidney. See *Su Wen* chapter 23. ② Spitting liquid. See *Su Wen* chapter 33.

唾血　①咳血，因邪伤肺络所致。出《素问·咳论》。②吐血，唾，吐。出《素问·腹中论》。

唾血（tuò xuè）　① Coughing up of blood，caused by pathogen qi that attacks the lung meridian and channels. See *Su Wen* chapter 38. ② Spitting blood. *Tuò* means to spit. See *Su Wen* chapter 40.

唾痛咒病　古代精神疗法之一。用恶毒、轻薄之语言来唾骂咒疾病。亦祝由之例。痛，指疾病。出《灵枢·官能》。

唾痈咒病（tuò yōng zhòu bìng）
cursing disease A kind of ancient psychotherapy by cursing disease with vicious, frivolous words. It is an example of *zhu you* therapy. *Yōng* means disease. See *Ling Shu* chapter 73.

婴儿风 八风之一，指由东方刮来的风。出《灵枢·九宫八风》。

婴儿风（yīng ér fēng） *ying er wind* One of the eight winds coming from the East. See *Ling Shu* chapter 77.

婴筋 颈部两侧的筋。出《灵枢·寒热病》。

婴筋（yīng jīn） **neck sinew** Sinews on both sides of the neck. See *Ling Shu* chapter 21.

移精变气 言运用某种方法转移病人的情志精神之所注，从而改变其气血紊乱的病理状态，达到治疗疾病的目的。具体如祝由疗法。有现代精神疗法的意义。出《素问·移精变气论》。

移精变气（yí jīng biàn qì） **to shift the essence and change qi** Use some method to divert the attention of the patient's emotions and spirits, so as to change the pathological state of qi and blood disorders as well as achieve the purpose of treating diseases, for example, the *zhu you* therapy, which is the same as modern psychotherapy. See *Su Wen* chapter 13.

移精变气论 《素问》篇名。移，转移。精，精神情志。变，变动。气，藏气。移精变气，即通过转移患者的精神情志，以调节藏气，达到治病的目的。此篇首论移精变气的祝由疗法，后言色诊、脉诊、问诊的重要意义，强调"神"之得失对预后的决定作用。

移精变气论（yí jīng biàn qì lùn） **Discussion on Shifting the Essence and Changing the Qi** Chapter name in *Su Wen*. *Yí* means to transfer, *jīng* means emotions and spirits, *biàn* means to change, *qì* refers to the storage of *qi*. By transferring the patient's emotions and spirits, the storage of *qi* is regulated and the purpose of treating diseases is achieved. This chapter first discusses the significance of *zhu you* therapy for changing the emotions and spirits as well as changing qi, and then the significance of color diagnosis, pulse diagnosis, and interrogation. It emphasizes the decisive role of the gains and losses of spirit on prognosis.

偶　即偶方。古之复方或组方药味成复数者。为七方之一。出《素问·至真要大论》。

偶（ǒu）　**paired** It refers to even-ingredient prescriptions，or to say，prescriptions with ingredients which are even in number. It is one of the seven kinds of prescriptions. See *Su Wen* chapter 74.

偶之制　偶方的组方制度。出《素问·至真要大论》。（1）复方。见《素问》王冰注。（2）方剂药味成双数者，属阴。见《素问直解》。（3）方剂之主要作用有两个方面者。见《内经评文》。

偶之制（ǒu zhī zhì）　Organization system of the even-ingredient prescriptions. See *Su Wen* chapter 74.（1）Compound. See *Su Wen* annotated by Wang Bing.（2）Prescriptions with even-numbered ingredients, pertaining to yin. See *Su Wen Zhi Jie*（*Direct Interpretation on Su Wen*）.（3）The main effect of the prescription has two aspects. See Literary Review of *Nei Jing*（*Huang Di's Internal Classic*）.

偶刺　十二刺法之一。偶，双数。即胸腹与后背配穴成双进行针刺，又称"阴阳刺"，可治心痹一类疾病。宜从傍斜刺，以免刺伤内脏。出《灵枢·官针》。

偶刺（ǒu cì）　**paired needling** One of the twelve needling methods. *ǒu* means even numbers. Acupuncture is performed in pairs of acupoints in the chest，abdomen and back，also called yin-yang needling. This method can cure heart impediment and other diseases. It is advisable to needle from the side to avoid puncturing the internal organs. See *Ling Shu* chapter 7.

偏历　经穴名。手阳明大肠经之络穴。在腕背横纹桡侧端上陷者中。出《灵枢·经脉》。

偏历（piān lì）　**Pian Li（LI 6）** An acupoint pertaining to the large intestine meridian of hand *yangming*. *Piān lì* is in the upper indentation at the radial end of the transverse veins on the dorsal aspect of the wrist. See *Ling Shu* chapter 10.

偏风　病名。出《素问·风论》。（1）风邪偏中于人体某脏某部而得的风证之总称，包括"五脏风"，以及脑风、目风、漏风、内风、首风、泄风、肠风等。（2）即偏枯，详该条。见《素问》王冰注。

偏风(piān fēng) Disease name. See *Su Wen* chapter 42. (1) Hemilateral wind. The general name of wind syndromes caused by wind pathogens invading a certain part of the body's internal organs, including wind syndromes of the five viscera, as well as brain wind, eye wind, leakage wind, endogenous wind, wind of the head, venting wind, and intestinal wind. (2) Paraplegia. See "偏枯" for detail. See *Su Wen* annotated by Wang Bing.

偏枯 病证名。偏，偏于身半。枯，肢体废而日久萎缩。偏枯即今称半身不遂。出《素问·生气通天论》《灵枢·热病》。

偏枯(piān kū) **paraplegia** Disease name. *Piān* means half. *Kū* means atrophy of the body. *Piān kū* means paraplegia. See *Su Wen* chapter 3 and *Ling Shu* chapter 23.

偏痹 病证名。半侧肢体酸疼沉重麻木之证。出《素问·本病论》。参"痹"条。

偏痹(piān bì) **hemilateral limb impediment** Name of disease which belongs to the syndrome of hemilateral limb soreness and numbness. See *Su Wen* chapter 73. See "痹".

假者反之 假，假象。反，与正相对，即与一般常规相反。病有真假，如见假寒假热之病，治疗当用不同于一般常规方法的反治法，如以寒治寒，以热治热。出《素问·五常政大论》。

假者反之(jiǎ zhě fǎn zhī) **anti-treatment** *Jiǎ* means false appearance. *Fǎn* means contrary to general. There are true and false diseases. For example, for false cold and false febrile disease, the anti-treatment should be different from the conventional methods, such as treating cold with cold and treating heat with heat. See *Su Wen* chapter 70.

得气 ① 针刺术语。即针感。指进针后，施以一定手法，在针下产生沉紧等感应，病人有酸、麻、重、胀等感觉，或沿经脉路线向远处放射的现象。这是针刺取得疗效的重要条件之一。出《灵枢·终始》《素问·离合真邪论》。② 指治病时，须根据天时气候并五脏五味苦欲所宜而用药，方为得调气之要领。出《素问·至真要大论》。

得气(dé qì) ① Acupuncture term. After the needle insertion, a certain technique is applied to produce a sense of tightness. The patient may have feelings of acidity，numbness，weight，swelling，or radiation to the extremities along the meridian's route. This is one of the important effects of acupuncture. See *Ling Shu* chapter 9 and *Su Wen* chapter 27. ② When treating the disease，the medicine should be taken according to the weather and the condition of five viscera as well as the rule of five tastes. This is the key of adjusting the qi. See *Su Wen* chapter 74.

得守　指脏气内守，协调之意。出《素问·脉要精微论》。

得守（dé shǒu）　**obtaining guard** Refers to the coordination of the visceral qi. See *Su Wen* chapter 17.

脚跳坚　症状名。指下肢膝以下部位有跳动及强硬感。出《灵枢·经筋》。

脚跳坚（jiǎo tiào jiān）　**stiff and beating feeling of lower limbs** Syndrome name. See *Ling Shu* chapter 13.

脖胦　穴位名。脖（bó 勃）胦（yāng 央），肓的原穴，即任脉的气海穴。一名下肓。在脐下一寸五分。见《灵枢·九针十二原》。

脖胦（bó yāng）　**Bo Yang（CV 6）** Name of an acupoint. Original acupoint of BL 43，also called the Qi Hai（CV 6）or Xia Huang（CV 6）point in the conception vessel. It located at 5 inches under the umbilicus. See *Ling Shu* chapter 1.

脱气　脱，脱失，耗脱的意思。脱气，与气脱义同，可见面色苍白，四肢厥冷，大汗淋漓，脉微欲绝等症候。出《灵枢·血络论》。

脱气（tuō qì）　**qi collapse** *Tuō* means losing. *Tuō qì*，sometimes recorded as *qì tuō*，is manifested with pale complexion，cold limbs，sweating，and faint pulse. See *Ling Shu* chapter 39.

脱肉　形容极度消瘦。出《素问·三部九候论》《素问·疟论》。

脱肉（tuō ròu）　**shedding of the flesh** Extreme emaciation. See *Su Wen* chapter 20 and 35.

脱血　大量失血之谓，包括呕血、吐血、衄血、便血以及女子血崩等。出《素问·平人气象论》《素问·腹中论》。

脱血（tuō xuè）　**blood desertion** Massive blood loss，including hematemesis，spitting blood，nosebleed，hematochezia and metrorrhagia in woman. See *Su Wen* chapter 18 and chapter 40.

脱色　面色突然苍白无华, 常为昏仆时伴随证候。见《素问·刺禁论》。

脱色（tuō sè）　**pale countenance** Pale facial complexion, always with the symptom of sudden syncope. See *Su Wen* chapter 52.

脱疽　病名。又名脱疽。发于足趾, 呈现黑色者, 热毒深重, 局部坏死, 急治之。不愈, 则急截之。否则可危及生命。出《灵枢·痈疽》。

脱疽（tuō yōng）　**sloughing welling abscess** Name of disease which starts on the toes and appears black, with severe heat toxin and local necrosis. This disease should be treated at an early stage quickly. If not cured, the lesion must be urgently cut away, otherwise it is life-threatening. See *Ling Shu* chapter 81.

脱营　病证名。由于先贵后贱, 心屈神伤, 志郁不伸, 导致营血虚衰的病证。出《素问·疏五过论》。

脱营（tuō yíng）　**exhaustion of nutrient qi** Disease name. Deficiency of nutrient-blood caused by sorrow and distress due to decline of living condition or social status. See *Su Wen* chapter 77.

逸者行之　治法。逸, 安逸。言气血凝滞的病症, 用行气活血的方法治疗。出《素问·至真要大论》。

逸者行之（yì zhě xíng zhī）　**treating stagnation by moving it** *Yi* means easy and comfortable. Treatment method in which the syndrome of qi and blood stagnation or disorders are treated with the method of activating qi and blood. See *Su Wen* chapter 74.

猛疽　病名。为发于咽喉之痈疽。由于毒势猛烈急速, 易塞咽喉而死, 故名。出《灵枢·痈疽》。

猛疽（měng jū）　**subcutaneous ulcer** Disease name. Refers to gangrene in the throat. Due to its violent and rapid poisonous nature, it is prone to plugging the throat and claiming lives, hence the name. See *Ling Shu* chapter 81.

馌　古噎字, 形容咽喉部犹如物堵, 而不得呼吸之状。出《灵枢·刺节真邪》。

馌（yē）　The ancient Chinese character of "噎"; the description of the situation of choking. See *Ling Shu* chapter 75.

凑理　即腠理, 见该条。出《素问·生气通天论》。

十一画

凑理(còu lǐ)　**striae and interstice**
The grain of skin and the texture of the subcutaneous flesh. See *Su Wen* chapter 3.

毫针　九针之一。长三寸六分，针尖细小，用针轻缓，留针稍长，治疗寒热痛痹，应用最广，又不伤正气。出《灵枢·九针十二原》。

毫针(háo zhēn)　**filiform needle**
One of the nine needles which is 3.6 cun long with a small tip. It is necessary that this kind of needle is applied with gentle force and remain slightly long on the surface of the human body. It is most widely used for treating pain or impediment caused by cold or heat and it does not hurt healthy qi. See *Ling Shu* chapter 1.

痔　病名。痔疮。出《素问·生气通天论》。

痔(zhì)　**hemorrhoids** Disease name. See *Su Wen* chapter 5.

痏　痏(wěi 委)。① 针刺计数单位。出《素问·刺腰痛》。② 指穴位。出《灵枢·热病》。③ 灸后瘢痕。引申为灸的次数。出《素问·刺腰痛》。④ 针孔。出《灵枢·邪气藏府病形》。

痏(wěi)　① The counting unit of needling. See *Su Wen* chapter

41. ② Acupoints. See *Ling Shu* chapter 23. ③ Scar after moxibustion. It is also used to count the number of moxibustion applications. See *Su Wen* chapter 41. ④ Pinhole. See *Ling Shu* chapter 4.

疵疽　病名。发于膝部的疽，见症外形漫肿，皮色不变，坚硬，发寒热。出《灵枢·痈疽》。

疵疽(cī jū)　**blemish swelling**
Name of disease in which there is a swollen carbuncle on the knee，unchanged in skin color，and hard. The patient always feels hot or cold. See *Ling Shu* chapter 81.

疵痈　病名。发于肩、臑的痈。出《灵枢·痈疽》。

疵痈(cī yōng)　**blemish abscess**
Name of disease in which an abscess starts from the shoulders and biceps. See *Ling Shu* chapter 81.

痎疟　痎(jiē 皆)。在此统指疟疾。即间歇发作的以寒战高热为特征的一类病证。又因此病往往迁延日久，致人瘦弱。出《素问·生气通天论》。

痎疟(jiē nüè)　**malaria** A disease characterized by intermittent high fever and chills which often lasts for a long time，making people thin and weak. See *Su Wen* chapter 3.

商　五音之一。五行属金,为西方秋金之音。运气学说以五音代表五运,以五音建运,则商为金运。出《素问·阴阳应象大论》。

商(shāng)　*shang* One of the five tones, pertaining to the metal phase. It is the tone of the western autumn metal. The school of five movements and six qi uses the five tones to represent and establish the five movements, thus *shang* means the movement of metal. See *Su Wen* chapter 5.

商丘　经穴名。足太阴脾经之经穴。在足内踝下前微陷者中。出《灵枢·本输》。

商丘(shāng qiū)　**Shang Qiu (SP 5)** An acupoint pertaining to the spleen meridian of foot *taiyin*. It is located at the indentation under the medial ankle. See *Ling Shu* chapter 2.

商阳　经穴名。又名绝阳。属手阳明大肠经,在示指桡侧指甲角旁约十分之一寸处。出《灵枢·本输》。

商阳(shāng yáng)　**Shang Yang (LI 1)** An acupoint pertaining to the large intestine meridian of hand *yangming*. Shang Yang (LI 1) is located at about one-tenth of an inch next to the corner of the nail on the radial side of the index finger. See *Ling Shu* chapter 2.

着痹　着,重着、留着之意。为痛处重滞固定的痹证。因风寒湿三邪之中,湿气偏胜,湿性滞着,故痛处固定。出《素问·痹论》。

着痹(zhuó bì)　**staying impediment** *Zhuó* is an adjective that means lingering or fixing, and refers to the impediment syndrome with pain lingering or fixing in a certain region. See *Su Wen* chapter 43.

粗工　医技粗糙的医生。出《素问·移精变气论》。

粗工(cū gōng)　**doctors with poor expertise** See *Su Wen* chapter 13.

焫　①烧的意思。出《素问·气交变大论》。②火灸法。《灵枢·痈疽》。

焫(ruò)　① Burn. See *Su Wen* chapter 69. ② Fire moxibustion. See *Ling Shu* chapter 81.

清气　①清阳之气。出《素问·阴阳应象大论》。②由胃化生的水谷精微中的轻清部分。出《灵枢·动输》。③清肃之气,为秋季气候的特征。出《素问·五常政大论》。④寒湿之气。出《灵枢·小针解》。

清气（qīng qì）　① The qi of clear yang. See *Su Wen* chapter 5. ② The light and clear part in the essence of the water and grain transformed and generated by the stomach. See *Ling Shu* chapter 62. ③ The qi of light and metal，and a characteristic of the autumn climate. See *Su Wen* chapter 70. ④ The qi of cold and dampness. See *Ling Shu* chapter 3.

清阳　① 指人体中轻清、上升的精微物质，有濡养上七窍的作用。出《素问·阴阳应象大论》。② 指卫气。出《素问·阴阳应象大论》。③ 指水谷精气。出《素问·阴阳应象大论》。④ 指自然界中轻清的阳气。出《素问·阴阳应象大论》。

清阳（qīng yáng）　① The light and clear essence in the human body，which has the function of nourishing the seven apertures in the human head. See *Su Wen* chapter 5. ② The defensive qi. See *Su Wen* chapter 5. ③ The essence of water and grain. See *Su Wen* chapter 5. ④ The light yang qi in nature. See *Su Wen* chapter 5.

清者温之　治法。病性清凉的，应用温热的方法治疗。出《素

问·至真要大论》。

清者温之（qīng zhě wēn zhī）　**to treat cool-natured diseases with warm methods** Treatment method of applying warmth/heat to treat cold-natured diseases. See *Su Wen* chapter 74.

清浊相干　清气属阳主升，浊气属阴主降。清阳浊阴互相干扰，以致升降失常，气机逆乱。出《灵枢·五乱》《灵枢·阴阳清浊》。

清浊相干（qīng zhuó xiāng gàn）　**the interference between the clear and turbid** Clear qi pertains to yang and always ascends whereas turbid qi pertains to yin，and always descends. Clear yang and turbid yin interfere with each other causing circuits and qi disorder. See *Ling Shu* chapter 34 and 40.

清厥　清，通清，冷之义。厥，厥逆。清厥，逆冷的意思。出《素问·藏气法时论》。

清厥（qīng jué）　**adverse flow of cold qi** "清" is the same as "清"，which means cold. *Jué* means inverse. *Qīng jué* means the adverse flow of cold qi. See *Su Wen* chapter 22.

淋　病名。小便淋沥不畅。出《素问·刺法论》。

淋(lín) **strangury** Disease name. Poor urination. See *Su Wen* chapter 72.

淋露 出《灵枢·官针》。① 指小便或经水淋沥不断。见《素问识》。② 作疲困解。

淋露(lín lù) See *Ling Shu* chapter 7. ① Continuous urination or menstruous blood. See *Su Wen Zhi*（*Understanding Su Wen*）. ② Tired and sleepy feeling.

渊腋 经穴名。属足少阳胆经。在腋中线上,当第五肋间隙处。一说在第四肋间隙。出《灵枢·经脉》《灵枢·痈疽》。

渊腋(yuān yè) **Yuan Ye（GB 22）** An acupoint that pertains to the gallbladder meridian of foot *shaoyang*. Yuan Ye（GB 22）is located at the midaxillary line，at the fifth intercostal space. See *Ling Shu* chapter 10 and 81.

淫气 ① 邪气。出《素问·痹论》。② 滋养。出《素问·经脉别论》。

淫气(yín qì) ① Pathogenic qi. See *Su Wen* chapter 43. ② Nutrients. See *Su Wen* chapter 21.

淫邪 ① 邪恶。出《素问·上古天真论》。② 泛指各种邪气。出《灵枢·九针论》《素问·八正神明论》。

淫邪(yín xié) ① Pathogen. See *Su Wen* Chapter 1. ② Various kinds of pathogenic qi. See *Ling Shu* chapter 78 and *Su Wen* chapter 26.

淫邪发梦 《灵枢》篇名。淫邪,泛指各种致病邪气。该篇主要论述了邪气淫溢内脏,以致魂魄飞扬,卧不得安而多梦的机理,指出各种梦境的发生,与脏腑的虚实有关,治疗以补虚泻实为原则,故名。

淫邪发梦(yín xié fā mèng) **Dreams due to Invasion of Pathogenic Factors** Chapter title in *Ling Shu*. *Yín xié* refers to various kinds of pathogenic qi that leads to disease. This chapter mainly discusses the mechanism of pathogenic qi that fills the internal organs and drives the spirit and soul out to make the patients restless and excessively dreaming at night. It points out that this is related to the deficiency and excess of the viscera. Treatment focuses on reducing excess and tonifying deficiency，hence the name.

淫泺 泺(luò 洛)。① 酸痛无力貌。出《素问·骨空论》。② 病变浸淫发展,逐渐加重。出《灵枢·厥病》。

淫泺（yín luò） ① Aching pain and acratia. See *Su Wen* chapter 60. ② Disease which develops and gradually deteriorates. See *Ling Shu* chapter 24.

液 ① 指津液中较稠厚，流动性较小的部分。由水谷所化生，灌注于骨节、脑髓、脏腑等组织，有濡养作用。出《灵枢·决气》《灵枢·口问》。② 指由五脏气化所产生的泪、汗、唾、涕、涎。出《素问·宣明五气》。

液（yè） ① The thicker，less fluid part of body fluids. It is transformed and generated by water and grain and perfused in tissues such as bone joints，brain marrow，and viscera，functioning as nourishing. See *Ling Shu* chapter 28 and chapter 30. ② The sweat，tears，salivation，nasal discharge and slabber produced by the qi transformation of the five viscera. See *Su Wen* chapter 23.

液门 经穴名。手少阳三焦经之荥穴。在小指次指间陷者中。出《灵枢·本输》。

液门（yè mén） **Ye Men（SJ 2）** An acupoint pertaining to the triple *jiao* meridian of hand *shaoyang*，and located at the

indentation of the second joint of the little finger. See *Ling Shu* chapter 2.

液脱 突然大量亡失津液。多因暴吐泻、多尿所致。出《灵枢·决气》。

液脱（yè tuō） **liquid collapse** A sudden loss of fluids mostly due to vomiting，diarrhea，or polyuria. See *Ling Shu* chapter 30.

惊则气乱 惊则神气散乱。出《素问·举痛论》。

惊则气乱（jīng zé qì luàn） **Fright causes disorder of qi.** See *Su Wen* chapter 39.

惊者平之 治法。出《素问·至真要大论》。① 惊悸，扰动不安一类病证，应用镇静安神之法治疗。见《类经·论治四》。② 因感触异常之声象而得的恐一类情志病，可用常闻常见之法，使之适应而趋平静。

惊者平之（jīng zhě píng zhī） Treatment method that originated in *Su Wen* chapter 74. ① For startled，disturbed，and other types of diseases, calming methods are used to treat. See *Lei Jing（Classified Classic）*"On Treatment Chapter 4". ② Panic caused by abnormal sounds or images can be adjusted and calmed down with exposure therapy.

惋　惋（wǎn 宛），郁结之意，在此指热内郁。出《素问·阳明脉解》。

惋（wǎn）　**pent-up** The stagnation of the inner heat. See *Su Wen* chapter 30.

寅申之纪　指纪年地支是寅、申之年，为少阳相火司天。纪，纪年。出《素问·六元正纪大论》。

寅申之纪（yín shēn zhī jì）　**the year of Yin or Shen** The calendar year when the earth branch is *Yin* or *Shen* and the *shaoyang* phase fire dominates the year. *Jì* means to record the year. See *Su Wen* chapter 71.

宿度　星宿运行的规律。出《素问·离合真邪论》。

宿度（sù dù）　**constellation law** The law of the movement of constellations. See *Su Wen* chapter 27.

密语　古籍名，即《玄珠密语》，已佚。出《素问·刺法论》。

密语（mì yǔ）　**Secret Word** Ancient book name, which has been lost in history. See *Su Wen* chapter 72.

谋风　八风之一，指由西南方刮来的风。出《灵枢·九宫八风》。

谋风（móu fēng）　*mou* **wind** One of the eight winds coming from the Southwest. See *Ling Shu* chapter 77.

谏议之官　指脾。脾主思虑，有协助心君决定意志的作用，故名。出《素问·刺法论》。

谏议之官（jiàn yì zhī guān）　**the officer of suggestion** The spleen dominates thinking and has the function of making decisions. Hence the name. See *Su Wen* chapter 72.

弹而怒之　言针刺虚证应用补法时的辅助手法。进针前用手弹其穴，以使气随脉络胀满如怒起，然后进针。出《素问·离合真邪论》。

弹而怒之（tán ér nù zhī）　**flicking manipulation** Auxiliary techniques when applying tonification needling techniques on deficiency syndromes. Before inserting the needles，flick the acupoints with the hand to make the qi swell along the meridians，and then insert the needles. See *Su Wen* chapter 27.

随　① 针刺方法之一。即迎随补泻法中的补法，针刺时针尖方向与经脉走向一致。出《灵枢·九针十二原》《灵枢·终始》。② 柔顺。出《素问·五常政大论》。

随（suí）　① Acupuncture method which is part of the directional

十一画

tonification and draining method. The direction of the needle tip is consistent with the direction of the meridian during acupuncture. See *Ling Shu* Chapter 1 and 9. ② Compliance. See *Su Wen* chapter 70.

颐　指目下齿上,颧鼻之间的部位。出《素问·至真要大论》。

颐(zhuō)　Refers to the area above the teeth under the eyes and between the cheekbone and nose. See *Su Wen* chapter 74.

隐白　经穴名。足太阴脾经之井穴,在足大趾内侧端。出《灵枢·本输》。

隐白(yǐn bái)　**Yin Bai (SP 1)** An acupoint that pertains to the spleen meridian of foot *taiyin*, and is located at the medial end of the toe. See *Ling Shu* chapter 2.

隐曲　见《素问·阴阳别论》《素问·风论》《素问·至真要大论》。① 男子前阴。② 指二便。③ 曲折难言的隐情。④ 人体俯首曲身。

隐曲(yǐn qū)　See *Su Wen* chapter 7, 42, and 74. ① Male genitals. ② Urine and stool. ③ The indescribable truth. ④ The human body bent over.

隐疹　皮肤瘙痒发疹。《素问·

四时刺逆从论》。

隐疹(yǐn zhěn)　**urticaria** Itchy skin rash. See *Su Wen* chapter 64.

颈动脉　指人迎动脉。出《灵枢·刺节真邪》。

颈动脉(jǐng dòng mài)　**man's prognosis artery** See *Ling Shu* chapter 75.

颈脉　即人迎脉,属足阳明经。出《素问·平人气象论》。

颈脉(jǐng mài)　**man's prognosis pulse** Pertains to meridian of foot *yangming*. See *Su Wen* chapter 18.

颈痈　病名。发于颈部之痈疡。初起者可针刺以散留止之气血,至气盛血聚化脓,可用砭石排泻之。出《素问·病能论》。

颈痈(jǐng yōng)　**neck carbuncle** Name of a disease in which a carbuncle develops on the neck. Little ones can be treated by acupuncture to disperse the stagnated qi and blood. However, if the qi is filled with blood and transformed into pus, then vermiculite is used to excrete it. See *Su Wen* chapter 46.

绳　面颊外侧耳前部位。面部色诊用以了解背部状况。出《灵枢·五色》。

绳(shéng)　**sheng** Anterior part of the cheek in front of the ear. Facial skin color inspection of this part can used to know the condition of the back. See *Ling Shu* chapter 49.

维厥 病症名。出《灵枢·邪气藏府病形》。（1）四肢厥逆之谓。见《类经·脉色十九》。（2）维指阴维脉，阳维脉。维厥为阴维阳维经气厥逆。见《灵枢注证发微》。

维厥（wéi jué） **linking reversal** Disease name. See *Ling Shu* chapter 4. (1) Cold limbs. See *Lei Jing* (*Classified Classic*) "Pulse and Color Chapter 19".

（2）*Wéi* refers to the *yinwei* meridian and the *yangwei* meridian. *Wéi jué* means the reversing qi of the *yinwei* meridian and the *yangwei* meridian. See *Ling Shu Zhu Zheng Fa Wei* (*Annotation and Elaboration on Ling Shu*).

维筋 左右相交维系某部分功能运动的筋。出《灵枢·经筋》。

维筋（wéi jīn） **linking sinew** The left and right intersecting sinews maintain a certain part of the functional movement. See *Ling Shu* chapter 13.

十二画

喜　① 七情之一。喜为心志，大喜则伤心。出《素问・举痛论》。② 善于。出《灵枢・癫狂》。

喜（xǐ）　① One of the seven emotions. Joy is the emotion of the heart. Overjoy hurts the heart. See *Su Wen* chapter 39. ② To be good at something. See *Ling Shu* chapter 22.

喜则气下　下，下坠、下陷。喜之太过，神气涣散下陷。出《素问・调经论》。

喜则气下（xǐ zé qì xià）　**Overjoy causes qi descendance.** *Xià* means to descend. Overjoy causes the descending of essence qi. See *Su Wen* chapter 62.

喜则气缓　喜则使人精神振奋，心情和缓，气机通利。但狂喜暴乐，亦可令人精神涣散，心气弛缓，出现心神异常的症状。出《素问・举痛论》。

喜则气缓（xǐ zé qì huǎn）　**Overjoy causes slackness of qi.** Joy inspires one's spirit, calms emotions, and makes the movement of qi easier. However, overjoy can also make people lose their spirits, relax and slow down their heart qi, and have abnormal symptoms of the heart. See *Su Wen* chapter 39.

喜伤心　心藏神，喜乐过极则心气弛缓，精神涣散，心悸、失眠，甚至精神错乱。出《素问・阴阳应象大论》《素问・五运行大论》。

喜伤心（xǐ shāng xīn）　**Overjoy damages the heart.** The heart stores spirit. Overjoy causes the heart qi to become loose, and the heart spirit scatters triggering palpitations, insomnia, and even insanity. See *Su Wen* chapter 5 and chapter 67.

喜胜忧　喜为心火之志，忧为肺金之志，火能克金，故云喜胜忧。又，忧则气机郁结，喜则气和志达，气机通利；喜可胜忧。这是一种"以情制情"的治疗方法。见《素问・阴阳应象大论》《素问・五运行大论》。

喜胜忧（xǐ shèng yōu）　**joy prevails over anxiety** Joy is the emotion of heart fire, and anxiety is the emotion of lung metal, thus fire can restrain metal. In addition，worry causes stagnation of circuits and qi，whereas joy makes free circuits and qi, so joy can restrain worry. This is a kind of psychological treatment method of restraining emotions with emotions. See *Su Wen* chapter 5 and 67.

援物比类　援，援引，引用。援物比类，即引用相类似的事物做比方，来说明医学的道理，为古人常用的思维方式和说理方法。出《素问·示从容论》。

援物比类（yuán wù bǐ lèi）**cited things as analogy** Similar things are cited as an analogy to explain the principles of medicine，the way of thinking and the reasoning commonly used by the ancients. See *Su Wen* chapter 76.

揆度　① 推测，度量。出《素问·玉版论要》。② 古医籍名。已佚。出《素问·病能论》。

揆度（kuí duó）　① Speculate；conjecture. See *Su Wen* chapter 15. ② An ancient medical book which has been lost in history. See *Su Wen* chapter 46.

散　① 脉来散乱不敛之象。揭示正气虚衰。出《素问·脉要精微论》。② 分散，与聚相对。出

《灵枢·五色》。③ 散行、散布。出《灵枢·经脉》。④ 耗散。出《素问·脉要精微论》。⑤ 指消散结聚的治疗方法。出《素问·至真要大论》。⑥ 指正气涣散的病证。出《素问·至真要大论》。⑦ 指散热。出《素问·生气通天论》。⑧ 疏散。出《素问·藏气法时论》。

散（sàn）　① The dissipated pulse，revealing a weakness in the healthy qi. See *Su Wen* chapter 17. ② Dispersal. See *Ling Shu* chapter 49. ③ Scatter. See *Ling Shu* chapter 10. ④ Dissipation. See *Su Wen* chapter 17. ⑤ The treatment of dissipative coalescence. See *Su Wen* chapter 74. ⑥ Refers to syndromes that lack healthy qi. See *Su Wen* chapter 74. ⑦ Heat dissipation. See *Su Wen* chapter 3. ⑧ Evacuation. See *Su Wen* chapter 22.

散下　针刺手法。针刺入皮肤后，向上、下、左、右不同方向刺之。适用于病情轻缓者。出《素问·诊要经终论》。

散下（sàn xià）　**dispersing manipulation** Acupuncture method. After the needle penetrates the skin，needle it upward，downward，left，and right. Applicable to those with mild diseases. See *Su Wen* chapter 16.

散阴颇阳 散,散乱。颇,偏,不正。言脉象散乱无常。出《素问·方盛衰论》。

散阴颇阳(sàn yīn pō yáng) **Yin disperses and yang increases.** Refers to the disperse pulse manifestation. See *Su Wen* chapter 80.

散者收之 治法。言精气耗散一类病症,如自汗,盗汗,久泻,崩漏,遗尿等,用收敛固涩法治疗。出《素问·至真要大论》。

散者收之(sàn zhě shōu zhī) **To treat dispersion with astringent** Treatment method. Syndromes of the dispersion of essence qi, such as spontaneous sweating, night sweats, chronic diarrhea, metrorrhagia, enuresis, etc., can be treated with astringent methods. See *Su Wen* chapter 74.

散俞 散布于经络之俞穴,用以出血。出《素问·诊要经论》。

散俞(sàn shū) **scattered acupoints** Acupoints scattered on meridians are used to stop bleeding. See *Su Wen* chapter 16.

散脉 出《素问·刺腰痛》。(1)足太阴经在小腿的支脉。见《素问》王冰注。(2)足阳明经在膝部的别络。见《素问识》。

散脉(sàn mài) See *Su Wen* chapter 41.（1）Branches of the foot *taiyin* meridian in the calf. See *Su Wen* annotated by Wang Bing.（2）Branches of the meridian of foot *yangming* in the knee. See *Su Wen Zhi* (*Understanding Su Wen*).

募 募,脏腑十二经脉经气结聚于胸腹部特定的腧穴,称为募穴。共有十二募穴。其名称是:中府(肺),期门(肝),日月(胆),章门(脾),京门(肾),天枢(大肠),膻中(心包),巨阙(心),中脘(胃),石门(三焦),关元(小肠),中极(膀胱)。出《素问·通评虚实论》。

募(mù) **front-*mu* points** The qi of the twelve meridians accumulate at specific points on the chest and abdomen. These points are called front-mu acupoints. They include 12 acupoints:LU 1 (Lung), LA 14 (Liver), GB 24 (Gallbladder), LR 13 (Spleen), GB 25 (Kidney), ST 25 (Large intestine), CV 17 (Pericardium), CV 14 (Heart), CV 12 (Stomach), CV 5 (Triple *jiao*), CV 4 (Small intestine), CV 3 (Bladder). See *Su Wen* chapter 28.

募原 肠胃外的膏膜。又称膜

原。出《灵枢·百病始生》。

募原(mù yuán)　**membrane source** The outer membrane of the intestine and stomach. See *Ling Shu* chapter 66.

募筋　募，通膜。膜筋，即筋膜。出《灵枢·邪客》。

募筋(mù jīn)　"募" is the same as "膜"."膜筋" is also written as "筋膜". See *Ling Shu* chapter 71.

楗　股骨。出《素问·骨空论》。

楗(jiàn)　**thigh bone** See *Su Wen* chapter 60.

厥　病证名。由于气机厥逆所引起的病证的总称，可因不同的表现而有不同名称：① 指以手足热或寒一类病证，即热厥、寒厥。由肾阴肾阳虚衰所致。出《素问·厥论》。② 昏厥，即突然昏倒不省人事之病证。《内经》有煎厥、薄厥、大厥、尸厥等证。各详该条。出《素问·厥论》。③ 指阴阳气机逆乱。出《素问·厥论》《素问·奇病论》《素问·解精微论》。

厥(jué)　Name of diseases, or a general name of the syndromes, caused by qi reversal, which may have different names due to different manifestations. ① heat or cold syndromes of foot and hand, such as heat syncope and cold syncope caused

by kidney yin and yang deficiency. See *Su Wen* chapter 45. ② syncope, namely, syndromes of sudden unconsciousness. *Huang Di's internal classic* includes boiling reversal, sudden syncope, coma and dead syncope. See *Su Wen* chapter 45. ③ reversal of the movement of yin and yang qi. See *Su Wen* chapter 45, 47 and 81.

厥大气　阴阳气血逆乱的厥证。出《素问·刺法论》。

厥大气(jué dà qì)　**reversal of qi and blood and disorder of yin and yang** Reversal syndrome featuring the reversal of qi and blood as well as the disorder of yin and yang. See *Su Wen* chapter 72.

厥气　① 逆乱之气。出《素问·阴阳应象大论》。② 指寒气。出《素问·至真要大论》。

厥气(jué qì)　① Reversing qi. See *Su Wen* chapter 5. ② Cold qi. See *Su Wen* chapter 74.

厥心痛　病证名。厥，逆之义。因五脏气机逆乱而致的心痛。包括肾心痛、胃心痛、脾心痛、肝心痛、肺心痛等多种心窝部疼痛之疾病。出《灵枢·厥病》。

厥心痛(jué xīn tòng)　**reversal heartache** Disease name, Jue refers to reversal. The heartache due to the reversal of the movement of qi of the five viscera, including reversal heart pain caused by kidney, stomach, spleen, liver and lung disease. See *Ling Shu* chapter 24.

厥头痛　病证名。由经气逆乱，上干头脑而致的头痛。出《灵枢·厥病》。

厥头痛（jué tóu tòng）　**reversal headache** Disease name of the headaches caused by the reversal of qi that invades the head and brain. See *Ling Shu* chapter 24.

厥论　《素问》篇名。厥：指阴阳气血逆乱而引起的病证。此篇较全面地论述了厥证的分类、病因病机及证治，故名。

厥论（jué lùn）　**Discussion on Jue-Syndrome** Chapter title in *Su Wen*. *Jué*, the name of the syndromes caused by the reversal of qi and blood as well as the disorder of yin and yang, this chapter comprehensively discusses the classification, etiology, pathogenesis, and treatment of *jue* syndromes, hence the name.

厥阴　① 指一阴。出《素问·经脉别论》。② 指二阴交尽。指阴历九、十月。出《素问·至真

要大论》《灵枢·阴阳系日月》。③ 单指或统指手、足厥阴心包、肝及其经脉。出《灵枢·经脉》《素问·诊要经终论》。④ 六气中之风气，主木。出《素问·五常政大论》《素问·六元正纪大论》。

厥阴（jué yīn）　① One yin. See *Su Wen* chapter 21. ② The lunar calendar's September and October. See *Su Wen* chapter 74 and *Ling Shu* chapter 41. ③ Refers to the hand, foot *jueyin* pericardium, liver and its meridians. See *Ling Shu* chapter 10 and *Su Wen* chapter 16. ④ Wind qi, one of the six factors in nature that dominates the wood phase. See *Su Wen* chapter 66 and 70.

厥阴之政　即厥阴司天之政。见该条。出《素问·六元正纪大论》。

厥阴之政（jué yīn zhī zhèng）　*jueyin* **dominates the celestial qi** See "厥阴司天之政". See *Su Wen* chapter 66.

厥阴之复　运气术语。复，即六气偏胜情况下而产生的复气。此指太阴湿土之气偏胜至一定程度，厥阴风木之气来复、气候变为多风、雨水湿度相对减少、尘土飞扬等。人体多见肝气偏胜之病。出《素问·至真要大论》。

厥阴之复（jué yīn zhī fù）　**retali-**

atory qi of *jueyin* A term in the five circuits and six qi theory. This refers to damp earth qi of the greater yin being particularly strong. The climate becomes windy, humidity decreases and it is dusty everywhere. Liver disease with prevalent liver qi is more common to see. See *Su Wen* chapter 74.

厥阴之胜 运气术语。指厥阴风木偏胜之气。如厥阴司天在泉之时风气偏盛,气候多风,人体多见肝气偏胜之肝病。出《素问·至真要大论》。

厥阴之胜(jué yīn zhī shèng) prevailing of *jueyin* A term in the five circuits and six qi theory. It refers to the qi of jueyin pertaining to wind and wood. For example, when wind qi is prevalent as *jueyin* dominates celestial qi and earth qi, it is windy in nature, and liver disease with prevalent liver qi is more common to see. See *Su Wen* chapter 74.

厥阴之厥 六经厥之一。乃足厥阴肝经气逆所致。症见少腹肿痛,腹胀,大小便不利,阴囊收缩等。出《素问·厥论》。

厥阴之厥(jué yīn zhī jué) qi-reversal of *jueyin* One of the six

meridian qi-reversals. It is caused by the reversal of qi of the liver meridian of foot *jueyin*. Symptoms include swelling and pain in the abdomen, bloating, unfavorable stools, and scrotal contraction. See *Su Wen* chapter 45.

厥阴风化 运气术语。化,制化,制则生化之意。根据五行原理,厥阴风木之气,可以制约湿土之气,从而维持自然气候的正常,有利于万物的生长化成。出《素问·六元正纪大论》。

厥阴风化(jué yīn fēng huà) transformation of *jueyin* A term in the five circuits and six qi theory. *Huà* means restraining and transforming. According to the rule of the five elements, qi of *jueyin* pertaining to wind and wood can restrain the qi of wet spleen earth to maintain a normal climatic condition, which is conducive to the growth and formation of everything. See *Su Wen* chapter 71.

厥阴司天 运气术语。指上半年由厥阴风木之气主事时的气候病候等情况。凡纪年地支逢巳、亥之年,均属厥阴风木司天。该年上半年气候偏温,风气偏胜,雨量减少。木能克土,临床多见脾病。出《素问·五常政大论》。

厥阴司天（jué yīn sī tiān）*jueyin dominates celestial qi* A term in the five circuits and six qi theory. It refers to the climatic and disease conditions when the qi of *jueyin* pertaining to wind and wood is in charge in the first half of the year. The years of which the Earthly Branches are *si* and *hai* have *jueyin* pertaining to wind and wood as the dominant celestial qi. In the first half of the year, the climate is warmer, the wind is milder, and there is less rainfall. Wood can restrain earth, thus clinically speaking, spleen diseases are more common to see. See *Su Wen* chapter 70.

厥阴司天之政 指厥阴风木司天的气候、物候及疾病流行情况。凡逢纪年地支是巳、亥的年份为厥阴风木司天。其特点是：厥阴主风、主温，气候上该年上半年偏温，风气偏胜，雨量减少。物候以麻、麦、谷类植物生长良好，毛虫、羽虫生育良好，介虫生育不利。临床多见肝盛侵脾犯胃的症状。政，主事、施政之意。出《素问·六元正纪大论》。

厥阴司天之政（jué yīn sī tiān zhī zhèng）**the condition when *jueyin* dominates celestial qi** Refers to the climate, phenology, and disease conditions when *jueyin*, pertaining to wind and wood, is the dominant celestial qi. The years when the Earthly Branches are *si* and *hai*, *jueyin* pertaining to wind and wood is the dominant celestial qi. In these years, *jueyin* dominates wind and warmth, the climate is warmer in the first half of the year, wind prevails, and the rainfall decreases. In these years, hemp, wheat, and cereal plants grow well, caterpillars and birds also grow well, whereas cypris grow badly. Symptoms of the liver invading the spleen and stomach are common to see. Zhèng here means dominating or administrating. See *Su Wen* chapter 71.

厥阴在泉 运气术语。指下半年由厥阴风木之气主事时的气候物候等情况。凡纪年地支逢寅、申之年，均属厥阴风木在泉。该年下半年气候多风、偏热。其所生成的食物或药物，在气味上也偏于温热。而具有清凉作用的药食物则生长不良。出《素问·五常政大论》。

厥阴在泉 (jué yīn zài quán)　*Jueyin* dominates terrestrial qi. A term in the five circuits and six qi theory. Refers to the climate and phenology dominated by the qi of *jueyin* pertaining to wind and wood in the second half of the year. The years when the Earthly Branches were *yin* and *shen* indicates that *jueyin* is the terrestrial qi. In the second half of the year，the climate is windy and hot. The food or medicine it produces is usually warm in smell and flavor. The food or medicine which is cool in nature grows poorly. See *Su Wen* chapter 70.

厥阴厥逆　十二经厥之一。为足厥阴肝经气逆之证。症见腰痛，少腹满，小便不利，谵语等。出《素问·厥论》。

厥阴厥逆 (jué yīn jué nì)　*jueyin reversal* One of the twelve meridian reversals that pertains to the syndrome of qi-reversal of the liver meridian of foot *jueyin*. Symptoms include lower back pain，abdomen fullness，unfavorable urination，impeded speech，etc. See *Su Wen* chapter 45.

厥疝　为腹中有气逆乱之证。出《素问·五藏生成》。① 因肾气上逆。见《素问》王冰注。② 因脾气逆于中。见《素问集注》。

厥疝 (jué shàn)　Abdominal qi-reversal. See *Su Wen* chapter 10. ① Kidney qi-reversal. See *Su Wen* annotated by Wang Bing. ② Spleen qi-reversal. See *Su Wen Ji Zhu*（*Collected Annotation of Su Wen*）.

厥逆　① 由于气逆所生的病证，如膺肿、颈痛、胸满、腹胀等。出《素问·腹中论》。② 十二经经气逆乱所致之病证，如太阴厥逆、少阴厥逆之类。出《素问·厥论》。③ 由寒邪犯脑所致之头痛。出《素问·大奇论》。

厥逆 (jué nì)　① Symptoms due to qi reversal，such as swelling，neck pain，chest fullness，abdominal distension and so on. See *Su Wen* chapter 40. ② Syndromes caused by the qi reversal of the twelve meridians，such as the qi reversal in greater yin or lesser yin. See *Su Wen* chapter 45. ③ Headaches caused by cold pathogens invading the brain. See *Su Wen* chapter 48.

厥热病　由热邪厥逆所致的病。见发热、头痛、眼部脉络抽动、鼻出血等。出《灵枢·热病》。

厥热病 (jué rè bìng)　**reversal fe-**

brile diseases Diseases caused by the reversal of heat pathogens. Symptoms include fever, headaches, vascular eye twitch, nosebleeds, etc. See *Ling Shu* chapter 23.

厥病　《灵枢》篇名。厥，逆也。此篇主要论述了由厥逆导致的九种厥头痛和六种厥心痛的不同症状和针刺方法，故名。

厥病（jué bìng）　*Jue* Syndrome Chapter title in *Ling Shu*. *Jué* means reverse. This chapter mainly discusses the different syndromes and acupuncture methods of the nine kinds of reversal headaches and six kinds of reversal heartaches, hence the name.

厥痹　自感逆气由下肢上升至腹的病证。出《灵枢·寒热病》。

厥痹（jué bì）　reversal impediment Symptoms of reversal qi rising from the lower limbs to the abdomen. See *Ling Shu* chapter 21.

雄黄　药名。性味苦辛温，有毒。有解毒消肿，杀虫之功。是古人用以预防疫疠的小金丹的组成之一。出《素问·刺法论》。

雄黄（xióng huáng）　realgar (*Realgar*) Name of a medicine which has a bitter, warm and pungent flavor. It is toxic and has the function of detoxification and swelling, an insecticidal effect. It is one of the constituents of the Xiao Jin Dan that the ancients used to prevent epidemics. See *Su Wen* chapter 72.

颊　面部两侧，在颧弓下耳前方处。出《素问·刺热》。

颊（jiá）　cheek The area on both sides of the face, in front of the lower ear of the zygomatic arch. See *Su Wen* chapter 32.

颊车　经穴名。属足阳明胃经，别名曲牙。在耳下曲颊端陷者中。出《灵枢·经脉》。

颊车（jiá chē）　Jia Che (ST 6) Acupoint name pertaining to the stomach meridian of foot *yangming*. It is located at the indentation under the ear of the buccal side. See *Ling Shu* chapter 10.

悲　七情之一。悲哀。出《素问·举痛论》。

悲（bēi）　sorrow One of the seven emotions. See *Su Wen* chapter 39.

悲则气消　消，通销，销蚀之义。悲哀气郁，销蚀正气。出《素问·举痛论》。

悲则气消（bēi zé qì xiāo）　Sorrow causes qi consumption. "消" is as the same as "销", which means consumption. Sorrow causes qi stagnation and consumes healthy qi. See *Su Wen* chapter 39.

悲胜怒　悲为肺金之志,怒为肝木之志,金能克木,故云悲胜怒。又,怒则气上,悲则气消,故悲可制怒。这是一种"以情制情"的心理治疗方法。出《素问·阴阳应象大论》《素问·五运行大论》。

悲胜怒（bēi shèng nù）　**Sorrow overcomes anger.** Sorrow is the emotion of lung metal, and anger is the emotion of liver wood, therefore metal can restrain wood, or sorrow can restrain anger. Also, anger will cause the qi to rise, whereas sorrow will cause the qi to be consumed. This is one of the psychological treatment methods of restraining emotions with emotions. See *Su Wen* chapter 5 and 67.

紫金　即金箔。性味辛平有毒。炼后入药有镇惊解毒作用。是古人用以预防疫疠的小金丹的组成之一。出《素问·刺法论》。

紫金（zǐ jīn）　**purple gold** Refers to the goldleaf. Pungent and toxic in flavor. After being refined, it has analgesic and detoxifying effects. It is one of the constituents of the Xiao Jin Elixir that the ancients used to prevent epidemics. See *Su Wen* chapter 72.

暑　①是夏季炎热的气候。出《素问·五运行大论》。②病因。为六淫之一。暑为阳邪,多在夏季致病,易耗津伤气。出《素问·生气通天论》。③病名。夏天为暑热之邪所伤的病变。出《素问·热论》。

暑（shǔ）　① Hot climate in summer. See *Su Wen* chapter 67. ② Etiology. One of the six kinds of pathogenic qi. Summer is a yang pathogen, and usually causes diseases in summer, in which body fluids and qi are easily consumed. See *Su Wen* chapter 3. ③ Disease name of those caused by summer pathogens in summer. See *Su Wen* chapter 31.

瞤（rún 音闰）,肌肉掣动。出《素问·气交变大论》《素问·六元正纪大论》。

瞤（rún）　**muscle tremor** See *Su Wen* chapter 70 and *Su Wen* chapter 72.

跗　足背。出《灵枢·骨度》。

跗（fū）　**acrotarsium.** See *Ling Shu* chapter 14.

跗上　足背上冲阳穴处。出《素问·疟论》。

跗上（fū shàng）　**dorsal aspect of**

the foot at the area of Chong Yang acupoint Area around the ST 42 acupoint. See *Su Wen* chapter 35.

跗属 足背前后所附属的组织，包括踝关节等。出《灵枢·骨度》。

跗属（fū shǔ） **attached foot** Tissue attached to the back of the foot，including the ankle. See *Ling Shu* chapter 14.

遗 ① 指病邪遗留未尽，热病迁延不愈。因病中或病邪将退之时多食所致。出《素问·热论》。② 失禁的意思。出《灵枢·九针论》。

遗（yí） ① Pathogen qi lingers and febrile disease lasts. It is caused by overeating when recovering from disease. See *Su Wen* chapter 31. ② Incontinence. See *Ling Shu* chapter 78.

遗矢 矢通屎，即大便。遗矢为大便失控遗出。出《素问·咳论》。

遗矢（yí shǐ） **fecal incontinence** "矢" is the same as "屎"，which refers to the stool. Fecal incontinence refers to uncontrolled excretion of stool. See *Su Wen* chapter 38.

遗溲 溲，小便。遗溲即小便失控而自遗。出《素问·刺腰痛》。

遗溲（yí sōu） **remaining urine** Incontinence of urine. See *Su*

Wen chapter 41.

遗溺 即遗尿。多由肾气不摄，膀胱失约所致。出《灵枢·九针论》。

遗溺（yí nì） **enuresis** Mostly caused by lack of kidney qi and the bladder losing control. See *Ling Shu* chapter 78.

蛟蛕 指蛔虫。蛕（jiāo 交）。出《灵枢·厥病》。

蛟蛕（jiāo huí） **roundworm** See *Ling Shu* chapter 24.

喘 ① 呼吸急促。出《素问·五藏生成》。② 指脉象。形容脉来急促，躁动如喘。出《素问·五藏生成》。③ 指局部的明显搏动。出《素问·举痛论》。

喘（chuǎn） ① Shortness of breath. See *Su Wen* chapter 10. ② Refers to a rapid，agitated pulse manifestation. See *Su Wen* chapter 10. ③ Refers to a local abnormal pulse. See *Su Wen* chapter 39.

喘鸣 呼吸急促，喉中鸣响。出《素问·阴阳别论》。

喘鸣（chuǎn míng） **wheezing dyspnea** Shortness of breath，and ringing in the throat. See *Su Wen* chapter 7.

喘逆 呼吸急促，上逆一类病证。由各种原因阻碍气机升降所致。出《素问·脉要精微论》。

喘逆（chuǎn nì）　**panting counterflow** Syndromes such as shortness of breath and qi reversal due to various reasons hindering the rising of the movement of qi. See *Su Wen* chapter 17.

喘息　① 呼吸气息。出《素问·阴阳应象大论》。② 呼吸气促。出《灵枢·杂病》。

喘息（chuǎn xī）　① Breath. See *Su Wen* chapter 5. ② Shortness of breath. See *Ling Shu* chapter 26.

喘喝　呼吸急促,发出喝喝之声。出《素问·生气通天论》。

喘喝（chuǎn hē）　**wheezing asthma** Taking short breaths, making the sound of he-he. See *Su Wen* chapter 3.

喉中　指廉泉穴,属任脉经。在颈部颔下,结喉上四寸中央。出《灵枢·卫气失常》。

喉中（hóu zhōng）　**Hou Zhong** (CV 23) Refers to Lianquan acupoint pertaining to the conception vessel and located at the center below the neck, four *cun* up from the throat. See *Ling Shu* chapter 59.

喉吤　吤,《脉经》作"介"。喉介,喉中如有物梗塞。出《灵枢·邪气藏府病形》。

喉吤（hóu jiè）　**throat obstruction** "吤" is written as "介" in the Mai Jing（*Cannon of Pulse*）. Something is stuck in the throat. See *Ling Shu* chapter 4.

喉痹　病名。指咽喉不利肿痛,音嘶等病证。出《素问·阴阳别论》《素问·咳论》。

喉痹（hóu bì）　**throat impediment** Disease name. Refers to syndromes such as swelling and sore throat, and hoarseness. See *Su Wen* chapter 7 and 38.

黑尸鬼　指水疫之邪。出《素问·本病论》。

黑尸鬼（hēi shī guǐ）　**black corpse ghost** Refers to pathogens coming from water-pestilence. See *Su Wen* chapter 73.

黑脉　肾脉。黑为肾之色,故称。出《素问·五藏生成》。

黑脉（hēi mài）　**black meridian** Kidney meridian of which the black color pertains to the kidney, hence the name. See *Su Wen* chapter 10.

黑眼　指瞳孔外围之黑色部分,即虹膜,与肝相应。出《灵枢·大惑论》。

黑眼（hēi yǎn）　**black eyes** Refers to the black part around the pupil, or the iris which corresponds to the liver. See *Su Wen* chapter 80.

骭　小腿胫骨。出《灵枢·经脉》。

骭（gàn）　**calf tibia** See *Ling Shu* chapter 10.

骭厥　病证名。骭（gàn 干），足胫骨。足阳明经气厥逆而出现种种病候称为骭厥。见上高而歌，弃衣而走，贲响腹胀等症。出《灵枢·经脉》。

骭厥（gàn jué）　**tibia reversal** Disease name. *Gàn* means tibia. It is a disease of the foot *yangming* meridian caused by qi reversal. Patients have symptoms like climbing to high places and singing, walking away without clothes，borborygmus and abdominal distension. See *Ling Shu* chapter 10.

锋针　九针之一，长一寸六分，三面有口，锐而锋利，后人称"三棱针"用于刺络放血，治热毒痈疡或顽固性疾病。出《灵枢·九针十二原》。

锋针（fēng zhēn）　**lance needle** One of the nine types of acupuncture needles. It is 1.6 *cun* long and has three sides of sharp edges. The later generations named it the three-edged needle and used it for releasing blood from the collaterals to cure heat toxins, welling-abscesses and sores, and some

obstinate diseases. See *Ling Shu* chapter 1.

锐骨　突起明显而锐的高骨。① 掌后腕部小指侧的高骨。出《灵枢·本输》。② 肘部内侧的高骨。出《灵枢·经筋》。

锐骨（ruì gǔ）　**The protuberant bone.** ① The protuberant bone on the wrist close to the palm by the side of the little finger. See *Ling Shu* chapter 2. ② The protuberant bone by the inner side of elbow. See *Ling Shu* chapter 13.

锐疽　病名。发于尾骶部的疽。形大色赤坚硬，其位在尾骶尖端，故名。后世称谓鹳口疽。出《灵枢·痈疽》。

锐疽（ruì jū）　**pilonidal disease** Disease name of a carbuncle that is located at end of the tailbone，big, red and hard. See *Ling Shu* chapter 81.

锐眦　外侧眼角。出《灵枢·癫狂》。

锐眦（ruì zì）　**outer canthus** See *Ling Shu* chapter 22.

锐掌　掌后高骨。出《灵枢·经脉》。

锐掌（ruì zhǎng）　**the bulged bone at the end of the palm** See *Ling Shu* chapter 10.

短　短脉。脉应指部位短，按寸不及关。揭示气血不足或气滞之象。出《素问·脉要精微论》。

短（duǎn）　**short pulse** The palpating area at the wrist where one can feel the pulse is short. This means that when feeling *cun* pulse, one cannot feel *guan* at the same time. It reveals insufficiency of qi and blood，or qi stagnation. See *Su Wen* chapter 17.

短虫　蛲虫。出《素问·脉要精微论》。

短虫（duǎn chóng）　**roundworm.** See *Su Wen* chapter 17.

短则气病　短，指脉形短于本位。为气血不足或气滞之病象。出《素问·脉要精微论》。

短则气病（duǎn zé qì bìng）　**Short pulse-feeling area indicates qi dificiency.** *Duǎn* refers to the touching area at the wrist where one can feel the pulse is short，revealing insufficiency of qi and blood，or qi stagnation. See *Su Wen* chapter 17.

短针　泛指各种针具。出《素问·宝命全形论》。

短针（duǎn zhēn）　**short needle** Generally，it refers to all kinds of needles for acupuncture. See *Su Wen* chapter 25.

短刺　刺法之一。进针时略略摇动针体而慢慢深入，在近骨处将针上下提插，似摩骨状，用治骨痹等深部病痛。出《灵枢·官针》。

短刺（duǎn cì）　**short needling** One of the needling methods which involves inserting a needle into the skin slowly and then shaking the needle slightly while pushing it deep into the skin，and then maneuvering it up and down when the needle is close to the bone as if massaging the bone to cure bone paralysis and so on. See *Ling Shu* chapter 7.

智　①智慧。在深思熟虑后，恰当地处理事物的能力之谓。出《灵枢·本神》。②聪明，有见识的人。出《素问·上古天真论》。③神志，意识。出《灵枢·热病》。

智（zhì）　① Wisdom. A kind of ability to deal with things with deliberation. See *Ling Shu* chapter 8. ② Intelligence，or people with vision. See *Su Wen* chapter 1. ③ Spirit and awareness. See *Ling Shu* chapter 23.

犊鼻　经穴名。属足阳明胃经，又称外膝眼。在膝关节前外侧大筋凹陷处。出《素问·气穴论》。

犊鼻（dú bí）　**Du Bi（ST 35）** An acupoint that pertains to the stomach meridian of foot *yang-*

ming，located at the anterolateral indentation of the knee's large sinew. See *Su Wen* chapter 58.

筋　① 五体之一。是联系全身骨节肌肉的筋腱韧带的总称。细分之，附于骨节的称筋，包于肌肉之外的称筋膜。出《灵枢·经脉》。筋质柔韧坚劲，有约束保护骨骼肌肉的作用，与人体活动关系最大。为肝脏所主，赖肝血濡养而柔韧。出《素问·宣明五气》。② 青色脉络。出《灵枢·水胀》。③ 经筋。是十二经脉连属于肢体外周筋肉的体系。出《灵枢·经筋》。④ 指代肝。出《灵枢·大惑论》。

筋（jīn）　① As one of five body constituents，sinew is the general name for all the sinews and ligaments. More specifically，those which adhere to bones are named sinews，and those which cover the muscles are named sinew membranes. See *Ling Shu* chapter 10. Sinews are strong and flexible. They regulate and protect the bones，which are of utmost importance for human movement. They are governed by the liver and nourished and softened by liver blood. See *Su Wen* chapter 23. ② Black col-

laterals. See *Ling Shu* chapter 57. ③ Meridian sinew，the meridians that connect the sinews on the periphery of the human body. See *Ling Shu* chapter 13. ④ Refers to the liver. See *Ling Shu* chapter 80.

筋之府　出《素问·脉要精微论》。见"膝者筋之府"条。

筋之府（jīn zhī fǔ）　house of sinews See *Su Wen* chapter 17. Also see term "膝者筋之府".

筋之精为黑眼　肝主筋，筋之精即肝之精。黑眼，即眼中的虹膜部分，能反映肝的生理病理状态。出《灵枢·大惑论》。

筋之精为黑眼（jīn zhī jīng wèi hēi yǎn）　essence of sinew is the black eye (iris) Black eye is the iris which reflects the physiological and pathological condition of the liver. See *Ling Shu* chapter 80.

筋生心　亦五脏相生，肝生心之意。出《素问·阴阳应象大论》。

筋生心（jīn shēng xīn）　sinew engenders heart It is the same as liver engendering the heart according to the five-viscera generation theory. See *Su Wen* chapter 5.

筋纽　筋相结之处。出《灵枢·九宫八风》。

筋纽（jīn niǔ）　**sinew knot** The knots that sinews connect. See *Ling Shu* chapter 77.

筋脉　也称筋膜。包括现代所称之肌腱、韧带等。出《素问·生气通天论》。

筋脉（jīn mài）　**sinew membrane** Modern medicine includes sinews，ligaments，etc. See *Su Wen* chapter 3.

筋度　度，度数。指筋的长短度数。出《素问·通评虚实论》。

筋度（jīn dù）　**sinew measurement** *Dù* refers to the measurement of the length of sinews. See *Su Wen* chapter 28.

筋痹　病证名。五体痹之一。病发于春季的痹证。因春主筋，故名。出《素问·痹论》。

筋痹（jīn bì）　**sinew paralysis** One of the five-body impediments occuring in spring which governs the sinews. See *Su Wen* chapter 43.

筋溜　病名。溜亦作瘤。由邪气结聚于筋，致筋屈而不能伸之病。出《灵枢·刺节真邪》。

筋溜（jīn liū）　**sinew tumor** "溜" is the same as "瘤". Pathogen qi gathers in sinews to curve them from being straightened. See *Ling Shu* chapter 75.

筋膜　指筋。出《素问·平人气象论》。

筋膜（jīn mó）　**sinew** See *Su Wen* chapter 18.

筋瘘　病名。鼠瘘之属。出《灵枢·经筋》。

筋瘘（jīn lòu）　**sinew fistula** Disease name. One kind of tuberculous fistula. See *Ling Shu* chapter 13.

筋躄　足不能行。出《灵枢·热病》。

筋躄（jīn bì）　**foot cripple** See *Ling Shu* chapter 23.

筋癫疾　病证名。癫疾之一种。因症有身体蜷缩挛急，脉大等，故名。出《灵枢·癫狂》。

筋癫疾（jīn diān jí）　**sinew epilepsy** A kind of epilepsy which manifests itself with a curling and cramping body and surging pulse. See *Ling Shu* chapter 22.

脂　大肠。出《灵枢·淫邪发梦》。

脂（zhí）　**big intestine** See *Ling Shu* chapter 43.

腓　又称腨。小腿肚。出《灵枢·寒热病》。

腓（féi）　**calf** The same as "腨" （shuàn）. See *Ling Shu* chapter 21.

腘　肘、膝后丰厚突起之肌肉。出《素问·玉机真藏论》。

腘（jùn）　*jun* The muscle that bulges at the back of the elbows and knees. See *Su Wen*

chapter 19.

膕肉　肌肉积聚之处。出《灵枢·卫气失常》。

膕肉（jùn ròu）　*jun* flesh The place that muscles gather. See *Ling Shu* chapter 59.

腄　臀部。出《素问·脉解》。

腄（shuí）　hip See *Su Wen* chapter 49.

脾　① 五脏之一。位居中焦，具有运化水谷，输布精微，化生气血的重要功能。其为胃行其津液，后世称为"生化之源""后天之本"。其经脉为足太阴脾经，与足阳明胃经相表里，五行配属为土，分主四时（一说长夏）。其在体为肉，在志为思，在液为涎，在窍为口，在味为甘，病理特征为湿。出《素问·太阴阳明论》《素问·灵兰秘典论》。② 脾之精气。出《素问·阴阳应象大论》。③ 足太阴脾经的经气。出《灵枢·本输》。④ 脾的运化功能。出《素问·太阴阳明论》。⑤ 脾在面部的望诊部位（鼻准头）。出《灵枢·五色》。

脾（pí）　① Spleen. It is one of the five viscera located in the middle *jiao* and functions as the organ that transforms water and grain, dissipates essence and generates qi and blood. The spleen generates liquid for the stomach, hence considered as the origin of generation and the foundation of nurtured life in later medical books. It pertains to the spleen meridian of foot *taiyin* and has interior and exterior relationships with the stomach meridian of foot *yangming*. It pertains to the earth phase and governs the four seasons (also called late summer). It corresponds to flesh according to the constitutions, thought to wills, saliva to liquids, mouth to orifices, sweet to flavors, and dampness to physiological characteristics. See *Su Wen* chapter 29 and 8. ② Essence qi of the spleen. See *Su Wen* chapter 5. ③ Meridian qi in the spleen meridian of foot *taiyin*. See *Ling Shu* chapter 2. ④ The transporting and transforming functions of the spleen. See *Su Wen* chapter 29. ⑤ Nose tip, which is the corresponding part on the face of the spleen. See *Ling Shu* chapter 49.

脾之大络　十五别络之一，穴名大包，其络从渊腋下三寸处分出，散布于胸胁部。出《灵枢·经脉》。

脾之大络（pí zhī dà luò）　the

large collateral of the spleen
One of the fifteen connecting
collaterals. It starts from Da
Bao （SP 21） and scatters
around the chest and rib-side.
See *Ling Shu* chapter 10.

脾不主时　脾属土位居中央,灌
溉于四藏,四时之中皆有土气,
每季之末各十八日为其旺时而
不独主一个时季。出《素问·
太阴阳明论》。

脾不主时（pí bù zhǔ shí）　**spleen
has no dominant season** The
spleen pertains to the earth element which is located at the
center of the five elements and
nurtures the other four viscera.
It exists in all four seasons and
dominates the latter 18 days of
each season. See *Su Wen* chapter
29.

脾气　① 指脾的精气,可滋养肌
肉、四肢乃至全身脏腑经络。
与口相通。出《灵枢·本神》。
② 脾的运化功能。出《素问·
经脉别论》。

脾气（pí qì）　① Essence qi of the
spleen，which can nourish mus-
cles，limbs and even the viscera
and bowels and meridians of
the whole body，communicating
with the mouth. See *Ling Shu*
chapter 8. ② The transporting

and transforming functions of the
spleen. See *Su Wen* chapter 21.

脾风　病名。风邪传变过程中由
肝传脾,或风邪直接内伤于脾
而出现多汗恶风,身体怠惰乏
力,不欲食,黄疸,发热等症状
的病证。出《素问·风论》《素
问·玉机真藏论》。

脾风（pí fēng）　**spleen wind** Disease name，of one which is
caused by wind pathogens that
transfer from the liver to the
spleen or go straight into spleen
and lead to excessive sweating，
aversion to wind，fatigue and
lack of strength，lack of appe-
tite，jaundice，fever，etc. See
Su Wen chapter 19 and 42.

脾风疝　疝病之一。由脾脏功能
失调,湿邪下注阴囊,而致肿坠
顽癫病。出《素问·四时刺逆
从论》。

脾风疝（pí fēng shàn）　**spleen
wind hernia** The malfunction of
the spleen causing dampness to
fall down into the scrotum and
thus leading to distention. See
Su Wen chapter 64.

脾为之使　使,役使之意。言脾的
运化功能。出《素问·刺禁论》。

脾为之使（pí wèi zhī shǐ）　**spleen
acts as the envoy** Refers to the
spleen's function of transporting

and transforming. See *Su Wen* chapter 52.

脾为阴中之至阴　根据阴阳五行原理,阴阳中又有阴阳可分。出《灵枢·阴阳系日月》。

脾为阴中之至阴(pí wèi yīn zhōng zhī zhì yīn)　**Spleen pertains to extreme yin among the five viscera.** According to the theory of the five elements, there are different levels of yin and yang. See *Ling Shu* chapter 44.

脾为涎　涎(xián 贤),口液,五液之一,出于口,口为脾之窍,故云。出《素问·宣明五气》。《灵枢·九针论》作"脾主涎"。

脾为涎(pí wèi xián)　**Spleen forms saliva.** *Xián* refers to saliva, one of the five kinds of fluids. It comes from the mouth which is the orifice where the spleen opens at. See *Su Wen* chapter 23. In *Ling Shu* chapter 78, this term is recorded as "脾主涎".

脾心痛　病证名。厥心痛之一。由脾气厥逆犯心所致,症见心痛如锥刺甚剧。出《灵枢·厥病》。

脾心痛(pí xīn tòng)　**reversal heartache caused by spleen disorder** Name of a disease. It is one of the reversal heartaches, which caused by the reversal of spleen qi attacking the heart and manifesting as heart pain as if pierced by thorn. See *Ling Shu* chapter 24.

脾生肉　脾主肌肉,脾气有生养肌肉的生理功能。见《素问·阴阳应象大论》。

脾生肉(pí shēng ròu)　**Spleen nourishes muscles.** The spleen governs the muscles, or generates and nourishes the muscles. See *Su Wen* chapter 5.

脾主口　脾受水谷,口纳五味,故主口。又唇之四白乃脾藏精气在外反映之处。故云。出《素问·阴阳应象大论》。

脾主口(pí zhǔ kǒu)　**Spleen governs mouth.** The spleen receives water and grain, while the mouth tastes the five flavors, hence to say the spleen governs the mouth. Moreover, the Four Whites (white muscles around mouth) reflect the essence qi contained in the spleen, hence to say that spleen governs mouth. See *Su Wen* chapter 5.

脾主长夏　此以五行学说归纳脏腑与季节时日的关系及治法。长夏主土属中央。足太阴脾是土脏,为己土、阴土;足阳明胃与脾相表里,为戊土、阳土,故治法相同。出《素问·藏气法时论》。

脾主长夏（pí zhǔ cháng xià）

Spleen governs late summer. The five element theory summarizes the relationship between the viscera and the seasons and their corresponding treatments. The late summer governs the earth element which is located in the middle of the five elements. The meridian of spleen foot *taiyin* is a viscus pertaining to earth, namely *Ji* earth branch (*Ji* is the sixth of the ten celestial stems) or yin-type earth branches; the meridian of stomach foot *yangming*, which is interiorly and exteriorly related to the spleen, pertains to *wu* earth branch (*wu* is the fifth of the ten heavenly branches), or yang-type earth branches. They share the same treatment methods. See *Su Wen* chapter 22.

脾主为胃行其津液者也 脾与胃相连，脏腑相合，相辅相成。胃主受纳腐熟水谷，化生精微津液，必赖脾气的输布运行，而后能布行于肢体周身。出《素问·太阴阳明论》。

脾主为胃行其津液者也（pí zhǔ wèi wèi xíng qí jīn yè zhě yě）

Spleen governs movement of stomach liquid. The spleen connects with the stomach, each assisting the other. The stomach contains and decomposes water and grain to generate essence and liquid, which are transported and distributed to all over the body by spleen qi. See *Su Wen* chapter 29.

脾主肉 主，掌管、主持之意。脾通于五脏，而五脏元真之气皆会通于肌肉腠理，故脾所主之外合为肉。出《素问·宣明五气》。

脾主肉（pí zhǔ ròu） **Spleen governs flesh.** *Zhǔ* means to govern or dominate. The spleen transports and distributes essence and qi to the five viscera, and the five viscera transport essence and qi to the flesh and interstices, hence to say the spleen governs flesh. See *Su Wen* chapter 23.

脾主肌 出《灵枢·九针论》。义同"脾主肉"，见该条。

脾主肌（pí zhǔ jī） **Spleen governs muscles.** See *Ling Shu* chapter 78. See "脾主肉".

脾主吞 吞，指反胃吞酸。言脾之病。出《灵枢·九针论》。《素问·宣明五气》作"脾为吞"。

脾主吞(pí zhǔ tūn)　Spleen disease leads to acid regurgitation. *Tūn* refers to nausea and acid regurgitation，diseases caused by malfunction of the spleen. See *Ling Shu* chapter 78. *Su Wen* chapter 23 records it as "脾为吞".

脾主身之肌肉　出《素问·痿论》。义同"脾主肉"，参该条。

脾主身之肌肉(pí zhǔ shēn zhī jī ròu)　Spleen dominates muscles all over the body. See *Su Wen* chapter 44. The same as "脾主肉".

脾主涎　义同"脾为涎"，参该条。出《灵枢·九针论》。

脾主涎(pí zhǔ xián)　Spleen dominates saliva. It is the same as "脾为涎". See *Ling Shu* chapter 78.

脾合肉　合，配合之意。出《灵枢·五色》。义同"脾主肉"，参该条。

脾合肉(pí hé ròu)　Spleen coordinates flesh. *Hé* means coordinate. See *Ling Shu* chapter 49. It is the same as "脾主肉".

脾合胃　合，配合之意。足阳明胃经与足太阴脾经相为表里，脾与胃以膜相连，两者功能上有密切联系。出《灵枢·本输》。

脾合胃(pí hé wèi)　Spleen coordinates stomach. *Hé* means to coordinate. The stomach meridian of foot *yangming* is interiorly and exteriorly related to the spleen meridian of foot *taiyin*，and the spleen is connected to the stomach by a membrane，which means that the spleen and stomach are closely related to each other in function. See *Ling Shu* chapter 2.

脾足太阴之脉　即足太阴脾经。为十二经脉之一。其循行路线从足大趾尖端(隐白穴)开始，沿大趾内侧赤白肉分界处，上行过大趾本节后的核骨，上行足内踝前方，再上腿肚，沿胫骨的后方，穿过足厥阴肝经的前面，进入腹部，属于脾，络于胃，穿过横膈，挟咽两旁，连于舌根，散于舌下。一支从胃部上行，通过横膈，注于心中(接手少阴心经)。出《灵枢·经脉》。

脾足太阴之脉(pí zú tài yīn zhī mài)　spleen meridian of foot *taiyin* One of the twelve meridians which starts from the tip of the big toe（YinBai point，SP 1) and goes upwards along the middle line of the inner side of the big toes，then passes the round bone of the big toe to the border part of the inner side of the ankles, goes along the calf and the posterior side of the shin bone, then across the liver meridian of foot *jueyin* and finally into the abdomen. There, it pertains to the spleen, connects to the stomach, and penetrates the diaphragm to the both sides of the throat, connects to the root of the tongue and finally scatters to the underside of the tongue. The other branch starts from the stomach, goes upwards, and penetrates the diaphragm to the both sides of the throat, connects to the root of the tongue and finally scatters to the underside of tongue. A branch goes upward from the stomach and penetrates the diaphragm until stretches into the heart (connecting the heart meridian of hand *shaoyin*). See *Ling Shu* chapter 10.

脾应肉　应，应合之意。出《灵枢·本藏》。与"脾主肉"义同，见该条。

脾应肉(pí yīng ròu)　**Spleen corresponds with flesh.** See *Ling Shu* chapter 47. It is the same as "脾主肉".

脾者主为卫　卫，护卫脏腑之意。

脾运化水谷，濡养脏腑，长养肌肉。出《灵枢·师传》。

脾者主为卫(pí zhě zhǔ wèi wèi)　**spleen as the guardian of viscera** *Wèi* means guard. The spleen transforms and transports water and grain so as to nurture the viscera and muscles. See *Ling Shu* chapter 29.

脾和则口能知五谷矣　出《灵枢·脉度》。

脾和则口能知五谷矣(pí hé zé kǒu néng zhī wǔ gǔ yǐ)　**Spleen functions well and men enjoy meals.** See *Ling Shu* chapter 17.

脾胀　病证名。五脏胀之一。症见善哕，肢体烦重，卧不安。出《灵枢·胀论》。

脾胀(pí zhàng)　**spleen distention** Disease name pertaining to visceral distension, manifested as having hiccups, heavy limbs, and restlessness when lying down. See *Ling Shu* chapter 35.

脾疟　五脏疟之一。症见畏寒、腹痛、肠鸣、汗出等。出《素问·刺疟》。

脾疟(pí nüè)　**spleen malaria** Pertains to visceral malaria and manifests as aversion to cold, abdominal pain, borborygmus, sweating, etc. See *Su Wen* chapter 36.

十二画

脾咳　五脏咳之一。证候特点为咳而单侧胁痛。出《素问·咳论》。

脾咳（pí ké）　**spleen cough** One of the five types of visceral cough and manifests as pain at either side of the rib area. See *Su Wen* chapter 38.

脾脉代　脾有胃气的正常脉象。出《素问·宣明五气》。

脾脉代（pí mài dài）　**regular intermittent pulse** The normal pulse when the spleen contains stomach qi. See *Su Wen* chapter 23.

脾神失守　犹言脾失去了正常的功能。出《素问·本病论》。

脾神失守（pí shén shī shǒu）　**Spleen loses its spirit.** The spleen loses its normal function. See *Su Wen* chapter 73.

脾恶湿　恶（wù 误），厌憎之意。脾主肌肉，本为湿土而喜燥，湿胜则气滞，有碍运化，并伤肌肉，为肿为痿，故脾恶湿。见《素问·宣明五气》。

脾恶湿（pí wù shī）　**Spleen has aversion to dampness.** *Wù* means aversion. The spleen governs the muscles, prefers dryness and has aversion to dampness. Dampness blocks qi and hence hinders the transforming and transporting functions of the spleen thus causing swelling or paralysis of the muscles. See *Su Wen* chapter 23.

脾病不能为胃行其津液　胃主化生津液和水谷精气，脾主运化，脾病则不能将胃化生的津液和水谷精气输布全身，而产生肢体不用等病证。出《素问·太阴阳明论》。

脾病不能为胃行其津液（pí bìng bù néng wéi wèi xíng qí jīn yè）　**Spleen malfunctions and unable to transport fluid for the stomach.** The stomach governs the generation of body fluids and essence of water and grain, while the spleen dominates the transformation and transportation of them. When disease occurs in the spleen, it is difficult to transfuse fluid and essence of water and grain to all over the body, hence causing difficulty for the limbs to move. See *Su Wen* chapter 29.

脾病而四支不用　支，通肢。四肢的活动，依赖胃气滋养以为用，但胃气必赖脾的运化功能，才能通过经脉达于四肢。如脾病失于运化，则四肢筋骨肌肉得不到水谷精微的滋养，日久可成为四肢不用之证。出《素问·太阴阳明论》。

脾病而四支不用(pí bìng ér sì zhī bù yòng) **Spleen disease causes the difficulty of movement in the four limbs.** "支" is the same as "肢". The movement of the four limbs relies on stomach qi, which，in turn，transfuses into the four limbs through the transformation and transportation of the spleen. When disease occurs in the spleen，the malfunction of the transforming and transporting functions fail to nurture the muscles，bones，and flesh of the four limbs，hence leading to the difficulty of movement in the four limbs. See *Su Wen* chapter 29.

脾腧 经穴名。属足太阳膀胱经。在十一椎下两旁各一寸五分处。出《灵枢·背腧》。

脾腧(pí shū) **Pi Shu (BL 20)** Pertains to the urinary bladder meridian of foot *taiyang*. It is located under the eleventh rib，1.5 *cun* apart from the spine. See *Ling Shu* chapter 51.

脾痹 病证名。五脏痹之一。由肌痹病久不愈，反复感受风寒湿之邪，发展而成。症见四肢疲软无力，咳嗽，呕吐涎沫，胸咽部感到痞塞等。出《素问·痹论》。

脾痹(pí bì) **spleen impediment** Pertains to visceral impediment and develops from chronic muscle impediment. It is repeatedly affected by the wind，cold，and dampness pathogens. Symptoms include weak and powerless limbs，cough，drool foaming at the mouth，oppression in the chest and throat，etc. See *Su Wen* chapter 43.

脾瘅 病名。瘅，热。由脾热而生口中味甘之病。脾属土，其味甘，脾热则其津上泛，故口中觉甜。病起于嗜食肥甘。出《素问·奇病论》。

脾瘅(pí dān) **spleen heat** Disease name. *Dān* means heat. Spleen heat leads to a sweet taste in the mouth. Spleen pertains to earth，which has a sweet flavor. Heat increases the liquid in the spleen，hence the patient tastes sweetness. The disease is caused by excessive intake of fat and sweet food. See *Su Wen* chapter 47.

脾藏肉 出《素问·调经论》。义同"脾主肉"。见该条。

脾藏肉(pí cáng ròu) **Spleen governs flesh.** See *Su Wen* chapter 62. See "脾主肉".

脾藏肌肉之气也 脾主肌肉之

义。出《素问·平人气象论》。

脾藏肌肉之气也(pí cáng jī ròu zhī qì yě) **spleen maintains muscle qi** The spleen dominates the muscles. See *Su Wen* chapter 18.

脾藏意　脾与精神活动有一定关系。意,指记忆能力。心主血脉而生脾土,故意藏于脾。出《素问·宣明五气》。

脾藏意(pí cáng yì) **Spleen stores will.** The spleen has some relationship with mental activities such as memory. The heart governs the blood and vessels and generates the spleen earth element, hence will is contained in the spleen. See *Su Wen* chapter 23.

腋　腋窝,胁上际、肩关节下方的窝状部。出《灵枢·经筋》。

腋(yè) **armpit** The pit between the fossa of the supracostal and lower side of the shoulder joint. See *Ling Shu* chapter 13.

腕　指前臂及手掌之间的部位。出《灵枢·本输》。

腕(wàn) **wrist** The part between the forearm and the palm. See *Ling Shu* chapter 2.

腕骨　① 手腕部骨骼的总称,由八块小骨(古称六块)组成的一个整体,介于前臂桡骨和手掌掌骨之间。出《灵枢·本输》。② 足第一蹠趾关节骨突。出《灵枢·本输》。③ 穴位名。手太阳小肠经之原穴,在手掌尺侧第五掌骨与腕骨构成关节部上方的凹陷中。出《灵枢·本输》。

腕骨(wàn gǔ)　① Wrist bone. The general name of wrist bones, in total 8 small bones (or 6 in ancient classics) as a whole between the forearm radius and the metacarpals. See *Ling Shu* chapter 2. ② Osteoid process of the first metatarsophalangeal joint of the foot. See *Ling Shu* chapter 2. ③ The name of acupoint SI 4 which pertains to the small intestine meridian of hand *taiyang*, located at the ulnar side of the palm, the pit in the joint formed by the fifth metacarpal bone and carpal bone. See *Ling Shu* chapter 2.

飧泄　病证名。水和饭曰飧,水注曰泄。即完谷不化之泄泻。出《素问·阴阳应象大论》。

飧泄(sūn xiè) **diarrhea with undigested food** Disease name. *Sūn* refers to water and grain, and *xiè* means watery diarrhea. See *Su Wen* chapter 5.

然谷　经穴名。足少阴肾经之荥

穴。在足内踝前大骨下陷者中。出《灵枢·本输》。

然谷（rán gǔ）　**Ran Gu（KI 2）** The brook point of the kidney meridian of foot *shaoyin*, located at the small pit at the downwards inner ankle bone. See *Ling Shu* chapter 2.

然骨　① 骨骼部位名。内踝前突起的舟骨粗隆部。出《灵枢·经脉》。② 指然骨穴。出《素问·缪刺论》。

然骨（rán gǔ）　① The name of a bone. Tuberosity of the navicular front projection of the medial malleolus, or scaphoid tuberosity. See *Ling Shu* chapter 10. ② The name of the acupoint Ran Gu（KI2）. See *Su Wen* chapter 63.

痞　以气闭胀满为主的病证。出《素问·六元正纪大论》。

痞（pǐ）　**stuffiness** Disease which mainly manifests as qi blockage and a feeling of fullness. See *Su Wen* chapter 71.

痟瘦　即消瘦。出《灵枢·经水》。

痟瘦（xiāo shòu）　**Emaciation** See *Ling Shu* chapter 12.

痟心　出《素问·经脉别论》。痟（yuān 渊），注有两义。① 心酸疼。见《素问》王冰注。② 心烦闷。见《素问识》。

痟心（yuān xīn）　See *Su Wen* chapter 7. *Yuān*, according to annotations, has two levels of meaning. ① Heart sore. See *Su Wen* annotated by Wang Bing. ② Vexation and oppression. See *Su Wen Zhi*（*Understanding Su Wen*）.

痤　病名。今称为痤疮，较粉刺为大，有时顶有小脓疱，可形成脂瘤或疖肿。多因汗出当风，汗液为寒气薄于肤腠郁久而成。出《素问·生气通天论》。

痤（cuó）　**acne** Disease name. Acne is usually bigger than comedo and has a pustule on the top. It might progress into a lipoma or boil and is usually induced from sweat binding in the interstices. See *Su Wen* chapter 3.

痤痱　痤，痤疮、小节。痱，暑疹。今称痱子。由汗出遇湿，致阳气发越受遏，郁于肤腠而成。出《素问·生气通天论》。

痤痱（cuó fèi）　**pock pimples** *Cuó* refers to acne and *fèi* refers to summer papule, or heat rash in today's language. It is induced from yang qi binding in the interstices when sweat is lingering with dampness. See *Su Wen* chapter 3.

痫 病名。即癫痫。表现为发作性昏厥，抽搐，口吐白沫，醒后一如常人。出《素问·大奇论》。

痫（xián） **epilepsia** Manifested as paroxysmal fainting, convulsion, foaming at the mouth, and returning to normal after waking up. See *Su Wen* chapter 48.

痫惊 病证名。出《素问·通评虚实论》。（1）癫痫瘈疭。见《素问集注》。（2）指惊风。见《素问识》。（3）痫为癫痫，惊为震惊。见《素问直解》。

痫惊（xián jīng） **epilepsia shock** Disease name. See *Su Wen* chapter 28.（1）Epileptic convulsion. See *Su Wen Ji Zhu* (*Collected Annotation of Su Wen*).（2）Fright wind. See *Su Wen Zhi* (*Understanding Su Wen*).（3）*Xián* refers to epilepsia and *Jīng* refers to shock. See *Su Wen Zhi Jie* (*Direct Interpretation on Su Wen*).

痫厥 癫痫发作时神志异常，突然昏厥。出《素问·大奇论》。

痫厥（xián jué） **epilepsia syncope** Sudden syncope when epilepsia occurs. See *Su Wen* chapter 48.

痫瘈 癫痫发作时出现的肢体抽搐。出《素问·大奇论》。

痫瘈（xián chì） **epilepsia con-** vulsion Convulsion when epilepsia occurs. See *Su Wen* chapter 48.

痟 疾病。出《素问·刺法论》。

痟（ē） **disease** See *Su Wen* chapter 72.

痛痹 病证名。为疼痛较剧烈之痹证。因风寒湿三邪之中，寒邪独胜，客于筋骨肌肉之间，凝聚不散，阳气不行，致局部组织绌急挛缩，故疼痛较剧。出《素问·痹论》。

痛痹（tòng bì） **pain impediment** Disease name. Refers to an impediment with drastic pain. Among the three pathogenic factors, namely, wind, cold and dampness, cold is more likely to linger in the sinews, muscles and flesh to impede yang qi, which may lead to tissue palpitation and cause drastic pain. See *Su Wen* chapter 43.

善忘 即健忘。出《灵枢·大惑论》。

善忘（shàn wàng） **forgetfulness** See *Ling Shu* chapter 80.

道 ① 规律、法则。出《素问·阴阳应象大论》。② 方法。出《素问·至真要大论》。③ 路径。出《灵枢·忧恚无言》。④ 道理。出《素问·气交变大论》。⑤ 针孔。出《素问·调经论》。⑥ 医学理论。出《素问·宝命全形论》。

道（dào）　① Laws. See *Su Wen* chapter 5. ② Method. See *Su Wen* chapter 74. ③ Route. See *Ling Shu* chapter 69. ④ Truth and reason. See *Su Wen* chapter 69. ⑤ The needle path. See *Su Wen* chapter 62. ⑥ Medical theories. See *Su Wen* chapter 25.

焠　烧灼。出《灵枢·寿夭刚柔》。

焠（cuì）　**burn** See *Ling Shu* chapter 6.

焠针　焠（cuì 翠），烧灼。以火烧针而后刺之，又称焠刺。出《素问·调经论》。

焠针（cuì zhēn）　**red-hot needling** *Cuì* refers to burning. *Cuì zhēn*, or named *cuì cì*, which refers to burning the needle before needling. See *Su Wen* chapter 62.

焠刺　九刺法之一。用烧红的针快速刺入穴位的一种方法，用治寒痹、瘰疬、阴疽等病症。出《灵枢·官针》。

焠刺（cuì cì）　**red-hot needling** One of the nine needling methods. Needling the acupoints quickly with burning red needles to treat cold impediment, scrofula and yin flat-abscess, etc. See *Ling Shu* chapter 7.

湿　① 潮湿的气候。为六气之一，是长夏所主的气候，五行属土。出《素问·阴阳应象大论》。② 病因。湿邪为六淫之一。出《素问·阴阳应象大论》。③ 病机。出《素问·至真要大论》。④ 病证。即水气停滞，出现浮肿胀满的一类病证。出《素问·至真要大论》。⑤ 涩滞。出《灵枢·大惑论》。湿，即涩。皮肤涩滞，分肉之间不滑利。⑥ 运气概念中的六气之一。出《素问·天元纪大论》。⑦ 指脾胃（土）。出《素问·至真要大论》。

湿（shī）　① Damp weather, one of the six qi, governed by the long summer and pertaining to earth. See *Su Wen* chapter 5. ② The pathogenic cause, damp pathogens, one of the six pathogens. See *Su Wen* chapter 5. ③ Pathogenesis. See *Su Wen* chapter 74. ④ Syndrome of the disease manifested as swelling and distension caused by the stagnation of water qi. See *Su Wen* chapter 74. ⑤ Rough and stagnated. See *Ling Shu* chapter 80. The skin is rough and the seams of the flesh are unsmooth. ⑥ One of the six qi in terms of the doctrine of the five circuits and six qi theory. See *Su Wen* chapter 66. ⑦ Stomach and spleen（earth phase）. See *Su Wen* chapter 74.

湿气　① 潮湿的气候。出《素问·五常政大论》。② 湿邪。出《素问·痹论》。③ 运气概念中的太阴湿土。出《素问·天元纪大论》。

湿气（shī qì）　① Damp weather. See *Su Wen* chapter 70. ② Damp pathogens. See *Su Wen* chapter 43. ③ Damp earth of *taiyin* according to the doctrine of the five movements and six qi theory. See *Su Wen* chapter 66.

湿化　气候从湿的变化。出《素问·至真要大论》。

湿化（shī huà）　Dampness formation See *Su Wen* chapter 74.

湿以润之　出《素问·五运行大论》。

湿以润之（shī yǐ rùn zhī）　to moisten the dampness See *Su Wen* chapter 67.

湿令　令，时令。湿令，潮湿气候所主的时令。农历六月，长夏为湿气所主时令。出《素问·六元正纪大论》。

湿令（shī lìng）　damp season *Lìng* refers to the lunar seasons. This term refers to the season governed by damp weather，usually in the lunar month of June

when dampness governs the late summer. See *Su Wen* chapter 71.

湿伤肉　脾主肉而恶湿，故湿甚则肉伤。出《素问·阴阳应象大论》《素问·五运行大论》。

湿伤肉（shī shāng ròu）　**Dampness damages flesh.** The spleen governs the flesh and has aversion to dampness. Hence excessive dampness will damage the flesh. See *Su Wen* chapter 5 and 67.

湿毒　由湿气郁积成毒，可致人于病。出《素问·五常政大论》。

湿毒（shī dú）　**damp toxin** Dampness gathers and turns out to be toxins that cause diseases. See *Su Wen* chapter 70.

湿胜则濡泻　濡泻，大便清稀。湿气胜则脾胃受困，失于健运，水谷不分，下注大肠，形成泄泻。见《素问·阴阳应象大论》《素问·六元正纪大论》。

湿胜则濡泻（shī shèng zé rú xiè）　**Excessive dampness leads to diarrhea.** *Rú xiè* refers to loose stools. Excessive dampness impedes the spleen and stomach，hence the transportation of the spleen malfunctions，water and grain are mixed and poured down to the large intestine causing diarrhea. See *Su Wen* chapter

5 and 71.

湿胜则濡泄　出《素问·六元正纪大论》。见"湿胜则濡泻"条。

湿胜则濡泄（shī shèng zé rú xiè）See *Su Wen* chapter 71. See "湿胜则濡泻".

湿淫　偏盛的湿气。见《素问·至真要大论》。

湿淫（shī yín）　**excessive dampness** Refers to relatively excessive damp qi. See *Su Wen* chapter 74.

温气　① 温热的气候。出《素问·至真要大论》。② 阳气。出《灵枢·百病始生》。

温气（wēn qì）　① Warm weather. See *Su Wen* chapter 74. ② Yang qi. See *Ling Shu* chapter 66.

温厉　即温疫。厉，通疠。出《素问·六元正纪大论》。

温厉（wēn lì）　**epidemic or pestilence** "厉" is the same as "疠". See *Su Wen* chapter 71.

温衣　令穿衣服温暖以保护阳气。出《素问·汤液醪醴论》。

温衣（wēn yī）　**warm clothes** To wear warm clothes to protect yang qi. See *Su Wen* chapter 14.

温者清之　治法。温热病应用清凉的方法治疗。出《素问·至真要大论》。

温者清之（wēn zhě qīng zhī）**treating warm with cold** Treatment method in which cold methods are applied to treat warm diseases. See *Su Wen* chapter 74.

温疟　病名。以先热后寒为发作特点的疟病，并见肌肉消瘦等症。病因病机由冬季感受风寒，病藏于肾，至春温夏著，阳气发泄，邪随外出，疟遂发作。出《素问·疟论》。

温疟（wēn nüè）　**warm malaria** Disease name. Refers to malaria manifested as heat followed by coldness, along with the symptoms like muscle wasting. The reason and mechanism of the disease lies in winter coldness that is hidden in the kidney and breaks out in the spring and summer when the warm yang qi is released and the pathogenic qi follows. See *Su Wen* chapter 35.

温疠　病名。为疫疠温瘴之类，属烈性传染病。为火郁所致。出《素问·本病论》。

温疠（wēn lì）　**warm plague** Disease name. A kind of deadly epidemic usually caused by fire stagnation. See *Su Wen* chapter 73.

温疫　病名。为感受天时不正之气而发的急性传染性疾病。出《素问·刺法论》。

温疫（wēn yì） **warm epidemic** Disease name. Refers to acute epidemics caused by abnormal seasonal qi in nature. See *Su Wen* chapter 72.

温病 病名。泛指发于春季的外感急性热病。其特点为起病急，传变快，热象盛，易伤阴。出《素问·热论》。

温病（wēn bìng） **warm disease** Disease name. Refers to acute exogenous warm diseases occuring in spring that usually feature acute occurrence，rapid progress，excessive heat and deficiency of yin. See *Su Wen* chapter 31.

滑 ① 脉象。其脉往来滑利，如珠走盘，可以见于正常人，揭示气血充盈。亦主实热，风疝，新病，痰饮，食积，妊娠等。出《灵枢·邪气藏府病形》《素问·玉机真藏论》《素问·四时刺逆从论》《素问·平人气象论》。② 尺部皮肤滑利，多主风病。出《灵枢·论疾诊尺》。

滑（huá） ① Pulse manifestation. The pulse feels smooth as if pearls are running across a plate. It is the pulse of healthy people who have an abundance of blood and qi. Sometimes this pulse is found in patients who suffer from excessive heat，wind-hernia，new diseases，phlegm and retained fluid，indigestion，pregnancy，etc. See *Ling Shu* chapter 4 and *Su Wen* chapter 18，19，and 64. ② The slippery skin of the Chi part on the wrist usually indicating wind diseases. See *Ling Shu* chapter 74.

溲 出《灵枢·本神》。① 指小便。见《素问》王冰注。② 指大小便。见《太素·藏府》。

溲（sōu） See *Ling Shu* chapter 8. ① Urine. See *Su Wen* annotated by Wang Bing. ② Urine and stool. See *Tai Su*（*Classified Study on Huang Di Nei Jing*）"Viscera and Bowels".

溲血 今称尿血。出《素问·痿论》。

溲血（sōu xuè） **urinating blood** See *Su Wen* chapter 44.

游针 指进针后，针下脉气的感传，犹似针之游行。出《素问·气穴论》。

游针（yóu zhēn） **moving needle** After the insertion of a needle，the qi of the pulse moves as if the needle moves. See *Su Wen* chapter 58.

游部 游行部位。指少阳经脉，出入于太阳阳明，游行于内外阴阳之间。出《素问·阴阳类论》。

游部（yóu bù）　**floating part** The place where the *shaoyang* meridian moves in and out of *taiyang* and *yangming* and moves between the inner yin and outer yang. See *Su Wen* chapter 79.

寒　①寒冷的气候，属冬令所主，五行属水。出《素问·阴阳应象大论》。②病因名。寒邪。为六淫之一，属阴邪。出《素问·热论》《素问·疟论》。③病机名。出《素问·至真要大论》。④症状名。肢体寒冷。出《灵枢·官能》。⑤寒冷的饮食物。出《素问·风论》。⑥治法，指寒凉法。出《素问·至真要大论》。⑦证候名。指寒证。出《素问·至真要大论》。

寒（hán）　① Cold weather, governed by winter and pertaining to the water element. See *Su Wen* chapter 5. ② Cold pathogen, the name of the cause of the disease. One of the six pathogens that pertains to yin. See *Su Wen* chapter 31 and chapter 35. ③ The name of the disease mechanism. See *Su Wen* chapter 74. ④ Symptom name. Refers to cold limbs. See *Ling Shu* chapter 73. ⑤ Cold food and drink. See *Su Wen* chapter 42. ⑥ Treatment method, treating disease with coldness. See *Su Wen* chapter 74. ⑦ Syndrome name. Refers to a cold syndrome. See *Su Wen* chapter 74.

寒中　即中气虚寒，多见泄泻、腹胀之类病症。出《素问·金匮真言论》。

寒中（hán zhōng）　**cold parapoplexy** Refers to the deficiency of middle qi, usually found in diarrhea and abdominal distention, etc. See *Su Wen* chapter 4.

寒气　①寒邪，六淫之一。见"寒邪"条。出《素问·痹论》。②寒冷的气候，六气之一。出《素问·至真要大论》。

寒气（hán qì）　① Cold pathogen, one of the six excesses. See "寒邪". See *Su Wen* chapter 43. ② Cold weather, one of the six qi. See *Su Wen* chapter 74.

寒邪　六淫之一，属阴邪。其性凝滞。主收引，罹病多寒热、疼痛等症。出《灵枢·痈疽》。

寒邪（hán xié）　**cold pathogen** As one of the six excesses, it pertains to yin with the characteristic of stagnating and may cause contractures and tautness which leads to alternate cold and heat and pain. See *Ling Shu* chapter 81.

十二画

寒因热用 反治法。出《素问·至真要大论》。(1)指用药反佐。即寒性药剂中佐以少量温热药作引子,以治大热证。见《素问注证发微》。(2)指服药反佐。如以寒药治热病用热服法。见《类经·论治四》。(3)现代一般据下文"塞因塞用,通因通用",径改为"寒因寒用"。为反治法。即真热假寒证,用寒药治疗。

寒因热用(hán yīn rè yòng) **to treat heat with cold** Paradoxical treatment. (1) Treat with paradoxical medicine. Use a small amount of warm medicines as conductor to treat great heat. See *Su Wen Zhu Zheng Fa Wei* (*Annotation and Elaboration on Su Wen*). (2) Taking medicine in the contrary way. Such as taking a hot decoction when treating heat with cold. See *Lei Jing* (*Classified Classic*) "On Treatment Chapter 4". (3) In modernity, it has been changed into "treating cold with cold" according to the context " treating obstructive disease with tonic drugs, treating discharging diseases with purgatives". It is a kind of paradoxical treatment. Treating true heat and false cold with cold medicines.

寒则气收 寒主收引,寒邪外束,腠理闭密,阳气不能宣达,故谓气收。出《素问·举痛论》。

寒则气收(hán zé qì shōu) **Cold causes qi to contract.** Cold pathogens close the interstices and impede yang qi from dispersing. See *Su Wen* chapter 39.

寒则血凝泣 出《素问·离合真邪论》。见"邪之入于脉也"条。

寒则血凝泣(hán zé xuè níng qì) **Cold causes blood stasis.** See *Su Wen* chapter 27. See "邪之入于脉也".

寒伤血 人之血气喜温而恶寒,寒伤则血气凝涩不畅。出《素问·阴阳应象大论》《素问·五运行大论》。

寒伤血(hán shāng xuè) **Cold impairs blood.** Qi and blood in the human body are in favor of warmth and detest cold. Thus cold leads to the stagnation of qi and blood. See *Su Wen* chapter 5 and 67.

寒者热之 治法。寒病应用温热之法治疗。出《素问·至真要大论》。

寒者热之(hán zhě rè zhī) **to treat cold with heat** Treatment method, treating cold disease with heat.

See *Su Wen* chapter 74.

寒府 ① 经穴名。膝阳关穴别名。属足少阳胆经。在膝外侧,阳陵泉直上三寸,股骨外上髁边缘凹陷中。出《素问·骨空论》。② 寒气集中的季节。出《素问·六元正纪大论》。

寒府(hán fǔ) ① The name of acupoint GB 33 pertaining to the gallbladder meridian of foot *shaoyang* and located at the small pit of the margin of the external epicondyle of the femur on lateral side of the knees, three *cun* above Yang Ling Quan (GB 34). See *Su Wen* chapter 60. ② The season when cold qi gathers. See *Su Wen* chapter 71.

寒疟 病名。以先寒后热为发作特点的疟病。发时先畏寒栗起毛竖,伸欠、寒战鼓颔,腰脊俱痛,移时寒已,高热,头痛如破,渴欲饮冷。如此每日或间日、间数日一作。病因病机为夏伤盛暑,于汗出腠疏之时感受暑气水寒,至秋汗出遇风,致邪伏营卫,随营卫之昼夜运行而发作。出《素问·疟论》。

寒疟(hán nüè) **cold malaria** Disease name. Patients first feel cold and then heat. When it occurs, patients first feel cold and their hairs stand up, they stretch themselves and yawn, then shiver with chattering jaws, followed by waist pain and a backache. When the feeling of cold disappears, fever comes. Patients have severe headaches and are thirsty for cold water. The alternating cold and heat occurs daily, or every other day, or every few days. The causes and pathogenesis lie in summer heatstroke, which is induced by cold pathogens that enter the sweating interstices in hot summer. Then in autumn, when patients sweat in the wind, the pathogens enter and hide in the nutrient and defense qi, along with the circulation of which, cold malaria occurs. See *Su Wen* chapter 35.

寒疡 寒性的疡疽。出《素问·气交变大论》。

寒疡(hán yáng) **cold ulceration** The sore and flat ulcerations that are caused by coldness. See *Su Wen* chapter 69.

寒毒 暴烈的寒邪。出《素问·五常政大论》。

寒毒(hán dú) **cold toxin** See *Su Wen* chapter 70.

寒政 寒冷的气候布行。政,施政。出《素问·六元正纪大论》。

十二画

寒政（hán zhèng）　**cold dominating** *Zheng* means governing. See *Su Wen* chapter 71.

寒胜则浮　浮，浮肿。寒气胜则阳气不行，气化失利，水液停留，发为浮肿。见《素问·阴阳应象大论》《素问·六元正纪大论》。

寒胜则浮（hán shèng zé fú）　**Excessive cold causes edema.** Excessive cold impedes the movement of yang qi. That leads to the retention of liquids in the human body and finally causes swelling. See *Su Wen* chapter 5 and 71.

寒热　① 症状名。指畏寒发热之症。出《素问·生气通天论》。② 指疾病的性质或寒或热。出《素问·五常政大论》。③ 病邪名。指寒邪、热邪。出《灵枢·百病始生》。④ 寒凉与温热。出《素问·阴阳应象大论》。⑤《灵枢》篇名。该篇主要讨论瘰疬病的病因病机及诊治等。因其病因由寒热毒气稽留于经脉之间，病症多伴发寒热，故以"寒热"名篇。

寒热（hán rè）　① Symptom name. Patients have fever and a fear of cold. See *Su Wen* chapter 3. ② The characteristic of disease, cold or hot. See *Su Wen* chapter 70. ③ Pathogen name, cold and heat. See *Ling Shu* chapter 66. ④ Cold and warmth. See *Su Wen* chapter 5. ⑤ Chapter title in *Ling Shu*. This chapter mainly discusses the causes and pathogenesis of scrofula. The major cause is toxic qi lingering in the meridians. Symptoms are accompanied by the feeling of cold and heat，hence named "cold and heat".

寒热俞　治疗寒热病的俞穴。出《素问·气穴论》。

寒热俞（hán rè shū）　**cold-heat acupoints** Refers to the acupoints that treat cold and febrile diseases. See *Su Wen* chapter 58.

寒热病　① 病证名。指寒热交作之病。出《素问·三部九候论》。②《灵枢》篇名。该篇着重讨论了皮寒热、肌寒热、骨寒热以及骨痹、体惰、厥痹、热厥、寒厥等多种杂病的临床表现和针刺手法。但以前三种寒热病冠于篇首，故以名篇。

寒热病（hán rè bìng）　① Syndrome name which is manifested as alternating heat and cold. See *Su Wen* chapter 20. ② Chapter title in *Ling Shu*. This chapter mainly discusses the clinical manifestations and acupuncture treatments of heat and cold in the skin，muscles，and bones，along with bone impediment，body sluggishness，reversal impediments，heat reversals，cold reversals and so on. The heat and cold in the skin，muscles，and bones are discussed at first，hence the name.

寒厥　病证名。主症为手足肘膝以下寒冷。乃自恃体壮，秋冬入房太甚，耗竭精气，并伤肾阳，阳气衰，不能温煦四肢所致。出《素问·厥论》。

寒厥（hán jué）　cold reversal Disease name，which major symptoms are feeling cold in the limbs and under elbows and knees. It always occurs in patients who are robust and have too much sex in autumn and winter. The essence qi is exhausted，kidney yang is damaged，and yang qi declines which makes it difficult to warm the four limbs. See *Su Wen* chapter 45.

寒痹　病名。又名痛痹。寒邪留经之痹证。症见疼痛，皮肤麻木不仁。出《灵枢·寿夭刚柔》《灵枢·贼风》。

寒痹（hán bì）　cold impediment Disease name，also called pain impediment and is caused by

cold pathogens lingering in the meridians with such symptoms as pain and paralysis of the skin. See *Ling Shu* chapter 6 and 58.

寒鼽　流清涕。出《素问·本病论》。

寒鼽（hán qiú）　running nose See *Su Wen* chapter 73.

窗笼　① 即足少阳胆经之听宫穴。出《灵枢·根结》。见"听宫"条。② 指耳。《灵枢·卫气》。

窗笼（chuāng lóng）　① Name of acupoint SI 19 pertaining to the gallbladder meridian of foot *shaoyang*. See *Ling Shu* chapter 5. See "听宫". ② Ear. See *Ling Shu* chapter 52.

颏中　颏（è呃），鼻梁上眉心下的部位。出《灵枢·经脉》。

颏中（è zhōng）　middle forhead *È*（颏）is located at the middle the eyebrows above the nose bridge. See *Ling Shu* chapter 10.

强者泻之　治法。强，亢盛的意思。邪气亢盛的，要用泻法治疗。出《素问·至真要大论》。

强者泻之（qiáng zhě xiè zhī） **The exuberance of pathogens must be drained.** Treatment method. *Qiáng* means excess. Patients who have exuberant pathogen qi must be drained. See *Su Wen* chapter 74.

疏五过论　《素问》篇名。疏（shù树），注疏、解释；五过，指诊治时的五种过失。此篇从病人的生活环境、饮食起居、精神状态、脉搏变化、个体差异等多方面，解释分析了医生在诊治时的五种过失，提出了医生应具备的素质。

疏五过论（shù wǔ guò lùn）　**Discussion on Five Errors Frequently Made in Diagnosis** Chapter title in *Su Wen*. *Shù* means to comment and explain. *Wǔ guò* refers to five kinds of mistakes made in diagnosis. This chapter analyzes and explains five diagnostic mistakes of doctors in five aspects, environment, diet, mental stage, pulse changes, and individual constitutions, hence putting forward the qualities of a qualified doctor.

隔　① 病证名。指太阳经气郁滞，二便不通的病证。出《素问·阴阳别论》。② 阻隔，阻塞。出《素问·至真要大论》。

隔（gé）　① Syndrome name. Fecal and urinary stoppage caused by blockage in the *taiyang* meridian. See *Su Wen* chapter 7. ② Blockage or stoppage. See *Su Wen* chapter 74.

隔肠　由于气机升降不利，肠道阻隔而不大便。出《素问·至真要大论》。

隔肠（gé cháng）　**blocked large intestine** When the movement of qi is impeded, the intestines are blocked and the bowels are unable to loosen. See *Su Wen* chapter 74.

絮针　古代一种缝絮之针，针身圆直，如筒状，较粗大。出《灵枢·九针论》。

絮针（xù zhēn）　**cotton needle** A kind of thick needle with a cylindrical body used for sewing clothes or quilts. See *Ling Shu* chapter 78.

皴揭　皴（cūn村），皮肤皴裂。揭（qì弃）皮肤因皴裂而掀起。出《素问·六元正纪大论》。

皴揭（cūn qì）　**skin chap** *cūn*（皴）refers to skin chap. *qì*（揭）refers to skin torn off. See *Su Wen* chapter 71.

缓　即缓方，为七方之一。指组方药物气味薄，作用缓和的方剂。适用于病轻或慢性病调理。出《素问·至真要大论》。

缓（huǎn）　**mild formula** One of the seven kinds of prescriptions. Mild formulas containing lightly-flavored material medica with mild effects mainly applied to light and chronic diseases. See

Su Wen chapter 74.

缓筋 见《灵枢·百病始生》。① 腹内之筋。见《灵枢集注》。② 足阳明筋。见《太素·邪传》。

缓筋（huǎn jīn） See *Ling Shu* chapter 66. ① Mild sinews in the abdomen. See *Ling Shu Ji Zhu*（*Collected Annotation of Ling Shu*）. ② Sinews of foot *yangming*. See *Tai Su*（*Classified Study on Huang Di Nei Jing*）"On Pathogen".

十三画

魂　精神活动的一种形式，如梦幻恍惚之类。属阳，藏于肝，肝的藏血功能正常，则魂有所舍。出《灵枢·本神》。

魂（hún）　ethereal soul A form of essence-spirit activity, such as dreaming and absent-mindedness. It pertains to yang and is stored in the liver. If the liver's function of storing blood is normal, then the soul has its storage place. See *Ling Shu* chapter 8.

魂魄飞扬　魂魄，这里代指精神活动。魂魄飞扬，此指因内外各种病因，导致精气离脏，精神不能内守的状况。出《灵枢·本神》。

魂魄飞扬（hún pò fēi yáng）**Ethereal soul and corporeal soul flies away.** The ethereal soul and corporeal soul refer to essence-spirit activity. Due to various internal and external disease causes, essence cannot be kept inside and leaves the viscera. See *Ling Shu* chapter 8.

魂魄不散　魂魄，这里代指精神活动。魂魄不散，即精神内守，注意力高度集中的意思。出《灵枢·终始》。

魂魄不散（hún pò bù sàn）**Ethereal soul and corporeal soul are concentrated.** The ethereal soul and corporeal soul refers to essence-spirit activity. It means the inner guarding of essence-spirit and intense concentration. See *Ling Shu* chapter 9.

鼓胀　①指心腹胀满，妨碍正常进食之病证。出《素问·腹中论》。②指身肿腹大，腹部皮肤呈青黄色，青筋暴露，即后世所谓之臌胀。出《灵枢·水胀》。

鼓胀（gǔ zhàng）　① It refers to the syndrome of fullness in the abdomen, which prevents essential eating. See *Su Wen* chapter 40. ② The body is swollen combined with a large abdomen, with blue-yellow abdominal skin and prominent veins, which are the so-called tympanites in later generations. See *Ling Shu* chapter 57.

蒐茹　药名，即茜草。气味苦寒，入肝经，能止血治崩，又能和血通经。出《素问·腹中论》。

蒐茹(lú rú)　**Radix Rubiae** Medicine name. Radix Rubiae is bitter-cold in flavor，and enters the liver meridian，stops bleeding and stem flooding，as well as harmonizes the blood and unblocks the meridian. See *Su Wen* chapter 40.

颐　部位名。位于面部二侧，口角处下方，颔的外上方，腮部的前下方。出《素问·刺热》。

颐(yí)　**lower cheek** Body part located at the two sides of the face，below the corner of the mouth，above the outside of the jaw，and below the front of the cheek. See *Su Wen* chapter 32.

蕠藗草根　药物名。出《灵枢·痈疽》。蕠，即菱；藗，即连翘。菱与连翘二草之根，皆有解毒作用。

蕠藗草根(lín qiào cǎo gēn)　**the root of fructus forsythiae and trapa bispinosa roxb** Medicine name. The root of fructus forsythiae and trapa bispinosa roxb have the function of detoxifying. See *Ling Shu* chapter 81.

禁服　《灵枢》篇名。禁，禁诫；服，服从，针刺治病原理十分精深，对此则既要有所禁诫，又应服从。

禁服(jìn fú)　**Inheritance of Knowledge Accumulated in History** Chapter title in *Ling Shu*. *Jìn* means commandment and *fú* means obedience. The principle of acupuncture treatment is profound，for which there should be some commandments and obedience.

禁数　禁刺的几个部位。为肝、肺、心、肾、脾、胃、鬲肓之上及七节之傍，均属脏腑要害，为禁刺之处。出《素问·刺禁论》。

禁数(jìn shù)　**forbidden acupuncture part** Several parts which are forbidden to perform acupuncture：the liver，lung，heart，kidney，spleen，stomach，upper part of the cardio-diaphragmatic interspace，and the vicinity of the seventh thoracic vertebra，the vital parts of the viscera and bowels. See *Su Wen* chapter 52.

雷气通于心　雷气，指火气。心为火脏，同气相求，故雷气通于心气。出《素问·阴阳应象大论》。

雷气通于心(léi qì tōng yú xīn)　**thunder qi coordinates with the heart** Thunder qi refers to the qi of the fire element. The heart is a viscera pertaining to the fire element. The same qi is more likely to gather together, therefore thunder qi coordinates with the heart. See *Su Wen* chapter 5.

雷公 传说中上古时代的医家，为黄帝之臣，精于针灸术。出《素问·疏五过论》。

雷公（léi gōng） **Lei Gong** A prestigious doctor in the remote ages, and one courtier of Huang Di（Yellow Emperor）who was skilled in acupuncture. See *Su Wen* chapter 77.

输 ① 音义同腧（shù），指腧穴。出《灵枢·经筋》。② 五腧穴中的输穴。出《灵枢·邪气藏府病形》。③ 运输，输注的意思。出《素问·经脉别论》。

输（shù） ① Acupoints. See *Ling Shu* chapter 13. ② The stream point of the five transport points. See *Ling Shu* chapter 4. ③ Transportation. See *Su Wen* chapter 21.

输刺 ① 九刺之一。输，即输穴。指选用五腧穴及脏腑背俞穴折针刺法。出《灵枢·官针》。② 与十二经相应的十二刺之一。指直入直出，取穴少，刺之深，而留针久的针法，治疗气盛而热之病。出《灵枢·官针》。③ 与五脏相应的五刺之一。直入直出，深刺至骨，用治与肾相应的骨痹。出《灵枢·官针》。

输刺（shū cì） ① One of the nine needling methods. Refers to the needling method applied on the five transport points and transport points of the viscera and bowels. See *Ling Shu* chapter 7. ② One of the twelve needling methods in accordance with the twelve meridians. It refers to the needling of straight inserting in and out with few acupoints and deep insertion as well as long time retention. This is used to treat febrile diseases caused by qi exuberance. See *Ling Shu* chapter 7. ③ One of the five needling methods in accordance with the five viscera, operated by straight inserting in and out with the needle deep into bone. This is used to treat bone impediment pertaning to kidney. See *Ling Shu* chapter 7.

输脉 背部联系脏腑的经脉和输穴。出《灵枢·百病始生》。

输脉（shū mài） **back meridian** Meridian vessels and acupoints on the back that connect with the viscera and bowels. See Ling Shu chapter 66.

督脉 奇经八脉之一。其循行路线，起源于小腹内，从会阴部向

十三画

后,行于脊里正中,上至内府,入于脑,上头顶,下额,至鼻柱及上齿。前后与任脉、冲脉相通,又与足太阳、足少阴相合;联系心、肾、脑。督脉能总一身之阳,故又称为"阳脉之海"。出《素问·骨空论》。

督脉(dū mài)　**governor vessel** One of the eight extra meridians. Its route originates in the lower abdomen, from the perineum back to the middle of the spine, up to the six bowels, into the brain and head, and down to the forehead, the nasal septum and upper teeth. The governor vessel is connected with conception vessel and thoroughfare vessel in the front and back as well as connected with foot *taiyang* meridian and foot *shaoyin* meridian. It connects the heart, kidney and brain. The governor vessel can govern the yang of whole body, so it is also called the sea of yang meridians. See *Su Wen* chapter 60.

督脉之别　十五别络之一,穴名长强。其络夹脊旁肌肉上向项部,散布于头上;下边当肩胛两侧,分支走向足太阳经,通贯脊旁肌肉。出《灵枢·经脉》。

督脉之别(dū mài zhī bié)　**the divergence meridian of the governor vessel** One of the fifteen meridian divergences, and also the name for acupoint Chang Qiang. The upper side of DU 1 flows along the paraspinal muscles up to the neck and spreads over the head; the lower side flows both sides of the scapula, and the branches go to the foot greater yang meridian, connecting the paraspinal muscles. See *Ling Shu* chapter 10.

跷　① 跷脉。见该条。《素问·经脉别论》:"跷前卒大,取之下俞。"② 举跷。出《素问·针解》。

跷(qiáo)　① Heel vessel. See "跷脉" for detail. See *Su Wen* chapter 21. ② Lift the heel. See *Su Wen* chapter 54.

跷脉　奇经八脉之一,左右成对,分为阴跷脉和阳跷脉。跷脉从下肢内、外侧分上行头面,具有交通一身阴阳之气和调节肢体肌肉运动的功能。阴阳跷脉交会于目内眦,入属于脑,故有濡养眼目和司眼睑开合的作用。出《灵枢·脉度》。

跷脉(qiáo mài)　**heel vessel** One of the eight extraordinary meridians, left and right paired. It is divided into yin heel vessel and yang heel vessel. The heel

十
三
画

vessel goes up to the head and face from the inner side and outside of the lower limbs and has the function of communicating between the qi of yin and yang and regulating the muscle movements of the limbs. The yin-yang heel vessel meets in the eyes and pertains to the brain，so it has the effect of nourishing the eyes and governing the opening and closing of the eyelids. See *Ling Shu* chapter 17.

嗌　即咽。出《素问·阴阳应象大论》。

嗌（ài）　**Pharynx** See *Su Wen* chapter 5.

蜀椒　药名，即川椒、花椒。性味辛热，有小毒。有温中散寒止痛作用。出《灵枢·寿夭刚柔》。

蜀椒（shǔ jiāo）　**pericarpium zanthoxyli** Medicine name. Pericarpium Zanthoxyli is pungent and warm in flavor and has minor toxicity. It has the function of warming the middle and dissipating the cold as well as relieving pain. See *Ling Shu* chapter 6.

颓疝　出《素问·阴阳别论》。① 睾丸纵缓之证。见《素问》王冰注。② 小腹牵引睾丸疼痛。

见《类经·疾病六》。③ 颓即顽，颓疝为睾丸大而不疼。见《素问》吴崑注。

颓疝（tuí shàn）　See *Su Wen* chapter 7. ① Swelling of the scrotum. See *Su Wen* annotated by Wang Bing. ② Scrotum pain due to traction by the lower abdomen. See *Lei Jing*（*Classified Classic*）" On Diseases Chapter 6". ③ Enlarged scrotum without pain. See *Su Wen* annotated by Wu Kun.

愁忧恐惧则伤心　愁忧恐惧，均为过度的情志活动。劳伤心神，故谓伤心。见《灵枢·邪气藏府病形》。

愁忧恐惧则伤心（chóu yōu kǒng jù zé shāng xīn）　**intense worry or dread impairing the heart** Intense worry or dread is excessive emotional activity，overconsuming the heart. See *Ling Shu* chapter 4.

筩　音义同"筒"。指中空如筒的针。出《灵枢·四时气》《灵枢·九针论》。

筩（tǒng）　**hollow** Refers to a hollow needle. See *Ling Shu* chapter 19 and 78.

鼠仆　出《素问·刺禁论》。① 鼠鼷部，在腹股沟处。见《新校正》。② 指鼠鼷与仆参之间的部位。见《素问集注》。

鼠仆（shǔ pū）　See *Su Wen* chapter 52. ① Groin. See *Su Wen* chapter 52. See *Xin Jiao Zheng*（*New Revisions of Su Wen*）. ② The part between the groin and acupoint BL 61. See *Xin Jiao Zheng*（*New Revisions of Su Wen*）.

鼠瘘　病名。瘰疬溃破后，流出脓水，久不收口，形成瘘管，犹如鼠穴，故称鼠瘘。出《素问·骨空论》《灵枢·寒热》。

鼠瘘（shǔ lòu）　**mouse fistula** Disease name, in which after the scrofula is ruptured, pus flows out, and the wound does not close for a long time, forming a fistula, like a mouse hole, thus called mouse fistula. See *Su Wen* chapter 60 and *Ling Shu* chapter 21.

微　① 脉象。脉来微细无力，按之欲绝。出《素问·方盛衰论》。② 微弱。出《素问·诊要经终论》《素问·脉要精微论》。③ 指病轻微。出《素问·调经论》。

微（wēi）　① Pulse manifestation. Faint pulse that comes weak and impalpable. See *Su Wen* chapter 80. ② Weakness and faintness. See *Su Wen* chapter 16 and 17. ③ Mild disease. See *Su Wen* chapter 62.

微风　风邪中于肌肉，肌肉蠕动的病证。病轻浅，故曰微风。出《素问·调经论》。

微风（wēi fēng）　**mild stroke** Wind pathogens invade the muscles, showing symptoms of muscle peristalsis. The disease is moderate, thus called mild stroke. See *Su Wen* chapter 62.

微动四极　四极，四肢。言轻微的运动四肢，使阳气流通运行，以消除因阳气阻遏所致的水肿。出《素问·汤液醪醴论》。

微动四极（wēi dòng sì jí）　**slightly move the limbs** Slightly move the limbs to promote the flow of yang qi and eliminate the edema caused by the obstruction of yang qi. See *Su Wen* chapter 14.

微者逆之　治法。病势较轻，病情较单纯，症状与病机相符者谓之微，治疗应用与症状性质相反的药物，属于正治法。如寒者热之，热者寒之。出《素问·至真要大论》。

微者逆之（wēi zhě nì zhī）　**mild conditions are treated by counteraction** Treatment method. The disease is mild, the condition is simple, and the symptoms are consistent with the pathogenesis. Applying medicine that has the opposite properties of the symptoms is called routine treatment，like treating cold with heat or treating heat with cold. See *Su Wen* chapter 74.

颔　下巴。出《素问·疟论》。

颔（hàn）　**jaw** See *Su Wen* chapter 35.

腠理　① 泛指皮肤肌肉和脏腑之纹理。出《素问·阴阳应象大论》。② 皮肤汗孔。出《素问·举痛论》。

腠理（còu lǐ）　① The texture of the skin，muscles，and viscera. See *Su Wen* chapter 5. ② Sweat pores. See *Su Wen* chapter 39.

腰者肾之府　肾有两枚，居于下焦两侧腰中，故腰为肾之府。若腰部酸痛，转动不便，多与肾有关，是肾气衰败之兆。出《素问·脉要精微论》。

腰者肾之府（yāo zhě shèn zhī fǔ）　**the waist as the house of kidneys** There are two kidneys on both sides of the waist in the lower *jiao*，therefore the waist is known as the house of the kidneys. A sore and hard rotation of the waist are mostly related to the kidney，meaning a debilitation of kidney qi. See *Su Wen* chapter 17.

腰俞　经穴名。属督脉经。在骶部中线，当骶管裂孔中。别名背解、髓空、腰户、腰柱、髓俞。出《素问·缪刺论》。

腰俞（yāo shū）　**Yao Shu（DU 2）** Acupoint name. DU 2 pertains to the governor vessel，and is located in the hiatus sacralis. It is also named Bei Jie，Sui Kong，Yao Hu，Yao Zhu，and Sui Shu. See *Su Wen* chapter 63.

腨　即腓。小腿肚。《灵枢·寒热病》："腓者，腨（shuàn 涮）也。"

腨（shuàn）　**calf** See *Ling Shu* chapter 21.

腨肠　即小腿肚，今称腓肠。出《素问·刺禁论》。

腨肠（shuàn cháng）　**calf** See *Su Wen* chapter 52.

腨痟　小腿肚。痟（yuān 渊），酸痛。即小腿肚酸痛。出《素问·阴阳别论》。

腨痟（shuàn yuān）　**sore calf** See *Su Wen* chapter 7.

腹中论　《素问》篇名。主要论述腹中之病，故名。

腹中论（fù zhōng lùn）　**Discussion on Abdominal Disorders** Chapter title in *Su Wen*. It mainly discusses abdominal diseases, hence the name.

腧　① 通"输"，泛指腧穴。出《灵枢·经筋》。② 为五腧穴之一。

脉气似水流由浅向较深处灌注者称腧,十二经脉各有一腧,分别靠近腕、踝关节。出《灵枢·九针十二原》。

腧(shù)　① Acupoint. "腧" is the same as "输". Refers to the acupoint. See *Ling Shu* chapter 13. ② One of the five transport points. Pulse qi which flows like water moving from the shallower to the deeper is called transporting，each of the twelve meridians have one transport point，close to the wrist and ankle respectively. See *Ling Shu* chapter 1.

鲍鱼　药名,味辛臭温平无毒,能通血脉,益阴气,补肝利肠。主治瘀血、血痹等。出《素问·腹中论》。

鲍鱼(bào yú)　**abalone** A medicine name. Abalone is warm in flavor and smells fetid without toxicity. It can unblock meridians and blood vessels，nourish yin qi，tonify the liver and soothe the intestinal tract，mainly used to treat static blood and blood impediment. See *Su Wen* chapter 40.

解　① 关节缝隙,亦称"骨解"。出《素问·骨空论》。② 通懈,作弛缓解。出《素问·生气通天论》。③ 解散。出《灵枢·九针十二原》。④ 滑利。出《灵枢·大惑论》。⑤ 理解。出《素问·著至教论》。⑥ 融化。出《素问·脉解》。

解(jiě)　① Joint gap. Also called bone gap. See *Su Wen* chapter 60. ② Relaxation. "解" is the same as "懈"，refer to flabby. See *Su Wen* chapter 3. ③ To dissolve. See *Ling Shu* chapter 1. ④ Smooth. See *Ling Shu* chapter 80. ⑤ To understand. See *Su Wen* chapter 75. ⑥ To melt. See *Su Wen* chapter 49.

解㑊　病证名。身体困倦,懈怠无力的病证。解,同懈。㑊(yì亦),同亦,变易,异于正常。出《灵枢·论疾诊尺》。

解㑊(xiě yì)　*xie yi* Disease name，or the syndrome of feeling drowsy and weak. "解" is the same as "懈"；"㑊" is the same as "亦". See *Ling Shu* chapter 74.

解脉　足太阳经别行之脉。出《素问·刺腰痛》。

解脉(jiě mài)　**divergence meridian** The divergence meridian of foot greater yang. See *Su Wen* chapter 41.

解剖　用器械剖割尸体,以了解人体内部各器官的位置、形态、构造及其相互关系。出《灵

十
三
画

枢·经水》。

解剖（jiě pōu）　**anatomy** Using devices to cut corpses in order to know the position，shape，structure and interrelationship of various organs inside the human body. See *Ling Shu* chapter 12.

解惑　① 五节刺法之一，用以治疗反复颠倒，迷惑无常之病。出《灵枢·刺节真邪》。② 解释疑惑。出《素问·举痛论》。

解惑（jiě huò）　① One of the five needling methods used to treat repeatedly falling down episodes and perplexing diseases. See *Ling Shu* chapter 75. ② Explain doubts. See *Su Wen* chapter 39.

解㑊　解，即懈。懈㑊，肢软倦怠乏力。出《素问·痹论》。

解㑊（xiè duò）　**sluggish limbs** Limb weakness and fatigue. See *Su Wen* chapter 43.

解㑊　解，通懈，弛而不收。㑊，通惰，疲而无力。形容肢体筋骨极度疲软无力，懒于动作。出《素问·诊要经终论》。

解㑊（xiè duò）　**flaccidity of limbs** "解" is the same as "懈", which refers to flabby. "㑊" is the same as "惰", which refers to weak. Limbs，sinews and bones are

extremely weak，and too lazy to move. See *Su Wen* chapter 16.

解溪　经穴名。属足阳明胃经。在冲阳穴后一寸五分。出《灵枢·本输》。

解溪（jiě xī）　**Jie Xi（ST 41）** An acupoint pertaining to the stomach meridian of foot *yangming* located 1.5 *cun* behind ST 42. See *Ling Shu* chapter 2.

解精微论　《素问》篇名。解，解释。精微，精深微妙的道理。此篇主要解释哭泣涕泪之病，关系阴阳水火神志的变化，其道理精深微妙，故名。

解精微论（jiě jīng wēi lùn）　**Discussion on the Elucidation of Abstruse Theory** Chapter title in *Su Wen*. This chapter mainly explains the disease of crying，snivelling and tearing，which are related to the change of yin，yang，water，fire and mind. The theory behind this chapter is profound and subtle，hence the name.

瘃　瘃（zhú 逐），病名，即冻疮。出《灵枢·阴阳二十五人》。

瘃（zhú）　**frostbite** Disease name. See *Ling Shu* chapter 64.

痱　病名。以四肢瘫痪为主要症状的病证。出《灵枢·热病》。

痱（féi）　*fei* Disease name in

十三画

which the main symptom is becoming quadriplegic. See *Ling Shu* chapter 23.

痹　① 痹闭不通之病机。出《素问・宣明五气》。② 病证名。泛指肢体酸痛麻疼之证。出《素问・痹论》《素问・金匮真言论》《灵枢・寿夭刚柔》。

痹（bì）　① Pathogenesis of impediment and obstruction. See *Su Wen* chapter 23. ② Disease name. Syndromes of limb soreness. See *Su Wen* chapter 4, Chapter 43 and *Ling Shu* chapter 6.

痹气　痹，不通之义。痹气指由于阳虚阴盛，而致正气不能畅通，营卫凝涩，寒湿之邪留滞的一类病证。出《素问・逆调论》。

痹气（bì qì）　impediment qi Refers to the syndrome that, due to yang deficiency and yin debilitation, healthy qi cannot flow smoothly, and nutrient-defense is astringent, thus the pathogen of cold-dampness remains. See *Su We*n chapter 34.

痹论　《素问》篇名。此篇系统地论述了痹证的病因、病机、分类、症候、治法和预后。故名。

痹论（bì lùn）　**Discussion on Bi-Syndrome** Chapter title in *Su Wen*. This chapter systematically

discusses the disease cause, pathogenesis, classification, symptoms, treatment methods and prognosis of impediment syndromes. Hence the name.

痹热　即热痹。由于体质偏于阳盛阴虚，虽感受风寒湿之阴邪，但外邪不能伤人体之阳，化而为热，故为热痹。出《素问・痹论》。

痹热（bì rè）　**impediment heat** Because the body constitution pertains to exuberant yang and deficient yin, although wind and cold-damp pathogens are contracted, the external pathogens cannot hurt the yang of the human body, and turns into heat, thus causing heat impediment. See *Su Wen* chapter 43.

痹厥　病证名。肢体酸重疼痛麻木与手足逆冷为主症。出《素问・金匮真言论》《素问・五藏生成》。

痹厥（bì jué）　**impediment reversal** Disease name, of which the main symptoms are soreness and numbness of the body and reversal cold of the limbs. See *Su Wen* chapter 4 and 10.

痹躄　痹，肢体酸重麻木之痹证。躄（bì 必），足不能行，或拘挛，或痿弱，皆能致此。出《素问・玉版论要》。

痹躄(bì bì) **impediment limbs** A kind of impediment syndrome with symptoms of soreness and numbness in the body. Bì means "the feet can't walk", and spasms or leg flaccidity can both cause this syndrome. See *Su Wen* chapter 15.

瘘 病证名。筋脉肌肉萎弱,废而不用。出《素问·瘘论》。

瘘(wěi) **wilting** Disease name, in which the sinews and muscles are wilted and disfunctional. See *Su Wen* chapter 44.

瘘论 《素问》篇名。此篇以五脏所合五体的理论,分别论述了瘘躄、脉瘘、筋瘘、肉瘘、骨瘘等病证的病因病机、症状及治疗。故名。

瘘论(wěi lùn) **Discussion on Flaccidity** Chapter title in *Su Wen*. Based on the theory of the five viscera combining with the five body parts, this chapter discusses the causes of disease, pathogenesis, symptoms and treatment methods of syndromes such as limb wilting, vessel wilting, sinew wilting, fleshy wilting and bone wilting. Hence the name.

瘘厥 瘘,四肢瘘废不用。厥,四肢厥冷,或气机逆乱之证。出《素问·四气调神大论》。

瘘厥(wěi jué) **wilting reversal** *Wěi* means the disfunction of the limbs and *jué* means the reversal of cold limbs or qi reversal syndrome. See *Su Wen* chapter 2.

瘘痹 病证名。表现为肢节痹痛、瘘弱无力,足不任身的病证。出《素问·气交变大论》。

瘘痹(wěi bì) **wilting impediment** Disease name, of which the main symptoms are impediment pain, weakness of the limbs, and losing control of the feet. See *Su Wen* chapter 69.

瘘躄 瘘,瘘弱不用。躄(bì 闭),两下肢俱废。瘘躄,在此统指四肢瘘废不用的病证。病起于五脏气热,津液不兴,肺热叶焦,津液不布,四肢筋骨失养。出《素问·瘘论》。

瘘躄(wěi bì) **wilting limbs** Syndrome of the dysfunction of the limbs. Heat in the five viscera causes a lack of fluids and humor, and heat in the lung, in turn, prevents the lung to distribute fluid, thus the limbs are unable to be nourished. See *Su Wen* chapter 44.

瘅 ①(dàn)即热。出《素问·举痛论》。②(dǎn)通疸,即黄疸。出《素问·玉机真藏论》。

瘅（dàn/dǎn）　①（dàn）Heat. See *Su Wen* chapter 39. ②（dǎn）Jaundice. "瘅" is the same as "疸". See *Su Wen* chapter 19.

瘅疟　（瘅，dān）病名。以但热不寒为发作特点的疟病，并见消瘦脱肉，少气烦闷，手足发热，欲呕吐等症。病因病机为素体阳盛，肺有郁热，感受风寒之邪后，邪随热化，故症见但热不寒。出《素问·疟论》。

瘅疟（dān nüè）　**pure-heat malaria** Malaria, characterized by a fever without cold. The main symptoms are emaciation, shedding of the flesh, shortness of breath, depression, heat in hands and feet, and vomiting, etc. The cause and pathogenesis of malaria are yang debilitation of the body and stagnated heat in the lung. When contracting a wind-cold pathogen, the pathogen will be transformed by heat, and thus is characterized by a fever without cold. See *Su Wen* chapter 35.

瘅热　①（瘅，dān）病证名。指温热病。出《灵枢·论疾诊尺》。②病机。瘅，（dān）即热，热甚则津伤。出《素问·举痛论》。

瘅热（dān rè）　① Disease name. Warm disease. See *Ling Shu* chapter 74. ② Pathogenesis. *Dàn* means pure heat, which will hurt fluid and humor. See *Su Wen* chapter 39.

廉泉　经穴名。属任脉。别名本池，舌本。在颔下结喉上，舌本下中点处。出《素问·刺疟》。

廉泉（lián quán）　**Lian Quan（ST 42）** Acupoint name pertaining to the conception vessel. It is located above the Adam's apple, on the middle point below the tongue base. See *Su Wen* chapter 36.

新洛　九宫之一，又名乾宫，居西北之位，主立冬、小雪、大雪三节气。出《灵枢·九宫八风》。

新洛（xīn luò）　*xin luo* One of the nine palaces, also called Qian palace. *Xīn luò* is located in the north-west, governing three solar terms: Beginning of Winter（19th solar term）, Slight Snow（20th solar term）and Great Snow（21st solar term）. See *Ling Shu* chapter 77.

意　① 记忆、意念。意为脾所主，以营气为物质基础。出《灵枢·本神》。② 臆断。出《灵枢·逆顺肥瘦》。③ 情状。出《灵枢·周痹》。

意（yì） ① Memory and thought, dominated by the spleen and which takes nutrient qi as its material base. See *Ling Shu* chapter 8. ② Assumption. See *Ling Shu* chapter 38. ③ Situation and condition. See *Ling Shu* chapter 27.

阙 两眉之间的部位,面部色诊用以测候肺的功能状况。出《灵枢·五色》。

阙（què） **glabella** the region between the two eyebrows; facial inspection uses it to measure the function of the lung. See *Ling Shu* chapter 49.

数 ①（shuò 朔）数脉。脉来急速,一息五至以上。主热证。数而有力为实热;数而无力为虚热。出《素问·阴阳别论》。②（shuò 朔）多,屡。出《素问·风论》。③（shù 树）方法,规则,技术。出《灵枢·邪客》《素问·上古天真论》。④（shù 树）指五行的生成之数。出《素问·六元正纪大论》。⑤（shǔ 暑）推测。出《素问·阴阳离合论》。⑥（shǔ 暑）清楚,明了。出《灵枢·百病始生》。⑦（shù 树）次数,引申为限度。出《灵枢·经筋》。

数（shuò） ① Rapid pulse, which comes at least five times during one breath, indicates heat syndromes. A strong rapid pulse means excess heat; a weak rapid pulse means deficient heat. See *Su Wen* chapter 7. ②（shuò） many. See *Su Wen* chapter 72. ③（shù） Method; rule; technique. See *Ling Shu* chapter 71 and *Su Wen* Chapter 1. ④（shù） Given numbers of the five elements. See *Su Wen* chapter 71. ⑤（shǔ） Speculation. See *Su Wen* chapter 6. ⑥（shǔ） Clear; understandable. See *Ling Shu* chapter 66. ⑦（shù） Number of times; limit. See *Ling Shu* chapter 13.

数则烦心 数,（shuò 朔）数脉。脉来急速,一息五至以上。指热证。出《素问·脉要精微论》。

数则烦心（shuò zé fán xīn） **Rapid pulse indicates heat syndrome.** A rapid pulse which comes more than five times during one breath indicates a heat syndrome. See *Su Wen* chapter 17.

煎厥 ① 指由于阳盛阴虚,入夏阳气鸥张导致的昏厥。出《素问·生气通天论》。② 指由于大怒,肝之阳气暴张而致的昏厥。出《素问·脉解》。

煎厥（jiān jué） ① Fainting due

to yin deficiency and yang exuberance in summer，when yang
qi in nature is excessive. See *Su
Wen* chapter 3. ② Fainting caused
by anger and exuberant liver
yang. See *Su Wen* chapter 49.

煴 没有火熖之火。出《灵枢·
寿夭刚柔》。

煴（yùn）　**fire without flame** See
Ling Shu chapter 6.

满者泄之　治疗原则。邪气满盛
之实证，应用宣泄邪气的泻法
治疗。原指针刺而言，亦适用
于其他各种疗法。出《素问·
宝命全形论》《灵枢·九针十
二原》。

满者泄之（mǎn zhě xiè zhī）　**to
drain the excess** Treatment principle. For an excess syndrome
of exuberant pathogen，the
draining method that purges
the pathogen should be taken.
Originally，it was an acupunture
technique；later，it became applicable to other therapies. See
Su Wen chapter 25，and *Ling
Shu* chapter 1.

满病　胀满一类病证。出《素问·
异法方宜论》。

满病（mǎn bìng）　**full disease**
Disease of distention and fullness. See *Su Wen* chapter 12.

溪　肌肉会合之处。出《素问·

气穴论》。

溪（xī）　**small muscular convergence** The place where muscles
converge. See *Su Wen* chapter 58.

溪谷　出《素问·气穴》。① 指
大、小分肉之纹理界畔。见《素
问集注》。② 指大小骨节。见
《类经·经络八》。

溪谷（xī gǔ）　See *Su Wen* chapter
58. ① Small or large interspace
of muscles. See *Su Wen Ji Zhu*
（*Collected Annotation of Su
Wen*）. ② Small or large sclero-
mere. See *Lei Jing*（*Classified
Classic*）"Meridians and Collaterals Chapter 8".

溜　① 滑，指脉象滑利。出《素
问·阴阳别论》。② 通"流"。
出《灵枢·小针解》。

溜（liū）　① Slippery pulse condition. See *Su Wen* chapter 7.
②"溜"is the same as"流".
See *Ling Shu* chapter 3.

溜脉　溜，流之义。凡经脉流行
于目部或耳部等者均称为溜
脉。出《素问·刺禁论》。

溜脉（liū mài）　**flowing pulse** *Liū*
means flowing. Meridians that
run around eyes or ears are
called flowing pulse. See *Su
Wen* chapter 52.

溏泄　大便稀薄。出《素问·气
交变大论》。

溏泄（táng xiè） **sloppy diarrhea** Loose stools. See *Su Wen* chapter 69.

溢阳 三阳之气溢于人迎脉，而见人迎脉盛于寸口脉四倍，脉形大而且数的脉象。又称"格阳""外格"，是阴气格阳于外，阴阳将要离决之象，预后极差。出《灵枢·禁服》。参"格阳""外格"条。

溢阳（yì yáng） **excessive yang** The qi of three yang is exuberant at the wrist pulse, and the pulse condition of the *cun kou* is four times as large and rapid as the carotid pulse. It shares the same meaning of "格阳" and "外格". It is the syndrome of yin repelling yang to the outside when yin and yang are about to depart，and the prognosis is very poor. See *Ling Shu* chapter 48. See "格阳" and "外格".

溢阴 三阴之气盛溢于寸口脉，而见寸口盛于人迎四倍，大而且数的脉象。又称"内关""关阴"。出《灵枢·终始》。参"内关""关阴"条。

溢阴（yì yīn） **excessive yin** The qi of triple yin is exuberant at the *cun kou* pulse, and the pulse condition of the wrist is four times as large and rapid as the carotid pulse. Also called "exuberant yang repelling yin". See *Ling Shu* chapter 9. See "内关" and "关阴".

溢饮 病症名。溢，满而外流。溢饮，因渴甚暴饮，水饮溢于肌肉皮肤以及肠胃间隙而致肿胀的病证。出《素问·脉要精微论》《灵枢·邪气藏府病形》。

溢饮（yì yǐn） **subcutaneous fluid retention** Disease name，when body swelling occurs due to thirst and overdrinking, causing water to overflow into the muscles, skin and gastrointestinal spaces. See *Su Wen* chapter 17 and *Ling Shu* chapter 4.

溓水 出《素问·阴阳类论》。① 指冬初之时。见《素问识》。② 三秋之时。见《素问集注》。

溓水（lián shuǐ） See *Su Wen* chapter 79. ① Early winter. See *Su Wen Zhi*（*Understanding Su Wen*）. ② The three months autumn. See *Su Wen Ji Zhu*（*Collected Annotation of Su Wen*）.

溺 ① 溺（niào 尿），同尿，即小便。出《灵枢·五癃津液别》。② 溺（nì 逆），淹没的意思。出《素问·方盛衰论》。③ 排小便。出《素问·诊要经终论》。

溺（niào/nì）　① Urination. See *Ling Shu* chapter 36. ② Submergence. See *Su Wen* chapter 80. ③ To urinate. See *Su Wen* chapter 16.

溺孔　排尿之孔道，在女子又名廷孔，男子则涵于阴茎之中。出《素问·骨空论》。

溺孔（nì kǒng）　**urinating hole** The urinary channel, is also known as the Ting hole in women, and in men is contained in the penis. See *Su Wen* chapter 60.

溺血　即尿血，由热结膀胱所致。出《素问·气厥论》。

溺血（nì xiě）　**urinating blood** Hematuria, caused by heat stagnated in the bladder. See *Su Wen* chapter 37.

惛痛　惛（xù 蓄），《针灸甲乙经》《太素》并作蓄，积聚之意。惛痛，痛聚于某处，形容痛处固定不移。出《灵枢·周痹》。

惛痛（xù tòng）　**accumulated pain** In *Zhen Jiu Jia Yi Jing*（*Classic of Acupuncture and Moxibustion*）and *Tai Su*（*Grand Plain*）, *xù* means accumulation. Accumulated pain means that a fixed pain stays in a certain part. See *Ling Shu* chapter 27.

塞因塞用　反治法。如证见痞塞，缘于气虚运化无力者，当用补药以治之。出《素问·至真要大论》。

塞因塞用（sāi yīn sāi yòng）　**to treat the stopped by stopping** Paradoxical treatment. Syndromes such as stuffiness and fullness，which are caused by qi deficiency as well as poor transportation and transformation，should be treated with tonification. See *Su Wen* chapter 74.

寝汗　睡眠时汗出。出《素问·藏气法时论》。

寝汗（qǐn hàn）　**sleeping sweat** See *Su Wen* chapter 22.

谨和五味　谨，慎重，小心。和，调和。五味，泛指饮食物。甘苦酸辛咸五味分走五脏，饮食应谨慎地调和五味，不可偏嗜某一性味，以防损伤脏气。出《素问·生气通天论》。

谨和五味（jǐn hé wǔ wèi）　**to balance the five kinds of flavours** The five kinds of flavors refers to food and drink. Sweet，bitter，sour，pungent，and salty affect the five viscera respectively. Thus, diets should be carefully balanced, and one should not be partial to a certain flavour, in case that hurts the viscera qi. See *Su*

Wen chapter 3.

辟阴 指肾病传脾。出《素问·阴阳别论》。① 辟，放辟。辟阴，指阴水扩散。见《类经·疾病六》。② 辟，邪辟，相对于正而言，肾水反侮脾，属反常传变，故称辟阴。见《素问》吴崑注。

辟阴（pì yīn） Kidney disease transmits to the spleen. See *Su Wen* chapter 7. ① *Pì* means transmission，and *pì yīn* means the transmission of yin water. See *Lei Jing*（*Classified Classic*）"On Diseases Chapter 6". ② *Pì* means pathogens，in contrast to healthy qi. Kidney water rebels to the spleen，is an abnormal transmission，so it is called *pì yīn*. See *Su Wen* annotated by Wu Kun.

十四画

髦　泛指较长的体毛。出《灵枢·经脉》。

髦（máo）　**long body hair** See *Ling Shu* chapter 10.

墙基　指面部四旁的骨骼。出《灵枢·寿夭刚柔》。

墙基（qiáng jī）　**wall footing** The bones around the face. See *Ling Shu* chapter 6.

綦针　古代缝制衣帛用的长针。出《灵枢·九针论》。

綦针（qí zhēn）　**long sewing-needle** A long needle for sewing clothes in ancient times. See *Ling Shu* chapter 78.

暮世　暮，晚。暮世，即后世。出《素问·移精变气论》。

暮世（mù shì）　**later generations** See *Su Wen* chapter 13.

蔽　耳门。出《灵枢·五色》。

蔽（bì）　**ear gate** Porus acusticus internus. See *Ling Shu* chapter 49.

皶　面部的粉刺。多因劳汗当风，寒气薄之，汗液凝于肤腠而生。出《素问·生气通天论》。

皶（zhā）　**acne on the face** Mostly caused by sweat blown by the wind while laboring and the cold qi of the wind that condenses sweat on the skin. See *Su Wen* chapter 3.

酸入肝　与"酸生肝"同理。见《素问·宣明五气》《素问·至真要大论》。见"酸生肝"条。

酸入肝（suān rù gān）　**sour enters liver** The same as sour engenders the liver. See *Su Wen* chapter 23 and 74. See "酸生肝".

酸生肝　酸为五味之一，根据五行理论，酸与肝同属木行，故酸味入口，先入肝而滋养肝木。见《素问·阴阳应象大论》。

酸生肝（suān shēng gān）　**Sour engenders the liver.** Sour is one of the five flavours. According to five element theory, the sour flavour and the liver pertain to the wood element, thus sour first enters the liver and tonifies liver wood. See *Su Wen* chapter 5.

酸伤筋　酸入肝，肝与筋相合，酸味固能滋养肝木，但若太过则能伤筋。见《素问·阴阳应象大论》。

酸伤筋（suān shāng jīn）　**Sour damages the sinews.** Sour enters the liver, and the liver is related to the sinews, thus over-tonifying the liver by sour flavours could damage the sinews. See *Su Wen* chapter 5.

酸走筋　酸入肝而肝主筋,故酸味走筋。酸性收,过于酸则筋挛不舒而伤筋。出《素问·宣明五气》《灵枢·五味论》。

酸走筋(suān zǒu jīn)　**Sour runs through the sinews.** The sour flavor enters the liver and the liver dominates the sinews, therefore sour runs through the sinews. The sour flavor has a contracting nature, thus ingesting too much sour would hurt the sinews by over-contracting them. See *Su Wen* chapter 23 and *Ling Shu* chapter 63.

雌黄　药名。性味辛平,有毒。具有杀虫虱、止身痒的作用,治疗疮疥、虫积、癫痫等症。是小金丹方的主药之一。此方古人用来预防疫疠。出《素问·刺法论》。

雌黄(cí huáng)　**orpiment** Medicine name. Orpiment has a pugent-warm flavor and is toxic. It has an insecticidal and antipruritic effect, and can treat sores, worms, and epilepsy. It is one of major medicines of Xiao Jin Dan formula which was used by ancient people to prevent epidemics. See *Su Wen* chapter 72.

瞑　目闭合。出《素问·刺热》。

瞑(míng)　**eyes closing** See *Su Wen* chapter 32.

骷骨　出《灵枢·师传》。① 膝骨。见《类经·藏象二十九》。② 改骷为骶。骨之端为骶,指胸骨下端之骨。一言骶为锁骨。见《灵枢集注》《灵枢注证发微》。

骷骨(kū gǔ)　See *Ling Shu* chapter 29. ① Kneecap. See *Lei Jing*（*Classified Classic*）" Viscera and Bowls Chapter 29". ② "骷" should be written into "骶". The end of the bone is *kū*, which refers to the bone at the lower end of the sternum. Others think that ku is the clavicle. See *Ling Shu Ji Zhu*（*Collected Annotation of Ling Shu*）and *Ling Shu Zhu Zheng Fa Wei*（*Annotation and Elaboration on Ling Shu*）.

骶　尾骶骨。位于脊椎末端。出《素问·刺热》。

骶(dǐ)　**sacrum and coccyx** Located at the end of the spine. See *Su Wen* chapter 32.

锃针　"九针"之一。长三寸半,

针尖如黍粟形，圆而微尖，用于按摩经脉，流通气血，为按压穴位用具。近人有称为"推针"者。出《灵枢·九针十二原》。

锃针（shí zhēn） **spoon needle** One of the nine classical needles which is 3.5 inches long, with a millet-like needle shape, round and slightly pointed. It is used to massage meridians, circulate qi and blood, and is also a kit for pressing acupoints. Some people call it push needle in recent times. See *Ling Shu* chapter 1.

颓 脊椎骨。颓（zhuī 椎）同椎。出《灵枢·经别》。

颓（zhuī） **spine** See *Ling Shu* chapter 11.

僦贷季 为传说中远古时代的医学家，据说是另一著名医学家岐伯的老师，故又称之为"先师"。出《素问·移精变气论》。

僦贷季（jiù dài jì） **Jiu Daiji** A medical expert in ancient times and was said to be the teacher of another famous medical expert Qi Bo, so he was also called the first teacher. See *Su Wen* chapter 13.

鼻孔 鼻腔与外界相通的孔道。出《灵枢·经脉》。

鼻孔（bí kǒng） **nostril** The opening between the nasal cavity and the outside. See *Ling Shu* chapter 10.

鼻洞 病名。即鼻渊，见该条。出《灵枢·忧恚无言》。

鼻洞（bí dòng） **nasal hole** Disease name. See "鼻渊" for detail. See *Ling Shu* chapter 69.

鼻息肉 鼻内息肉。出《灵枢·邪气藏府病形》。

鼻息肉（bí xī ròu） **nasal polyp** Polyp in the nose. See *Ling Shu* chapter 4.

鼻渊 病名。以浊涕腥臭，头胀鼻塞鼻酸为主症。由胆热循经上犯所致。出《素问·气厥论》。

鼻渊（bí yuān） **sinusitis** Disease name, of which the main symptoms are turbid nasal discharge, fullness in the head, nasal obstruction, and an irritating sensation in the nose, and are all caused by upward invading gallbladder heat. See *Su Wen* chapter 37.

鼻窒 鼻塞。出《素问·五常政大论》。

鼻窒（bí zhì） **rhinobyon** See *Su Wen* chapter 70.

鼻槁腊 症状名。槁，腊，均干之意。鼻槁腊即鼻干燥。出《灵枢·寒热病》。

鼻槁腊（bí gǎo là） **dried-meat

十
四
画

nose Symptom name. Dryness of the nose. See *Ling Shu* chapter 21.

鼻隧 鼻腔孔道。鼻为肺之窍,肺与大肠相表里,故鼻隧与大肠相应。出《灵枢·师传》。

鼻隧(bí suì) **nasal passages** Nasal foramen. The lung opens at the nose, in addition, the lung and the large intestine are exteriorly and interiorly related to each other, so the nasal passages corresponds to the large intestine. See *Ling Shu* chapter 29.

魄 神的一部分,为与生俱来的本能的动作和感觉功能。属阴,藏于肺。出《灵枢·本神》。

魄(pò) **corporeal soul** As part of the spirit and vitality, the corporeal soul is instinctual in movement and sensory function, and pertains to yin, while being stored in the lung. See *Ling Shu* chapter 8.

魄门 肛门。魄通粕,传送糟粕之门。出《素问·五藏别论》。

魄门(pò mén) **anus** "魄" is the same as "粕". Refers to the gate used to transport dregs. See *Su Wen* chapter 10.

魄门亦为五藏使 魄门,即肛门。使,役使之意。肛门有排泄粪便的功能,肛门启闭还赖五脏之气的调节。如心神之主宰,肺气之宣肃,脾气之升提,肝气之条达,肾气之固摄皆与肛门功能有关。其启闭又能影响五脏气机之升降。故魄门功能常反映五脏之状况。出《素问·五藏别论》。

魄门亦为五藏使(pò mén yì wéi wǔ zàng shǐ) **Anus is governed by five viscera.** The anus has the function of excreting feces, and the opening and closing of the anus depends on the regulation of the five viscera. The domination of the mind and spirit, the diffusion of lung qi, the upbearing of spleen qi, the free coursing of liver qi, and the containing of kidney qi are all related to anal function. Its opening and closing affects the circuits and qi of the five viscera. Therefore, the function of the anus often reflects the status of the five viscera. See *Su Wen* chapter 10.

魄汗 出《素问·生气通天论》《素问·阴阳别论》《素问·通评虚实论》《素问·至真要大论》等篇。① 自汗。见《素问识》。② 肺藏魄,主皮毛,汗出于皮毛,故亦称魄汗。见《素问

十
四
画

注证发微》。③ 阴汗。见《素
问》吴崑注。

魄汗（pò hàn）　See *Su Wen*
chapter 3，7，28，and 74.
① Spontaneous sweating. See
Su Wen Zhi（*Understanding Su
Wen*）. ② Lung stores the corporeal soul and dominates the
skin and（body）hair；sweat
comes from the skin. Thus it is
called corporeal soul perspira-
tion. See *Su Wen Zhu Zheng Fa
Wei*（*Annotation and Elaboration on Su Wen*）. ③ Genital
sweating. See *Su Wen* annotated
by Wu Kun.

膜　体内的膜状组织，如筋膜、耳
膜、肓膜等。出《素问・痹论》。

膜（mó）　**membrane** Membrane
tissues in the body，such as fas-
cia，eardrums，and membrane
tissues between the five viscera.
See *Su Wen* chapter 43.

膜原　又作募原。泛指胸腹肠胃
间之脂膜。出《素问・举痛论》。

膜原（mó yuán）　**membrane source**
Refers to the lipid membrane
between the intestines and the
stomach in the abdomen. See
Su Wen chapter 39.

膜胀　症状名，指胸腹部的胀满。
出《素问・阴阳应象大论》。

膜胀（chēn zhàng）　**inflated full-**
ness Refers to distention and
fullness in the abdomen. See
Su Wen chapter 5.

膈　① 横膈。出《灵枢・经脉》。
② 阻隔。出《灵枢・四时气》。

膈（gé）　① Diaphragm. See *Ling
Shu* chapter 10. ② Obstruction.
See *Ling Shu* chapter 19.

膈中　病名。症见食后又吐出。
出《灵枢・邪气藏府病形》。

膈中（gé zhōng）　**obstruction in
middle** Disease name. Vomiting
after eating. See *Ling Shu*
chapter 4.

膈俞　经穴名。属足太阳膀胱
经。八会穴之血会。在第七椎
下，两旁各一寸五分处。出《灵
枢・背腧》。

膈俞（gé shū）　**Ge Shu（BL 17）**
Acupoint name pertaining to
the bladder meridian of foot
taiyang. It is the blood meeting
point of the eight meeting points,
and is located under the seventh
vertebrae，1.5 *cun* away on each
side. See *Ling Shu* chapter 51.

膈洞　出《灵枢・根结》。① 膈，
为膈气虚弱。洞，谓洞泄无禁。
见《太素・经脉根结》。② 膈，
为上下不通之膈症。见《灵枢
注证发微》。

膈洞（gé dòng）　See *Ling Shu*
chapter 5. ① The qi of the dia-

phragm is weak with symptoms of purgation. *Tai Su*（*Classified Study on Huang Di Nei Jing*）"The Root of Meridians and Collaterals". ② Syndrome of obstruction between the upper and lower. See *Ling Shu Zhu Zheng Fa Wei*（*Annotation and Elaboration on Ling Shu*）.

膀胱 六腑之一。位于下焦，贮藏与排泄小便为其主要功能。出《素问·灵兰秘典论》。

膀胱(páng guāng) **bladder** One of the six bowels. The bladder is located in the lower *jiao* and has the function of storing and excreting urination. See *Su Wen* chapter 8.

膀胱不约为遗溺 溺(niào 尿)，同尿。约，约束。膀胱主贮存和排泄小便，如膀胱气虚，不能约束，发为遗尿。出《灵枢·九针论》。

膀胱不约为遗溺(páng guāng bù yuē wéi yí niào) **Failure retention of bladder causes enuresis.** The bladder stores and excretes urine. Syndromes such as bladder qi deficiency, which means the bladder can't be restrained, will cause enuresis. See *Ling Shu* chapter 78.

膀胱足太阳之脉 即足太阳膀胱经，为十二经脉之一。其循行路线从目内眦(睛明穴)开始，向上经过额部，交会于巅顶(百会穴)。一支从巅顶至耳上角。再一支从巅顶入里络脑，返出下行项后，沿肩胛骨内侧，挟脊柱两旁，直达腰中，进入脊柱两旁的肌肉(膂)，入腹腔，络于肾，属于膀胱。再一支从腰部沿脊柱两旁下行，穿过臀部，直入膝腘窝中。再一支从左右肩胛，挟脊柱，由内部下行至环跳骨处，沿股外侧后缘内而下，会合前一支脉于膝弯内(腘内)，由此下行至小腿肚(踹)，出外踝骨之后方，沿小趾本节后圆骨至小趾外侧端(接足少阴肾经)。出《灵枢·经脉》。

膀胱足太阳之脉(páng guāng zú tài yáng zhī mài) **bladder meridian of foot *taiyang*** One of the twelve meridians which starts from the inner canthus（Acupoint BL 1），passes upward through the forehead，and meets at the parietal（Acupoint DU 20）. One part of this meridian goes from the parietal to the top corner of the ear. Another enters from the parietal to the brain collaterals，and returns to the neck back，goes along the inside of the scapula,

十四画

follows the spine sides, reaches the waist, enters the muscles (backbone) on both sides of the spine and then the abdomen along the kidney collaterals. This part of the meridian pertains to the bladder. Another one descends from the waist along the spine sides, through the hips, and straight into the knee popliteal fossa. Another runs from the left and right shoulder blades, goes along the spine, from the inside to the kneecap, down the lateral posterior edge of the leg, and joins the previous meridian in the knee bend (inside the popliteal). Then, from there, it descends to the calf, comes out from the back of the lateral anklebone along the posterior round bone of the little toe to the lateral end (connected to the kidney meridian of foot *shaoyin*). See *Ling Shu* chapter 10.

膀胱胀　病症名。六腑咳之一。症见少腹胀满而小便不利。出《灵枢·胀论》。

膀胱胀（páng guāng zhàng）
bladder distension Disease name. One of the six types of bowel coughs, of which the main

symptom is abdominal fullness with poor urination. See *Ling Shu* chapter 35.

膀胱咳　六腑咳之一。由肾咳不愈传变而成。证候特点为咳而小便随遗。出《素问·咳论》。

膀胱咳（páng guāng ké）　**bladder cough** One of the six types of bowel coughs transmitted and transmuted by an uncured kidney cough. The main symptom is coughing with enuresis. See *Su Wen* chapter 38.

豪针　豪通毫。即毫针。多用刺婴儿疾病。出《灵枢·逆顺肥瘦》。参"毫针"条。

豪针（háo zhēn）　**filiform needle** "豪" is the same as "毫". Mainly used to treat infant diseases. See *Ling Shu* chapter 38. See "毫针".

膏　①指水谷精气中稠厚的部分。其内渗于骨空，有滑润关节、补益脑髓等作用。出《灵枢·五癃津液别》。②油脂。出《灵枢·经筋》。③脏腑的膏膜。出《灵枢·九针十二原》。④肌肉、皮肤松弛不坚之人。出《灵枢·卫气失常》。⑤肥甘厚味的食品。出《灵枢·根结》。⑥用油脂涂擦。出《灵枢·经筋》。

膏（gāo）　① It refers to the thick part of water and grain's essence. It infiltrates into the bone space and has the function of smoothing joints and tonifying marrow. See *Ling Shu* chapter 36. ② Grease. See *Ling Shu* chapter 13. ③ Membrane of the five viscera and six bowels. See *Ling Shu* chapter 1. ④ People with loose skin and muscles. See *Ling Shu* chapter 59. ⑤ Fatty and spicy food. See *Ling Shu* chapter 5. ⑥ Rubbing with grease. See *Ling Shu* chapter 13.

膏人 体质名,指皮肤纵缓,肌肉松弛下垂者。出《灵枢·卫气失常》。

膏人(gāo rén) *gao*-type people Name of constitution,which refers to people with loose skin and sagged muscles. See *Ling Shu* chapter 59.

瘈瘲 瘈(chì 赤),音义同瘛,为筋脉急而牵引。瘲(zòng 纵),筋脉缓而伸展。一急一缓,一引一伸,谓之瘈瘲,即抽搐之义。出《素问·诊要经终论》。

瘈瘲(chì zòng) convulsions *Chì* means sinews get pulled rapidly, *Zòng* means sinews get stretched slowly. Pull and stretch are called *chì zòng*,that is,the meaning of convulsions. See *Su Wen* chapter 16.

瘄 同疹。皮肤发出的红色小点如粟米。由热伏营血所致。出《素问·刺法论》。

瘄(zhěn) eruption Visible red lesions of the skin,resembling millet seeds,and caused by hidden heat in the nutrient blood. See *Su Wen* chapter 72.

瘄疟 病名。同痎疟,详见该条。出《素问·刺法论》。

瘄疟(jiē nüè) old malaria Disease name for the same disease as the long-lasting malaria. See that term for detail. See *Su Wen* chapter 72.

癀阴 病证名。癀同癫(tuí 颓)。即阴囊肿大之癫疝。出《灵枢·五色》。

癀阴(tuí yīn) decadent yin Disease name which manifests with the swelling of the scrotum. See *Ling Shu* chapter 49.

癀疝 病名。又名颓疝,为疝之一种。症状为男子小腹有块,下冲阴囊,疼痛。出《灵枢·邪气藏府病形》。

癀疝(tuí shàn) incarcerated hernia Disease name,which is also called the swelling of the scrotum,and of which the main symptom is a lump in the lower abdomen affecting the scrotum,and causing pain. See

Ling Shu chapter 4.

痨癃　病名。出《灵枢·邪气藏府病形》。① 作颓癃。癃，小便不畅利之谓。见《太素·五藏脉诊》。② 即痨癃疝。见《类经·疾病三》。参"痨癃疝"条。

痨癃（tuí lóng）　Disease name. See Ling Shu chapter 4. ① Difficult urination. Tai Su（Classified Study on Huang Di Nei Jing）"Pulse Diagnosis Based on Five viscera". ② Difficulty and pain in urination. See Lei Jing（Classified Classic）"On Diseases Chapter 3". See "痨癃疝".

瘦人　为体质瘦弱，肤色少泽，气血不足的一类人。其体质特点：皮薄，色淡，肌瘦而骨骼棱角分明，薄唇，言语时唇动轻捷，其血清气滑，气血易脱。出《灵枢·逆顺肥瘦》。

瘦人（shòu rén）　thin people It refers to a group of people with weak constitutions，less skin complexion as well as insufficient qi and blood. Its constitutional characteristics：thin skin，light complexion，thin muscles with angular bones and thin lips，their lips move swiftly when speaking. They have slippery qi and clear blood，which

both collapse easily. See Ling Shu chapter 38.

瘖　即暗，失音。出《素问·奇病论》。

瘖（yīn）　mute Loss of voice. See Su Wen chapter 47.

瘖门　即哑门，督脉经穴名。又名舌厌、舌横，在项后风府各一寸，入发际五分，项中央。出《素问·气穴论》。

瘖门（yīn mén）　Yin Men（DU 15）Pertains to the governor vessel and is located 1 cun from either side of Feng Fu（DU 16）at the center of the back of the neck，half into the hairline. See Su Wen chapter 58.

瘰　病名。出《素问·生气通天论》。① 指鼠瘰。见《类经·疾病五》。② 马刀挟瘰。按马刀为结核生于腋下，挟瘰为结核生于颈旁。即今之瘰病。见《素问集注》。③ 久疮不愈，脓水淋漓之谓。

瘰（lòu）　Disease name. See Su Wen chapter 3. ① Mouse fistula. See Lei Jing（Classified Classic）"On Diseases Chapter 5". ② Sabre-beadstring scrofulae. The saber scrofulae develops under the armpit，and the beadstring scrofulae beside the neck. That is called scrofulous today. See *Su Wen Ji Zhu* (*Collected Annotation of Su Wen*). ③ Sores that do not heal for a long time with dripping pus.

瘕　病名。瘕，假之义，指腹中聚散无常之结块，故又名聚。出《素问·大奇论》。《内经》有疝瘕、虫瘕、水瘕、虑瘕等名，详各条。

瘕（jiǎ）　**aggregation** Disease name which refers to an impermanent aggregation-accumulation lump in the abdomen. See *Su Wen* chapter 48. There are lower abdominal colic aggregations，worm aggregations，water aggregations，and large intestinal aggregations in *Huang Di's Internal Classic*. See corresponding terms for detail.

膂　指脊柱骨及两旁之肌肉。出《素问·疟论》。

膂（lǚ）　**backbone** Refers to vertebra and the muscles on its both sides. See *Su Wen* chapter 35.

膂筋　脊内之筋。出《灵枢·百病始生》。

膂筋（lǚ jīn）　**backbone sinew** Sinews in the spine. See *Ling Shu* chapter 66.

精　① 指水谷精气。出《素问·经脉别论》。② 泛指体内的阴精。出《素问·金匮真言论》。③ 特指生殖之精。出《灵枢·本神》。④ 指精神、情志。出《素问·移精变气论》。⑤ 旺盛，强健。出《素问·生气通天论》。⑥ 即指气。出《素问·阴阳应象大论》。⑦ 指清爽，与昏昧相对。出《灵枢·营卫生会》。⑧ 指精细，精微。出《素问·汤液醪醴论》。⑨ 正。出《灵枢·本神》。⑩ 即睛。出《素问·四气调神大论》。⑪ 运行流利。出《素问·八正神明论》。⑫ 指男子的精液。出《灵枢·本神》。⑬ 眼睛具有的视觉功能。出《灵枢·大惑论》。

精（jīng）　① Essence qi from water and grain. See *Su Wen* chapter 7. ② Yin essence in the body. See *Su Wen* chapter 4. ③ The essence of reproduction. See *Ling Shu* chapter 8. ④ Refers to spirit and mood. See *Su Wen* chapter 13. ⑤ Exuberant；sturdy. See *Su Wen* chapter 3. ⑥ Qi. See *Su Wen* chapter 5. ⑦ Clear-minded，as opposed to fuzzy-headed. See *Ling Shu* chapter 18. ⑧ Micro；subtle. See *Su Wen* chapter 14. ⑨ Rightness. See *Ling Shu* chapter 8. ⑩ Eyes. See *Su Wen* chapter 2. ⑪ Run fluently. See

Su Wen chapter 26. ⑫ Male semen. See Ling Shu chapter 8. ⑬ The visual function of the eyes. See Ling Shu chapter 80.

精之窠为眼　脏腑之精气皆注于目之故。见《灵枢·大惑论》。

精之窠为眼（jīng zhī kē wéi yǎn）**eye as the nest of essence** The essence qi of the five viscera and six bowels pour through the eye. See Ling Shu chapter 80.

精气　① 生殖之精。出《素问·上古天真论》。② 自然界的清气。出《素问·上古天真论》。③ 脏腑精气。出《灵枢·大惑论》。④ 水谷精气。出《灵枢·小针解》。⑤ 指正气。出《素问·通评虚实论》。

精气（jīng qì）　① The essence of reproduction. See Su Wen chapter 1. ② Clear qi in nature. See Su Wen chapter 1. ③ Essence qi in the five viscera and six bowels. See Ling Shu chapter 80. ④ Essence qi in water and grain. See Ling Shu chapter 3. ⑤ Healthy qi. See Su Wen chapter 28.

精气夺则虚　出《素问·通评虚实论》。见"邪气盛则实"条。

精气夺则虚（jīng qì duó zé xū）**Lack of essential qi causes deficiency syndromes.** See Su Wen chapter 28. See "邪气盛则实" for detail.

精明　① 指眼神。出《素问·脉要精微论》。② 指眼睛。出《素问·脉要精微论》。③ 指精气神明。出《素问·脉要精微论》。

精明（jīng míng）　① Refers to the expression in one's eyes. See Su Wen chapter 17. ② Eyes. See Su Wen chapter 17. ③ Refers to essence qi and spirit. See Su Wen chapter 17.

精明之府　出《素问·脉要精微论》。见"头者精明之府"条。

精明之府（jīng míng zhī fǔ）**house of bright essence** See Su Wen chapter 17. See "头者精明之府".

精神　① 指精气与神明。出《素问·生气通天论》。② 指人的生命功能活动。出《灵枢·本藏》。③ 神志，心神。出《素问·徵四失论》。④ 神采。出《素问·解精微论》。

精神（jīng shén）　① Essence qi and spirit. See Su Wen chapter 3. ② Human life activities. See Ling Shu chapter 47. ③ Mind and spirit. See Su Wen chapter 78. ④ Expression. See Su Wen chapter 81.

精脱　精的突然亡失。出《灵枢·决气》。

十四画

精脱（jīng tuō）　**essence collapse** Loss of essence within a short time. See *Ling Shu* chapter 30.

精液　泛指精血津液。出《素问·六元正纪大论》。

精液（jīng yè）　**essence liquid** Refers to essence，blood，fluid and humor. See *Su Wen* chapter 71.

漏　① 流泪不止。出《素问·刺禁论》。② 漏泄。见《素问·刺禁论》。

漏（lòu）　① Unceasing lacrimation. See *Su Wen* chapter 52. ② Leakage. See *Su Wen* chapter 52.

漏风　病名。病起于饮酒后中于风邪。因汗多好漏，故名。出《素问·风论》。

漏风（lòu fēng）　Disease name for leaking wind. A wind syndrome caused by the invasion of wind after drinking because sweat leaks easily，hence the name. See *Su Wen* chapter 42.

漏泄　病证名。指热饮食而过多汗出。由于卫气不能固密腠理，复外伤于风邪，致汗泄如漏。出《灵枢·营卫生会》。

漏泄（lòu xiè）　**leakage** Disease name. Refers to excessive sweating due to eating too much hot-natured food. Because of the ina-bility of defensive qi to consolidate and secure the interstices，together with the contraction of the wind pathogen，sweating like leakage occurs. See *Ling Shu* chapter 18.

漏病　出《素问·著至教论》。① 指大小便不禁。见《新校正》。② 指下出脓血。见《素问》王冰注。

漏病（lòu bìng）　See *Su Wen* chapter 75. ① Refers to faecal and urinary incontinence. See *Xin Jiao Zheng*（*New Revisions of Su Wen*）. ② Genital bleeding with pus. See *Su Wen* annotated by Wang Bing.

瞀　① 昏眩。出《素问·至真要大论》。② 目不明。出《素问·玉机真藏论》。

瞀（mào）　① Dizzy. See *Su Wen* chapter 74. ② Blurred vision. See *Su Wen* chapter 19.

鹜溏　病证名。鹜（wù 务），鸭。鹜溏，形容大便稀溏如鸭便。出《素问·至真要大论》。

鹜溏（wù táng）　**duck-stool diarrhea** Disease name. Refers to loose stools that look like a duck's. See *Su Wen* chapter 74.

缨脉　缨，冠带。缨脉指颈部两侧靠近冠带通过部位的动脉，属足阳明胃经。出《素问·通评虚实论》。

缨脉（yīng mài） **tassel vessel** The arteries on both sides of the neck close to the submandibular space，and which pertain to the stomach meridian of foot *yangming*. See *Su Wen* chapter 28.

缪传 病邪不当传变而传之。出《素问·缪刺论》。

缪传（miù chuán） **wrong transmission** Refers to the incorrect transmission and transmutation of pathogens. See *Su Wen* chapter 63.

缪刺 缪，交错，不同之意。病在左而刺右之大络，病在右而刺左之大络的刺络法，与左取右，右取左，刺其大经的巨刺法不同。出《素问·缪刺论》《素问·汤液醪醴论》。

缪刺（miù cì） **contralateral needling** When the disease is on the left side of the body，and needling occurs on the right collateral，and vice versa. It is different from contralateral meridian needling which considers the meridians rather than the collaterals as the needling position. See *Su Wen* chapter 14 and 63.

缪刺论 《素问》篇名。缪（miù 谬）通谬，交错。缪刺，左病取右，右病取左的一种针刺方法。此篇主要论述了缪刺法的概念及临床应用，提出只有络病而经不病者，才可用缪刺法的原则。故名。

缪刺论（miù cì lùn） **Discussion on Contralateral Needling Therapy** Chapter title in *Su Wen*. "缪" is the same as "谬"，here it means contralateral. Contralateral needling is an acupuncture method which takes the contralateral part to needle. This chapter mainly discusses the concept and clinical application of contralaterally needling，and proposes that it can only be used on those who have collateral disease without meridian disease. Hence the name.

十五画

髯 生于双颊的胡须。出《灵枢·阴阳二十五人》。

髯（rán） **whiskers** Beards growing on both cheeks. See *Ling Shu* chapter 64.

黅天之气 黅（jīn 今），黄色。古代天文学家在心、尾、角、轸诸宿间看到的黄色之气。其中心、尾二宿当东方偏北之甲位，角、轸二宿当东南方己位。《内经》以此说明"天干纪运"的方法，即黄属土，故土运主甲己年。出《素问·五运行大论》。

黅天之气（jīn tiān zhī qì） **the qi of yellow heaven** *Jīn* means yellow. The yellow qi that ancient astronomers saw in the heart mansion, tail mansion, horn mansion, and chariot mansion. The heart mansion and tail mansion are located at the *Jia* position in the northeast, and the horn and chariot mansion are located at the *Ji* position in the southeast. *Nei Jing* (*Internal Classic*) explains the method of using the ten Heavenly Stems to record the motions of the stars, that is, yellow pertains to earth, so the earth motion dominates the year of *Jia* and *Ji*. See *Su Wen* chapter 67.

蕤宾 阳六律之一，为角音，即木音。出《素问·本病论》。

蕤宾（ruí bīn） *rui bin* One of the six yang tonalities in ancient Chinese music, also named *Jue* tone, that is, the tone of wood phase. See *Su Wen* chapter 73.

蕃 蕃，同藩。藩篱之义，指颊后耳门部位。出《灵枢·五色》。

蕃（fān） **fence** Refers to the posterior auricular region of the cheek. See *Ling Shu* chapter 49.

横骨 泛指横置的骨骼。① 枕骨。出《素问·骨空论》。② 舌根部的软骨。出《灵枢·忧恚无言》。③ 耻骨。出《素问·气府论》。④ 锁骨。出《素问·骨空论》。

横骨（héng gǔ） It broadly refers to the horizontally-laid bones. ① Occipital bone. See *Su Wen* chapter 60. ② Cartilage at the base of the tongue. See *Ling Shu* chapter 69. ③ Pubic bone. See

Su Wen chapter 47. ④ Clavicle.
See Su Wen chapter 60.

横脉　横斜而行之经脉、络脉。
出《素问·刺症》。① 足太阴经
在足内踝前斜行而过之脉。见
《素问》王冰注。② 横行之络
脉。见《素问集注》。

横脉（héng mài）　The meridians,
vessels and collaterals running
horizontally or obliquely. See
Su Wen chapter 36. ① The
foot *taiyin* meridian that passes
obliquely in front of the medial
malleolus. See Su Wen annotated by Wang Bing. ② The collaterals running horizontally. See
Su Wen Ji Zhu（Collected Annotation of Su Wen）.

横络　横行之络脉。出《灵枢·
刺节真邪》。

横络（héng luò）　**transverse collateral** The collaterals running
horizontally. See Ling Shu
chapter 75.

颣　通颔。出《灵枢·癫狂》。

颣（hàn）　**chin** "颣" is the same as
"颔". See Ling Shu chapter 22.

瞋目　瞋（chēn 琛），张目。瞋目
指张目不寐。出《灵枢·寒热病》。

瞋目（chēn mù）　**glare** Keep one's
eyes open without sleep. See
Ling Shu chapter 21.

暴注　泄泻如水下注之突发者。

出《素问·至真要大论》。

暴注（bào zhù）　**sudden diarrhea**
Manifested with diarrhea as if
water is pouring down on one-
self. See Su Wen chapter 74.

暴厥　病证名。突然昏厥。见
《素问·大奇论》。

暴厥（bào jué）　**sudden reversal**
Disease name. Sudden fainting.
See Su Wen chapter 48.

暴瘖　病证名。突然失音。出
《灵枢·寒热病》。

暴瘖（bào yīn）　**sudden mute**
Disease name. Sudden loss of
voice. See Ling Shu chapter 21.

踝　① 足踝。小腿下端近足跟处
两侧之骨突起部分。内侧为内
踝，外侧为外踝。出《素问·三
部九候论》。② 手腕后小指侧
突起之高骨。出《灵枢·经脉》。

踝（huái）　① Ankle. Boney pro-
trusions on both sides of the
lower leg near the heel. The
medial side is called the medial
malleolus and the lateral side is
called the lateral malleolus. See
Su Wen chapter 20. ② The high
bone protruding from the side
of the little finger behind the
wrist. See Ling Shu chapter 10.

踝厥　足太阳经循行足踝，该经
经气厥逆而出现种种病候，称
为踝厥。出《灵枢·经脉》。

踝厥（huái jué）　**ankle reversal** The foot meridian of *taiyang* runs along the ankle. Syndromes caused by reversal of ankle qi are called ankle reversal. See *Ling Shu* chapter 10.

骹　剑突下方左右胁肋部分。出《灵枢·本藏》。

骹（jiāo）　**pastern** The left and right lateral thorax under the xiphoid process. See *Ling Shu* chapter 47.

骸　① 泛指骨骼躯体。出《灵枢·天年》。② 骨名。出《素问·骨空论》。（1）胫骨。见《类经·经络十九》。（2）膝骨。见《素问直解》。

骸（hái）　① Refers to the skeleton and body. See *Ling Shu* chapter 54. ② Bone name. See *Su Wen* chapter 60. (1) Tibia. See *Lei Jing* (*Classified Classic*) "Meridians and Collaterals Chapter 19". (2) Kneecap. See *Su Wen Zhi Jie* (*Direct Interpretation on Su Wen*).

骸厌　骸，胫骨。骸厌，指胫骨上端外侧近膝之陷空处，属足少阳经。出《素问·气穴论》。

骸厌（hái yàn）　*hai yan Hái* means tibia. *Hái yàn* refers to the hollow part of the lateral upper tibia near the knee, which per-

tains to the *shaoyang* meridian. See *Su Wen* chapter 58.

骸关　① 膝关节。出《素问·骨空论》。② 指阳关穴。出《素问·骨空论》。

骸关（hái guān）　① Knee joint. See *Su Wen* chapter 60. ② The name of acupoint Yang Guan (GB 33). See *Su Wen* chapter 60.

骱　足胫，俗称小腿。出《素问·脉要精微论》。

骱（héng）　**shank** See *Su Wen* chapter 17.

镇星　土星，为五大行星之一，与五行中的土，五脏中的脾相通应。出《素问·金匮真言论》。

镇星（zhèn xīng）　**saturn** One of the five planets, corresponding to the earth in the five elements and the spleen in the five viscera. See *Su Wen* chapter 4.

僻邪　指邪气。《灵枢·本神》曰："僻邪不至，长生久视。"《素问·六节藏象论》又作"邪僻"，参见该条。

僻邪（pì xié）　**unusual pathogen**. See *Ling Shu* chapter 8. In *Su Wen* chapter 9 it was called "邪僻", see "邪僻" for detail.

德化政令灾变　此以施政时的某些概念，以类比气候变化的不同功用。德化政令，指在五方五气四时气候下生物及人体的正常变化。灾变,为异常情况下的变异灾伤。德,恩惠。指自然气候对生物的恩德。化,万物的生化。政,行施职能,发挥作用。令,时令。灾,灾害。变,变异。出《素问·气交变大论》。

德化政令灾变(dé huà zhèng lìng zāi biàn) **moral, change, governance, season, catastrophe and altering** This is to use some concepts of governance to compare the different effects of climate change. The "moral, change, governance and season" refers to the normal changes of living things and human bodies under the climate of five orientations, five qi and four seasons. Catastrophe refers to a mutation disaster under abnormal conditions. In detail, moral refers to the kindness of nature to creatures. Change refers to the growing and transforming of all things. Governance refers to the executive function. Season and catastrophe refers to the abovementioned meaning. See *Su Wen* chapter 69.

德全不危　言全面掌握养生之道,才不致有衰老的危害。出《素问·上古天真论》。

德全不危(dé quán bú wēi)　so-phistication ensuring health A comprehensive understanding of life nurturing will prevent aging. See *Su Wen* chapter 1.

徵　五音之一。五行属火,为南方夏火之音。运气学说将五音代表五运,以五音建运,则徵(zhǐ纸)为火运。出《素问·阴阳应象大论》。

徵(zhǐ)　*zhi* One of the five tones pertaining to the fire element. It is the tone of summer fire in the south. The theory of the five circuits and six qi uses the five tones to represent the five circuits. Thus, *zhǐ* is fire circuit. See *Su Wen* chapter 5.

徵四失论　《素问》篇名。徵(chéng),同惩,惩戒之意。本篇主要指由于医生精神不专与学业不精而造成诊治的四种过失,提出来惩戒或论证,以引起重视。故名。

徵四失论(chéng sì shī lùn)　**Discussion on the Four Therapeutic Errors** Chapter title in *Su Wen*. This chapter mainly discusses the four kinds of faults in diagnosis and treatment caused by doctors' lack of concentration and incompetence of ability, which are brought forward to focus special attention on. Hence the name.

膝者筋之府　府为聚物之处，筋联络全身骨节，维护人身行动的协调，其中尤以膝胭之筋为最，故称膝为筋之府。如屈伸不利或曲身不能直，附物而行，则为筋坏之兆。出《素问·脉要精微论》。

膝者筋之府（xī zhě jīn zhī fǔ）**Knees are houses of sinews. A house is the place where things get together. Sinews connect the joints of the whole body to maintain the coordination during body movements，of which the sinews of the knee and popliteal area are the most important，thus the knee is called the house of sinews. If one cannot bend and stretch flexibly and needs to hold something to walk，that is a sign of sinew problems. See *Su Wen* chapter 17.

膝解　解，骨缝。指膝之关节缝。出《素问·骨空论》。

膝解（xī jiě）**knee sutura** It refers to the joint gap of the knee. See *Su Wen* chapter 60.

膝膑　膝盖骨。出《素问·刺禁论》。

膝膑（xī bìn）**patella** See *Su Wen* chapter 52.

摩　治法。即按摩。详见该条。见《素问·至真要大论》。

摩（mó）**massage** Treatment method. See "按摩" for detail. See *Su Wen* chapter 74.

瘛　筋脉抽掣。出《素问·玉机真藏论》。

瘛（chì）**convulsive** Convulsive tendon and sinews. See *Su Wen* chapter 19.

瘛疭　抽搐、抽风一类病证。筋脉挛急曰瘛，筋脉弛缓为疭，手足筋脉伸缩抽动不止谓瘛疭。出《素问·诊要经终论》。

瘛疭（chì zòng）**convulsion and spasms** Syndromes of convulsions. The spasm of tendons and sinews is called *chì*. The relaxation of tendons and sinews is called *zòng*. Stretching and twitching of the limbs，tendons and sinews without stopping are called *chì zòng*. See *Su Wen* chapter 16.

瘛挛　筋脉挛急拘缩一类疾病。瘛，同瘛。出《灵枢·邪气藏府病形》。

瘛挛（chì luán）**convulsion and contraction** Diseases of tendons and sinews with convulsions or contractions. See *Ling Shu* chapter 4.

瘨　出《素问·腹中论》。①同癫。见《素问》吴崑注。②同䐜，即腹胀。见《素问识》。③《针灸甲乙经》瘨作疽。

瘨（diān） See *Su Wen* chapter 40. ① Mental disorder. See *Su Wen* annotated by Wu Kun. ② Abdominal fullness. See *Su Wen Zhi* （*Understanding Su Wen*）. ③ Recorded as "疽" in the *Zhen Jiu Jia Yi Jing* （*Classic of Acupuncture and Moxibustion*）.

瘜肉 病证名。在此指附肠而生之肿块。出《灵枢·水胀》。

瘜肉（xī ròu） **polyp** Disease name, or a protruding growth in the intestines. See *Ling Shu* chapter 57.

瘠 体虚而瘦。出《素问·五常政大论》。

瘠（jí） **lean** Thin and weak. See *Su Wen* chapter 70.

颜 额。又称庭。出《灵枢·五色》《素问·刺热》。

颜（yán） **forehead** Also called *Ting*. See *Ling Shu* chapter 49 and *Su Wen* chapter 32.

懊憹 心烦不可名状。出《素问·六元正纪大论》。

懊憹（ào náo） **annoyed** Vexed. See *Su Wen* chapter 71.

憎风 即恶风。出《素问·藏气法时论》。

憎风（zēng fēng） **hating wind** Aversion to wind. See *Su Wen* chapter 22.

谵妄 谵言乱语,妄见幻觉。出《素问·气交变大论》。

谵妄（zhān wàng） **delirium** A mental disturbance characterized by confusion, disordered speech and hallucinations. See *Su Wen* chapter 69.

谵言 病中说胡话。因热盛神明受扰所致。出《素问·热论》。

谵言（zhān yán） **delirious speech** Disordered speech in delirium, due to the bright spirit having been harassed by exuberant heat. See *Su Wen* chapter 31.

谚谙 经穴名。足太阳膀胱经穴名,在肩髆内廉,挟第六椎下两旁各三寸处。出《素问·骨空论》。

谚谙（yì xī） **Yi Xi（BL 45）** An acupoint pertaining to the bladder meridian of foot *tai-yang*, located on the upper back, at the same level as the inferior border of the spinous process of the six thoracic vertebra, 3 *cun* lateral to the posterior median line. See *Su Wen* chapter 60.

十六画

髭 口上胡须。出《灵枢·阴阳二十五人》。

髭（zī） **moustache** Beard on mouth. See *Ling Shu* chapter 64.

颞颥 出《灵枢·热病》。① 颅骨的一部分。即颞骨，又称鬓骨，在头部两侧眉后、耳前部位，太阳穴当其处。见《类经·针刺四十》。② 穴名，为脑空穴之别名，属足少阳胆经，是足少阳与阳维脉的会穴。位于枕部，在风池穴直上，与枕外隆凸上缘相平处。见《类经·针刺四十》。

颞颥（niè niè） See *Ling Shu* chapter 23. ① Tempora. Part of the skull. The temporal bone, located behind the eyebrows on both sides of the head and in front of the ears, next to the acupoint EX-HN5. See *Lei Jing*（*Classified Classic*）"Needling Chapter 40". ② Another name for acupoint GB 19 and the meeting point of the *yangwei* meridian and the gallbladder meridian of foot *shaoyang*. GB 19 is on the head, at the same level as the superior border of the external occipital protuberance, directly superior to GB 20. See *Lei Jing*（*Classified Classic*）"Needling Chapter 40".

薄 治法。出《素问·至真要大论》。① 指挤压、压迫的治疗方法。见《素问集注》。② 指逐渐消去病邪的侵蚀法。见《素问》吴崑注。③ 指搜迫隐蔽之邪。见《类经·论治四》。

薄（bó） Treatment method. See *Su Wen* chapter 74. ① Refers to treatment involving compressing and squeezing. See *Su Wen Ji Zhu*（*Collected Annotation of Su Wen*）. ② Erosion methods that gradually eliminate pathogens. See *Su Wen* annotated by Wu Kun. ③ Refers to hunting for hidden pathogens. See *Lei Jing*（*Classified Classic*）"Chapter 4 Treatment".

薄厥 病名。薄，迫也，厥，突然昏倒不省人事的病证。病由大怒、阳气暴张、气血上迫神明所致，症见昏厥，筋脉弛纵等。见《素问·生气通天论》。

薄厥（bó jué） **flopping syncope**

Disease name of acute characteristic characterized by sudden fainting，caused by great anger and triggering yang qi to overspread and force the qi and blood to distress the spirit. The main symptoms are fainting as well as loose meridians and sinews. See *Su Wen* chapter 3.

颠疾　① 颠通癫。颠疾，属精神异常之病。出《灵枢・颠狂》。② 指癫痫病。出《素问・奇病论》。③ 头顶头部之疾，颠通巅。出《灵枢・邪气藏府病形》。

颠疾（diān jí）　① "颠" is the same as "癫". Refers to a disease that is classified as a mental disorder. See *Ling Shu* chapter 22. ② Malcomitial. See *Su Wen* chapter 47. ③ Diseases at the apex of the head. "颠" is the same as "巅" in ancient Chinese. See *Ling Shu* chapter 4.

橛骨　即尾骶骨，又称穷骨、尻骨。出《素问・骨空论》。

橛骨（jué gǔ）　**coccyx** See *Su Wen* chapter 60.

霍乱　病名。因邪在中焦，吐泻交作，挥霍之间，已致撩乱，病势急暴故名。出《素问・通评虚实论》。

霍乱（huò luàn）　**cholera** Disease name. A disease characterized

by the sudden onset of simultaneous vomiting and diarrhea with the pathogen existing in the middle *jiao*. The progression of the disease is fast，hence the name. See *Su Wen* chapter 28.

踹　小腿肚。

踹（chuài）　**calf** See *Ling Shu* chapter 10.

踵　① 足跟。出《素问・刺腰痛》。② 追随。引申为继承、因袭。出《灵枢・玉版》。

踵（zhǒng）　① Heel. See *Su Wen* chapter 41. ② To follow. Extending into inheritance. See *Ling Shu* chapter 60.

器　① 泛指事物之形。出《素问・六微旨大论》。② 指胃肠等有贮纳作用的脏器。出《素问・六节藏象论》。

器（qì）　① The shape of things. See *Su Wen* chapter 68. ② Viscera and bowels that have the function of storage，such as the stomach and intestine. See *Su Wen* chapter 9.

噫　症状名。俗称嗳气。出《素问・宣明五气》。① 胃气上逆，多见于饱食之后。见《素问集注》。② 气闭郁而叹气。见《素问经注节解》。

噫（yī）　Symptom name，also called eructation. See *Su Wen*

十六画

chapter 23. ① Stomach qi counterflowing or ascending, always seen after meal. See *Su Wen Ji Zhu* (*Collected Annotation of Su Wen*). ② Melancholy sigh caused by blocked qi. See *Su Wen Jing Zhu Jie Jie* (*Annotation and Explanation of Su Wen*).

黔首　先秦时代对百姓的称谓。出《素问·宝命全形论》。

黔首（qián shǒu）　**populace** The name of the common people in the pre-Qin era. See *Su Wen* chapter 25.

赞刺　十二刺法之一。赞，助也。刺入浅而多次刺，是局部多针浅刺出血的针法，用治痈肿、丹毒等症。出《灵枢·官针》。

赞刺（zàn cì）　**repeated shallow needling** One of the twelve needling methods. An ancient needling method characterized by multiple shallow needle insertions causing bleeding. It is mainly used for treating symptoms such as abscesses and erysipelas. See *Ling Shu* chapter 7.

篡　篡（cuàn 窜）。前后阴间的会阴部。出《素问·骨空论》。

篡（cuàn）　**perineum** The perineum of the external genitalia and the anus. See *Su Wen* chapter 60.

鼽　鼻塞流涕。出《素问·金匮真言论》。

鼽（qiú）　**rhinallergosis** Nasal obstruction with a running nose. See *Su Wen* chapter 4.

鼽骨　鼽（qiú 求）通頄，即颧骨。出《素问·气府论》。

鼽骨（qiú gǔ）　**cheekbone** "鼽" is the same as "頄", and refers to the cheekbone. See *Su Wen* chapter 59.

衡络之脉　即带脉。出《素问·刺腰痛》。

衡络之脉（héng luò zhī mài）　**belt vessel** See *Su Wen* chapter 41.

膲理　三焦纹理。膲，通焦。出《灵枢·岁露论》。

膲理（jiāo lǐ）　**texture of the triple *jiao*** "膲" is the same as "焦". See *Ling Shu* chapter 79.

䕌　形容物之下垂貌。此指全身或局部肢体困疲无力，甚则不能举动的病证。系因胃气素弱，诸脉不足，加之强力入房，元气虚而不复所致。出《灵枢·口问》。

䕌（duǒ）　**hanging down** Describes the hanging of objects. It refers to a disease in which the whole body or part of the body is tired and weak，and even unable to move. It is caused by weak stomach qi，insufficient pulse qi，coupled with source qi deficiency due to sexual intercourse.

See *Ling Shu* chapter 28.

瘰疬　病名。为生于颈部或腋下之结核，推之不移，小者为瘰，大者为疬，破溃后不易收口，可形成瘘管，为顽固的外科疾病。出《灵枢·寒热》。

瘰疬（luǒ lì）　**scrofula** Chronic inflammation of the cervical lymph nodes, growing on the neck or oxter. Scrofulas are difficult to bind up after rupture and can form fistulas, which are stubborn surgical diseases. See *Ling Shu* chapter 70.

癃　病证名。小便不利。出《素问·宣明五气》。

癃（lóng）　**difficult urination** Disease name. Difficulty urinating or anuria. See *Su Wen* chapter 23.

癃闭　大小便不通。

癃闭（lóng bì）　**difficult urination and defecation** Difficulty in urination and defecation.

壅骨　拇指本节后的第一掌骨。又称手鱼骨。出《灵枢·邪客》。

壅骨（yōng gǔ）　**styloid process of radius** First metacarpal bone behind the thumb section. Also called the hand's fishbone. See *Ling Shu* chapter 71.

燔针　即火针。用火烧红针尖部而后用之。多用于痹症，痈疡，瘰疬等病。出《素问·调经论》

《灵枢·官针》。

燔针（fán zhēn）　**fire needling** An acupuncture technique involving the swift pricking of diseased parts with a red hot needle, mainly used for diseases such as impediment, abscesses, ulcers, and scrofula. See *Su Wen* chapter 62, and *Ling Shu* chapter 7.

燔针劫刺　进针后以火烧使暖，以此劫散邪气。出《素问·调经论》。

燔针劫刺（fán zhēn jié cì）　**fire needling to eliminate the pathogen** Using fire to warm needles after insertion, which could eliminate pathogens. See *Su Wen* chapter 62.

燔治　用火烧制的药物治疗。出《素问·缪刺论》。

燔治（fán zhì）　**fire treatment** Using flame-treated medicine. See *Su Wen* chapter 63.

颡大　① 头维穴别名，属足阳明胃经，在额角发际，挟本神两旁各一寸五分处。见《灵枢识》。② 指大迎。见《类经·经络三十》。③ 部位名。指颃颡，即上腭与鼻相通的孔窍处。见《灵枢集注》。

颡大（sǎng dà）　① Another name for acupoint Tou Wei (ST 8). ST 8 pertains to the stomach meridian of foot *yangming*. It is in the depression between the midpoint of the inferior border of the zygomatic arch and the mandibular notch. See *Ling Shu Zhi* (*Understanding Ling Shu*). ② Da Ying (ST 5) Acupoint.

See *Lei Jing* (*Classified Classic*) "Meridians and Collaterals Chapter 30". ③ Nasopharynx. The orifice where the palate joins up with the nose. See *Ling Shu Ji Zhu* (*Collected Annotation of Ling Shu*).

十七画

戴眼 双目仰视而固定。为足太阳膀胱经气绝之表现。出《素问·三部九候论》。

戴眼(dài yǎn) **hyperphoria with fixed eyeballs** The manifestation of qi exhaustion in the bladder meridian of foot *taiyang*. See *Su Wen* chapter 20.

藏 ①（cáng）储藏、潜藏。出《素问·五藏别论》《素问·四气调神大论》。② 深，里。出《素问·长刺节论》。③（zàng）指五脏。出《素问·咳论》。④ 五脏六腑内脏之总称。出《素问·灵兰秘典论》。

藏(cáng/zàng) ① Storage. See *Su Wen* chapter 2 and *Su Wen* chapter 11. ② Deep；inner. See *Su Wen* chapter 55. ③ Refers to five viscera. See *Su Wen* chapter 38. ④ General name for the five viscera and six bowels. See *Su Wen* chapter 8.

藏气 ① 五脏之气，出《素问·藏气法时论》。②（藏，cáng）冬令所主闭藏之气，五行属水，故又称水之藏气。出《素问·五常政大论》。

藏气(zàng qì) ① The qi of the five viscera. See *Su Wen* chapter 22. ② The storing qi of the winter，which pertains to the water element，thus also called "the storing qi of water". See *Su Wen* chapter 70.

藏气法时论 《素问》篇名。藏气，五脏之气。法，效法。藏气法时，指五脏之气，相应于天地四时，故治疗疾病时，要效法天地四时的变化规律。此篇根据五行的生克规律，阐述了五脏病证发展变化的一般规律，强调五脏之气与四时的关系，提出了法时而治的原则。故名。

藏气法时论(zàng qì fǎ shí lùn) **Discussion on the Association of the Zang Qi with the Four Seasons** Chapter title in *Su Wen*. The qi of the five viscera corresponds to the four seasons. Therefore，when treating diseases，it is necessary to follow the rule of the four seasons in nature. This chapter explains the general rule of the development and transformation of the five viscera syndromes based on the interrelationship of the five elements，emphasizes the relationship between the five viscera's qi and the four seasons，and proposes the principle of treatment according to the season. Hence the name.

藏化　寒化。寒主闭藏故尔。出《素问·六元正纪大论》《素问·至真要大论》。

藏化（cáng huà）　**storage transformation** Transforming into cold. Cold means to close and store. See *Su Wen* chapter 71 and 74.

藏会　指背部俞穴，是脏气聚会之处。出《素问·长刺节论》。

藏会（zàng huì）　**viscera meeting** Refers to the transport acupoints，where the viscera qi meets. See *Su Wen* chapter 55.

藏府　即脏腑。总指人体的内脏组织器官，包括五藏、六府、奇恒之府等。见《素问·金匮真言论》《灵枢·邪气藏府病形》。

藏府（zàng fǔ）　**viscera and bowels** Refers to the internal organs of the human body，including the five viscera，six bowels and extraordinary organs. See *Su Wen* chapter 4 and *Ling Shu* chapter 4.

藏府之风　为五脏六腑风证之统称。由五脏所主之时中于风邪，或风邪侵袭五脏六腑的俞穴，循经入里所致。出《素问·风论》。

藏府之风（zàng fǔ zhī fēng）　**wind of the viscera and bowels** The general name for wind syndromes in the five viscera and six bowels，which is caused by seasonal wind pathogens of that which the viscera corresponds，or by wind pathogens invading the transport acupoints of the viscera and bowels and entering the interior along the meridians. See *Su Wen* chapter 42.

藏政　指以封藏为特点的气候、物候现象布行。政，施政。出《素问·五常政大论》。

藏政（cáng zhèng）　**storing governance** *Cáng* refers to the distribution of climate and phenological phenomena characterized by storing. *Zhèng* means governance. See *Su Wen* chapter 70.

藏俞　俞，指井、荥、俞、经、合五腧穴。五脏之五腧穴谓藏俞，左右共五十穴。出《素问·气穴论》。

藏俞（zàng shū）　**viscera transport acupoints** Refers to the five transport acupoints including the well points，brook points，stream points，river points and sea points. The five transport acupoints of the five viscera are called viscera transport acu-points，with a total of 50 acu-points on the left and right. See *Su Wen* chapter 58.

藏俞五十穴　五脏各有五腧穴，左右相合，计五十穴。出《素问·气穴论》(见表 4)。

表4　藏俞五十穴

脏＼俞	井(木)	荥(火)	俞(土)	经(舍)	合(水)
肝	大敦	行间	太冲	中封	曲泉
心	少冲	少府	神门	灵道	少海
脾	隐白	大都	太白	商丘	阴陵泉
肺	少商	鱼际	太渊	经渠	尺泽
肾	涌泉	然谷	太溪	复溜	阴谷

藏俞五十穴 (zàng shū wǔ shí xué) **fifty transport acupoints of the five viscera** Each viscera has five transport acupoints which are divided into left and right parts，totaling 50 acu-points. See *Su Wen* chapter 58 (See Table 4).

Table 4　Fifty Transport Acupoints of the Five Viscera

Viscera ＼ transport acu-points	well (wood)	brook (fire)	stream (earth)	river (metal)	sea (water)
Liver	Da Dun (LR 1)	Xing Jian (LR 2)	Tai Chong (LR 3)	Zhong Feng (LR 4)	Qu Quan (LR 8)
Heart	Shao Chong (HT 9)	Shao Fu (HT 8)	Shen Men (HT 7)	Ling Dao (HT 4)	Shao Hai (HT 3)
Spleen	Yin Bai (SP 1)	Da Du (SP 2)	Tai Bai (SP 3)	Shang Qiu (SP 5)	Yin Ling Quan (SP 9)

续　表

transport acupoints / Viscera	well (wood)	brook (fire)	stream (earth)	river (metal)	sea (water)
Lung	Shao Shang (LU 11)	Yu Ji (LU 10)	Tai Yuan (LU 9)	Jing Qu (LU 8)	Chi Ze (LU 5)
Kidney	Yong Quan (KI 1)	Ran Gu (KI 2)	Tai Xi (KI 3)	Fu Liu (KI 7)	Yin Gu (KI 10)

藏脉　手足三阴三阳脏腑之经脉。出《素问·热论》。

藏脉(cáng mài)　**viscera vessel** Hand and foot triple yin meridians and vessels. See *Su Wen* chapter 31.

藏度　藏,泛指脏腑等内脏。度,度数。指内脏的长短大小度数。出《素问·方盛衰论》。

藏度(zàng dù)　**viscera measure** The measurement of length of the internal organs. See *Su Wen* chapter 80.

藏真　五脏所藏之真气,以胃气为代表。出《素问·平人气象论》。

藏真(zàng zhēn)　**viscera genuineness** Genuine qi stored in the five viscera, which is represented by stomach qi. See *Su Wen* chapter 18.

藏虚　指内脏虚。出《素问·八正神明论》。

藏虚(zàng xū)　**visceral deficiency** See *Su Wen* chapter 26.

藏象　藏,指藏于体内,具有一定

形态的脏腑器官。象,指脏腑机能表现于外的各种征象。出《素问·六节藏象论》。

藏象(zàng xiàng)　**visceral manifestation** *Zàng* refers to the viscera and bowels that are stored in the body and have a certain form. *Xiàng* refers to various manifestations in which visceral functions are manifested externally. See *Su Wen* chapter 9.

藏寒生满病　因内脏受寒,寒伤阳气,失于温运而生胀满一类病变。出《素问·异法方宜论》。

藏寒生满病(zàng hán shēng mǎn bìng)　**Cold viscera and bowels cause fullness disease.** Diseases such as distension and fullness are caused by internal viscera and bowels suffering from cold pathogens, where cold pathogens hurt yang qi, and then the viscera and bowels lose the function of warming and transporting. See *Su Wen* chapter 12.

藏腧　脏腑在背部的腧穴。出《灵枢·官针》。

藏腧（zàng shū）　**visceral transport acupoint** Acupoints on the back of the body where the qi of the viscera is infused. See *Ling Shu* chapter 7.

翳　障蔽之谓。此指目疾所引起的障膜。出《素问·本病论》。

翳（yì）　**corneal opacity** Cloudy opacity of the cornea caused by eye disease. See *Su Wen* chapter 73.

龋　蛀牙。出《素问·缪刺论》。

龋（qǔ）　**cavities** See *Su Wen* chapter 63.

龋齿　病名。牙齿蛀蚀，时时疼痛。出《灵枢·论疾诊尺》。

龋齿（qǔ chǐ）　**dental cavities** Disease name. Refers to the decay of teeth with frequent pain. See *Ling Shu* chapter 74.

瞳子　即瞳孔，又称瞳神、眸子。为目中黑睛中央之圆孔，随光线的变化而展缩，属肾。出《灵枢·大惑论》。

瞳子（tóng zǐ）　**pupil** The opening at the center of the iris, which shrinks and stretches with the change of light and pertains to the kidney. See *Ling Shu* chapter 80.

嚏　喷嚏。为机体驱邪外出的生理反射。出《灵枢·口问》《素问·宣明五气》。

嚏（tì）　**sneezing** Physiological reaction when the body eliminates pathogenic factors. See *Ling Shu* chapter 28 and *Su Wen* chapter 23.

髁　即髁骨，又名髋骨。出《素问·刺腰痛》。

髁（kē）　**innominate bone** It refers to the hipbone. See *Su Wen* chapter 50.

髁骨　即髋骨。出《素问·刺腰痛》。

髁骨（kē gǔ）　**hipbone** See *Su Wen* chapter 41.

髀　股部，即大腿部。出《灵枢·骨度》。

髀（bì）　**the upper half of the thigh** Huckle. See *Ling Shu* chapter 14.

髀厌　髋关节部位，即髀枢之中。其中有环跳穴。出《素问·气穴论》。

髀厌（bì yàn）　**hip region** Refers to the region of the greater trochanter. *Huan Tiao*（GB 30）is located in this region. See *Su Wen* chapter 58.

髀阳　大腿、股部外侧。出《灵枢·经脉》。

髀阳（bì yáng）　**thigh yang** lateral thigh. See *Ling Shu* chapter 10.

髀枢　髀（bì 婢），大腿；枢，枢机、

转轴。指股骨头与髋臼构成的髋关节。出《灵枢·经脉》。

髀枢(bì shū) **thigh pivot** Refers to the hip joint formed by the femoral head and acetabulum. See *Ling Shu* chapter 10.

髀骨 大腿骨、股骨。出《素问·骨空论》。

髀骨(bì gǔ) **femur** Femur. See *Su Wen* chapter 60.

膻中 ① 胸中,宗气积聚之处。出《灵枢·海论》。② 心包络。出《素问·灵兰秘典论》《灵枢·胀论》。③ 穴位名。在两乳间正中部,属任脉。出《灵枢·根结》。

膻中(dàn zhōng) ① Center of the chest，where the ancestral qi accumulates. See *Ling Shu* chapter 33. ② Pericardium. See *Su Wen* chapter 8, and *Ling Shu* chapter 35. ③ The name of acupoint Dan Zhong (CV 17). CV 17 is located between the two breasts and pertains to the conception vessel. See *Ling Shu* chapter 5.

膺 胸前两侧肌肉隆起处。出《灵枢·经别》。

膺(yīng) **pectoral muscle** Inflating muscles on both sides of the chest. See *Ling Shu* chapter 11.

膺中 ① 胸中。出《素问·气府论》。② 胸之中央一行,为任脉

经过之部位。出《素问·气府论》。

膺中(yīng zhōng) ① Center of the chest. See *Su Wen* chapter 59. ② The central line of the chest where the conception vessel passes. See *Su Wen* chapter 59.

膺中外俞 胸膺部之俞穴,指云门、中府二穴。出《灵枢·五邪》。

膺中外俞(yīng zhōng wài shū) **acupoints on the chest** Refers to acupoint Zhong Fu (LU 1) and Yun Men (LU 2). See *Ling Shu* chapter 20.

膺俞 ① 即中府穴,在胸外上方,平第一肋间隙,胸正中线旁开六寸处。或于云门下一寸,乳上三肋间陷者中。见《素问·水热穴论》。② 泛指胸膺部的俞穴,左右共十二穴。见《素问·气穴论》。参"膺俞十二穴"条。

膺俞(yīng shū) ① Zhong Fu (LU 1) located on the anterior thoracic region，at the same level as the first intercostal space，lateral to the infraclavicular fossa，6 *cun* lateral to the anterior median line. See *Su Wen* chapter 61. ② Generally refers to the chest acupoints，with a total of 12 acupoints on the left and right. See *Su Wen* chapter 58. See "膺俞十二穴".

膺俞十二穴 胸膺部的十二个俞

穴。出《素问·气穴论》。

膺俞十二穴（yīng shū shí èr xué）
twelve acupoints on the chest
See *Su Wen* chapter 58.

麋衔　药名。一名薇衔。味苦平，微寒，主治风湿。与泽泻、白术合方治疗饮酒中风者。出《素问·病能论》。

麋衔（mí xián）　**herba pyrolae**
Medicine name of which the flavor is warm and bitter, and is slightly cold in nature. It is mainly used to treat wind-dampness, and also combined with Rhizoma Alismatis and Rhizoma Atractylodis Macro-cephalae to treat wind strokes caused by inebriation. See *Su Wen* chapter 46.

燥　①正常的气候。为六气之一，是秋季所主的气候，五行属金。出《素问·阴阳应象大论》。②病因。燥邪为六淫之一。出《素问·至真要大论》。③伤津耗液的病证。可见口干、鼻燥、唇焦、便结等。出《素问·阴阳应象大论》《素问·至真要大论》。④有燥湿作用的治法。出《素问·至真要大论》。⑤运气概念中六气之一。出《素问·天元纪大论》。

燥（zào）　① Normal climate. One of the six qi, in which the climate is dominated by autumn, and pertains to the metal element. See *Su Wen* chapter 5. ② Cause of disease. Dryness as one of the six excesses. See *Su Wen* chapter 74. ③ Syndromes which damage fluid, and of which the main symptoms are dry mouth, dry nose, parched lips and constipation. See *Su Wen* chapter 5 and 74. ④ Drying dampness treatment. See *Su Wen* chapter 74. ⑤ One of the six qi in the theory of five movements and six qi. See *Su Wen* chapter 66.

燥气　六气之一，为秋季所主的气候，五行属金。出《素问·天元纪大论》。

燥气（zào qì）　**dryness qi** One of the six qi which is dominated by autumn and pertains to the metal phase. See *Su Wen* chapter 66.

燥化　①运气学说中，当阳明燥金当令时，气候干燥。出《素问·至真要大论》。②用性燥的药物法除湿邪。出《素问·六元正纪大论》。

燥化（zào huà）　① In the theory of five circuits and six qi, when *yangming* dryness metal dominates, the climate is characterized by dryness. See *Su Wen* chapter 74. ② Eliminating dampness with dry-flavored medicine. See *Su Wen* chapter 71.

燥者润之　治法。凡病气干燥的,应用润泽的方法治疗。出《素问·至真要大论》。

燥者润之(zào zhě rùn zhī)　**to moisten dryness** Treatment which uses the moistening method to treat diseases with dryness pathogens. See *Su Wen* chapter 74.

燥者濡之　言津液不足一类干燥病症,如口渴,皮肤皲裂,大便干燥等,应用滋阴生津法治疗。出《素问·至真要大论》。

燥者濡之(zào zhě rú zhī)　**to smoothen dryness** Diseases of dryness with insufficient fluid and humor, such as thirst, chapped skin and dry stools, should be treated by nourishing yin and engendering fluid. See *Su Wen* chapter 74.

燥毒　暴烈的燥气。出《素问·五常政大论》。

燥毒(zào dú)　**dryness toxicity** Violent dryness qi. See *Su Wen* chapter 70.

燥政　干燥的气候流行。政,施政。出《素问·五常政大论》。

燥政(zào zhèng)　**climate of dryness** A dry climate. *Zhèng*

means dominating. See *Su Wen* chapter 70.

燥胜则干　燥气胜则内外津液干涸,出现口干、舌少津,皮肤干燥等津液亏损的临床表现。见《素问·阴阳应象大论》《素问·六元正纪大论》。

燥胜则干(zào shèng zé gàn)　**domination of dryness brings about deficiency of fluid** If dryness prevails, the internal and external body fluids will dry up, resulting in clinical manifestations of body fluid loss such as a dry mouth, a tongue with less fluid, dry skin, etc. See *Su Wen* chapter 5 and 71.

燥胜寒　燥从热生,故胜寒。临床上寒犯经络成痹,每用温燥之品散寒除痹。出《素问·阴阳应象大论》《素问·五运行大论》。

燥胜寒(zào shèng hán)　**dryness overcomes cold** Dryness arises from heat, thus restraining the cold. Clinically, cold invading the meridians and collaterals will cause impediment diseases, thus warm and dry medicine should be used to dissipate cold and eliminate impediment. See *Su Wen* chapter 5 and 67.

燥淫　偏盛的燥气,即燥邪。出《素问·至真要大论》。

燥淫（zào yín）　**dryness excess** Excessive dryness pathogens. See *Su Wen* chapter 74.

濡泄　病证名。泄泻如水，多因湿盛所致。又名濡泻。出《素问·六元正纪大论》。

濡泄（rú xiè）　**watery diarrhea** Disease name，in which the diarrhea is like water，and is mostly caused by excessive dampness. See *Su Wen* chapter 71.

濡泻　濡，湿。濡泻，湿胜而大便水泻。出《素问·阴阳应象大论》。

濡泻（rú xiè）　**watery diarrhea** Dampness prevails and the stools are watery. See *Su Wen* chapter 5.

蹇膝　蹇（jiǎn 简），涩滞不滑利之谓。蹇膝，言膝关节伸屈不利。出《素问·骨空论》。

蹇膝（jiǎn xī）　**lameness knee** *Jiǎn* means difficulty in movement. *Xī* means knee. *Jiǎn xī* means difficulty in extension and flexion of the knee joint. See *Su Wen* chapter 60.

臂　① 从肩到腕的部分，俗称胳膊。出《灵枢·五色》。② 疑"贲"之误。出《灵枢·经筋》。

臂（bì）　① The body part from the shoulder to the wrist，commonly known as the arm. See *Ling Shu* chapter 49. ② It is suspected that"贲"was mistakenly written as"臂". See *Ling Shu* chapter 13.

臂骨　臂肘下的桡骨和尺骨。出《灵枢·经脉》。

臂骨（bì gǔ）　**bone of arm** The radius and ulna under the elbow. See *Ling Shu* chapter 10.

臂厥　手太阴、手少阴均循行下臂，两经经气厥逆发生种种病候，称为臂厥。见《灵枢·经脉》。心手少阴之脉是动则病嗌干心痛，渴而欲饮，是为臂厥。

臂厥（bì jué）　**arm reversal** Meridians of hand *taiyin* and hand *shaoyin* both follow the lower arm，and diseases caused by qi reversal in both meridians are called arm reversal. See *Ling Shu* chapter 10.

十七画

十八画

醪药　即药酒，又称醪酒。见《素问·血气形志》。

醪药（láo yào）　**medicinal liquor** See *Su Wen* chapter 24.

醪酒　药酒，又称醪药。古人用以治病之深重者。出《素问·玉版论要》。

醪酒（láo jiǔ）　**medicinal liquor** The ancient people used it to cure severe diseases. See *Su Wen* chapter 15.

醪醴　五谷制成的甘浊之酒，古人用以治病。醪为浊酒，醴为甜酒。出《素问·汤液醪醴论》。

醪醴（láo lǐ）　**sweet and unstrained liquor** Liquor made from five cereals and used by ancient people to cure diseases. *Láo* means unstrained liquor，li means sweet liquor. See *Su Wen* chapter 14.

蹠跛　蹠（zhí 职），足不能行。破（bǒ 匡），一足偏废。出《素问·通评虚实论》。

蹠跛（zhí bǒ）　**lame** *Zhí* means the feet cannot walk. *Bǒ* means one foot losing its function. See *Su Wen* chapter 28.

髃　即髃骨，参该条。出《灵枢·经筋》。

髃（yú）　**acromion scapulae** See term "髃骨" for detail. See *Ling Shu* chapter 13.

髃骨　① 锁骨与肩胛冈之结合部，又称肩端骨，相当于肩髃（yú 娱）穴部位。出《素问·气府论》。② 穴位名。即肩髃穴，属手阳明大肠经。出《素问·水热穴论》。

髃骨（yú gǔ）　① The junction of the clavicle and the shoulder blade，equivalent to the area of acupoint Jian Yu（LI 15）. See *Su Wen* chapter 59. ② The name of acupoint Jian Yu（LI 15）pertaining to the large intestine meridian of hand *yangming*. See *Su Wen* chapter 61.

髃骨之会　即肩髃穴，在锁骨肩峰端与肱骨大结节之间。出《素问·气府论》。

髃骨之会（yú gǔ zhī huì）　**meeting of acromion scapulae** Refers to Jian Yu（LI 15）acupoint located between the acromion at the end of the clavicle and the greater tuberosity humerus. See *Su Wen* chapter 59.

髃骬 胸骨剑突部，又名鸠尾。出《灵枢·骨度》。

髃骬（hé yú） **sternal xiphoid process** Also called dovetail. See *Ling Shu* chapter 14.

髂 即髂骨。出《素问·长刺节论》。

髂（qià） **ilium** See *Su Wen* chapter 55.

髂髎 指髂骨两侧的居髎穴。属足少阳胆经，在章门下八寸三分，监骨上陷者中。出《素问·长刺节论》。

髂髎（qià liáo） **Qia Liao（GB 29）** Pertaining to the gallbladder meridian of foot *shaoyang* and located at the indentation above the ilium, 8.3 *cun* below Zhang

Men（LR 13）. See *Su Wen* chapter 55.

癩疝 病名。指睾丸肿胀，不痛不痒之症。一作㿉疝、㿗疝。见《素问·脉解》。

癩疝（tuí shàn） **swelling of the scrotum** Disease name. Refers to scrotum swelling with no symptoms of pain and itching. See *Su Wen* chapter 49.

癩癃疝 包括两种病证：癩疝，即阴器肿胀。癃，小便不能。出《素问·脉解》。

癩癃疝（tuí lóng shàn） **swelling of the scrotum and dysuria caused by hernia** Includes two diseases: swelling of the scrotum and difficult urination. See *Su Wen* chapter 49.

十八画

十九画

巅 ① 部位名。头顶部。出《素问·骨空论》。② 病名。巅、癫通,即癫痫。出《素问·奇病论》。③ 指头部。出《素问·方盛衰论》。

巅(diān) ① Area at the top of the head. See *Su Wen* chapter 60. ② Disease name,"巅" is the same as "癫", known as epilepsy. See *Su Wen* chapter 47. ③ Refers to the head. See *Su Wen* chapter 80.

巅疾 ① 头部疾患。出《素问·方盛衰论》。② 癫痫。出《素问·奇病论》。③ 癫狂病。出《素问·阴阳类论》。

巅疾(diān jí) ① Diseases of the head. See *Su Wen* chapter 80. ② Epilepsy. See *Su Wen* chapter 47. ③ Depressive psychosis. See *Su Wen* chapter 79.

髆 通膊。膀子,上臂靠近肩的部分。出《素问·骨空论》。

髆(bó) **upper limb** "髆" is the same as "膊". The part of the upper limb near the shoulder. See *Su Wen* chapter 60.

髋 髋骨。髀上的大骨,连接两股之端。俗称胯骨。出《素问·骨空论》。

髋(kuān) **innominate bone** The large bone at the upper area of the thigh connects the ends of two sections. Commonly known as the hipbone. See *Su Wen* chapter 60.

二十画

躁 ① 指脉象。脉率数急，一息六至。多见于温热病中。出《素问·平人气象论》。② 躁动不安的症状。出《素问·痹论》《素问·至真要大论》。③ 动。出《素问·阴阳应象大论》。

躁（zào） ① An agitated pulse, which is one that feels rapid and rushing, and comes six times within one breath, usually indicating warm diseases. See *Su Wen* chapter 18. ② Symptoms of restlessness. See *Su Wen* chapter 43 and 74. ③ Movement. See *Su Wen* chapter 5.

躁悸 躁扰心悸。出《素问·气交变大论》。

躁悸（zào jì） **agitated palpitations** Palpitations caused by agitation. See *Su Wen* chapter 69.

衊 出《素问·气厥论》。① 汗孔出血。见《圣济总录》。② 血污。见《素问直解》。

衊（miè） See *Su Wen chapter* 37. ① Hemorrhage coming from the sweat pores. *Sheng Ji Zong Lu*（*Comprehensive Recording of Sage-like Benefit*）. ② Bloodiness. See *Su Wen Zhi Jie*（*Direct Interpretation on Su Wen*）.

灌汗 见《素问·脉要精微论》。① 汗出灌以冷水，致汗郁皮腠。② 形容汗多之状。

灌汗（guàn hàn） See *Su Wen* chapter 17. ① Cold water being poured on the skin when one is sweating causes the sweat to stagnate in the skin interstices. ② Polyhidrosis.

二十一画

髓　奇恒之府之一。由水谷精微及肾精化合而成的膏状物质，注于骨腔，集于脑，有充骨补脑的作用。髓生于肾，与肾关系密切。出《素问·阴阳应象大论》《素问·脉要精微论》《灵枢·海论》《灵枢·五癃津液别》。

髓（suǐ）　**marrow** One of the extraordinary organs，it is a creamy substance formed by the combination of water and grain's essence and kidney essence，existing in the bone cavities and converging in the brain. Marrow is born in the kidney and has the function of nourishing the bones and the brain. It is closely related to the kidney. See *Su Wen* chapter 5 and 17；*Ling Shu* chapter 33 and 36.

髓之府　出《素问·脉要精微论》。见"骨者髓之府"条。

髓之府（suǐ zhī fǔ）　**house of marrow** See *Su Wen* chapter 17. See "骨者髓之府".

髓孔　即骨空、骨孔。出《素问·骨空论》。参"骨空"条。

髓孔（suǐ kǒng）　**bone interval** See *Su Wen* chapter 60. See "骨空".

髓生肝　五脏相生肾生肝之意。出《素问·阴阳应象大论》。

髓生肝（suǐ shēng gān）　**marrow engendering the liver** The kidney engenders the liver，while marrow pertains to the kidney，hence to say marrow engenders the liver. See *Su Wen* chapter 5.

髓空　① 经穴名。指腰俞穴。属督脉经，在第二十一椎下间。出《素问·水热穴论》。② 经穴名。指风府穴。属督脉经，在项后正中线，后发际一寸处。出《素问·骨空论》。

髓空（suǐ kōng）　① An acupoint name，Yao Shu（DU 2）. It pertains to the governor vessel，and is located below the 21st intervertebral space. See *Su Wen* chapter 61. ② An acupoint name，Feng Fu（DU 16）. It pertains to the governor vessel，and is located at the midline posterior to the neck，1 *cun* from the posterior hairline. See

Su Wen chapter 60.

髓海　四海之一，即脑，为髓所汇聚之所。出《灵枢·海论》《素问·五藏生成》。

髓海（suǐ hǎi）　**sea of marrow** One of the four seas. Refers to the brain，where marrow converges. See *Ling Shu* chapter 33，*Su Wen* chapter 10.

癫狂　《灵枢》篇名。癫，癫疾，包括癫证和痫证；狂，狂证。此篇重点讨论了癫狂病的病因、症状和治疗方法。故名。

癫狂（diān kuáng）　**Mania** Chapter title in *Ling Shu*. *Dian* means *dian* disease，including depressive psychosis and epilepsy. *Kuang* means manic psychosis. This chapter focuses on the causes，symptoms and treatment methods of these kinds of diseases. Hence the name.

癫病　指癫痫。出《素问·长刺节论》。

癫病（diān bìng）　**mania disease** Refers to epilepsy. See *Su Wen* chapter 55.

癫疾　即癫痫。是一种发作性神志异常的病变。出《灵枢·癫狂》。

癫疾（diān jí）　**epilepsy** A paroxysmal disease with symptoms of abnormal consciousness. See *Ling Shu* chapter 22.

蠡沟　经穴名。属足厥阴肝经。在小腿前内侧，足内踝上五寸。出《灵枢·经脉》。

蠡沟（lí gōu）　**Li Gou（LR 5）** LR 5 pertains to the liver meridian of foot *jueyin*，and is located on the medial anterior leg，five inches above the medial malleolus. See *Ling Shu* chapter 10.

二十一画

二十二画

囊纵　囊，指阴囊。纵，松弛。厥阴病解后，阴囊由收缩渐趋松弛。出《素问·热论》。

囊纵（náng zòng）　**scrotum laxity** After yin reversal disease is cured, the scrotum gradually relaxes from contraction. See *Ling Shu* chapter 31.

囊缩　阴囊上缩。为厥阴肝经受邪所致。出《素问·热论》。

囊缩（náng suō）　**shrinkage of the scrotum** Shrinkage of the scrotum, caused by pathogens invading the liver meridian of foot *jueyin*. See *Su Wen* chapter 31.

镵石　古代的石制针具，作外治用。出《素问·汤液醪醴论》《素问·宝命全形论》。

镵石（chán shí）　**chisel stone** Ancient stone needles, which were used for external treatment. See *Su Wen* chapter 14 and 25.

镵针　九针之一。长一寸六分，针头大，针尖锐利如箭头，用于浅刺，以泻肌表阳热。出《灵枢·九针十二原》。

镵针（chán zhēn）　**chisel needle** One of the nine classical needles. It is 1.6 *cun* long, with a large needle which is shaped like a sharp arrow. It is used for shallow needling to purge yang heat on the body surface and muscles. See *Ling Shu* chapter 1.

二十三画

颧　指眼外下方有骨隆起的部位。出《灵枢·五色》。

颧（quán）　**cheek** Refers to the part below the eye with bone protuberance. See *Ling Shu* chapter 49.

颧骨　眼眶外下方之高骨，左右各一。出《素问·刺热》。

颧骨（quán gǔ）　**cheek bone** The high bone below the orbit has one on each side. See *Su Wen* chapter 32.

参 考 书 目

［1］王庆其,陈晓.实用内经词句辞典［M］.上海：上海科学技术出版社,2017.

［2］李照国,刘希茹.黄帝内经素问：汉英对照［M］.西安：世界图书出版公司西安公司,2005.

［3］李照国,刘希茹.黄帝内经灵枢：汉英对照［M］.西安：世界图书出版公司西安公司,2008.

［4］Paul U. Unschuld. *Huang Di Nei Jing Ling Shu: The Ancient Classic on Needle Therapy The complete Chinese text with an annotated English translation*［M］. Berkeley, Los Angeles, London：University of California Press. 2016.

［5］Paul U. Unschuld. *Huang Di Nei Jing Su Wen: nature, knowledge, imagery in an ancient Chinese medical text, with an appendix, the doctrine of the five periods and six qi in the Huang Di Nei Jing Su Wen*［M］. Berkeley, Los Angeles, London：University of California Press. 2011.

［6］李照国.简明汉英黄帝内经词典［M］.北京：人民卫生出版社,2011.

［7］世界卫生组织（西太平洋地区）,北京大学第一医院中西医结合研究所.WHO西太平洋地区传统医学名词术语国际标准［M］.北京：北京大学医学出版社,2009.

［8］世界中医学会联合会.中医基本名词术语中英对照国际标准［M］.北京：人民卫生出版社,1999.

［9］左言富.新世纪汉英中医辞典［M］.北京：人民军医出版社,2004.

附　　录

附录1　《素问》篇目索引

Su Wen（Simple Conversation）

- 上古天真论篇第一

Chapter 1　Shanggu Tianzhen Lunpian：Theory on Ancient Ideas on How to Preserve Natural Healthy Energy

- 四气调神大论篇第二

Chapter 2　Siqi Tiaoshen Dalunpian：Major Discussion of Regulation of Spirit According to the Changes of the Four Seasons

- 生气通天论篇第三

Chapter 3　Shengqi Tongtian Lunpian：Discussion on the Interrelationship Between Life and Nature

- 金匮真言论篇第四

Chapter 4　Jingui Zhenyan Lunpian：Discussion on the Important Ideas in the Golden Chamber

- 阴阳应象大论篇第五

Chapter 5　Yinyang Yingxiang Dalunpian：Major Discussion on the Theory of Yin and Yang and the Corresponding Relationships Among all the Things in Nature

- 阴阳离合论篇第六

Chapter 6　Yinyang Lihe Lunpian：Separation and Combination of Yin and Yang

- 阴阳别论篇第七

Chapter 7　Yinyang Bie Lunpian：Separate Discussion on Yin and Yang

● 灵兰秘典论篇第八

Chapter 8　Linglan Midian Lunpian：Discussion on the Secret Cannons Stored in Royal Library

● 六节藏象论篇第九

Chapter 9　Liujie Zangxiang Lunpian：Discussion on the Six-six System and the Manifestations in the Viscera

● 五藏生成篇第十

Chapter 10　Wuzang Shengchengpian：Discussion on Various Relationships Concerning the Five Viscera

● 五藏别论篇第十一

Chapter 11　Wuzang Bielunpian：Different Discussion on the Five Viscera

● 异法方宜论篇第十二

Chapter 12　Yifa Fangyi Lunpian：Discussion on Different Therapeutic Methods for Different Diseases

● 移精变气论篇第十三

Chapter 13　Yijing Bianqi Lunpian：Discussion on Shifting the Essence and Changing the Qi

● 汤液醪醴论篇第十四

Chapter 14　Tangye Laoli Lunpian：Discourse on Decoctions and Wines

● 玉版论要篇第十五

Chapter 15　Yuban Lunyao Pian：Discussion on the Jade Inscription

● 诊要经终论篇第十六

Chapter 16　Zhenyao Jingzhong Lunpian：Discussion on the Essentials of Diagnosis and the Exhaustion of the Twelve Meridians

● 脉要精微论篇第十七

Chapter 17　Maiyao Jingwei Lunpian：Discussion on the Essentials of Pulse

● 平人气象论篇第十八

Chapter 18　Pingren Qixiang Lunpian：Discussion on the Pulse Conditions of Healthy People

● 玉机真藏论篇第十九

Chapter 19　Yuji Zhenzang Lunpian：Discussion on Genuine-Zang Pulses

● 三部九候论篇第二十

Chapter 20　Sanbu Jiuhou Lunpian：Discussion on the Three Sections and Nine Indicators

● 经脉别论篇第二十一

Chapter 21　Jingmai Bielunpian：Special Discussion on Channels and Vessels

● 藏气法时论篇第二十二

Chapter 22　Zangqi Fashi Lunpian：Discussion on the Association of the Zang Qi with the Four Seasons

● 宣明五气篇第二十三

Chapter 23　Xuanming Wuqipian：Discussion on the Elucidation of Five Qi

● 血气形志篇第二十四

Chapter 24　Xueqi Xingzhipian：Blood，Qi，Physique and Emotion

● 宝命全形论篇第二十五

Chapter 25　Baoming Quanxing Lunpian：Discussion on Preserving Health and Protecting Life

● 八正神明论篇第二十六

Chapter 26　Bazheng Shenming Lunpian：The Theory of Spirit Brilliance in the Eight Directions

● 离合真邪论篇第二十七

Chapter 27　Lihe Zhenxie Lunpian：Discussion on the Separation and Combination of Zhen Qi（Genuine Qi）and Xie Qi（Pathogen Qi）

● 通评虚实论篇第二十八

Chapter 28　Tongping Xushi Lunpian：General Discussion on Xu（Deficiency）and Shi（Excess）

● 太阴阳明论篇第二十九

Chapter 29　Taiyin Yangming Lunpian：Discussion on *Taiyin* and *Yangming*

● 阳明脉解篇第三十

Chapter 30　Yangming Maijie Pian：Explanation of the *Yangming* Meridian

● 热论篇第三十一

Chapter 31　Relun Pian：Discussion on Heat

● 刺热篇第三十二

Chapter 32　Cire Pian：Discussion on Acupuncture Treatment of Febrile Diseases

● 评热病论篇第三十三

Chapter 33　Ping Rebing Lunpian：Comments on Febrile Diseases

● 逆调论篇第三十四

Chapter 34　Nitiao Lunpian：Discussion on Disharmony

● 疟论篇第三十五

Chapter 35　Nùelun Pian：Discourse on Malaria

● 刺疟篇第三十六

Chapter 36　Cinùe Pian：Discussion on Treatment of Malaria by Acupuncture

● 气厥论篇第三十七

Chapter 37　Qijuelun Pian：Discussion on the Reverse Flow of qi

● 咳论篇第三十八

Chapter 38　Kelun Pian：Discussion on Cough

● 举痛论篇第三十九

Chapter 39　Jutonglun Pian：Discussion on Pains

● 腹中论篇第四十

Chapter 40　Fuzhonglun Pian：Discussion on Abdominal Disorders

● 刺腰痛篇第四十一

Chapter 41　Ci Yaotong Pian：Discussion on Treatment of Lumbago with Acupuncture

● 风论篇第四十二

Chapter 42　Fenglun Pian：Discussion on Wind

● 痹论篇第四十三

Chapter 43　Bilun Pian：Discussion on Bi-Syndrome

erals

Changes of Qi Convergence

● 解精微论篇第八十一

Chapter 81　Jiejingwei Lunpian：Discussion on the Elucidation of Abstruse Theory

附录 2　《灵枢》篇目索引

Ling Shu（Spiritual Pivot）

● 九针十二原第一

Chapter 1　Jiuzhen Shi'eryuan：Nine Needles and Twelve Origins〔Openings〕

● 本输第二

Chapter 2　Benshu：Discussion on Acupoints

● 小针解第三

Chapter 3　Xiaozhenjie：Explanatory Remarks on the Small Needles

● 邪气藏府病形第四

Chapter 4　Xieqi Zangfu Bingxing：Symptoms of Viscera and Bowels Due to Attack of Pathogenic Factors

● 根结第五

Chapter 5　Genjie：Root and Knot

● 寿夭刚柔第六

Chapter 6　Shouyao Gangrou：Discussion on Long life，Short life，Sturdiness and Softness

● 官针第七

Chapter 7　Guanzhen：Application of Needles

● 本神第八

Chapter 8　Benshen：Basic State of Spirit

● 终始第九

Chapter 9　Shizhong：Beginning and Ending

● 经脉第十

Chapter 10　Jingmai：Channels and Collaterals